JRCALC

Clinical
Guidelines 2022

JRCALC

Clinical Guidelines 2022

Edited for JRCALC and AACE by

Dr Simon N Brown, Dr Alison Walker
and Cathryn James

**On behalf of the National Ambulance Service
Medical Directors Group**

Dr Fenella Wrigley and medical director colleagues

CLASS
PROFESSIONAL
PUBLISHING

Printing history

First edition published 2000, second edition 2004, third edition 2006
Fourth edition published 2013, reprinted 2014, 2015 (twice, Version 1.3)

The content for Reference Edition 1.3 and Pocket Book 1.2 was updated in January 2015
2016 edition published 2016, reprinted 2016 (Version 1.5)
JRCALC Clinical Practice Supplementary Guidelines 2017 published 2017. Reprinted 2018
2019 edition published 2019. Reprinted twice in 2019.
2022 edition published in 2022.

The authors and publisher welcome feedback from the users of this book.
Please contact the publisher:
Class Professional Publishing,
The Exchange, Express Park, Bristol Road, Bridgwater TA6 4RR
Telephone: 01278 427 800
Email: apps@class.co.uk
Website: www.classprofessional.co.uk

Class Professional Publishing is an imprint of Class Publishing Ltd

A CIP catalogue record for this book is available from the British Library
This edition: JRCALC Clinical Guidelines 2022 ISBN 9781801610230
ISSN 2514-6084

Also available: JRCALC Clinical Guidelines 2022 (eBook) ISBN 9781801610223

Printed in the UK by Hobbs the Printers Ltd.

Contents

Contents

Disclaimer

The Association of Ambulance Chief Executives and the Joint Royal Colleges Ambulance Liaison Committee have made every effort to ensure that the information, tables, drawings, algorithms and diagrams contained in these guidelines are accurate at the time of publication. However, the guidelines are advisory and have been developed to assist healthcare professionals, to make decisions about the management of the patient's health, including assessments and treatments. This advice is intended to support the clinical decision making process and is not a substitute for sound clinical judgement. The guidelines cannot always contain all the information necessary for determining appropriate care and cannot address all individual situations; therefore, individuals using these guidelines must ensure they have the appropriate knowledge and skills to enable suitable interpretation.

JRCALC has referenced NICE in these guidelines. NICE guidance is prepared for the National Health Service in England and is subject to regular review and may be updated or withdrawn. NICE has not checked the use of its content in these guidelines to confirm that it accurately reflects the NICE publications from which it is taken.

Users of these guidelines must always be aware that alterations after the date of publication cannot be incorporated into the printed edition.

The Association of Ambulance Chief Executives and the Joint Royal Colleges Ambulance Liaison Committee accepts no legal liability of whatever nature arising from or connected to, the accuracy, reliability, currency or completeness of the content of these guidelines.

Although some modification of the guidelines may be required by individual ambulance services, and approved by the relevant local clinical committees, to ensure they respond to the health requirements of the local community, the majority of the guidance is universally applicable to NHS ambulance services. Modification of the guidelines may also occur when undertaking research sanctioned by a research ethics committee.

Whilst these guidelines cover a range of paramedic treatments available across the UK they will also provide a valuable tool for a range of care providers. Many of the assessment skills and general principles will remain the same. All clinical staff must practise within their level of training and competence.

Updates to these guidelines will be published on the JRCALC apps which will always contain the most current content.

Foreword

Welcome to the JRCALC Clinical Guidelines 2022. It is three years since the last full print publication of JRCALC guidelines. During this time, we continued work throughout the pandemic to ensure guidance was reviewed, updated and newly developed guidance was issued so that we continue to provide the best possible care to our patients. We are aware that the majority of people now access guidance and information via the JRCALC apps, iCPG and JRCALC Plus, and this remains the preferred way of accessing current clinical guidance, particularly when needing guidance for direct patient care. However, we understand that people still want access to printed material, in particular students and for general use as a reference book.

In this 2022 print edition, one of the main changes we have undertaken is the removal of the medicines section. New guidelines are being added regularly and existing guidelines being expanded which, on a practical level means the size of the book is constantly growing; we want to keep the book a manageable size for users, and for it to reflect how the book is mostly used. Furthermore, it supports our recommendation that students and clinicians access the most current information for medicines via the apps. For all references to medicines with the book, please refer to the relevant medicine on the apps.

The apps give us the ability to publish updates to guidance in real-time and in the three years since the previous print edition, we have released a total of nine bundle updates, all of which are included in this book.

We have engaged with a number of patients, patients' representatives and patient organisations who have supported us and provided a new focus on the patient perspective when updating guidance. These include The Sickle Cell Society, The Addisons Disease support group and the National Poisons Information Service (NPIS-Toxbase).

Updated guidance has also been included following our support to the responses of a number of Coroners' Preventing Future Death (PFDs) rulings; and in response to recommendations from the Health Services Investigation Branch (HSIB), including specific guidance around the dangers of ingestion of button batteries and propranolol overdose.

We reviewed guidance for a number of conditions to reduce inequity in care for people with darker skin tones. As a result, we have new and updated guidance for the clinical assessment of people with darker skin tones including specific information on the recognition of cyanosis, anaemia, bruising in darker skin; individualised pain management; and in the maternity section relating to higher risks of dying during pregnancy or childbirth for women from Black and Mixed Ethnic background women.

New for this edition are updated guidelines on: resuscitation; clinical management of steroid-dependent patients; non-traumatic lower back pain; CBRN and special situations; interacting with patients with communication difficulties; presentations of acute behavioural disturbance; alcohol-use disorders; and vascular emergencies. Many more updates have been made across medical, trauma and general guidance, often in response to queries being raised and new evidence becoming available.

Throughout these guidelines, we have used the term 'woman, women or mother' in relation to the gynaecological and pregnancy related conditions that ambulance clinicians may be called to assess and manage. We would like to acknowledge that this term does not reflect the diverse range of patients that you may see with these conditions including those who identify as non-binary or transgender, and we commit to continually reviewing the use of language within the guidance to ensure inclusive language is used. We encourage clinicians to consider the terms they use when assessing all patients and to be mindful of drawing erroneous conclusions related to perceived gender related diagnoses.

On behalf of JRCALC, NASMeD and AACE, we would like to thank all those that have contributed to our guidelines, the committee members who acted as lead authors and the groups of expert and enthusiastic healthcare professionals who all gave so willingly of their time. We thank the many paramedics who are passionate about a particular condition and have been motivated and willing to assist us with our work. Our special thanks to Class Professional Publishing, in particular Rebecca Spatuzzi, Gaby Stocker and Emma Milman for their considerable expertise, knowledge and energy.

Dr ALISON WALKER

Chair, Joint Royal Colleges Ambulance Liaison Committee

Dr SIMON BROWN

JRCALC Clinical Guidelines Development Lead

CATHRYN JAMES

Clinical Support Manager for NASMeD and JRCALC

STEVE IRVING

Executive Officer, Association of Ambulance Chief Executives

Guideline Developers and Contributors

The authors and editors would like to thank everyone who has contributed to the JRCALC guidelines. Many people have given freely and generously of their time and expertise to help draft, develop and improve the guidelines. In particular, we wish to acknowledge the work of the members of the Joint Royal Colleges Ambulance Liaison Committee, the National Ambulance Service Medical Directors group, the Ambulance Lead Paramedics group, Ambulance Pharmacists Network and national groups for End of Life, Safeguarding and Maternity. Other contributors have come from a variety of multidisciplinary groups which include healthcare professionals, educators and patients.

EDITORIAL LEADS

Dr Simon N Brown, *GP and Assistant Medical Director, South Central Ambulance Service, JRCALC guideline lead,*

Cathryn James, *Clinical Support for NASMeD and JRCALC, AACE*

Steve Irving, *Executive Officer, AACE*

JRCALC Chair: Dr Alison Walker, *Medical Director, West Midlands Ambulance Service and Consultant in Emergency Medicine, Harrogate & District NHS FT*

NASMeD Chair: Dr Fenella Wrigley, *Chief Medical Officer, London Ambulance Service*

JRCALC COMMITTEE MEMBERS

Dr Mark Baxter, *The Royal College of Physicians of London*

Dr John Black, *NASMeD and Medical Director South Central Ambulance Service.*

Dave Bywater, *Ambulance Lead Paramedic Group*

Professor Charles D Deakin, *The Royal College of Anaesthetists*

Dr Tim Edwards, *Ambulance Lead Paramedic Group*

Dr Paul Ferguson, *The Royal College of Pathologists*

Mr Kim Hinshaw, *The Royal College of Obstetricians and Gynaecologists*

Dr Matt Inada-Kim, *The Royal College of Physicians of London*

Dr Kate Jefferies, *The Royal College of Psychiatrists*

Dr Tony Joy, *The Royal College of Emergency Medicine*

Dawn Kerslake, *The Royal College of Midwives*

Dr Dhushy Surendra Kumar, *The Royal College of Anaesthetists*

Dr John Madar, *The Royal College of Paediatrics and Child Health*

Dr Stuart Maitland-Knibb, *The Royal College of General Practitioners*

Amanda Mansfield, *The Royal College of Midwives*

Louise Maunick, *The Royal Pharmaceutical Society/ Ambulance Pharmacists Network*

Dr Elizabeth Miller, *The Royal Pharmaceutical Society/ Ambulance Pharmacists Network*

Dr Fionna Moore, *NASMeD and Executive Medical Director, South East Coast Ambulance Service*

Professor Tom Quinn, *The Royal College of Nursing*

Dr Julian Sandell, *The Royal College of Paediatrics and Child Health*

Mr Richard Steyn, *The Royal College of Surgeons*

Dr Simon Stockley, *The Royal College of General Practitioners*

Tony Stone, *The College of Paramedics*

Ian Teague, *National Education Network of Ambulance Services*

Andy Thurgood, *Faculty of Pre Hospital Care (RCSEd)*

Dr Darren Walter, *The Royal College of Emergency Medicine*

Professor Julia Williams, *The College of Paramedics*

Thanks to the Library and Knowledge Service for NHS ambulance services in England: Matt Holland

Class Publishing – Emma Milman, Rebecca Spatuzzi, Gaby Stocker, Mo Forman

GENERAL LIST OF MANY NAMES TO THANK

Dr Peter Aitken,

Paul Aitken-Fell,

Dr Belinda Allan,

Dr Lisa Anderson,

Dr Mark Anderson,

Dorothy Antrim,

Sally Arnold-Jones,

Chris Ashton,

Dr Jay Banerjee,

Dr Lucy Bates,

Helen Beaumont-Waters

Dr Christopher Bowles,

Annmarie Breslin,

Mr Marcus Brooks,

Claire Capito,

Sonia Chand,

Stephen Clarke,

Robert Cole,

Keith Colver,

Christian Cooper,

Richard Corrall,

Dr James Coulson,

Dr Phil Cowburn,

Shirmilla Datta,

Jenna Davies,

Dr Jon M Dickson,

Prof Tim Draycott,

Matthew Dunn,

Dr Ed England,

Lewis Ewington,

Mark Faulkner,

Dr David Fitzpatrick,

Craig Garner,

Dawne Garrett,

Guideline Developers and Contributors

Joanna Garrett,

Mr Paul Gibbs,

Dr Les Gordon,

James Gough,

Simon Grant,

Dr Richard Grunewald,

Rhys Hancock,

Jon Harvey,

Dave Hawkins,

Daniel Haworth,

Claire Henderson,

Amanda Hensman-Crook,

Dr Liz Herrieven,

Daniel Holland,

Dr Matthew House,

Andrew Humber,

Tim Jones,

Sharon Jordan,

Dr Partha Kar,

Michelle Knight,

Vicky Kypta,

Prof Paul Lewis,

Jaqualine Lindridge,

Carly Lynch,

Denice Mace,

Stephanie Michaelides,

Prof Ian Maconochie,

Dr Julian Mark,

Chris Martin,

Dr John Mcanaw,

Mr Alistair Mccleary,

Graham Mcclelland,

Scott Munro,

Barry Murphy-Jones,

Georgina Murphy-Jones,

Ann Murray,

Ian Mursell,

Jo Nevett,

Mr Roger Neuberg,

Nicky Nicol,

Edward O'brian,

Sue Oakley,

Prof Gavin Perkins,

Carl Powell,

Sue Putman,

Prof Markus Reuber,

Ashley Richardson,

Duncan Robertson,

Simon Rose,

Amy Sainsbury,

Alex Sharp,

Gary Shaw,

Steven Short,

Nick Sillett,

Neil Sinclair

Prof Niro Siriwardena,

Simon Standen,

Joanne Stonehouse,

Robert Taylor,

Lee Thompson

Jacqui Tomkins,

Dr Eddie Tunn,

Louise Walker,

Matt Ward,

Mark Whitbread,

Jason Wiles,

Ian Wilmer,

Caitlin Wilson,

Prof Mark Wilson,

Cathy Winter,

Tholi Wood,

Prof Jonathan Wyllie,

Dr Aarti Ullal,

Aimee Yarrington

Dr Shyam Balasubramanian,

Richard Berry,

Alice Breton,

Cherylene Camps,

Simon Chase,

Nikki Harvey,

Simon Hester,

Dr Paul Kelly,

Dr Colville Laird,

Mark Millins,

Jane Mitchell,

Tracy Nicholls,

Menai Owen-Jones,

Martin Parkinson,

Richard Pilbery,

Prof Sir Keith Porter,

Mike Smyth,

Alan Taylor,

Charles Till,

Sam Thompson,

Sarah Thompson,

Philip Tremewan,

Prof John Wass,

Kevin Webb,

James Wenman,

Katherine White,

Dave Whitmore

Guideline Development Methodology

The methodology used by JRCALC (Joint Royal Colleges Ambulance Liaison Committee) to develop the UK Ambulance Services Clinical Practice Guidelines is designed to comply with the criteria used by the AGREE II (Appraisal of Guidelines for Research and Evaluation in Europe) instrument. This process is a leading academic tool to identify good quality guidelines: http://www.agreetrust.org/

The purpose of the AGREE II, is to provide a framework to:

- assess the quality of guidelines
- provide a methodological strategy for the development of guidelines
- inform what information and how information ought to be reported in guidelines.

By adopting these principles, guidelines are developed that support safe decision making and high quality patient care.

Guideline Selection

JRCALC, NASMeD (National Ambulance Service Medical Directors) and the ALPG (Ambulance Lead Paramedic Group) will advise on those clinical guidelines which need updating and those clinical conditions which need a new guideline developing. These are then prioritised and assessed with regard to urgency and risk. Clinical topics can be identified through a variety of means including the monitoring of serious incidents within individual UK Ambulance Service Trusts, preventing future death reports issued by coroners and national service reconfigurations. In addition JRCALC provide extensive clinical expertise and advice on potential new developments to ensure that the guidelines capture latest best practice and future innovations and encourage further research into pre hospital care.

Feedback is welcome via JRCALC@AACE.org

Editorial Independence

No external funding has been received for the development of these guidelines and no competing or conflicting interests have been declared by those involved in their development.

Citing the JRCALC Guidelines

The JRCALC Guidelines are cited as:

Joint Royal Colleges Ambulance Liaison Committee, Association of Ambulance Chief Executives (2022) JRCALC Clinical Guidelines 2022. Bridgwater: Class Professional Publishing.

Update Analysis – 'What's changed?'

Note : The table below details updates to guidelines and new guidance since the 2019 Reference Edition was published.

Note : A number of additional guidelines have had minor changes, relating to consistency, and the assessment and management tables have been re-formatted.

Section 1	General Guidance
Acute Behavioural Disturbance	New guideline.
Alcohol-use Disorders	New guideline.
Domestic Abuse	Revised and updated with current legislation.
Duty of Care	This guideline has had a full review and update.
End of Life Care	This guideline has had a full review and update.
Human Factors	New guideline. Replaces the Human Factors in Cardiac Arrest guideline from the Resuscitation section. A smaller section on human factors remains in 'Out-of-Hospital Cardiac Arrest: Overview'
Pain Management in Adults	New wording around individualised pain management has been added.
Patients with Communication Difficulties	New guideline.
Safeguarding Adults at Risk	Guideline revised and updated with current legislation. Additional wording has been included to consider bruising in people with darker skin tones.
Safeguarding Children	Guideline revised and updated with current legislation. Additional wording has been included to consider bruising in people with darker skin tones.

Section 2	Resuscitation
Advanced Life Support	Reviewed and updated in line with RCUK 2021. Updated guidance on mechanical chest compression devices and use of ultrasound. Other key changes include: ▫ Addition of HOT approach: hypovolaemia, oxygenation (hypoxia) and tension pneumothorax. Blood sugar should remain an important consideration during cardiac arrest and should be undertaken as soon as practical. A precordial thump is no longer recommended for initial treatment of shockable rhythms, even if a defibrillator is not immediately available. ▫ In children where hypovolaemia is thought to be a contributory factor, give a fluid bolus of 10 ml/kg (N.saline (0.9%) or Hartmann's solution), repeated once if indicated. Seek appropriate medical opinion if further boluses are thought to be indicated. ▫ We suggest a starting energy of at least 150J, escalating to maximum output for refractory rhythms. ▫ Quickly shaving the chest prior to defibrillation not only ensures better electrical contact (and therefore defibrillation success) but is likely to reduce the risk of electrical arcing between pads which may trigger a fire. ▫ Laryngoscopy remains an important skill for visually inspecting the oropharynx in choking and should be part of ongoing competency assessments. ▫ Staff attending the arrest will need to be trained to provide support to the clinician that is performing the intubation, such as preparing and passing the equipment.

Update Analysis – 'What's changed?'

	• Waveform capnography should always be used when using a supraglottic device and BVM. • Once a tracheal tube is in place, continue continuous chest compressions with 10 gentle ventilations per minute. Avoid hyperventilation and high airway pressures during manual ventilation which adversely affect outcome.
Basic Life Support in Adults	Reviewed and updated in line with RCUK 2021. New wording added: *Use of a CPR feedback device allows optimisation of BLS delivery and assessment of performance.*
Basic Life Support in Children	Reviewed and updated in line with RCUK 2021. New wording added: *Remember that pulse checks may be unreliable and are prone to errors. The detection of circulation therefore should also include other intra-arrest parameters such as ETCO2, blood pressure and SpO2.*
Foreign Body Airway Obstruction	Reviewed and updated in line with RCUK 2021. Includes new guidance to highlight there will be occasions when a patient who has a DNACPR form may have a cardiac arrest that is considered unnatural and not in the envisaged circumstances and has a potentially reversible cause such as choking. All reversible causes should be considered. In these circumstances, resuscitation and rapid conveyance to hospital should be considered as the cause of the arrest is unrelated to their main clinical problem(s) and could be reversible.
Out-of-Hospital Cardiac Arrest: Overview	Reviewed and updated in line with RCUK 2021. New wording included: *Auditing and reviewing data downloads will help determine how quickly shocks are being delivered. Based on local data, decisions can be made as to whether to recommend using AED mode for the first shock in order to minimise shock delays. Local audit data can help inform the decision making process.*
Return of Spontaneous Circulation	The ROSC algorithm has been updated. Aim for a systolic blood pressure (SBP) > 100 mmHg. In patients with an adequate heart rate, attempt to achieve this with IV (or IO) fluids, together with IV (or IO) adrenaline.
Termination of Resuscitation and Verification of Death in Adults	Reviewed and updated in line with RCUK 2021. New section on advance care planning included and more guidance added to clarify decisions around ADRT, lasting power of attorney and DNACPR, expected and unexpected deaths. The decision to terminate resuscitation has been increased to 30 minutes from 20 minutes: *If, following ALS interventions, the patient has been persistently and continuously asystolic for 30 minutes and all reversible causes have been identified and corrected, resuscitation may be discontinued except in cases listed below:* • *pregnancy* • *hypothermic patients (where hypothermia is the primary cause of the cardiac arrest)* • *suspected drugs overdose/poisoning* • *infants, children and adolescents (i.e., all those < 18 yrs age) – refer to termination of resuscitation and verification of death in children.*
Termination of Resuscitation and Verification of Death in Children	New title replacing 'Death of a Child' guideline. Reviewed and updated in line with RCUK 2021. Includes guidance for children with care plans and for expected deaths.
Tracheostomy and Laryngectomy Emergency Pre-Hospital Management	Reviewed and updated in line with RCUK 2021. Algorithms have been reviewed and revised.

Update Analysis – 'What's changed?'

Section 3	Medical Emergencies
Allergic Reactions including Anaphylaxis	The guideline has been fully reviewed and updated to bring in line with 2021 RCUK guidance.
Altered level of consciousness	Updated appendix: The order of the Glasgow Coma Scale was corrected to Eyes, Verbal, Motor-EVM.
Asthma in Adults and Children	Clarification wording was added: *Asthma is rare in very young children (under 1 year) and other causes of wheeze (such as bronchiolitis or viral induced wheeze) should be considered.* This guideline was updated to include new medicines; Magnesium and Prednisolone.
Chronic Obstructive Pulmonary Disease	This guideline was updated to include reference to medicines; Prednisolone and Hydrocortisone.
Convulsions in Adults	Wording was added regarding treating focal motor seizures. A disparity between guidance has been addressed, regarding when convulsion in pregnancy should be considered as eclampsia.
Convulsions in Children	A clarification regarding a third dose of benzodiazepine was added; staff must seek senior clinical advice to consider a third dose. This change brought the Convulsions in Children guideline in line with Convulsions in Adults. The definition of convulsive status epilepticus (CSE) has been updated to follow the definition in the JRCALC Convulsions in Adults guideline.
Glycaemic Emergencies in Adults and Children	Table 3.57 was clarified: patients can be considered for discharge if their blood sugar is greater than 4 mmols. Removal of caution around fluids causing cerebral oedema in children and young adults. Revised wording around fluid administration in DKA.
Headache	New wording added to Key Points: *A tension-type headache is the most common symptom of mild carbon monoxide poisoning.*
Low Back Pain (Non-Traumatic)	New guideline.
Management of Resuscitation and Patients with Left Ventricular Assist Devices (LVADs)	Emergency contact numbers have been updated.
Medical Emergencies in Adults	Updated appendix: The order of the Glasgow Coma Scale was corrected to Eyes, Verbal, Motor-EVM. New wording around how to recognise cyanosis and anaemia in people with darker skin colour has been added to the assessment and management table. Images have been added of cyanosis and the conjunctiva in anaemia. New guidance on the use of the Clinical Frailty Scale (CFS) has been added, and guidance on steroid-dependent patient has been removed (see **new Steroid-dependent Patients** guideline).
Medical Emergencies in Children	Updated appendix: The order of the Glasgow Coma Scale was corrected to Eyes, Verbal, Motor-EVM.
Mental Capacity Act 2005 (England and Wales)	Revised and updated with current legislation. New flowchart for assessing mental capacity included with information around causative nexus.

Update Analysis – 'What's changed?'

Mental Health Presentation: Crisis, distress and Disordered Behaviour	Removal of risk levels mild, moderate, severe, extreme from the IPAP suicide risk levels Table 3.82. The NICE guideline on self-harm does not advise using risk assessment tools and scales for suicide and self-harm.
Overdose and Poisoning in Adults and Children	Irrigation time for corrosive injuries clarified as 20-60 minutes. Additional guidance on overdose of beta-blockers was added. The Specific Substance Management section was reviewed and updated, including an addition of sodium thiosulphate as an antidote for cyanide poisoning. Further guidance was added on button batteries and the risks of small, powerful magnets.
Respiratory illness in children	Clarification wording was added: *Asthma is rare in very young children (under 1 year) and other causes of wheeze (such as bronchiolitis or viral induced wheeze) should be considered.* *Salbutamol is not indicated in bronchiolitis. It will not benefit the condition and the resultant tachycardia may confuse subsequent clinical assessment in hospital.* Removal of modified Taussig croup score as it is no longer advised by NICE. Dexamethasone is now indicated for all children with croup, regardless of whether it is mild, moderate, or severe.
Sickle Cell Disease	This guideline has had a full review and update. Guidance on administration of opioids has been aligned with Pain Management in Adults Guideline.
Steroid-dependent Patients	New guideline.
Stroke/Transient Ischaemic Attack	This guideline has had a full review and update.
Vascular Emergencies	New guideline. Includes guidance on aortic aneurysm, aortic dissection, ischaemic limbs and diabetic foot problems. Contains guidance on AV fistula bleeds – this existing guidance has been moved from the trauma emergencies in adults overview.

Section 4	**Trauma**
Burns and Scalds	Irrigation time for chemical burns was clarified as a minimum of 20 minutes.
Falls in Older Adults	Section 6.4 on postural hypotension and the procedure of how to measure it was amended. New guidance on the use of the Clinical Frailty Scale (CFS) has been added.
Head Injury	New wording added: 'Following the results of the CRASH 3 trial, TXA should be administered to any patient aged 18 years and over who have a known or suspected head injury, with a GCS of 12 or less, where the injury has occurred within the last 3 hours.' The Assessment and Management of Head Injury algorithm was amended in line with JRCALC update on CRASH 3 trial.
Limb Trauma	Wording relating to administering prophylactic antibiotics within one hour of injury for open fractures was amended. New section and wording on crush injury and crush syndrome.

Update Analysis – 'What's changed?'

Trauma Emergencies in Adults	Updated appendix: The order of the Glasgow Coma Scale was corrected to Eyes, Verbal, Motor-EVM.
	Section on AV fistula bleeds was moved into a new guideline, Vascular Emergencies.
	New guidance on the assessment and management of hangings has been added.
	New guidance on the use of the Clinical Frailty scale (CFS) has been added.
	Wording on guidance for steroid-dependent patient has been removed (due to new Steroid-dependent Patients guideline).
Trauma Emergencies in Children	Updated appendix: The order of the Glasgow Coma Scale was corrected to Eyes, Verbal, Motor-EVM.
	The algorithm for the application of a tourniquet for catastrophic limb haemorrhage in children has been corrected, to be the same as adults.

Section 5	Maternity Care
	All mentions of 'premature baby' were changed to say 'preterm baby' to reflect current terminology.
Birth imminent	Updated wording to explain that the amniotic membranes should not be ruptured if they are visible during birth.
	New photographs were added to illustrate assessment and management of and 'en caul' birth.
	Updated wording due to changes to Misoprostol drug guideline.
	A disparity between guidance has been addressed, regarding when convulsions in pregnancy should be considered as eclampsia.
Care of the Newborn	Updated and inclusion of guidance for preterm babies in line with the British Association of Perinatal Medicine (BAPM) framework for practice: *Prehospital management of the baby born at extreme preterm gestation.*
	Guidance on 'comfort care' for babies known to be born before 22 weeks.
Maternity Care (including Obstetric Emergencies Overview)	A new section was added which includes guidance regarding at-risk patients.
	The guidance around female genital mutilation (FGM) was reviewed and updated.
	New guidance around waterbirths was added to the Special Cases section.
Newborn Life Support	Updated and algorithm revised in line with RCUK 2021.
Pregnancy Induced Hypertension (including Eclampsia)	A disparity between guidance has been addressed, regarding when convulsions in pregnancy should be considered as eclampsia.

Section 6	Special Situations
Chemical Biological Radiological Nuclear (CBRN) incidents including Hazardous Materials	New guidance in the Special Situations section. Includes Safety Triggers for Emergency Personnel (STEP) 1-2-3 Plus, CRESS tool (consciousness, respiration, eyes, secretion, skin), specific agents: nerve agents, cyanide, opiates, atropine toxicity, corrosive substances, Individual Chemical Exposure (ICE), ionising radiation and decontamination, illicit drugs lab.
DuoDote	This guideline has been removed and is now incorporated into the new CBRN guideline.

Update Analysis – 'What's changed?'

Major, Complex and High-Risk Incidents	Reviewed and updated by NARU. Principles of joint working diagram updated, inclusion of SORT. Removal of diagram of gunshot entry and exit wounds.
Police Incapacitants	Reviewed and updated by NARU. Updated guidance on Conducted Energy Devices (Tasers) and for their assessment, management and removal, updated assessment and management of irritant/incapacitant sprays, attenuating energy projectiles and batons.

List of Abbreviations

The glossary of terms listed below is designed to assist reading ease and is **NOT** provided as a list of short-hand terms. The Joint Royal Colleges Ambulance Liaison Committee reminds the user that abbreviations are not to be used in any clinical documentation.

Term	
AAA	Abdominal Aortic Aneurysm
ABCDE	A – Airway
	B – Breathing
	C – Circulation
	D – Disability
	E – Exposure and environment
ABD	Acute behavioural disorder
AC	Alternating Current
ACS	Acute Coronary Syndrome
ADHD	Attention Deficit Hyperactivity Disorder
ADRT	Advance Decision to Refuse Treatment
AED	Automated External Defibrillation
AHF	Acute Heart Failure
ALoC	Altered level of consciousness
ALS	Advanced Life Support
AMH	Adult Mental Health Services
AMHP	Approved Mental Health Professional
APC	Antero-Posterior Compression
APGAR	A – Appearance
	P – Pulse rate
	G – Grimace or response to stimulation
	A – Activity or muscle tone
	R – Respiration
ARDS	Acute Respiratory Distress Syndrome
ATMIST	A – Age
	T – Time of incident
	M – Mechanism
	I – Injuries
	S – Signs and symptoms
	T – Treatment given/immediate needs
ATP	Anti-Tachycardia Pacing
AV	Atrioventricular
AVPU	A – Alert
	V – Responds to voice
	P – Responds to pain
	U – Unresponsive

Term	
BBB	Bundle branch block
bd	Twice daily
BG	Blood Glucose
BIA	Best Interest Assessors
BiPAP	Bilevel Positive Pressure Ventilation
BLS	Basic Life Support
BM	Stick Measures blood sugar
BMI	Body mass index
BP	Blood Pressure
bpm	Beats per minute
BR	Breech
BSA	Body Surface Area
BTCS	Bilateral Tonic-Clonic Seizures
BTS	British Thoracic Society
BVM	Bag-Valve-Mask
BMV	Bag-mask ventilation
<C>ABCDE	<C> – Catastrophic haemorrhage
	A – Airway
	B – Breathing
	C – Circulation
	D – Disability
	E – Exposure and environment
CA	Cancer
CAMHS	Child and Adolescent Mental Health Services
CBRNE	Chemical, Biological, Radiological, Nuclear and Explosive
CBT	Cognitive Behavioural Therapy
CCF	Congestive cardiac failure
CCS	Central Cord Syndrome
CD	Controlled Drug
CES	Cauda Equina Syndrome
CEW	Controlled Electrical Weapon
CFR	Community first responder
CHD	Coronary Heart Disease
CHF	Congestive Heart Failure
CMHT	Community Mental Health Team
CMI	Combined Mechanical Injury
CNS	Central Nervous System
CO	Carbon monoxide
CO_2	Carbon dioxide

List of Abbreviations

COP	Code of Practice
COPD	Chronic Obstructive Pulmonary Disease
CPAP	Continuous Positive Airway Pressure
CPN	Community Psychiatric Nurse
CPP	Cerebral Perfusion Pressure
CPP	Coronary perfusion pressure
CPR	Cardiopulmonary Resuscitation
CPR-IC	CPR-induced consciousness
CRT	Capillary Refill Test
CRT	Cardiac Resynchronisation Therapy
CSA	Child Sexual Abuse
CSE	Child Sexual Exploitation
CSE	Convulsive status epilepticus
CT	Computerised Tomography
CVA	Cerebo Vascular Accident
DBS	Disclosure and Barring Service
DC	Direct Current
DIC	Disseminated Intravascular Coagulation
DKA	Diabetic Ketoacidosis
DM	Diabetes Mellitus
DNA	Deoxyribonucleic Acid
DNACPR	Do Not Attempt Cardio-Pulmonary Resuscitation
DoLS	Deprivation of Liberty Safeguards
DPA	Data Protection Act
DVT	Deep Vein Thrombosis
E	Ecstasy
EC	Enteric Coated
ECG	Electrocardiograph
ECT	Electro-convulsive therapy
ECMO	ECMO Extra-corporeal membrane oxygenation
ED	Emergency Department
EDD	Estimated Date of Delivery
EF	Ejection fraction
EMS	Emergency Medical Services
EOC	Emergency Operations Centre
ERC	European Resuscitation Council
ESC	European Society of Cardiology
ET	Endotracheal
ETA	Expected Time of Arrival
EtCO$_2$	Exhaled (end-tidal) carbon dioxide
EUPD	Emotionally unstable personality disorder

FAST	**F** –	Face
	A –	Arms
	S –	Speech
	T –	Test
FBAO	Foreign Body Airway Obstruction	
FC	Febrile Convulsions	
FEV	Forced Expiratory Volume	
FGM	Female genital mutilation	
FLACC	**F** –	Face
	L –	Legs
	A –	Activity
	C –	Cry
	C –	Consolability
FII	Fabricated or Induced Illness	
FGM	Female Genital Mutilation	
FVC	Forced Vital Capacity	
g	Grams	
GBS	Group B Strep Infection	
GCS	Glasgow Coma Scale	
GDPR	General Data Protection Regulations 2018	
GI	Gastrointestinal	
GP	General Practitioner	
GTN	Glyceryl Trinitrate	
GUM	Genito-urinary medicine	
HART	Hazardous Area Response Team	
HCP	Healthcare Professional	
HFpEF	Heart failure with preserved ejection fraction	
HFrEF	Heart failure with reduced ejection fraction	
HIV	Human Immunodeficiency Virus	
HME	Heat moisture exchanger	
HPV	Human papillomavirus	
HNSCC	Head and neck squamous cell carcinoma	
HR	Heart Rate	
HSE	Health and Safety Executive	
HVS	Hyperventilation Syndrome	
IA	Impaired awareness	
IBS	Irritable Bowel Syndrome	
ICD	International Classification of Diseases	
ICD	Implantable Cardioverter Defibrillator	
ICE	Infant Cooling Evaluation	

List of Abbreviations

ICP	Intracranial Pressure
IGIV	Immunoglobulin Intravenous
IHD	Ischemic Heart Disease
ILCOR	International Liaison Committee on Resuscitation
IM	Intramuscular
IMCA	Independent Mental Capacity Advocates
IO	Intraosseous
IPAP	**I** – Intent
	P – Plans
	A – Actions
	P – Protection
IQ	Intelligence Quotient
ISVA	Independent Sexual Violence Adviser
ITD	Impedance threshold device
ITU	Intensive Care Unit
IV	Intravenous
IVC	Inferior Vena Cava
J	Joule
JESIP	Joint Emergency Services Interoperability Programme
JRCALC	Joint Royal Colleges Ambulance Liaison Committee
JVP	Jugular Venous Pressure
kg	Kilogram
kPa	Kilopascal
kV	Kilovolt
LBBB	Left Bundle Branch Block
LC	Lateral Compression
LMA	Laryngeal Mask Airway
LMP	Last Menstrual Period
LOC	Level of Consciousness
LPA	Lasting Power of Attorney
LSD	Lysergic Acid Diethylamide
LVAD	Left ventricular assist device
LVF	Left Ventricular Failure
LVSD	Left ventricular systolic dysfunction
MAOI	Monoamine Oxidase Inhibitor antidepressant
MAPPA	Multi-Agency Public Protection Arrangements
MAP	Mean Arterial Pressure

MBRRACE	Mothers and Babies: Reducing Risk through Audits and Confidential Enquiries
MCA	Mental Capacity Act
mcg	Microgram
mCPR	Mechanical chest compression devices
MDMA	Methylene Dioxymethamphetamine
MECC	Making Every Contact Count
mg	Milligram
MH	Mental Health
MHA	Mental Health Act
MHSOP	Mental Health Services for Older People
MI	Myocardial Infarction
MINAP	Myocardial Ischaemia National Audit Project
ml	Millilitre
mmHG	Millimetres of Mercury
mmol	Millimoles
mmol/l	Millimoles per Litre
MOI	Mechanisms of Injury
MSC	**M** – Motor
	S – Sensation
	C – Circulation
msec	Millisecond
MTC	Major Triage Centre
NARU	National Ambulance Resilience Unit
Neb	Nebulisation
NEET	Not in Education, Employment or Training
NEWS	National Early Warning Score
NG	Nasogastric
NHS	National Health Service
NICE	National Institute for Health and Care Excellence
NiPPV	Non-invasive Positive Pressure Ventilation
NLS	Newborn Life Support
NPA	Nasopharyngeal airway
NPCC	The National Police Chiefs Council
NPIS	National Poisons Information Service
NSAID	Non-Steroidal Anti-inflammatory Drug
NSTEMI	Non-ST Segment Elevation Myocardial Infarction

List of Abbreviations

O$_2$	Oxygen
OHCA	Out of Hospital Cardiac Arrest
OOH	Out of Hours
OPA	Oropharyngeal Airway
ORS	Oral Rehydration Salt
P	Parity
PaO$_2$	Partial pressure of oxygen
PCO$_2$	Measure of the Partial Pressure of Carbon dioxide
PE	Pulmonary Embolism
PEaRL	Pupils Equal and Reacting to Light
PEA	Pulseless Electrical Activity
PEF	Peak Expiratory Flow
PEFR	Peak Expiratory Flow Rate
PHECG	Pre-hospital 12-lead electrocardiogram
PHTLS	Pre-hospital Trauma Life Support
PIH	Pregnancy Induced Hypertension
PNES	Psychogenic non-epileptic seizures
POM	Prescription Only Medicine
PPCI	Primary Percutaneous Coronary Intervention
PPE	Personal Protective Equipment
PPH	Post-Partum Haemorrhage
pr	Per Rectum
PTSD	Post-traumatic Stress Disorder
PreSep	Prehospital Early Sepsis Detection
PRESS	Prehospital Recognition of Severe Sepsis
PSM	Patient Specific Medication
PSP	Patient specific protocol
prn	When required medication
PV	Per Vaginam
pVT	Pulseless ventricular tachycardia
RAID	Rapid Assessment, Interface and Discharge
RBBB	Right bundle branch block
RCT	Randomised Controlled Trial
ReSPECT	Recommended Summary Plan for Emergency Care and Treatment
ROLE	Recognition Of Life Extinct
ROSC	Return of Spontaneous Circulation
RR	Respiratory Rate
RSV	Respiratory Syncytial Virus
RTC	Road Traffic Collision
RVF	Right Ventricular Failure

RVP	Rendezvous Point(s)
SAD	Supraglottic Airway Device
SARC	Sexual Assault Referral Centre
SaO$_2$	Oxygen Saturation Of Arterial Blood
SBAR	**S** – Situation
	B – Situation
	A – Assessment
	R – Recommendation
SBI	Serious Bacterial Infection
SBP	Systolic Blood Pressure
SC	Subcutaneous
SCENE	**S** – Safety
	C – Cause including MOI
	E – Environment
	N – Number of patients
	E – Extra resources needed
SCI	Spinal Cord Injury
SGA	Supraglottic airway
SOB	Shortness of breath
SOBOE	Shortness of breath on exertion
SOCRATES	**S** – Site
	O – Onset
	C – Character
	R – Radiation
	A – Associated symptoms
	T – Time
	E – Exacerbation
	S – Severity
SOP	Standard operating procedure
SORT	Special Operations Response Team
SpO$_2$	Oxygen Saturation Measured With Pulse Oximeter
SSRIs	Selective Serotonin Re-Uptake Inhibitors
STEMI	ST Segment Elevation Myocardial Infarction
STI	Sexually transmitted infections
SUDEP	Sudden Unexpected Death in Epilepsy
SUDI	Sudden Unexpected Death in Infants
SUDICA	Sudden Unexpected Death in Infants, Children and Adolescents
SVT	Supraventricular Tachycardia
T1DM	Type 1 diabetes mellitus
TARN	Trauma Audit Research Network

List of Abbreviations

Term	
TBI	Traumatic Brain injury
TBSA	Total Body Surface Area
TEP	Tracheoesophageal Puncture
TIA	Transient Ischaemic Attack
TLoC	Transient loss of consciousness
TOBY	Total Body Hypothermia for Neonatal Encephalopathy
URTI	Upper Respiratory Tract Infection

Term	
UTI	Urinary Tract Infection
VF	Ventricular Fibrillation
VS	Vertical Shear
VT	Ventricular Tachycardia
VTE	Venous Thromboembolism
WHO	World Health Organisation

1

General Guidance

Consent in Pre-hospital Care

1. Consent in Pre-hospital Care

- The laws and guidance that relate to consent to assessment, treatment, care and other interventions are different in the countries and/or jurisdictions that constitute the UK.

- Therefore, these guidelines do not offer guidance on obtaining consent beyond the general advice in this statement; the Joint Royal Colleges Ambulance Liaison Committee (JRCALC) advises strongly that readers should seek specific guidance on consent from their ambulance services, Trusts or other relevant employers.

- JRCALC advises that obtaining consent in ways that are lawful in the jurisdiction in which each reader works is fundamental to meeting patients' legal and ethical rights in determining what happens to them and to their own bodies. Therefore, it is important to ensure that you always act in the patient's best interest and that you have legally valid consent to conduct assessments, treatments or interventions, and provide care.

- Consent must be obtained from each patient or their legally valid representative (defined according to the law in the relevant country or jurisdiction) prior to conducting examinations or treatment, or providing care.

- Ensure that you provide patients with the appropriate information to enable them to comprehend the assessment, treatment or interventions being proposed. This means that in order for the patient to provide informed consent, they must be able to understand not only the assessment, treatment and interventions to be carried out, but also the consequences of such actions.

- In pre-hospital situations, it is not uncommon for patients to refuse assessment, care or treatment. Although patients may refuse, there may be, depending on the circumstances, continuing moral duties and legal responsibilities for ambulance clinicians to provide further intervention, particularly if life-threatening risk is involved. Again, ambulance clinicians are advised to obtain advice from their employers about circumstances of this nature so the actions they take are appropriate to the legal jurisdiction in which they are working.

- When communicating with other healthcare professionals, discussion should include information about the patient's ability to consent.

Domestic Abuse

1. Introduction

- Domestic violence and abuse is any incident or pattern of incidents of controlling, coercive or threatening behaviour, violence or abuse between those aged 16 or over who are or have been, intimate partners or family members regardless of gender or sexuality. The abuse can encompass, but is not limited to, psychological, physical, sexual, financial and emotional harm.

- Controlling behaviour is a range of acts designed to make a person subordinate and/ or dependent by isolating them from sources of support, exploiting their resources and capacities for personal gain, depriving them of the means needed for independence, resistance and escape and regulating their everyday behaviour.

- Coercive behaviour is an act or pattern of acts of assault, threats, humiliation and intimidation or other abuse that is used to harm, punish or frighten the victim.

- Domestic abuse is the most prevalent form of violence against women and girls.

- Pre-hospital healthcare practitioners are in a key position to identify domestic abuse and to initiate support and safety for victims.

- Domestic abuse is extremely distressing; managing such cases demands sensitive, non-judgemental medical and emotional care and an awareness of the forensic requirements.

- In December 2015, a new criminal offence of domestic abuse, 'coercive and controlling behaviour', came into force, making all domestic abuse a reportable crime. In April 2021, the Domestic Abuse Act 2021 came into force recognising children as victims and economic abuse as a form of domestic abuse, and introducing new measures to support victims.

- Patients are likely to be very distressed about the events surrounding domestic abuse. They may not want to involve anybody else, and may not consent to disclosure of information to other parties such as the police. Do not judge or give the appearance of judging the patient. Be kind and considerate, and allow the patient space and as much choice as possible about options for their treatment.

- There can be a complex but significant relationship between alcohol and drug use and domestic abuse perpetration.

- **Further care** – it is important to encourage all victims of domestic abuse to seek medical help and inform the police. Both will be able to provide physical, medical and emotional support.

- In cases of domestic abuse in adults with needs for care and support, refer to **Safeguarding Adults at Risk**.

- In cases of domestic abuse where children are present, involved or potentially affected by the emotional impact of domestic abuse, refer to **Safeguarding Children**.

2. Incidence

- In 2020, 5.5% of adults aged 16 to 74 years experienced domestic abuse in the 12 months prior. 18% of all offences recorded by the police in the year ending March 2021 were domestic abuse-related crimes. There were 362 domestic homicides recorded in the three-year period between year ending March 2018 and year ending March 2020.

- Women are significantly more likely than men to be victims and survivors of domestic abuse.

3. Severity and Outcome

The severity of the abuse can vary from verbal abuse to sustaining life-threatening injuries or death. The outcome of the abuse can lead to long-term psychological and physical effects.

Exposure to domestic abuse during childhood can have a profound effect on children's development and wellbeing.

4. Pathophysiology

- Domestic abuse is an incident or pattern of incidents of controlling, coercive or threatening behaviour, violence or abuse to those aged 16 or over. These types of abuse include: psychological, physical, sexual, financial and emotional harm.

- Domestic abuse also includes 'honour'-based violence, forced marriage and female genital mutilation (FGM); for FGM, also refer to **Safeguarding Adults at Risk** and **Safeguarding Children**.

5. Consent

- Clinicians should seek the consent of the adult to share information, unless doing so would increase the risk of harm. Whilst a capacitated adult is free to make an unwise or bad decision, the local authority and/or the police can take steps to protect them if they are at risk of abuse if they are being unduly influenced, coerced or intimidated.

- Information can be shared with other professionals, without the adult's consent, if the following apply:
  - There is an immediate risk of harm.
  - Other people are being put at risk (for example, letting friends who are abusive or exploitative into a shared living environment, where they may put other residents at risk).
  - A child is involved.
  - The alleged person causing harm has care and support needs and may also be at risk.
  - A crime has been committed.
  - Staff are implicated.

Domestic Abuse

Domestic Abuse

There will be times when an adult who has mental capacity decides to accept a situation considered as harmful or neglectful. Where this is the situation and they do not want any action to be taken, this does not preclude the sharing of information with relevant professional colleagues. This is to enable professionals to assess the risk of harm and be confident that the adult is not being unduly influenced, coerced or intimidated and is aware of all the options.

Poor handling of the consent process may result in a breakdown of trust between patients and clinicians, may result in opportunities to safeguard patients being missed and may also result in complaints from patients through the NHS complaints procedure or to professional bodies.

Where a person lacks the capacity to make a decision for themselves, any decision must be made in that person's best interests.

Remember that GDPR applies and you should only share relevant information to the safeguarding concern. Medical information not relevant should not be shared.

If the concern is a care concern and not safeguarding, then consent must be obtained. All consent discussions and decision should be recorded using your trust's reporting processes.

6. Assessment and Management

For the assessment and management of domestic abuse, refer to Table 1.1.

TABLE 1.1 – ASSESSMENT and MANAGEMENT of: Domestic Abuse

Assess <C>ABCD

If any **TIME-CRITICAL** features present major ABCD problems:

- Start correcting **<C>ABCD** problems.
- Undertake a **TIME-CRITICAL** transfer to nearest receiving hospital.
- Continue patient management en-route.
- Provide an ATMIST information call.

Assess

- Limit questions to those identifying the need for medical treatment, but allow the patient to talk and document what is said. **NB** It is not appropriate to probe for details of the abuse and it could affect the outcome of criminal investigations.
- Manage according to condition:
  - Acute injury – refer to **Trauma Emergencies in Adults** and **Trauma Emergencies in Children**.
  - Acute illness – refer to **Medical Emergencies in Adults** and **Medical Emergencies in Children**.

Indicators in the patient:

- Seems afraid or anxious to please their partner.
- Agrees with everything their partner says.
- Checks everything first with their partner.
- Talks about their partner's temper or jealousy.
- Has frequent injuries, often described as 'accidents'.
- Dresses in clothing designed to hide bruises or scars.
- Is restricted from seeing family and friends.
- Has limited access to money, credit cards etc.
- Has low self-esteem.
- Is depressed, anxious or has suicidal thoughts/action.

Approach

- Know and recognise risk factors, signs and presenting patterns of behaviour associated with domestic abuse.
- Facilitate privacy and do not do anything which could place the victim at further risk, such as making enquiries in earshot of the perpetrator.
- Use a sensitive and respectful manner but ask direct questions about relationships, risks and safety factors.
- Focus on your care but be mindful of your surroundings and the information that is being passed to you, both verbal and non-verbal.
- Consider cultural/religious issues.
- Where possible, accommodate the patient's requests.

Domestic Abuse

TABLE 1.1 – ASSESSMENT and MANAGEMENT of: Domestic Abuse *(continued)*

Remember that this may be the first time the victim has felt able to disclose risk to a professional, or even the only time they have ever had the opportunity.

- Where possible, avoid disturbing the scene.
- Where possible, and safe to do so, gain consent from the victim for referral to the police or a specialist domestic abuse service approved by your organisation's safeguarding lead.
- Multiagency input and assessment is essential in reducing the risk of domestic abuse. Follow your local protocols when referring to external agencies. If your local protocol recommends that you complete a DASH risk assessment, then always complete this face to face with the victim rather than retrospectively after the episode of contact has concluded.
- Obtain a safe contact number for the victim for other agencies to use to contact them without risk of alerting the perpetrator.

Criminal Offence/Forensic Examination

- Many forms of domestic violence are criminal offences and staff must report all serious crimes to the police, particularly if:
  - The patient has suffered from abuse involving a weapon/strangulation/smothering or has sustained a significant injury
  - The patient is in fear of the perpetrator
  - The abuse is escalating
  - The perpetrator is stalking the patient and/or
  - There is an immediate risk to the patient or any children in the household.
- Always attempt to gain consent from the victim to report to the police, but consent is not required if there is a public interest of other legal justification.
- Forensic examination may be required if a physical assault has taken place. Domestic abuse is a criminal offence and the police must be informed immediately (refer to **Sexual Assault**).

Transfer[1]

- Encourage all patients to attend further care.
- Refer the victim to an appropriate external service.
- Transfer patients to further care according to local guidelines.
- Where a patient is competent and refuses hospital treatment, advise them to seek further medical attention.
- If safe to do so, provide information on where the patient may seek further support in relation to domestic abuse.
- If children are involved, a safeguarding notification of concern must be made using local ambulance procedures.
- If the patient is transported to hospital, do not leave children in the care of the alleged perpetrator.
- Always try to speak to the patient alone to avoid placing them at further risk.
- Remember that consent is not always required from the patient to report the crime, particularly if the patient remains at risk.
- Share concerns at the receiving hospital.

[1]*In some areas, arrangements exist for patients to be examined and interviewed in police or other facilities.*

Documentation

- Complete the clinical record in great detail contemporaneously and document:
  - only facts, not personal opinion
  - what the patient says and in their own words
  - clinical findings with relevant timings
  - the ambulance identification number.
- A police statement may be required later.
- Consideration must be given with regard to leaving any documentation (such as a clinical record) with a victim, which could potentially increase the risk of harm.

Domestic Abuse

Domestic Abuse

- If staff suspect a crime has been committed resulting in harm to the patient, the police must be called.
- Always attempt to obtain consent from the patient before making a referral for them but recognise when consent is not required.
- Listen closely to the patient for disclosure, and document this on the patient record.
- If possible, take the patient away from the scene.
- Treatment should avoid disturbing evidence where possible.
- Take into account any information that is disclosed by children.
- Never leave a child with an alleged perpetrator if transporting the patient to hospital.
- Accommodate patient wishes where possible.

Further Reading

Other useful resources include:

Department of Health: Domestic violence and abuse. Professional guidance. https://www.gov.uk/government/uploads/system/uploads/attachment_data/file/211018/9576-TSO-Health_Visiting_Domestic_Violence_A3_Posters_WEB.pdf.

Women's Aid: Support for women to escape abuse. www.womensaid.org.uk.

Mankind Initiative: Information and support for male victims of domestic abuse or violence. https://www.mankind.org.uk.

LGBT+ Domestic Abuse Helpline: Support for LGBT+ people who have experienced abuse and violence. 0300 999 5428, www.broken-rainbow.co.uk.

Refuge. National helpline: 0808 2000 247, email: helpline@refuge.org.uk.

Foreign and Commonwealth Office: Forced marriage. www.fco.gov.uk/en/travel-and-living-abroad/when-things-go-wrong/forced-marriage.

Bibliography

1. HM Government. *Tackling Domestic Abuse Plan*. 2022. Available from: https://assets.publishing.service.gov.uk/government/uploads/system/uploads/attachment_data/file/1064427/E02735263_Tackling_Domestic_Abuse_CP_639_Accessible.pdf.

2. House of Common Library. *Briefing Paper 9233: The Role of Healthcare Services in Addressing Domestic abuse*. 2021. Available from: The role of healthcare services in addressing domestic abuse (parliament.uk).

3. Department of Health. *Responding to Domestic Abuse: A resource for health professionals*. 2017. Available from: https://www.gov.uk/government/publications/domestic-abuse-a-resource-for-health-professionals.

4. National Institute for Health and Clinical Excellence. *Domestic Violence and Abuse: Multi-agency working* (PH50). London: NICE, 2014. Available from: https://www.nice.org.uk/guidance/ph50/chapter/introduction.

5. Office for National Statistics. *Domestic Abuse Prevalence and Trends, England and Wales: Year ending March 2021*. 2021. Available from: https://www.ons.gov.uk/peoplepopulationandcommunity/crimeandjustice/articles/domesticabuseprevalenceandtrendsenglandandwales/yearendingmarch2021.

6. Home Office. *Multi-agency Statutory Guidance for Dealing with Forced Marriage*. 2022. Available from: https://www.gov.uk/government/publications/the-right-to-choose-government-guidance-on-forced-marriage/multi-agency-statutory-guidance-for-dealing-with-forced-marriage-and-multi-agency-practice-guidelines-handling-cases-of-forced-marriage-accessible#page25.

7. Edelson JL. The overlap between child maltreatment and women battering. *Violence Against Women* 1999, 5(2): 134–154.

8. Home Office, *Female Genital Mutilation: Resource pack*. 2021. Available from: https://www.gov.uk/government/publications/female-genital-mutilation-resource-pack/female-genital-mutilation-resource-pack.

9. McAfee RE. *Domestic Abuse as a Woman's Health Issue*. Chicago: Elservier Science Inc, 2001.

10. McWilliams M, McKiernan S. *Bringing It Out in the Open*. Belfast: HMSO, 1999.

11. NSPCC. *Domestic Abuse*. 2022. Available from: https://www.nspcc.org.uk/what-is-child-abuse/types-of-abuse/domestic-abuse.

Duty of Care

1. Introduction

- It is obvious that ambulance clinicians have a duty to provide care to their patients but establishing exactly how that duty applies during high-risk emergency situations can be challenging.

- The duty of care represents moral, professional and legal obligations. The moral obligation to provide care is a matter of individual and social conscience. The professional obligation arises from a clinician's professional registration and organisational procedures or national best practice guidelines. The legal obligation arises from several sources which are summarised below.

- It is particularly hard for ambulance clinicians to discharge their duty of care correctly at incidents where patients need clinical interventions but hazards expose responders to considerable risk.

2. Application

The duty of care applies to ambulance clinicians and managers in two fundamental ways:

1. Staff safety: The duty to keep yourself and your team safe.

2. Patient care: The duty to provide a reasonable standard of care to your patient.

Whilst the United Kingdom has three separate jurisdictions – England and Wales, Scotland and Northern Ireland – the duty of care principles are broadly consistent throughout.

3. Health and Safety Duties

- The Health and Safety at Work Act 1974 and associated regulations require ambulance clinicians to have a safe system of work. NHS ambulance services have a legal duty to implement and maintain safe systems of work for their employees, and in turn employees have a legal duty to comply with these systems.

- A safe system of work is usually achieved through:
  - Effective operating procedures
  - Staff competence (qualifications and training)
  - Fit for purpose equipment
  - Effective risk assessments.

- This means ambulance clinicians should:
  - Ensure they and their colleagues engage in approved activities which have procedures and controls in place to mitigate the risks
  - Ensure that they are competent to perform those activities (i.e. they have been suitably trained to do it and that training is up to date or current)
  - Ensure that they have the necessary equipment for those activities and the equipment being used is fit for purpose (i.e. appropriately maintained). This includes personal protective equipment (PPE)
  - Ensure that staff are aware of pre-existing generic risk assessments for the specific activity being undertaken and that subsequent dynamic risk assessments are used just prior to committing to the activity so that specific situational hazards and risks are considered.

- A safe system of work does not necessarily mean one which is free of risk. It is one where the risk is being appropriately managed or controlled. Given the nature of pre-hospital ambulance work, a level of risk exposure will need to be accepted.

- Safe systems of work must also be reviewed periodically and/or when the work activity or risk changes. NHS ambulance services must also implement appropriate monitoring/supervision to ensure compliance with the safe system of work.

4. The Tort of Negligence

- The emergency services (including police and fire and rescue services) do not generally owe a legal duty of care to individual members of the public except in certain, limited circumstances (*Hill v Chief Constable of West Yorkshire* [1989] AC 53 (HL)). Their duty is focused more on protecting the public 'at large'.

- The law will recognise a breach of duty by Police or Fire and Rescue Services if they have acted in a certain way in certain specific situations (*Caparo Industries Plc v Dickman* [1990] 2 AC 605).

- However, the NHS Ambulance Service has an established legal duty to provide a reasonable standard of care to patients without unreasonable delay. This is a positive duty which engages from the point at which the Ambulance Service accepts the emergency call and agrees to attend (*Kent v Griffiths* [2001] QB 36).

- A reasonable standard of care relates to clinical care that can be supported by a responsible body of medical opinion (*Bolam v Friern Hospital Management Committee* [1957] 2 All ER 118). The opinion relied upon must have a logical basis (*Bolitho v City and Hackney Health Authority* [1998] AC 232). With regard to the clinical practice of ambulance staff, these standards are set out in approved clinical practice guidelines and the standards set by relevant professional bodies.

- This puts the ambulance service in a position where the care provided or any unreasonable delay in the provision of care may need to be explained and legally justified to avoid liability. Failure to discharge this duty could expose the ambulance service to a charge of clinical negligence.

Duty of Care

5. Article 2 – The Right to Life

- It has been recognised that Article 2 of the Human Rights Act 1998 creates a positive duty on public sector organisations, including the NHS ambulance services, to do all they reasonably can to protect those they know, or ought to know, are at real and immediate risk (*Van Colle v CC of Hertfordshire* [2007] EWCA Civ 325).

- However, there may be occasions where it is justifiable not to act immediately to save someone's life. For example, ambulance clinicians are not under a duty to sacrifice their own life to save a patient.

- If you manage to effectively balance two fundamental duties of care by putting a safe system of work in place and avoiding any unreasonable delay in providing care to patients, then you will invariably discharge your obligations under Article 2.

6. Appendix – Duty of Care Aide Memoire

- The aide memoire depicted in Table 1.2 has been developed to assist you in applying the duty of care correctly.

TABLE 1.2 – Duty of Care Aide Memoire

Duty of Care Requirement		Steps to Take	Explanation
Duty of care to staff	Take all reasonable and practical steps to keep employees safe.	Perform approved activities and apply the controls specified in procedures. Ensure there is a generic risk assessment already in place. Ensure you are trained and competent to undertake the activity. Ensure the minimum equipment mandated by procedures is available and used (including your Personal Protective Equipment (PPE).	These are statutory duties under the Health and Safety at Work Act 1974 and associated regulatory provisions. These steps will help ensure you have a safe system of work. Most of these provisions should already be established prior to the incident.
Duty of care to the patient	Provide a reasonable standard of care without any unreasonable delay.	Undertake a dynamic risk assessment and determine the action you need to take as quickly as possible. Continually review the position and deliver care as soon as possible. If you need specialist support, make sure you request it as soon as possible.	This is an established duty at common law. It is a positive duty on the ambulance service to provide a reasonable standard of care without unreasonable delay. This duty is unique to healthcare professionals. The police and fire services have duties to the public at large but their duty to individual patients is largely discretionary (*Kent v Griffith* [2001] QB 36).
Article 2 right to life	Take steps to protect people from harm which may lead to loss of life.	Balance the two duties set out above.	If the correct balance is achieved (staff safety but also avoiding unreasonable delay in treating patients), this duty will be discharged. If the rescue is too dangerous for the responders, Art. 2 positive duties can be temporarily avoided.

Duty of Care

TABLE 1.2 – Duty of Care Aide Memoire *(continued)*

Duty of Care Requirement		Steps to Take	Explanation
Risk-assess the activity	Assess the risks for both staff and patients.	Supplement the pre-existing generic risk assessment with a dynamic risk assessment at the scene considering the situation and hazards. Mitigate the risks as best you can. The risk to patients must be included in that assessment. Regularly review the risk assessment.	If the activity is likely to result in death or serious injury to you or a member of your team despite the controls, do not commit. Statutory health and safety obligations provide justification for the temporary delay of care.
Multi-agency Joint Doctrine	Contribute to the joint risk assessment as part of JESIP and ensure a common understanding of the risks.	For complex incidents involving a multi-agency response, ensure there is a joint risk assessment using the JESIP tools. Ensure the ambulance service duty of care is considered as part of this joint risk assessment.	If the risk of death or serious injury to you or your team can be mitigated by a safe system of work, making the likelihood low but accepting some residual risk, you must avoid unreasonable delay in committing and providing emergency care. For complex or major incidents, ambulance commanders are responsible for balancing these principles.

KEY POINTS!

- The duty of care requires ambulance clinicians to achieve a careful balance. They must take reasonable steps to ensure they are as safe as is realistically possible, but they must also be prepared to accept some risk to deliver effective care to patients in the pre-hospital setting. They must also be sufficiently trained and experienced to act quickly where life is at risk.
- To do this they must:
    - Implement an approved safe system of work and associated procedures.
    - Avoid any unreasonable delays in providing emergency care to patients that require it.

SECTION 1 General Guidance

End of Life Care

1. Introduction

- Approximately 1% of the population of the UK die each year, which is about half a million people, and around 75% of these deaths are expected. This presents an opportunity to plan for an individual's death, to improve the quality of life remaining, to support those close to the patient, to provide symptom control and to establish preferences for care as an illness progresses.

- Palliative care is for people living with a progressive terminal illness where a cure is no longer possible. In addition to cancers, this encompasses conditions secondary to end organ failure, e.g. COPD, renal failure, liver failure, dementia, heart failure and motor neurone disease. Patients with progressive incurable illnesses may receive palliative care for weeks, months or years and include end of life care planning as their condition deteriorates.

- End of life care is considered for patients within the last year of life. As illness trajectories differ for each condition, end of life care may refer to the last few months, weeks or days of life.

- Ambulance clinicians increasingly encounter patients who are palliative and approaching their end of life, either whilst facilitating planned transfers or providing an emergency response to a sudden crisis.

- Due to an ageing population and an expected 17% increase in annual deaths by 2030, there will be an increasing demand for high-quality end of life care. This will be reflected in the workload of ambulance services.

- Unlike conventional areas of pre-hospital care, such as cardiac arrest and trauma, which aim to save life and rely on algorithms and clear parameters, end of life care seeks to provide supportive care using a holistic approach tailored to each individual. This presents unique challenges to ambulance clinicians insofar as there is no pre-existing relationship with the patient, there is limited or no knowledge of either their condition or treatment preferences and, based on limited information, **TIME-CRITICAL** decisions have to be made.

- People at the end of life may have contact with ambulance services on several occasions, for example when a complication occurs which creates a sudden health crisis or for an unrelated event such as a fall. Be aware of the underlying condition(s) and any advance care planning decisions that may be in place when administering care or seeking a referral or admission.

- Increasingly, calls to ambulance services may indicate that a person's condition is deteriorating; for example, in a person with COPD who is experiencing increased difficulty in breathing, ambulance clinicians may be the first point of contact for this individual. Ambulance clinicians need to be able to recognise signs, signals and clues that suggest it may be time to initiate discussions about end of life care and relay this information to the patient's GP, hospital or other appropriate health professional or organisations so that appropriate action can be taken.

2. Severity and Outcome

- The focus in managing end of life care situations should always be to enable a person to achieve care according to their preferences.

- For those who are nearing the terminal phase of illness, the aspirational outcome would be for that person to have a 'good death'; to die in a place of their choosing, with dignity and respect, without pain, in a calm and familiar atmosphere, surrounded by loved ones.

- Several acute presentations are reversible and require urgent treatment including transfer to the Emergency Department (ED) in order to improve an individual's prognosis or quality of life. However, sometimes a potential reversible condition may have been discussed previously between the patient and their care provider and following these discussions a 'ceiling of treatment' may have been agreed. If a ceiling of treatment has been set, remember the ceiling is for a certain treatment only: there is never a ceiling to care. Where possible, check that any previously agreed ceiling of treatment is still what the patient wants. Any patient with capacity is allowed to change their mind.

3. Management – Patients Who Are Not Expected to Die Within 72 Hours

- Establish the patient's wishes for their care, including their desire for interventions and preferred place of care.

- If the patient does not have the capacity for decision making, establish if an advance care plan, a Recommended Summary Plan for Emergency Care and Treatment (ReSPECT) or an Advance Decision to Refuse Treatment (ADRT) exists.

- Establish if a family member has Lasting Power of Attorney (LPA) for Health and Welfare. An LPA for Health gives a family member the legal right to refuse a treatment for the patient that has lost capacity, if they deem it not in that patient's best interests at that time. It does not however allow the Attorney to insist on any forms of treatment or conveyance to hospital.

- Consult with family members and carers but remember that the patient's best interests take precedence.

End of Life Care

- Access personalised care plans and follow directions where appropriate.
- **If not in the active stage of dying, determine:**
  - if there is a reversible cause for symptoms and manage as per guidance
  - if the patient's symptoms can be managed in their home environment or if hospital/hospice admission is required
  - if the patient has psychological, emotional or spiritual needs that would benefit from specialist support
  - if the patient requires additional social support at home or if hospital admission is necessary: Are family members exhausted? Can they manage to provide care? Is physical equipment required to support care at home? Seek out local services that may be able to assist with support.

3.1 Care Pathways

- Unless the patient clearly requires urgent hospital conveyance for a reversible condition, seek specialist advice to support decision making.
- Be aware of any wishes regarding future care that may have been recorded on an advance care plan, especially patients receiving palliative care and those with long-term conditions, such as COPD and dementia, however be aware that patients can change their mind and contradict what's in their care plan, if they have capacity, and then their current preference takes priority.
- Be prepared to ask the person/carer about possible end of life care planning and related issues.
- Contact the palliative care team using contact details in a personalised care plan.
- Contact the patient's GP, an out-of-hours GP or district nurse.
- Contact local palliative care pathways (e.g. rapid response teams or hospice-at-home services).
- Consider contacting a religious leader if appropriate.
- Consider referral to social services if appropriate.
- Consider contacting senior clinical support within your Trust.

3.2 Shared Decision Making

- Ambulance clinicians often become involved in the complex care of patients with whom they have had no prior contact. In managing end of life situations, where there may be a need to administer medicines for symptom control or facilitate the patient's preference with regard to the place of care, remember that the patient's existing care team will hold more information about them and have met them in person in the past. Shared decision making by contacting and discussing

cases with the patient's GP, an out-of-hours GP or local palliative care teams is invaluable.

3.3 Palliative Emergencies

Metastatic Spinal Cord Compression

Background

- Spinal cord compression due to direct pressure or collapse of a vertebral body due to spinal metastases can result in vascular injury, cord necrosis and neurological disability.

Signs and Symptoms

- Pain in thoracic or cervical spine and/or progressive, severe lumbar spinal pain.
- Pain aggravated by straining (passing stools, coughing or sneezing) or nocturnal pain preventing sleep.
- Limb weakness.
- Difficulty walking.
- Sensory loss or bladder or bowel dysfunction.
- Localised spinal tenderness.

Management

1. If any of the following **TIME-CRITICAL** features are present, undertake a **TIME-CRITICAL** transfer to nearest Emergency Department:
   - major ABCD problems
   - neurological deficit in lower limbs.
- Undertake a **TIME-CRITICAL** transfer to nearest Emergency Department.
- Provide patient management en-route.
- Provide an alert/information call.

2. Measure and record a pain score.
- Offer analgesia (refer to **Pain Management in Adults**).

3. Position supine with neutral spine alignment for patients with severe pain, neurological symptoms or signs of compression. Exceptions to this would be patients with severe COPD or heart failure who, due to co-morbidity, are unable to tolerate lying supine. In these cases the patient should be transferred in the most comfortable position for them.

NB There are no clear guidelines and there is a lack of evidence to advise the correct position for patients – adopt NICE guidelines, as in the pre-hospital phase it seems prudent to manage as if the spine is unstable until an MRI can confirm this.

4. Transfer to the nearest Emergency Department or to a specialist unit if advised by expert team.

Superior Vena Cava Compression

Background

- Occlusion of the superior vena cava due to either external compression or internal obstruction. This is most commonly caused by a tumour of the bronchus or lymphomas, or cancers of the breast, colon or oesophagus. Patients with lung, prostate

End of Life Care

End of Life Care

and breast cancer are at the greatest risk, with the thoracic spine most commonly affected.

- Severity of symptoms varies depending on the degree of obstruction but reflects the underlying venous congestion, laryngeal and cerebral oedema.

Signs and Symptoms

- Facial, neck or arm swelling, worse on lying down or bending over.
- Dilated veins on neck, chest and arms.
- Dyspnoea.
- Cough or hoarseness.
- Headache.
- Dizziness, confusion or lethargy.

Management

1. If any of the following **TIME-CRITICAL** features are present, undertake a **TIME-CRITICAL** transfer to the nearest Emergency Department:
   - major ABC problems
   - stridor or severe difficulty in breathing.
- Start correcting A and B problems.
- Undertake a **TIME-CRITICAL** transfer to the nearest Emergency Department.
- Provide patient management en-route.
- Provide an alert/information call.

2. Sit the patient upright or elevate the head.

3. If the patient is hypoxaemic, administer supplemental oxygen and aim for a target saturation within the range of 94–98% (refer to **Oxygen**).

(**NB** – Points 2 and 3 provide symptomatic relief.)

4. Transfer to the nearest Emergency Department or to a specialist unit if advised by an expert team.

Neutropenic Sepsis

NB Neutropenic sepsis can occur in patients who are undergoing treatment for curative cancer as well as patients receiving palliative care.

Background

- Neutropenic sepsis is a potentially fatal complication of treatments for cancer, such as chemotherapy or immunotherapy. Such treatments can suppress the ability of bone marrow to respond to infection.
- Patients that have received chemotherapy and anti-cancer treatments in the past 8 weeks are at particular risk (the highest risk is within the first 10 days after treatment).
- Consider use of the UKONS/Macmillan Primary Care Triage Pocket Tool to help identify patients at risk of deterioration

Disclaimer: Clinicians using the UKONS/Macmillan Primary Care Triage Tool are expected to use independent clinical judgement in the context of the presenting clinical circumstances to determine any

patient's care or treatment. UKONS and Macmillan do not guarantee, and accept no legal liability of whatever nature arising from or connected to, the accuracy, reliability, currency or completeness of the content of the above UKONS/Macmillan Primary Care Triage Tool.

Signs and Symptoms

- Classic signs of sepsis may be absent. A neutropenic patient at risk of sepsis can look deceptively well but deteriorate rapidly. A high index of suspicion is necessary, particularly in a patient who has recently undergone chemotherapy and has an increased temperature.
- Neutropenic patients are unable to produce the pus normally associated with skin infections.
- Minor illness or feels unwell.
- Vomiting and/or diarrhoea.
- Raised temperature. Fever may be absent in some infected patients who are dehydrated, severely shocked or taking steroids or NSAIDs.

Management

1. Treat suspected neutropenic sepsis as an acute medical emergency.

2. Manage as per sepsis guidelines.

3. Identify a patient alert card and contact local acute oncology team. Consider the patient's advance care plan, ReSPECT plan or ADRT. They may wish to remain at home. Otherwise, transfer to the nearest Emergency Department or to a specialist unit if advised by an expert team.

Hypercalcaemia

Background

- Hypercalcaemia (high calcium level) occurs in 20–30% of patients with cancer (most commonly in patients with bone secondaries from their cancer). Some patients may have repeated episodes of hypercalcaemia; ask them if they have had this before.

Signs and Symptoms

- Too much calcium in the blood interferes with brain function, resulting in alterations in mental status, confusion, fatigue, headache and lethargy. If left to accumulate, this can lead to unconsciousness, coma and ultimately death.
- Frequent urination and excessive thirst.
- Nausea, vomiting, diarrhoea/constipation.
- Palpitations and fainting.

Management

1. Transfer to the nearest Emergency Department or to a specialist unit if advised by an expert team. In some areas, treatment can be provided at home or in a day-hospice setting, therefore contact the acute oncology helpline or palliative care helpline for advice (if patient receiving palliative as opposed to curative treatment).

End of Life Care

Figure 1.1 – UKONS/Macmillan Primary Care Triage Pocket Tool. Reproduced with kind permission from UKONS and Macmillan.

3.4 Recognising the Last Year of Life

▪ End of life care is defined as care of a patient with any disease process who is thought to be in their last year of life. Care should always be delivered in accordance with a person's cultural, spiritual or religious beliefs wherever possible and where clinically appropriate.

▪ There are different tools used within palliative care to help identify patients that may be in their last year of life: these include the Gold

End of Life Care

Standards Framework (GSF) and the Supportive and Palliative Care Indicators Tool (SPICT). These tools include prompts such as use of the surprise question (GSF): 'Would you be surprised if this patient were to die in the coming months, weeks or days?'. It also provides both general indicators of decline and disease-specific indications that a patient may be in the last year of life. The SPICT tool asks the question 'Are there clinical indicators that the health of this person who has one or more progressive conditions is deteriorating?'. If yes, it is time to assess the person's holistic care needs and start planning future care with them.

- **General indications of the last year of life may include:**
  - Decreasing activity: functional performance status declining, limited self-care, in bed or a chair for half of the day and increasing dependence during most activities of daily living
  - Co-morbidity: this is regarded as the biggest predictive indicator of mortality and morbidity
  - General physical decline and increasing need for support
  - Advanced disease: unstable, deteriorating and complex symptom burden
  - Decreasing response to treatments and decreasing reversibility
  - Choice of no further active treatment
  - Progressive weight loss >10% in the past 6 months
  - Repeated unplanned and crisis admissions
  - Sentinel event, for example a serious fall, bereavement or transfer to nursing home.

- **Specific indicators may include:**
  - Cancer: metastatic disease. The Gold Standard Framework explains that 'the single most important predictive factor in cancer is performance status and functional ability'
  - COPD: disease is severe, recurrent hospital admissions, i.e. at least three in the last 12 months due to COPD, fulfils long-term oxygen therapy criteria, Medical Research Council (MRC) Dyspnoea Scale grade 4/5, shortness of breath after 100 metres and confined to house
  - Dementia: unable to walk without assistance, urinary and faecal incontinence, no consistently meaningful conversation and unable to undertake Activities of Daily Living (ADLs).

3.5 Care in the Last Few Days of Life

- A point comes when the person enters the 'dying phase'. Ambulance services are frequently called upon at this stage. This may be for planned transport, such as the rapid transfer of a person from clinical settings to their preferred place of death.

- Ambulance services are also frequently called during the dying phase because of an unexpected complication or a sudden deterioration in condition. Good call-handling procedures can help ascertain what outcome the person or carer wants and expects from ambulance services – to make the person comfortable, for example, and avoid unwanted hospital admission or attempts at resuscitation.

- Families and carers may sometimes wish for ambulance services to be called even where the patient themselves has indicated a preference to die at home or in their usual care setting, such as a care home. The reasons for this may be multi-factorial.

- At the scene, the focus must at all times be on providing the patient with the care and treatment that is in their best interests. Families and carers can be valuable sources of knowledge and expertise on this and should be kept informed. Ambulance clinicians must at the same time be alert to the possibility of differing views and/or resistance to following an agreed care plan or stated preference among families and carers, including GPs, and be prepared to manage these. Be aware that relatives and carers may be distressed by the situation, especially in the case of unexpected complications or sudden deterioration.

Management

- Focus on care and treatment that is in the patient's best interests.

- Try and establish the wishes of the patient but be aware of differing views or resistance to follow an agreed care plan among families and carers.

- Seek clinical decision support, i.e. shared decision making with medical colleagues, e.g. GP or palliative medicine team; or follow the patient's care plan (if appropriate).

- Recognise the signs that a patient is at the end of life and that lifesaving skills, interventions and clinical observations may not be appropriate.

3.6 Signs That a Patient Is at the Very End of Life

- It can sometimes be difficult to decide when someone is in the last few days or hours. However, some of the signs below may become noticeable:
  - Abnormal clinical observations
  - Breathing may become irregular (shallow with deep sighs), with pauses (apnoeic episodes)
  - Reduced conscious levels; sleeping more and at times being difficult to waken
  - Impaired vision and may develop a fixed stare
  - Confusion or agitation
  - Restlessness, pulling at the bed linen and having visions or hallucinations of persons or things that are not present
  - Loss of appetite

End of Life Care

- Loss of control of urine or bowels. The amount of urine may decrease or stop as death approaches
- Occasionally after death there may be a 'last sigh' or gurgling sound particularly on moving or rolling a patient. There is no need to become alarmed about this, as it is the normal pattern
- Secretions collect at the back of the throat that sound like a rattle. Respiratory secretions are common and often occur in the last 24–48 hours of life. These secretions may be the reason for the 999 call as family members fear their loved one is drowning or choking. It can be useful to explain when offering reassurance that secretions are a small amount of fluid (saliva) at the top of the larynx or voice box and that breathing through the secretions is therefore amplified; that the sound is not a build-up of fluid within the lungs; and that the patient is no longer able to clear their throat, hence the pooling of saliva
- Cool arms and legs as the circulation slows down. The face may become pale, and the feet and legs take on a purple-blue mottled appearance.

3.7 Care at and After Death

- Ambulance clinicians will often be on the scene at or shortly after the point of death. There may be occasions where it is clear that the patient is in the final stages of dying. If all reversible causes have been considered, then supportive care for the patient and the relatives/carers may be all that is required. If a DNACPR or ReSPECT form is not present, ambulance clinicians are not obliged to commence CPR where the person is known to be in the final stages of an irreversible condition and where CPR would be both inappropriate and unsuccessful. Refer to **Termination of Resuscitation and Verification of Death in Adults** and **Termination of Resuscitation and Verification of Death in Children**.

4. Symptom Management in End of Life Care

- There are several common symptoms that may present at the end of life; these are often referred to as breakthrough symptoms. Symptoms will vary for each individual and may be controlled through non-pharmacological and/or pharmacological approaches.

- If the patient has their own medicines present, these should always be used in preference to ambulance service medicines to manage breakthrough symptoms. Using a patient's own medicines at the prescribed dose is a safe course of action to assist with symptom relief.

- The use of communication skills should not be underestimated when providing good symptom management. Acknowledging a patient's situation along with explanation, reassurance and a calm approach are all beneficial.

4.1 Pain – Introduction

- Adequate pain management at the end of life is a right of the dying patient and the duty of all clinicians. This provides one of the most challenging tasks that the clinician will face and requires the treatment of the 'whole person' as well as the physical pain by adopting a biopsychosocial approach.

- Pain is present in approximately 70% of patients with advanced cancer, and 65% in patients with a non-malignant disease. However, due to the longevity and nature of the dying process it is likely that most patients nearing the end of life will feel pain at some stage. In 10% of patients, the pain is described as 'difficult' and may require a more in-depth investigation and pain management programme.

- Most of these patients who are suffering with complex pain have input/support from a palliative care team/clinic who, along with the patient's GP, have the responsibility of monitoring for changes in pain intensity and character, and adjusting the management strategy accordingly. For those not under the guidance of a pain specialist/clinic, it is advisable for the clinician to make a referral or to make contact with a doctor so that a long-term plan to manage the pain can be sought.

- Of patients in the last week of life, 35% describe their pain as 'severe' or 'intolerable', and should be treated as a medical emergency where the challenge is to provide comprehensive pain management in order to alleviate suffering.

- Be aware that not all people in the last days of life experience pain. If pain is identified, manage it promptly and effectively. Identify and treat any reversible causes of pain; examples of this may include urinary retention requiring catheterisation or patient repositioning/turning.

4.2 Assessment of Pain

- Pain is a complex, subjective and dynamic phenomenon, which is affected by the emotional context in which it is endured. In line with current JRCALC guidelines set out in **Pain Management in Adults** and **Pain Management in Children**, clinicians should pay particular attention to any psychological and sociological factors. Wherever possible, a patient self-assessment strategy should be used and only substituted when the patient is unable to do so. A patient-centred approach should take into account the patient's needs and preferences so that they may be able to make an informed decision about their care. For this, good communication and understanding is essential.

End of Life Care

TABLE 1.3 – Types of Assessment	
Medical assessment	▪ It is important to take the time to thoroughly assess patients at the end of life as there may be other underlying issues that need addressing.
	▪ As well as the usual assessments carried out in line with clinical training and local protocols, it is advisable to also check for pressure ulcers and review dressings as these may need attention. If the patient is catheterised, it may be worth asking if it is fitted comfortably or causing any issues. If possible, advise the patient to maintain a degree of movement as this helps to prevent muscle atrophy and joint stiffness.
Sociological assessment	▪ A sociological assessment builds upon the premise that no illness is experienced in isolation; in fact, the assumption is that people will rationalise what is happening to them within a social model and create a social construction that is based on their relationships, past experience and language. The sociological assessment should look at how the individual makes sense of the illness and the physical and social interactions that are affected as a result. This 'individualism' of the disease combined with the social factors cannot, and does not, fit into the biomedical model which lends its intellect mainly to the giving of drugs to treat a specific dysfunction. If left untreated, the sociological aspect of dying will affect both the medical and psychological states of the patient.
Psychological assessment	▪ For many patients nearing the end of life, the dying process will lead to various psychological problems, especially disorders such as depression and anxiety. These have long since been known to accompany chronic pain and long-term illness, with research showing that increased pain perception contributes to the variables seen in the development of the symptomatology of psychological disorders.
	▪ The general assumption is that pain perception, alongside cognitive behavioural traits, plays an important part in the symptomatology of chronic pain, and therefore patients suffering from more intense, more frequent and longer-lasting painful episodes are more likely to suffer severe depression.
	▪ A lack of treatment will only serve to increase the level of depression, which acts as a vicious circle that is degenerative in nature and contributes to, or even exacerbates, the psychological problems encountered.

▪ Many patients nearing the end of life live with a degree of persistent pain for which they may already be receiving treatment. This is termed 'background pain'. If a new pain or an increase in the severity of the background pain occurs, then this should be treated as a new condition and assessed as such. An increase in severity of background pain or a new pain is termed as 'breakthrough' or 'breakout' pain.

4.3 Management of Pain

Non-pharmacological Management of Pain

▪ Non-pharmacological treatment of end of life pain involves addressing many different issues.

▪ Patient position: As many palliative care patients spend considerable lengths of time in the same position it may be possible to help reduce levels of pain through movement and pillow placement. Always be aware of pressure areas and treat if required.

▪ Psychological, social and spiritual concerns: Although the clinicians' time with the patient is limited, studies have shown that addressing these areas will help to provide comfort for the patient.

The mental state is very important and will affect pain levels if left untreated.

▪ A good bed-side manner: Calm and reassurance may be all that the patient needs in some circumstances, and this plays a big role in caring for end of life patients.

Pharmacological Management of Pain

▪ Where pain is intense and opioids are already prescribed, morphine should be the first-line treatment for breakthrough pain (unless a patient has an anticipatory prescription chart for other analgesics). This should be administered in line with local protocols and as part of a multi-modal pain management strategy (i.e. to be administered alongside other analgesics like NSAIDs or paracetamol). Where the new pain is not intense, the WHO analgesic ladder should be followed. It is important that the baseline medication is checked FIRST before administering any medication. If morphine is not the baseline medication then it should not be used as a breakthrough; there may be a reason why another opioid has been chosen and morphine should be avoided. Use the opioid of choice for breakthrough.

End of Life Care

TABLE 1.4

Step 1 – (<3/10) non opioid +/– adjuvant
Step 2 – (3–6/10) opioid for mild to moderate pain +/– non opioid +/– adjuvant
Step 3 – (>6/10) opioid for moderate to severe pain +/– non opioid +/– adjuvant

- The use of subcutaneous morphine should be considered in end of life care patients not wishing to attend hospital. It is important to administer morphine cautiously so as to achieve a stable and satisfactory level of pain relief without any adverse effects. The use of intravenous paracetamol may also be used by the clinician and has shown to be good at relieving symptoms of bone pain (a pain which is often difficult to fully control using morphine alone). Refer to **Morphine Sulfate** and **Paracetamol**.

- Do not dilute the morphine, as more than 2 ml of fluid injected subcutaneously into the site of administration is not recommended.

- The effects of IM/SC morphine are evident after 15–20 minutes.

- For pain in the last days or hours of life when the patient is in the dying phase, morphine may be given with caution for patients with a systolic blood pressure of 90 mmHg or less.

- It is important to check for prior paracetamol and opioid use before administration (including transdermal analgesic patches) to avoid overdosing the patient. The minimum dose of paracetamol should not be less than 4 hours apart (6 hours in patients with renal impairment).

- Paracetamol should be administered over a 15-minute period.

- Check that if the patient has a syringe driver in situ:
  - it is connected to the patient
  - where it is infusing into the patient the infusion site is not red/inflamed and therefore likely to be affecting the absorption and effect of the opioid
  - the syringe driver or tubing is not leaking
  - it is 'running to time', as if the delivery of medication is slow then breakthrough symptoms may become evident, e.g. an increase in pain if an opioid syringe driver is leaking or running slowly.

- After any drug has been administered, it is good practice to inform the patient's own GP or palliative team.

- Be cautious if the patient is on a syringe driver. In such cases contact the patient's care provider prior to the administration of any analgesic. However, if the patient is written up for and has their own anticipatory prescription or 'just in case' (JIC) medications, and they are on a syringe driver, the prescribed PRN dose has likely been calculated taking the syringe driver dose into account, meaning the PRN dose is safe to administer whilst the syringe driver is running.

- Where pain relief medication is administered, the ambulance clinician should check the patient's response after each dose. If further analgesia is required and the anticipatory prescription allows, this should be administered according to the drug chart. Shared decision making with the patient's GP or palliative care team is recommended when giving repeat doses of analgesia.

4.4 Managing Breathlessness

- Breathing discomfort varies in intensity and may not be associated with hypoxia, tachypnoea or bradypnoea.

- Be aware that severe breathlessness often causes anxiety, which can then increase breathlessness further.

- Identify and, if appropriate, treat reversible causes of breathlessness in the dying person, for example pulmonary oedema or pleural effusion.

- Consider patient positioning.

- Consider non-pharmacological management of breathlessness in a person in the last days of life.

- Do **NOT** routinely start oxygen to manage breathlessness. Only offer oxygen therapy to people known or clinically suspected to have symptomatic hypoxia.

- Medications to manage breathlessness may include:
  - an opioid, e.g. Oramorph® or low-dose morphine sulphate.
  - a benzodiazepine, e.g. lorazepam or midazolam
  - a combination of an opioid and benzodiazepine.

Oxygen Administration

- There is no evidence that oxygen therapy relieves breathlessness, unless the patient suffers hypoxia. Considering its disadvantages, namely an invasive intervention requiring tubing and tanks, the risk of nosebleeds and the patient's psychological addiction to this 'umbilical cord', it cannot be recommended for routine use.[1] The British Thoracic Society (2017) has published guidelines on the use of oxygen in adults, which includes a review of oxygen use for the patient with breathlessness associated with palliative illness in the emergency care setting:[2]
  - 'Oxygen therapy for the symptomatic relief of breathlessness in palliative care patients is more complex than the simple correction of hypoxia.

End of Life Care

- Consider the following issues:
- Consider early involvement of palliative care specialists and physiotherapists.
- As breathlessness is a multifactorial sensation—a comprehensive assessment of contributing factors (such as anxiety) should be carried out.
- Low-dose opioids should be considered because they are effective for the relief of breathlessness in palliative care patients. Remember, oxygen is a cure for hypoxia, it is **NOT** a cure for breathlessness.
- A trial of a hand held fan or sitting by an open window to help relieve breathlessness is recommended prior to trial of oxygen.
- Oxygen use has to be tailored to the individual and a formal assessment made of its efficacy for improving quality of life for that person.
- Oxygen therapy should not be continued in the absence of patient benefit or where its disadvantages (e.g. discomfort of masks or nasal cannulae, drying of mucous membranes) outweigh any likely symptomatic benefit'. (BTS, 2017)

- As an ambulance clinician it is vital that you are mindful of the evidence which concludes that the use of a fan and low-dose opiates is as effective, if not more effective, than the administration of oxygen. The disadvantages often outweigh the benefit of administering oxygen in that if a patient feels that they cannot breathe and an ambulance clinician attends and administers oxygen, the patient may believe that they need oxygen therapy each time thereafter that they feel breathlessness. Even worse, the patient may fear that the thing they need to breathe is being taken away when you leave the house. This may result in the person feeling that they need an emergency response whenever they feel breathless.

Non-pharmacological Management of Breathlessness

- Positioning (various advice depending on position: sit upright, legs uncrossed, let shoulders droop, keep head up; lean forward).
- Relaxation techniques.
- Pursed-lips breathing. In pursed-lips breathing, people inhale through their nose for several seconds with their mouth closed, then exhale slowly through pursed lips for 4–6 seconds. This can help to relieve the perception of breathlessness during exercise or when it is triggered.
- Reduce room temperature.
- Cooling the face by using a cool flannel or cloth.
- Portable fan use or sitting near an open window. **NB** Portable fans are not recommended for patients with suspected or confirmed COVID-19.

Pharmacological Management of Breathlessness

- Oxygen (no evidence of benefit in the absence of hypoxia).
- Opioids may reduce the perception of breathlessness.
- Oramorph® if present. If patient has own Oramorph® refer to patient's prescribed dose on drug chart. If using ambulance service morphine, refer to dosage table 'Breathlessness End of Life – Oral' in the **Morphine Sulfate** guideline.
- Morphine SC/IM. If patient has own JIC medication, refer to patient's prescribed dose on drug chart. If using ambulance service morphine, refer to dosage table 'Breathlessness End of Life – SC/IM' in the **Morphine Sulfate** guideline.
- Other medications may also need to be administered for breathlessness and anxiety, such as lorazepam or midazolam.

4.5 Managing Nausea and Vomiting

- Consider likely causes of nausea or vomiting in the dying person. These may include:
  - Certain medicines that can cause or contribute to nausea and vomiting
  - Recent chemotherapy or radiotherapy
  - Psychological causes
  - Biochemical causes, e.g. hypercalcaemia
  - Raised intracranial pressure
  - Gastrointestinal motility disorder
  - Ileus or bowel obstruction.
- If the patient had previous, well-controlled nausea and vomiting using medicines via a syringe driver, consider reviewing the syringe driver to confirm it is not leaking and the infusion site is not inflamed (inflammation at the infusion site which might reduce absorption and therefore effectiveness of medication).
- Discuss the options for treating nausea and vomiting with the dying person and those important to them.
- Consider non-pharmacological methods for treating nausea and vomiting. For people in the last days of life with obstructive bowel disorders who have nausea or vomiting, medications used include:
  - Hyoscine butylbromide
  - Octreotide
  - Cyclizine
  - Haloperidol
  - Levomepromazine.
- See 4.8 – Patient's Own Medications.

End of Life Care

Non-pharmacological Management of Nausea and Vomiting

- Avoid eating or preparing food when patient feels sick or nauseous.
- Avoid fried foods or foods with strong smells.
- Small meals.
- Sip drinks slowly.

Pharmacological Management of Nausea and Vomiting

- Patient's own JIC medication prescribed for nausea/vomiting as per their medication chart.

4.6 Managing Anxiety, Delirium and Agitation

- Explore the possible causes of anxiety or delirium with the dying person and those important to them. Be aware that agitation in isolation is sometimes associated with other unrelieved symptoms or bodily needs, such as unrelieved pain, their positioning, medications, a full bladder or rectum, organ failure or infection.
- Consider non-pharmacological management of agitation, anxiety and delirium in a person in the last days of life, e.g. care for the patient in a well-lit room to avoid misinterpretation of shadow, ensure spectacles if used are clean, use short sentences. Consider calming music and environmental changes that may help.
- Consider any reversible causes of agitation, anxiety or delirium, for example psychological causes or certain metabolic disorders, such as renal failure or hyponatraemia.
- Medications used include:
  - Benzodiazepine to manage anxiety or agitation, e.g. lorazepam and midazolam
  - An antipsychotic medicine to manage delirium or agitation, e.g. haloperidol and levomepromazine.
- Seek specialist advice if the diagnosis of agitation or delirium is uncertain, if the agitation or delirium does not respond to antipsychotic treatment or if treatment causes unwanted sedation.
- See 4.8 – Patient's Own Medications.

Non-pharmacological Management of Managing Anxiety, Delirium and Agitation

- Identify and manage the possible underlying cause or combination of causes (pain, urinary retention, constipation, anxiety, breathlessness).
- Ensure effective communication and reorientation (for example explaining where the person is, who they are and what your role is) and provide reassurance for people diagnosed with delirium.
- Consider involving family, friends and carers to help with this.

- Where possible, ensure people at risk of delirium are cared for by family or carers who are familiar to the patient.
- Avoid moving people within and between rooms unless absolutely necessary.
- Ensure adequate lighting and consider environmental factors.

Pharmacological Management of Managing Anxiety, Delirium and Agitation

- Patient's own JIC medication prescribed for delirium as per their medication chart.
- Ambulance Service JIC Midazolam (**NB** This is only applicable to Trusts that have either a PGD that specifically allows Midazolam use in EoLC, or if a verbal order process is set up and authorised that allows for its use in EoLC). Refer to local guidance.

4.7 Managing Noisy Respiratory Secretions

- These can be associated with the disease process, or a result of excessive weakness in the patient and an inability to maintain their own airway through normal physiological procedures, such as coughing or clearing of the throat, resulting in a pooling of saliva.
- Assess for the likely causes of noisy respiratory secretions in people in the last days of life. Establish whether the noise has an impact on the dying person or those important to them. The noise associated with respiratory secretions can be a source of distress for carers.
- Ambulance clinicians may need to provide additional explanation and reassurance that although the noise can be distressing, it will not cause discomfort or distress to the patient.
- Repositioning the patient such that they are sitting up a little or laying on their side to aid postural drainage can be effective in managing secretions. Suctioning is not usually used or recommended.
- Be prepared to talk about any fears or concerns the patient or carers may have.
- Consider non-pharmacological measures to manage noisy respiratory or pharyngeal secretions, to reduce any distress in people at the end of life.
- Medications include:
  - Glycopyrronium bromide
  - Hyoscine butylbromide
  - Hyoscine hydrobromide.
- It is important to note that medications will not dry up existing secretions; positioning is the primary treatment to aid this. Medications may then be administered to help prevent a further build-up of secretions.
- See 4.8 – Patient's Own Medications.

End of Life Care

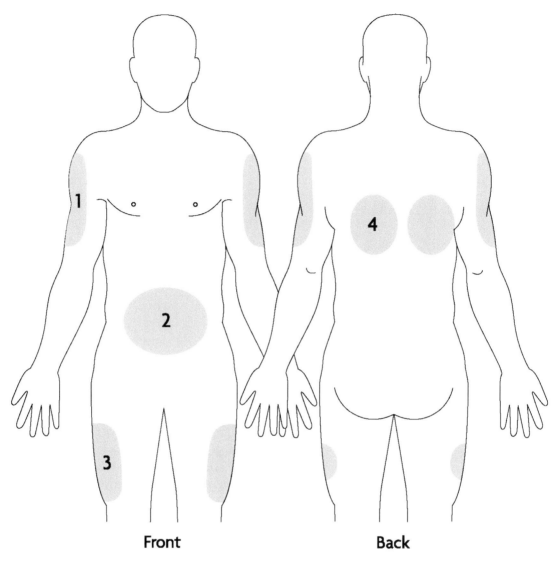

Front

1. The deltoid (upper arm)
2. The abdomen (avoid the umbilicus)

Back

3. The thigh
4. The scapula

Figure 1.2 – Sites for injection of intramuscular and subcutaneous administrations.

Non-pharmacological Management of Respiratory Secretions

- Positioning (sit up slightly if lying flat or onto side – postural drainage).
- Explanation/reassurance to relatives that noise is not causing distress or pain to patient.

Pharmacological Management of Respiratory Secretions

- Patient's own JIC medication prescribed for respiratory secretions as per their medication chart.

- Ambulance Service JIC Glycopyrronium or Hyoscine (if available).

4.8 Patients' Own Medications

Many more patients nearing the end of life are cared for at home in their final days/weeks with the express wish to remain at home. As part of their end of life care plan, they may have 'anticipatory' or 'just in case' medications.

Clinicians are permitted to administer these medications provided that:

SECTION **1** General Guidance

End of Life Care

- The clinician is competent in the method of administration. A person who administers a prescribed medicine is accountable for their own practice.

- A signed Medication Administration and Authorisation Record (MAAR) chart is present and authorised by an independent prescriber. (In some Trusts, local guidelines specific to EoLC medication administration are in place. Refer to local guidance.)

- The clinician has access to the relevant paperwork supplied with the 'just in case' medication, providing the necessary information on each drug's indication, dosage, adverse effects, signs and treatments for overdose.

- In law, anyone may follow a Patient Specific Direction (PSD), but some organisations may extend or limit those who are authorised to administer medicines under a PSD within their local medicines policies and governance arrangements. Always check local policy.

- Follow this best practice advice when working with 'just in case' medications:
  - Establish what medication the patient has already received, including drug name, dosage and time of administration.
  - Use shared decision making if appropriate; see 3.2 – Shared Decision Making.
  - Only administer via the prescribed route and the prescribed dose.
  - Consider reversible causes.
  - Consider if the patient is opioid naïve (not on regular opioids). Start on the lowest dose prescribed.
  - Check for and leave transdermal patches in situ.
  - Never alter syringe driver settings.
  - Talk to the patient, family and caregivers. Ask what helps ease their discomfort and what does not.

4.9 Documentation

- Ambulance clinicians **MUST** complete the administration chart that accompanies a patient's medication in addition to completing their own Trust documentation following the use of anticipatory or 'just in case' medications. This enables the specialist palliative team, district nurse or GP to see what medications have been administered. There are some self-explanatory pages at the back of the administration chart which should be filled in and signed to show the use of certain controlled medications, and also the current stock level. Always be mindful of the stock balance; fill out on the form when a medication is administered and arrange a GP follow-up if the stock is sufficiently depleted. Be particularly mindful of this when approaching a weekend or bank holiday when medication prescriptions can be harder to source. Proactive care ensures crisis management is minimised and makes a great deal of difference in the patient's experience in their last days or hours of life.

5. Considerations Relating to Medicine Administration Near the End of Life

- When administering medications at the end of life, there are additional factors that should be considered; this applies to both the patient's own and ambulance service medications. Shared decision making should always be considered prior to administration. Follow Trust guidelines relating to shared decision making.

5.1 Management of Opioid Overdose in End of Life Patients

- Opioid reversal in end of life patients is a specialist skill and should never be undertaken without advice and guidance from specialist palliative care teams.

- If the patient is opioid naïve, (not on regular opioids) then it is safe to reverse the opioid effect immediately (refer to **Naloxone Hydrochloride**). This is unlikely in end of life patients.

- It is important in the management of patients in pain that the signs of advanced progressive disease are not confused with those of opioid overdose.

- If the patient is taking regular opioids, the aim is to reverse the respiratory depression only:
  - Stop the opioid.
  - Administer oxygen if saturations <94%.
  - Give Naloxone until the respiratory status is satisfactory (>8 respirations per minute) – ensure the cannula is flushed after each administration. Refer to **Naloxone Hydrochloride**.
  - If IV access cannot be established or is not permitted (due to clinical grade of ambulance clinician), carry out IM administration. Refer to **Naloxone Hydrochloride**. Shared decision making should always be considered prior to administration.
  - The aim is for slow administration of the drug to avoid a surge of pain from complete antagonism of opioid.
  - If there is no response, consider other causes.

5.2 Naloxone Use in End of Life Care

- The use of naloxone in palliative care is not routinely practised and is only indicated in circumstances where a clinician suspects opioid-induced toxicity, from intentional or unintentional overdose. The aim is to reverse life-threatening

End of Life Care

respiratory depression only, e.g. if the respiratory rate is <8 breaths per minute and the patient is unconscious and/or cyanosed.

- Do not give Naloxone for opioid-induced drowsiness or reduced level of conscious if the respiratory rate is satisfactory or the patient is in the final dying stage.

- If the respiratory rate is ≥8 breathes per minute and the patient is easily rousable/not cyanosed, adopt a wait-and-see approach; consider reducing or omitting the next regular dose or discontinuing continuous parenteral administration.

- Patients on regular opioids for pain and symptom control can be physically dependent; naloxone given in too large a dose or too quickly can cause an acute withdrawal reaction and an abrupt return of pain that is difficult to control; this is also extremely distressing for patients with cancer or advanced progressive illness.

5.3 Opioid Administration in the Last Hours of Life

- The BMA Medical Ethics Today (2012) explains the use of opioids and sedatives in end of life care and the principle of double effect as follows: 'the principle of double effect allows doctors to provide medical treatment that has both good and bad effects, as long as the intention is to provide an overall good effect. They can give sedatives and analgesics with the intention of and in proportion to the relief of suffering, even if as a consequence the patient's life risks being shortened. The moral distinction is between intending and foreseeing harm. The intention of giving the drugs is to relieve pain and distress; the harmful but unintended effect is the risk of shortening life, which the doctor may foresee but not intend'.[49]

5.4 Death After Medicine Administration

- It must be recognised that the prognosis for patients receiving palliative care is poor and death is an expected consequence of their condition. It is entirely possible that a patient may die whilst in our care or shortly after an intervention we have provided. As ambulance clinicians we should be prepared for this, but it is also important to explain to any relatives or carers present that the purpose of any intervention, whether pharmacological or not, is to relieve symptoms, not advance death.

5.5. Renal Failure

- Prescribing at the end of life for patients with renal failure is complex, and advice should always be sought from the renal and palliative care specialists. Many of the medicines used for symptom control in end of life care are eliminated by the kidney to a greater or lesser degree. Morphine and diamorphine accumulate in even modest degrees of renal impairment; great care is needed to avoid opioid toxicity.

5.6. Syringe Drivers and Transdermal Patches

- If the patient has a syringe driver or transdermal patch in situ and suddenly experiences an increase in pain then some problem-solving is required.

- Assess:
  - When was the patch (Fentanyl or Buprenorphine) last changed and when should it have been changed? Some patches need to be changed every 7 days, whereas others require changing every 3 days.
  - Is the patch fully adherent to the skin? The dose of the drug depends on the surface area of the patch. If the patch is falling off, the dose of drug administered/absorbed will be reduced. Sometimes the patch can become dislodged due to body hair, sweating or movement. Take advice if the patch has been dislodged. Ensure safe disposal of any patches (these can be disposed of in a sharps box).
  - Is the syringe driver running properly? Is the battery light flashing? Is the battery still in? If not, take advice.
  - Is the syringe driver site (subcutaneous butterfly cannula) intact? Is there any evidence of it becoming dislodged or a significant amount of unabsorbed fluid being present around the cannula site? If so, take advice.

6. Staff Wellbeing and End of Life Care

- Managing a patient at the end of their life and supporting their families and carers is very distressing for all those involved. Opportunities for debriefing and/or counselling should be available for ambulance clinicians. Follow local procedures for post-critical incident debriefing and refer to **Staff Health and Wellbeing** for more guidance.

End of Life Care

End of Life Care

- **Providing adequate pain management at the end of life is a right of the dying patient and the duty of all clinicians.**
- **Acute or escalating pain is a medical emergency requiring a prompt response.**
- **Wherever possible, a patient self-assessment strategy should be used and only substituted when the patient is unable to do so.**
- **Pain is easier to prevent than to relieve.**
- **Where pain is intense and opioids are already prescribed, morphine should be the first line treatment for breakthrough pain.**
- **The presence (or absence) of a DNACPR order must not direct treatment options or discussion in a patient who is actively dying. In the absence of a valid DNACPR form, any ambulance clinician who has diagnosed a patient as dying is not obliged to commence CPR at the point of death. Remember that a DNACPR is not a legally binding document; it is a decision support tool to help guide clinicians as to whether CPR is appropriate. Refer to local guidelines on DNACPR orders, as many Trusts have clear guidance to help clarify queries such as forms from different areas, photocopies, etc.**
- **Patients' own just in case (JIC) medication may be administered by a trained clinician (refer to local guidance).**
- **Just in case medication carried by registered ambulance clinicians can be administered via a valid Patient Specific Direction or via a verbal order depending on your Trust. Local guidelines and policies must be adhered to.**

Further Resources

Visit https://www.respectprocess.org.uk for more information on caring for people when they do not have capacity to make or express choices.

Further important information and evidence in support of this guideline can be found in the Bibliography.

Bibliography

1. Kloke M, Cherny N. Treatment of dyspnoea in advanced cancer patients: ESMO Clinical Practice Guidelines. *Annals of Oncology* 2015, 26: 5.

2. British Thoracic Society. *Guidelines*. 2017. Available from: www.brit-thoracic.org.uk/standards-of-care/guidelines.

3. British Thoracic Society Emergency Oxygen Guideline Development Group. BTS guideline for oxygen use in adults and healthcare and emergency settings. *Thorax* 2017, 72(1): 1–90. Available from: https://www.brit-thoracic.org.uk/document-library/clinical-information/oxygen/2017-emergency-oxygen-guideline/bts-guideline-for-oxygen-use-in-adults-in-healthcare-and-emergency-settings/.

4. Colvin L, Forbes K, Fallon M. ABC of palliative care: difficult pain. *British Medical Journal* 2006, 332(7549): 1081–1083.

5. Vantafridda V, Ripamonti C, DeConno F, et al. Symptom prevalence and control during cancer patients' last day of life. *Journal of Palliative Care* 1990, 6: 7.

6. McCaffery M, Pasero CL. Assessment: underlying complexities, misconceptions, and practical tools. *Pain Clinical Manual*. 2nd edn. St Louis: Mosby, 1999, 35–102.

7. World Health Organization. *Cancer Pain Relief: With a Guide to Opioid Availability*. 2nd edn. Geneva, 1996.

8. Freidman DP. Perspectives on the medical use of drugs of abuse. *Journal of Pain Symptom Management* 1990, 51 suppl: S2–5.

9. Scottish Intercollegiate Guidelines Network. *Control of Pain in Adults with Cancer*. SIGN, 2008. Available from: https://www.sign.ac.uk/assets/sign106.pdf.

10. Quill TE, Brady RV. "You promised me I wouldn't die like this." A bad death as a medical emergency. *Arch Interim Med* 1995, 155: 1250.

11. Rudy TE, Kerns RD, Tuerk DC. Chronic pain and depression: toward a cognitive-behavioural medication model. *Pain* 1988, 35: 129–140.

12. Tan G, Jensen MP, Robinson-Whelen S, Thornby JI, Monga TN. Measuring control appraisals in chronic pain. *The Journal of Pain* 2002, 3(5): 385–393.

13. Turner JA, Dworkin SF, Manel LL, Huggins KH, Truelove EL. The roles of beliefs, catastrophizing, and coping in the functioning of patients with temporomandibular disorders. *Pain* 2001, 92: 41–51.

14. Fishbain DA, Cutler R, Rosomoff HL, Rosomoff RS. Chronic pain-associated depression: antecedent of consequence of chronic pain? A review. *Clinical Journal of Pain* 1979, 13(2): 116–137.

15. Poole H, White S, Blake C, Murphy P, Bramwell R. Depression in chronic pain patients: prevalence and measurement. *World Institute of Pain* 2009, 9(3): 173–180.

16. Morley S, Williams AC, Black S, A confirmatory factor analysis of the Beck Depression Inventory in chronic pain. *Pain* 2009, 99: 289–298.

End of Life Care

17. Leeds-Hurwitz W. Social construction of reality. In Littlejohn S, Foss, K. *Encyclopedia of Communication Theory*. Thousand Oaks, CA: SAGE Publications, 2009.

18. Bury M. Chronic illness as biographical disruption. *Sociology of Health and Illness* 1982, 4: 167–182.

19. Gonzales MJ, Pantilat SZ. Pain at the end of life. *Hospital Medicine Clinics* 2012, 1(1): 109–123.

20. National Institute for Health and Clinical Excellence. *Supportive and Palliative Care: The manual*. NICE, 2004. Available from: http://guidance.nice.org.uk/CSGSP/Guidance/pdf/English.

21. Patient UK. *Palliative Care*. Available from: http://patient.info/doctor/palliative-care.

22. Department of Health. *End of Life Care Strategy – Promoting high quality care for all adults*. DOH, 2008. Available from: https://www.gov.uk/government/publications/end-of-life-care-strategy-promoting-high-quality-care-for-adults-at-the-end-of-their-life.

23. Beauchamp TL, Childress JF. *Principles of Biomedical Ethics*. 6th edn. Oxford University Press, 2008.

24. European Court of Human Rights. *Convention for the Protection of Human Rights and Fundamental Freedoms (European Convention on Human Rights, as amended)* (ECHR), Article 2.

25. European Court of Human Rights. *Convention for the Protection of Human Rights and Fundamental Freedoms (European Convention on Human Rights, as amended)* (ECHR), Article 3.

26. European Court of Human Rights. *Convention for the Protection of Human Rights and Fundamental Freedoms (European Convention on Human Rights, as amended)* (ECHR), Article 8.

27. South Western Ambulance Service Trust. *Palliative Care Clinical Guideline*, 2014.

28. South Western Ambulance Service Trust. *Palliative Care Clinical Guideline*. 2014. Available from: http://www.swast.nhs.uk/.../Clinical%20Guidelines%20SWASFT%20staff/CG29.

29. Scottish Palliative Care Guidelines. Palliative Emergencies. 2014. Scotland: NHS Scotland View. Available from: https://www.palliativecareguidelines.scot.nhs.uk.

30. Health and Care Professions Council. *Standards of Conduct, Performance and Ethics: Your Duties as a Registrant*. London: Health Professions Council, 2003.

31. Blackmore S, Pring A, Verne J. *Predicting Death: Estimating the Proportion of Deaths That Are 'Unexpected'*. London: National End of Life Intelligence Network, 2011.

32. Department of Health. *End of Life Care Strategy. Promoting High Quality Care for All Adults at the End of Life*. London: HMSO, 2008.

33. Office for National Statistics. *Mortality in the United Kingdom*, 2010. London: Crown Copyright, 2012.

34. NHS England. *Actions for End of Life Care: 2014–16*. London: NHS England, 2014.

35. Gomes B, Higginson I. Where people die (1974–2030): past trends, future projections and implications for care. *Palliative Medicine* 2008, 22: 33–41.

36. National End of Life Care Programme. *The Route to Success in End of Life Care – Achieving quality in ambulance services*. London, 2012.

37. Leadership Alliance for the Care of Dying People. *One Chance to Get it Right. Improving people's experience of care in the last few days and hours of life*. London: Leadership Alliance for the Care of Dying People, 2014.

38. Robson P. Metastatic spinal cord compression: a rare but important complication of cancer. *Clinical Medicine* 2014, 14(5): 542–545.

39. Sui J, Fleming JS, Kehoe M. An audit of current practice and management of metastatic spinal cord compression at a regional cancer centre. *The Irish Medical Journal* 2011, 104(4): 111–114.

40. McLinton A, Hutchison C. Malignant spinal cord compression: a retrospective audit of clinical practice at a UK regional cancer centre. *British Journal of Cancer* 2006, 94: 486–491.

41. National Institute for Health and Care Excellence. *Metastatic Spinal Cord Compression. Diagnosis and management of adults at risk of and with metastatic spinal cord compression*. Manchester, 2008.

42. Watson M, Lucas C, Hoy A, et al. (eds). *Palliative Adult Network Guidelines*. Anglia, Kent and Medway, Mount Vernon, Northern Ireland, South East London, Surrey, West Sussex and Hampshire, Sussex Cancer Networks and Palliative Care Cymru Implementation Board, 2011.

43. McCurdy M, Shanholtz CB. Oncological emergencies. *Critical Care Medicine* 2012, 40(7): 2212–2222.

44. Samphao S, Eremin JM, Eremin O. Oncological emergencies: clinical importance and principles of management. *European Journal of Cancer Care* 2010, 19: 707–713.

45. Walji N, Chan AK, Peake DR. Common acute oncological emergencies: diagnosis, investigation and management. *Postgraduate Medical Journal* 2008, 84: 418–427.

46. Abner A. Approach to the patient who presents with superior vena cava obstruction. *Chest* 1993, 103: 394–397.

47. National Institute for Health and Care Excellence. *Neutropenic Sepsis: prevention and management of neutropenic sepsis in cancer patients*. Manchester, 2012.

48. Royal College of General Practitioners. *The National GSF Centre's Guidance for Clinicians to Support Earlier Recognition of Patients Nearing the End of Life*. 2011. Available from: https://www.goldstandardsframework.org.uk/cd-content/uploads/files/General%20Files/Prognostic%20Indicator%20Guidance%20October%202011.pdf.

49. BMA. *Medical Ethics Today*. 2012. Available from: https://www.bma.org.uk/advice/employment/ethics/medical-ethics-today.

50. Welsh Ambulance Service NHS Trust Clinical Guidelines. *Palliative Symptom Control Guidance for Welsh Ambulance Service Staff*, 2020.

Human Factors

1. Introduction

- Team resource management, a component of human factors, is a discipline that seeks to understand the interaction of humans, their work and the systems and environment they inhabit in order to utilise **ALL** available resources, both human and technological, to achieve safe and efficient clinical best practice.

- Effective leadership skills are vital when it comes to ensuring maximal efficiency, particularly at critical and life-threatening incidents, but most of the errors occur when there is a failure to establish leadership in the first place (refer to Table 1.5).

TABLE 1.5 – Leadership Skills: Good Practice	
States own position and acknowledges lead role	Supports team awareness
Coordinates and manages the scene	Actively listens to and acknowledges team suggestions
Motivates and coaches	Active and approachable
Guidelines and standard operating procedure (SOP) compliant	Adheres to Guidelines, SOPs or evidence base
Challenges deviation	Recognises and addresses errors
Encourages and utilises team around them	Shares tasks
Uses clear and inclusive communications	Involves the team in changes in the clinical and operational plans
Maintains situational awareness	Recognises own capacity to lead and manages this through delegation to increase 'band width' or hands over leadership to others appropriately
Maintains team focus and role allocation	Oversees task completion

2. Situational Awareness

- Situational awareness is made up of three elements:

  1 **Perception** – the understanding of where you and your team are in the environment around you.

  2 **Comprehension** – how this will impact on your ability to undertake the task at hand.

  3 **Projection** – what is likely to happen next.

- Although effective team resource management requires that everyone is situationally aware, the team leader will be best placed to focus on these three elements, sharing and implementing this mental model with the team.

- Failure to appreciate and act on any one of those elements within a critical situation may lead to situational awareness errors occurring.

3. Communication

- As well as strong leadership and shared situational awareness, an important indicator of team function is the extent and quality of communication. Effective leaders will utilise and encourage those around them, fostering an environment of respectful communications.

- In the early stages of a life-threatening situation or critical incident, team members' bandwidth may be predominantly utilised for technical tasks. As the team grows, its capacity for simultaneous activity increases. So too does the need for the team leader to establish a shared model of what the team must achieve and how it will go about doing so.

- This is where the need for clear and concise communications is vital. Effective communications should have clarity, brevity, empathy and an element of feedback for confirmation of instructions passed or decisions being made.

- There is strong evidence to support the use of checklists to improve clinical management and patient safety. No one can remember everything in every situation.

4. Clinical Decision Making

- Clinical decision making involves the assimilation of information leading to an appropriate course of action.

- There are many barriers to effective decision making, including time, incomplete facts, stress and seniority. These barriers can be overcome by utilising tools such as checklists and SOPs. Using the Page for Age, for example, will save time and reduce workload when calculating drug doses, and ensure accurate calculations.

- Trying to do too much yourself will only lead to cognitive overload – a high risk when dealing with life-threatening incidents.

- Stress can have positive and negative effects on our performance and, ultimately, some level of stress is necessary to achieve an ideal mental state for performance. However, very high levels

Human Factors

of stress are associated with disordered thinking and reduced motor control, which will hinder performance.

▪ Human factors can greatly influence the clinical effectiveness and efficiency of incident and patient management. Only by understanding these factors and applying principles of their management can the efficiency and effectiveness of patient care be optimised, leading to improved patient outcomes.

5. Managing Behaviours

▪ Clinically demanding situations can involve differing opinions on the right course of action. As discussed above, good communication, shared decision making and good situational awareness will aid in successful delivery of clinical interventions.

▪ Professional standards and behaviours in modern clinical practice should welcome and encourage challenge as part of a shared decision making model. Only by challenging the ideas of others in a structured and positive way can we learn as individuals and perform well as a team.

▪ Good team resource management (TRM) will respect that every individual has a voice, an opinion and should be heard. Good leaders will foster and empower staff to speak up and challenge interventions and actions being undertaken. Three steps for effective challenge for patient advocacy are:

– **Clarify** – Simply ask for clarification of the course of action being undertaken. Each clinician should be able to articulate at any time clinical rational for what they are doing

and why, which will improve team situational awareness.

– **Advocate** – If any course of action is deemed unjustified or if a more suitable alternative needs to be made apparent, any team member should feel empowered to speak up, advocate an alternative and initiate a professional conversation about the course of action being undertaken.

– **Intervene** – If during an incident, despite clarification and advocation being undertaken, the course of action is still unnecessary or dangerous (e.g. a clinician attempting to defibrillate a non-shockable rhythm), an intervention is required, whether physical or verbal, to prevent patient or clinician harm.

▪ With challenge comes potential conflict; the good aspects of correctly focused challenge will be beneficial:

– Challenge is the root of change.
– People learn and grow as a result of appropriate challenge.
– Challenge can provide diagnostic information about problem areas to improve.
– After challenge, a sense of achieved partnership working can be established.

▪ The key is maintaining sustained professional behaviours in the face of stress, and understanding that limiting conflict to that of positive challenge in all situations (fact based, SOP and clinical rationale driven) can lead to resolution avoiding interpersonal conflict (emotional, personality and frustration driven) which could lead to negative scene management or patient outcome.

Bibliography

1.   Resuscitation Council (UK). *Acute Care – Quality standards for CPR (2010).* London: Resuscitation Council UK, 2021. Available from: https://www.resus.org.uk/quality-standards/acute-care-quality-standards-for-cpr/#team.

2.   Resuscitation Council (UK). *ALS Course. Chapter 2: Human factors and quality in resuscitation.* Available from: https://lms.resus.org.uk/modules/m40-v2-decisions/10346/resources/chapter_2.pdf.

Pain Management in Adults

1. Introduction

- Relief of pain is one of the most important clinical outcomes in paramedic practice. Often, pain is the chief complaint that has resulted in seeking assistance. Apart from the humanitarian dimension, managing pain has several clinical benefits. Analgesia should be swiftly initiated as soon as clinically possible after arriving on scene. There is no reason to delay pain relief because of uncertainty with the definitive diagnosis. It does not affect later diagnostic efficacy, but may potentially aid in arriving at a prompt diagnosis, as patients are more cooperative when comfortable. Intense pain can modify the nervous system, leading to chronic persistent pain – a troublesome long-term problem with huge health and socioeconomic impacts.

- Barriers to effective pain management include:
  - patient factors (general condition, communication, cooperation)
  - knowledge and experience of the clinician
  - environment and available resources.

2. Assessment

- Pain is a complex and dynamic experience and all clinicians should place the requirements and needs of the individual at the forefront of all assessments. Ideally, multidisciplinary assessment ascertains the most appropriate and efficient course of treatment in both acute and chronic pain conditions, but limited resources in the pre-hospital environment can make comprehensive assessment a challenging task.

- The pain experience of individuals is influenced by bio-psycho-social factors, such as:
  - the nature of any underlying medical condition
  - age, gender, genetics
  - prior pain experience, culture, beliefs
  - environment and social conditions.

- When managing pain for any patient, clinicians should provide pain control interventions or administer analgesia and other treatments based on the needs of the individual patient. Clinicians should be aware of the risks of unconscious bias and should not manage any patient based on a stereotype based on age, gender, sexuality, ethnicity or any other characteristic. There are a wide range of expressed emotions in patients from all backgrounds. Care must be taken not to treat an individual in pain as 'stoical' or 'highly expressive' based on their perceived ethnic group or other characteristic as this may lead to either ineffective or excessive pain relief.

- Research indicates that patients from the Black ethnic groups and Mixed ethnic groups are less likely to be offered pain relief and this may lead to patient harm.

- Where there is a communication barrier of any kind, please use the locally available translation service or pre-hospital communication guide/app, and/or refer to **Patients with Communication Difficulties**.

- Treat the individual in front of you using a structured approach with a focused history and clinical examination, irrespective of your perception of their patient group.

- To ensure every patient receives appropriate pain relief, explore pain descriptors carefully, giving extra time to consider individual patient needs.

2.1 Measuring Pain

- Although different scoring systems are used to gauge the intensity of pain, patients' experiences cannot be objectively validated in the same way as other vital signs. JRCALC recommend the 0–10-point verbal numerical scale in which 0 refers to no pain and 10 is the worst imaginable pain. In most pre-hospital situations, this score is suitable to assess severity of pain and the response to treatment. As there is inter-individual variability, the trend in the scores is more important than the absolute value in assessing efficacy of treatment. Apart from initial assessment and scoring, subsequent periodic measurement after each intervention is a recommended practice. However, no pain assessment tool is set in stone and the patient's needs should always be considered above the findings of the assessment tool.

- Scoring can be difficult in patients with dementia, cognitive impairment, altered level of consciousness or communication difficulties. In these scenarios, pain is assessed through behavioural cues. Remember: no behaviour is unique to pain; behaviour is unique to individuals.[5]

- The prevalence of persistent pain in older adults is high, with the main causes originating as a result of degenerative changes. In both sexes, incidence of arthritis increases with age. Both osteoarthritis and osteoporosis are more common in women. Due to unmet healthcare needs, other concurrent medical conditions or poor compliance with medications, managing pain in older adults is often suboptimal. This has adverse effects on mood, sleep and activity. Ageing-related alteration to pharmacokinetics, pharmacodynamics and polypharmacy also contributes to poorly controlled pain. Older adults may not complain or effectively communicate their needs. In addition, they may also be living with dementia. The process of assessing older adults should be the same as for younger people, utilising numerical or pictorial pain assessment scales. The Abbey Pain Scale can be used to measure pain (refer to Figure 1.3).

Pain Management in Adults

Figure 1.3 – The Abbey Pain Scale.

2.2 Clinical Evaluation of Acute Pain

▪ Assessment and treatment of acute pain has to be immediate, with minimal interruption to other aspects of the patient's life. Poorly managed acute pain can result in certain changes in the nervous system, commonly described as 'plasticity', which predispose to development of chronic pain. Knowledge of exacerbating and relieving factors can complement pain management.

▪ A commonly used mnemonic in acute pain assessment is SOCRATES:

Pain Management in Adults

- **Site** (e.g. calf pain due to deep venous thrombosis; associated chest pain may be due to pulmonary embolism).
- **Onset** (acute onset or progressive worsening of an underlying condition).
- **Character** (aching pain with movements can be musculoskeletal; burning pain, pins and needles can be neuropathic).
- **Radiation** (back pain radiating to legs can be due to nerve root irritation; chest pain with radiation to the left arm can be due to angina).
- **Associated symptoms** (fever, chills, nausea may be due to infectious cause).
- **Time**/duration.
- **Exacerbation** and relieving factors (pain with movement may be musculoskeletal, pain associated with bowel and bladder disturbance may be due to abdominal problems).
- **Severity** (scoring tools to assess baseline intensity and monitor progress).

- All patients with pain should have at least two pain scores taken, the first one before the treatment and the subsequent measurements after the treatment is commenced. Scoring and systematic assessment increases awareness of pain management, reveals previously unrecognised pain and improves analgesic administration.

2.3 Clinical Evaluation of Chronic Pain

- Chronic pain is not prolonged acute pain. The experience of pain is influenced by 'bio-psycho-social' factors, such as medical condition, mood, sleep, beliefs and behaviour, as well as cultural and social factors.

- Patients with chronic pain may have heightened sensitivity of the nervous system and are prone to develop exacerbation episodes necessitating a call for urgent help.

- The fundamental principles of assessing these patients are the same as described above, but consideration should be given to psychological and social factors. The challenges for paramedics include seeing these patients for the first time and hence difficulty in obtaining a global picture, and limited resources/time to conduct a comprehensive assessment. This may result in disbelief of the patient's report of pain. Without precise knowledge of the patient's background medical history, malingering may be suspected and this impression may negatively affect the quality of care. A safer approach is to seek and accept the patient's self-report of their pain.

Examples of questions to assess patients with chronic pain

- How would you rate your pain on a 0 to 10 scale at the **present**, where 0 is 'no pain' and 10 is 'worst imaginable pain'?
- In the past 6 months, how intense was your **worst** pain, rated on a 0 to 10 scale?
- In the past 6 months, on **average**, how intense was your pain, rated on a 0 to 10 scale?
- In the past 6 months, how much has the pain interfered with your daily activities, rated on a 0 to 10 scale where 0 is 'no interference' and 10 is 'unable to carry on any activities'?
- In the past 6 months, how much has the pain changed your ability to take part in recreational, social and family activities where 0 is 'no change' and 10 is 'extreme change'?
- In the past 6 months, how much has the pain changed your ability to do housework where 0 is 'no change' and 10 is 'extreme change'?
- About how many days in the past 6 months have you been kept from your usual activities (work, school or housework) because of pain?

3. Management

- Whenever possible, treat the cause (for example, glyceryl trinitrate sublingual spray for angina and oxygen for sickle cell crisis). When the cause is not readily treatable or if it is not apparent, then other analgesic interventions are necessary.

- The pain relief options are:
  - psychological (e.g. reassurance, distraction)
  - physical (e.g. dressing burns wound, splinting fracture)
  - pharmacological (e.g. paracetamol, NSAID, morphine).

- 'Balanced analgesia' with a multimodal pain plan is recommended by JRCALC in pre-hospital pain management and involves administration of analgesics with different mechanisms of action. The synergistic effects should improve effectiveness while limiting the side effects. An example is the combination of paracetamol and morphine. Studies show that the dose of morphine can be reduced by 40–50% when administered alongside paracetamol or ibuprofen. This complementary effect not only offers a more effective pain solution for the patient, but will also improve safety when paramedics administer morphine. Often, a combination of pharmacological and non-pharmacological methods may be necessary; for example, Entonox, morphine or ketamine may be required to enable the application of a splint for fractures.

SECTION 1 General Guidance

Pain Management in Adults

Figure 1.4 – Pain pathway and treatment options.

- Treatment of acute pain may not follow the WHO analgesic ladder as closely as in other elective clinical scenarios. Initially, effective pain control is facilitated with stronger opioids and, wherever appropriate, local anaesthetic techniques. Entonox can be judiciously used for a short period until the other analgesics have had time to take effect. Once controlled, enteral options, such as regular oral opioid analgesics (codeine) and then simple analgesics (paracetamol, NSAID), are introduced.

- Any pain relief must be accompanied by careful explanation of the patient's condition and the pain relief methods being used. Understanding the basic sites of action of different analgesics will aid in choosing the optimal combinations.

3.1 Choice of Analgesics

Refer to Figure 1.5.

- Simple analgesics:
  - paracetamol, non-steroidal anti-inflammatory drugs (NSAIDs), e.g. ibuprofen, Diclofenac, Naproxen.
- Opioids:
  - codeine, morphine.
- Miscellaneous:
  - Entonox, Methoxyflurane, ketamine, local anaesthetic blocks.

3.2 Routes of Administration

- The oral route is mostly sufficient for mild to moderate pain. In severe pain, the intravenous route has the advantage of rapid onset and the dose can be titrated against analgesic effect. In a subgroup of patients, such as those suffering from sickle cell disease or requiring end-of-life care, intramuscular or subcutaneous injections, or the oral route, are appropriate and local Trust guidelines should be followed. In specific circumstances, the intraosseous route may be considered.

- The intranasal route of offering pain relief has many advantages over the traditional routes. It overcomes the cannulation barrier associated with the administration of opioid analgesia that has been shown to be a major problem in the young, the elderly, the shocked patient and the cognitively impaired. Studies looking at pain management in children have found that the intranasal route offers a kinder and less intrusive mechanism for drug delivery while at the same time offering the same level of analgesia as the intravenous route.

- Inhalational analgesia is particularly useful when venous access is not readily secured or when there is a need for immediate relief of severe pain. It can be used as the first analgesic while

Pain Management in Adults

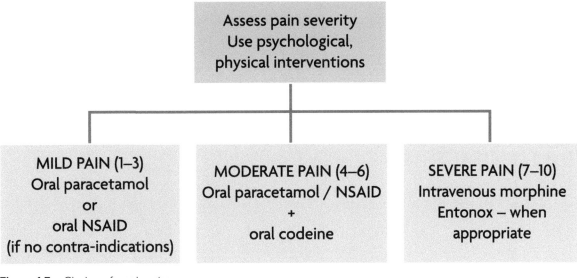

Figure 1.5 – Choice of analgesics.

Figure 1.6 – Routes of administration.

other pain relief is instituted, or in conjunction with other medications until satisfactory control is achieved. Inhalational analgesia is only for short-term use.

3.3 Chronic Pain[6,7]

- These patients are commonly on pain medications, such as gabapentin, pregabalin, amitriptyline and duloxetine, and a significant dose of opioids. Unlike acute pain management, complete resolution of symptoms can be challenging in 'acute on chronic' pain management. Understanding the complexity of chronic pain helps in handling the situation. Ensuring compliance to the prescribed chronic pain medications can help to avoid adding more medicines. Patients may be on a significant dose of opioids such as morphine, oxycodone, Fentanyl or buprenorphine patches. Recent

evidence throws light on the limitations of using stronger opioids in chronic pain management.

- If patients require intravenous morphine or inhalation of Entonox to help break the pain–spasm cycle and enable assessment, it is prudent to reiterate that this is only a short-term intervention for temporary relief; long-term exposure to opioids or Entonox can be potentially harmful.

- In general, the treatment plan for patients with chronic pain runs closely alongside the principle of 'start low and go slow' with regards to the analgesics. If clinical assessment did not identify any fresh cause for exacerbation of pain, reassurance, compliance with prescribed medicines, simple non-pharmacological interventions, such as a TENS machine, may minimise the need for transportation to the emergency department and instead facilitate

Pain Management in Adults

elective review with the general practitioner or the pain clinic.

- Modern medicine has heavily relied on the 'biomedical model', where clinicians regarded diseases as derangement in normal body structure and function that can be fixed with a drug or a procedure. We now recognise that the brain does not work in isolation, especially in pain. When managing chronic illnesses, the major shortcoming is lack of emphasis placed on the person as a whole. The bio-psycho-social model encompasses all the three important facets that influence pain experience, i.e. biological, psychological and social factors (refer to Table 1.7).

TABLE 1.7 – The Bio-psycho-social Model
Biological
Concerns itself with the biological aspects of the illness and is usually managed within the biomedical model. Although alleviating pain with good analgesics is still the main aim, it is equally important that clinicians do not reduce the problem of pain to simply labelling it as a broken or dysfunctional part of the body in isolation and apply a specific treatment for that cause.
Psychological
Explores the emotional aspect of the person and behaviour, or indeed the change in the behaviour that accompanies pain. Commonly, patients with persistent pain also have mental health issues such as anxiety and depression, either as a cause or as an association. Timely recognition of mental health difficulties and facilitating appropriate psychological support can avoid escalation into other complex long-term problems.
Social
Pain-related beliefs and behaviour could have social repercussions at home, work and in the wider society. Patients will rationalise what is happening to them within a social model, which will have impacts on their relationships, family, employment etc. In chronic pain, a social constructionist approach will help to develop a holistic treatment plan.

TABLE 1.8 – Non-pharmacological Methods of Pain Relief	
▪ **Physical**	▪ Cooling of burns can reduce the pain. Burns should not be cooled for longer than 20 minutes total time and care should be taken with large burns to avoid hypothermia.
	▪ Splintage and immobilisation of fractures provides pain relief as well as minimising ongoing tissue damage, bleeding and other complications.
	▪ Warm blankets can help to keep the patient comfortable and avoid hypothermia.
▪ **Psychological**	▪ Fear and anxiety worsen pain; reassurance and explanation can go a long way towards alleviation of pain.
	▪ Distraction makes pain easier to tolerate; simple conversation is the simplest form of distraction.

SECTION **1** General Guidance

Pain Management in Adults

TABLE 1.9 – Pharmacological Methods of Pain Relief (Refer to Specific Drug Protocols)

▪ **Oral analgesia**	▪ Paracetamol and ibuprofen may be used in isolation or together for the management of mild to moderate pain when used in appropriate dosages. It is important to assess the presence of contraindications to all drugs, including simple analgesics. Non-steroidal anti-inflammatory drugs are responsible for large numbers of adverse events, because of their gastrointestinal and renal side effects and their effects on asthmatics. Some ambulance services may also choose to add a paracetamol/codeine combination and/or other opioid-based oral analgesics to their formulary.
	▪ Oral morphine is useful for less severe pain but has the disadvantage of delayed onset, some unpredictability of absorption and having to be given in a set dose. It has the advantage of avoiding the need for intravenous access. It is widely used for patients with mild/moderate pain from injuries such as fractures.
▪ **Parenteral analgesia (intravenous, intramuscular, subcutaneous, intraosseous)**	▪ Morphine is approved for administration by paramedics. Intravenous morphine is a potent analgesic to manage acute pain, but has significant side effects. For satisfactory relief, in presentations such as severe musculoskeletal pain, co-administration of intravenous paracetamol should be considered. This will improve effectiveness while keeping the dose of morphine to a minimum. As with other opioids, effects of morphine are reversed with the opioid-antagonist naloxone. The person administering opioids should have the expertise and resources for maintaining airway, breathing and circulation, and have ready access to naloxone. Decisions to reverse the opioid's effect using naloxone should be made cautiously as this will return the patient to their pre-treatment pain level. Another common unpleasant side effect of opioids is nausea and vomiting, which may require administration of an antiemetic, such as ondansetron.
	▪ Intramuscular and subcutaneous injections are offered in special circumstances, such as patients with sickle cell disease or end-of-life care pathways as per pre-agreed local Trust guidelines. Occasionally, when the only available vascular access is the intraosseous route and the patient is in severe pain, intraosseous morphine can safely be administered with good effect.
▪ **Inhalational analgesia**	▪ Entonox (50% nitrous oxide, 50% oxygen) is a good analgesic for adults who are able to self-administer and who can rapidly be taught to operate the demand valve. It is fast acting but has a very short half-life, so the analgesic effect wears off rapidly when inhalation is stopped. It can be used as the first analgesic while other pain relief is instituted. It can also be used as part of a balanced analgesic approach, particularly during painful procedures such as splint application and patient movement. It is safest to avoid its use in situations such as head injuries (as it can raise intracranial pressure) and pneumothorax (or any other condition where air is trapped in the body).
	▪ Methoxyflurane (Penthrox) is an inhaled analgesic designed for self-administration. It can be used as a non-opioid alternative to morphine or in conjunction with morphine for very severe pain. Evidence has shown that methoxyflurane works well when combined with morphine and, therefore, morphine administration is encouraged at the earliest possible opportunity (as with Entonox) to work alongside methoxyflurane as part of a multi-modal approach to pain

(continued)

Pain Management in Adults

TABLE 1.9 – Pharmacological Methods of Pain Relief (Refer to Specific Drug Protocols) *(continued)*	
	management.[8] If methoxyflurane treatment has been initiated prior to the arrival of clinicians on scene, this should be continued providing the treatment is helping to manage pain and the clinician is confident in using methoxyflurane. It is particularly useful when venepuncture cannot be achieved or when there is a need for immediate relief of severe pain. It also has advantage over Entonox in patients with chest injuries/pneumothorax.
	Methoxyflurane is presented in 3 ml doses, which will provide analgesia for approximately 30 minutes with continuous inhalation, or up to 60 minutes with intermittent inhalation. Intermittent inhalation is recommended. A maximum dose of 6 ml per day is considered safe.

TABLE 1.10 – Methods That Require Appropriately Trained Practitioners	
Ketamine analgesia	Ketamine is an NMDA receptor antagonist with some action on opioid receptors. Depending upon the dose, it can produce analgesia, sedation or anaesthesia. It is particularly useful in serious trauma because it is less likely to significantly depress blood pressure or respiration compared to other agents. Ketamine is also useful in entrapments, where a person can be extricated with combined analgesic and sedative effects.
	When used in moderate to higher dosages, adults may experience unpleasant side effects, such as hallucinations and agitation. Ketamine produces salivation so careful airway management is important, although unnecessary interference should be avoided as laryngospasm may occasionally occur. Concurrent use of atropine may minimise excessive salivation.
Intranasal opioids (e.g. Fentanyl)	Evidence of its effectiveness in the emergency department has highlighted the potential of intranasal Fentanyl for helping paramedics treat severe pain where venous access is compromised. Studies have shown that intranasal Fentanyl compares with the analgesic standard set by intravenous administration. Also, due to the lack of significant histamine release with Fentanyl, the risk of hypotension is less; this is especially useful in trauma situations. The nasal mucosa offers a capillary-rich environment for absorption. In addition, the duration of action of 30 minutes offers greater control for the clinician. Intranasal Fentanyl at a dose of 1.5 mcg/kg, to a maximum of 100 mcg divided evenly between nares, appears to be a safe and effective analgesic in the pre-hospital management of acute severe pain and may be an attractive alternative to both oral and intravenous opiates.
Local anaesthetic techniques	There is limited room for regional nerve blocks because of the environment and the need to transport the patient to hospital in a timely manner. However, they can be effective in certain circumstances of severe pain and do not induce drowsiness or disorientation. Examples include femoral nerve/fascia iliaca block for lower limb injuries such as a fractured femur. Clinicians undertaking regional analgesia techniques must be suitably trained, and should be able to manage local anaesthetic toxicity.

Pain Management in Adults

> ### KEY POINTS!
>
> **Pain Management in Adults**
> - Timely management of pain has clinical benefits.
> - Pain relief does not affect later diagnosis.
> - Multimodal analgesia is effective and has to be tailored to both patient and practitioner variables.
> - Pain measurements and re-assessments will help to monitor progress.

Further Reading

Further important information and evidence in support of this guideline can be found in the Bibliography.[9,10,11,12]

Bibliography

1. Kennel J, Withers E, Parsons N, Woo H. Racial/ethnic disparities in pain treatment: evidence from oregon emergency medical services agencies. *Medical Care* 2019, 57(12): 924–929.

2. Lord B, Khalsa S. Influence of patient race on administration of analgesia by student paramedics. *BMC Emergency Medicine* 2019, 19(1): 32.

3. Hewes HA, Dai M, Clay Mann N, Baca T, Taillac P. Prehospital pain management: disparity by age and race. *Prehospital Emergency Care* 2018, 22(2): 189–197.

4. Young MF, Hern HG, Alter HJ, Barger J, Vahidnia F. Racial differences in receiving morphine among prehospital patients with blunt trauma. *The Journal of Emergency Medicine* 2013, 45(1): 46–52.

5. Alzheimer's Australia. *Pain and Dementia*. 2011. Available from: https://www.fightdementia.org.au/files/helpsheets/Helpsheet-DementiaQ andA16-PainAndDementia_english.pdf.

6. Von Korff M, Ormel J, Keefe FJ, Dworkin SF. Grading the severity of chronic pain. *Pain* 1992, 50: 133–149.

7. Scottish Intercollegiate Guidelines Network. *Management of Chronic Pain* (SIGN 136). Edinburgh: SIGN, 2013.

8. Bendall JC, Simpson PM, Middleton PM. Effectiveness of prehospital morphine, fentanyl, and methoxyflurane in pediatric patients. *Prehospital Emergency Care* 2011, 15(2).

9. Lo JC, Kaye DA. Benzodiazepines and muscle relaxants. *Essentials of Pharmacology for Anesthesia, Pain Medicine, and Critical Care*. New York: Springer, 2015: 167–178.

10. National Institute for Health and Care Excellence. *Diazepam*. Available from: https://bnf.nice.org.uk/drug/diazepam.html.

11. Lord B, Deveson M. Assessment and management of chronic pain in adults: implications for paramedics. *Journal of Paramedic Practice* 2011, 3(4): 166–172.

12. Pak SC, Micalos PS, Maria SJ, Lord B. Nonpharmacological interventions for pain management in paramedicine and the emergency setting: a review of the literature. *Evidence-Based Complementary and Alternative Medicine* 2015 (2015).

SECTION 1 General Guidance

Pain Management in Children

1. Introduction

- All children in pain need analgesia, regardless of age or situation, and when appropriate, analgesia should be administered as soon as clinically possible after arriving on scene, although this can be done en-route so as not to delay time-critical patients. There is no reason to delay relief of pain because of uncertainty with the definitive diagnosis.

- Pain is one of the commonest symptoms in patients presenting to ambulance services.

- Control of pain is important not only for humanitarian reasons but also because it may prevent deterioration of the child and allow better assessment.

- There is no excuse for leaving a child in pain because of a lack of necessary skills in the clinician. If necessary, suitable expertise should be sought to provide pain relief.

- Pain is a multi-dimensional construct (see below).

Pain consists of several elements:

- Treatment of the underlying condition.
- Non-pharmacological methods, including:
  - psychological support and explanation
  - physical methods, e.g. splinting.
- Pharmacological treatment.

Pain relief will depend on:

- Cause, site, severity and nature of the pain.
- Age of child.
- Experience/knowledge of the clinician.
- Distance from receiving unit.
- Available resources.

---

2. Assessment

- An assessment should be made of the requirements of the child. Pain is a complex experience that is shaped by gender, cultural, environmental, social and personal factors, as well as by prior pain experience. Thus the experience of pain is unique to the individual.

- It is important to remember that the pain a child experiences cannot be objectively validated in the same way as other vital signs. Attempts to estimate the child's pain should be resisted, as this may lead to an underestimation of the child's experience. Several studies have shown that there is a poor correlation between the patient's pain rating and that of the health professionals, with the latter often underestimating the patient's pain.

- Instead, ambulance clinicians need to seek and accept the child's self-report of their pain. This is reinforced by a popular and useful definition of pain: 'pain is whatever the experiencing person says it is, existing whenever they say it does'.

- All children in pain should have their pain assessed for its location, nature, severity and duration. Any factors related to, or that exacerbate or improve, the pain should also be assessed.

2.1 Pain scoring

- There is no validated method of pain scoring for children in the pre-hospital environment. It is suggested that, pending this, a method that has been validated in the paediatric emergency department (ED) setting is used. The Wong-Baker 'faces' (scoring 0 = no hurt, 1–2 = hurts little bit, 3–4 = hurts little more, 5–6 = hurts even more, 7–8 = hurts whole lot, 9–10 = hurts worst) (refer to Appendix 1) are useful for younger children. The FLACC scale is useful for preverbal children and may also be used for older children if needed (refer to Appendix 2).

- The trend in the scores is more important than the absolute value in assessing efficacy of treatment. Scoring will not be possible in all circumstances (e.g. cognitively impaired individuals, and those with communication difficulties or altered level of consciousness) and in these circumstances behavioural cues will be more important in assessing pain.

3. Management

- Analgesia should normally be introduced in an incremental way, with each agent being titrated to effect, considering timeliness, effectiveness and potential adverse events. Utilising a balanced analgesic approach will often allow improved efficacy with reduced side effects. Generally this should always include the non-pharmacological methods of treatment as a starting point and background to all pharmacological therapy (refer to Tables 1.11–1.14).

- However, it may be apparent from the assessment that it is appropriate to start with stronger analgesia because of the child's condition; for example, a child with bilateral fractured femurs is likely to require vascular access to provide circulatory replacement and will be in severe pain. It would, therefore, be inappropriate to only try paracetamol and ibuprofen and wait for them to work. Other agents including inhaled (entonox) and intravenous/transmucosal agents as part of a balanced analgesic approach would be indicated at an early stage (this may include paracetamol, opioids and ketamine when appropriate). This along with non-pharmacological methods of pain control would provide the best possible analgesia with a lower risk of side effects. However, in a child with a small superficial burn, one might try paracetamol with or without ibuprofen and, along with non-pharmacological methods, this may be

Pain Management in Children

adequate. The child will still require regular re-assessment and a change of approach if needed.

- Entonox should be given using an appropriate technique until the other drugs have had time to take effect, and if the child is still in pain. Administering analgesia in this stepwise, incremental way minimises the amount of potent analgesia that is required while still achieving adequate analgesia with fewer side effects.

- Any pain relief must be accompanied by careful explanation, involving the child, where possible, and the carer. Include details of the child's condition, the pain relief methods being used and any possible side effects.

TABLE 1.11 – Non-Pharmacological Methods of Pain Relief

Psychological

- Fear and anxiety worsen pain and a child-friendly environment (e.g. removing equipment which may cause fear and having toys or child-friendly pictures around) may go a long way towards alleviation of pain, as may keeping the patient comfortable (e.g. warm).

- The presence of a parent has been shown to reduce the unpleasantness of hospital emergency procedures more than any other single factor and there is no reason why this should not be true in the pre-hospital setting.

- Distraction (toys, stories, games etc.) is a potent analgesic – whatever is to hand may be used, but there is no substitute for forward planning.

Dressings

- Burns dressings that may cool, such as those specifically designed for the task or cling film, can alleviate the pain in the burnt or scalded child. Burns should not be cooled for more than 20 minutes total time and care should be taken with large burns to prevent the development of hypothermia.

Splintage

- Simple splintage of fractures provides pain relief as well as minimising ongoing tissue trauma, bleeding and other complications.

NB These should be part of all other methods of pain relief.

TABLE 1.12 – Pharmacological Methods of Pain Relief (Refer to Specific Drug Protocols)

Oral analgesia

- Initially administer either **paracetamol** or **ibuprofen** alone. Both are suitable first-line choices for treating mild to moderate pain in children.

- If the child does not respond to the first analgesic, recommend switching to the alternative alone. If the child has not responded sufficiently to appropriate doses of either drug alone, consider alternating paracetamol and ibuprofen. Care needs to be taken not to exceed the maximum dose of each drug in a 24-hour period.

- Evidence shows that the simultaneous use for the treatment of fever is not beneficial and does not reduce the fever duration over ibuprofen use alone. Alternating these agents may be suggested to carers to manage longer term pain in accordance with any pain plan.[2,3]

- **Oral morphine solution** may also prove very effective in the child with moderate to severe pain such as a fractured forearm (although in isolation this is not the ideal class of drug for musculoskeletal pain), but has the disadvantage of delayed onset, some unpredictability of absorption and having to be given in a set dose. It has the advantage of avoiding the need for intravenous access. Those with severe pain are best treated with an intravenous preparation, augmented with entonox if required.

Inhalational analgesia

- **Entonox (50% nitrous oxide, 50% oxygen)** is a good analgesic for children who are able to self-administer and who can rapidly be taught to operate the demand valve. It is rapid acting but has a very short half-life, so the analgesic effect wears off rapidly when inhalation is stopped. It can be used as the first analgesic whilst other pain relief is instituted. It can also be used in conjunction with morphine, particularly during painful procedures such as splint application and patient movement. Quite young children can use the system providing they can be taught to operate the demand valve, and the child's fear of the noise of the gas flow and the mask can be overcome. Flavoured (e.g. bubblegum) clear masks may help the child overcome the fear.

(continued)

Section 1 General Guidance

Pain Management in Children

Parenteral and enteral analgesia

- Morphine remains an important component for balanced analgesia and can be administered intravenously, intraosseously and orally (refer to **Morphine Sulfate**). Opioid analgesics should be given intravenously rather than intramuscularly to avoid erratic absorption when possible. When used in isolation for musculoskeletal pain, there may be an increased risk of side effects before achieving adequate analgesia, emphasising the need for a balanced analgesic approach. Therefore, other agents such as IV paracetamol should be considered (see medication sheets).

- As with the other opioids, morphine is reversed by naloxone. When administering opioids to children, ability to maintain airway/breathing/circulation and naloxone **MUST** be available and the required dose calculated in case urgent reversal is necessary. If clinically significant sedation or respiratory depression occurs following the administration of opioids, the child's ventilation should be assisted. Decisions to reverse the opioid effects using an opioid antagonist such as naloxone should be made cautiously as this may return the child to their pre-opioid pain level depending on dosage of naloxone given, which should therefore be titrated to desired effect.

- Intranasal opioids (morphine, diamorphine and fentanyl) are not currently approved for paramedic administration. Intranasal opioid analgesia is becoming used more frequently in hospital and has the advantage of potent, rapid action without needing parenteral administration. However, it is fairly difficult to prepare the appropriate dose and concentration in the pre-hospital context.

- In certain patients the subcutaneous routes may be used effectively, and these may be most appropriate for patient-specific protocols for groups of patients such as end of life and sickle cell disease. In the event of breakthrough pain with palliative care, advice should be sought from the patient's care team whenever possible.

- There is no evidence that metoclopramide is effective in relieving nausea induced by opioids. Children have a significant risk of dystonic reactions with metoclopramide and therefore this is not advised in these circumstances.

- Other anti-emetics (e.g. ondansetron) can be used for opioid-induced nausea and vomiting.

TABLE 1.13 – Pain Relief Which Requires Appropriately Trained Practitioners

Ketamine analgesia/anaesthesia

- Ketamine is particularly useful in entrapments where a child can be extricated with combined analgesic and sedative effects. At present, only appropriately trained practitioners may carry ketamine.

- Ketamine has a predominantly non-opioid mechanism of action. At higher doses, it can be used as a general anaesthetic agent. It is particularly useful in serious trauma because it may not significantly depress blood pressure or respiration depending on the particular patient (acute and chronic comorbidity) and the time since injury.

- Older children in particular may experience unpleasant emergence phenomena but these tend to be less common in the young, especially if appropriate analgesic doses are utilised and titrated to effect. Ketamine in higher doses (not often a problem with appropriate analgesic doses titrated to effect) produces salivation, so careful airway management is important, although unnecessary interference should be avoided as laryngospasm may occasionally occur. Atropine may be used with care concurrently to minimise hypersalivation.

Regional anaesthesia

- There is very limited room for regional nerve blocks because of the environment and the need to transport the child to hospital in a timely manner. However, they can be effective in certain circumstances of severe pain and do not induce drowsiness or disorientation. Femoral nerve blocks may be useful and provide good analgesia for a fractured femur. Clinicians undertaking regional anaesthesia must be suitably trained, prepared and experienced, and fully understand and have the mechanism to treat local anaesthetic toxicity in the pre-hospital environment.

Pain Management in Children

TABLE 1.14 – Pre-Hospital Analgesic Drugs Used in Children				
Drug	**Route**	**Pain severity**	**Advantages**	**Disadvantages**
Paracetamol	Oral (the rectal route is no longer recommended for analgesia) Intravenous	Mild–moderate (may be opioid sparing when used for more severe pain as better efficacy for musculoskeletal pain than opioids alone)	Readily accessible and well tolerated orally. Well-accepted antipyretic	Slow action when given orally. Inadequate and unpredictable plasma levels if given rectally
Ibuprofen	Oral (other IV NSAIDs are available but currently not available for paramedic use)	Mild–moderate (may be opioid sparing when used for more severe pain as better efficacy for musculoskeletal pain than opioids alone)	Moderately good analgesic, antipyretic and anti-inflammatory	Slow action. May cause bronchospasm in asthmatics. Caution in trauma and patients with regards to platelet and renal function
Entonox	Inhaled	Mild–moderate (may be opioid sparing when used for more severe pain as better efficacy for musculoskeletal pain than opioids alone)	Quick, dose self-regulating. Relative contra-indications are important	Fear of mask. Understanding, coordination and cooperation required. (Demand valves for younger children becoming more available. Cannot use free-flow if not scavenging in confined space, e.g. ambulance.)
Oral morphine	Oral	Moderate	Good analgesic for minor/moderate pain particularly of a visceral nature	May need to adjust dose of IV morphine if given subsequently. Reduced oral bioavailability. Slow action
Morphine	Intravenous Intraosseous Intramuscular Subcutaneous	Severe	Rapid onset. Reversed with naloxone (although requires care). Some euphoria	Not ideal as solo agent when used for musculoskeletal pain. Need access. Respiratory depression, vomiting. Controlled drug

(continued)

Pain Management in Children

TABLE 1.14 – Pre-Hospital Analgesic Drugs Used in Children *(continued)*

Drug	Route	Pain severity	Advantages	Disadvantages
Diamorphin[a]	Intranasal Intravenous Intraosseous	Moderate–severe pain particularly of visceral nature	Intranasal – quick and effective although logistically difficult in pre-hospital practice. Best efficacy if used with other agents (e.g. paracetamol)	As for morphine if given IV. More euphoria. Intranasal not currently approved for paramedics
Ketamin[b]	Intravenous Intramuscular Oral	Severe pain from either musculoskeletal or visceral aetiologies (excluding acute coronary syndromes)	Can be increased to general anaesthesia in experienced hands. Less respiratory and cardiovascular depression than other strong analgesic/anaesthetic drugs. Concerns re-raised ICP less clinically relevant than previously thought	Emergence phenomena, salivation, occasional laryngospasm (usually with higher doses, therefore small doses 0.1 mg/kg/dose for analgesia and titrate to effect). Comes in three different concentrations which may lead to confusion

[a] Currently not approved for general paramedic administration; doctor and suitably trained and authorised paramedic administration only.

[b] Currently not approved for general paramedic administration; doctor and suitably trained and authorised paramedic administration only.

4. Pain Relief Which Requires Appropriately Trained Practitioners

- These methods are included because it is necessary to know what can be done to reduce pain in children before hospital, if time and logistics allow. A suitably licensed and trained pre-hospital practitioner should be called early to the scene if it is thought that such assistance may be necessary. Hospital personnel may not all have these skills.

KEY POINTS!

Pain Management in Children

- All children in pain need analgesia.

- The method of pain relief used will depend on the cause, site, severity and nature of the pain, as well as the age of the child.

- Analgesia should be introduced incrementally and titrated to effect.

- Pain-scoring faces and the FLACC scale are useful for use with young children.

- A balanced analgesic approach to pain management consists of treating the cause wherever possible, and analgesia involving psychological, physical and pharmacological interventions (more than one agent, when possible, in smaller and titrated doses to achieve better analgesia with fewer side effects by acting at different areas involving the pain pathways).

- Balanced analgesia remains the objective and should be tailored according to both patient and practitioner variables.

SECTION 1 General Guidance

Pain Management in Children

APPENDIX 1 – The Wong-Baker FACES Pain Rating Scale

- The Wong-Baker Faces Scale is available from: http://wongbakerfaces.org/instructions-use.

- This rating scale is recommended for persons aged three years and older.

- **Instructions:** Point to each face using the words to describe the pain intensity. Ask the child to choose the face that best describes their own pain and record the appropriate number.

- Explain to the child that each face is for a person who feels happy because they have no pain (hurt) or sad because they have some or a lot of pain.

- Face 0 is very happy because they don't hurt at all.

- Face 2 hurts just a little bit.

- Face 4 hurts a little more.

- Face 6 hurts even more.

- Face 8 hurts a whole lot.

- Face 10 hurts as much as you can imagine, although you don't have to be crying to feel this bad.

- From Hockenberry MJ, Wilson D, Winkelstein ML: Wong's Essentials of Pediatric Nursing, ed. 7, St. Louis, 2005, p. 1259. Copyright, Mosby.

APPENDIX 2 – The FLACC Scale

- The **Face, Legs, Activity, Cry, Consolability scale** or **FLACC scale** is a measurement used to assess pain for children up to the age of seven years or individuals who are unable to communicate their pain. The scale is scored on a range of 0–10 with 0 representing no pain. The scale has five criteria which are each assigned a score of 0, 1 or 2.

TABLE 1.15 – The FLACC Scale			
Criteria	Score – 0	Score – 1	Score – 2
Face	No particular expression or smile	Occasional grimace or frown, withdrawn, uninterested	Frequent to constant quivering chin, clenched jaw
Legs	Normal position or relaxed	Uneasy, restless, tense	Kicking, or legs drawn up
Activity	Lying quietly, normal position, moves easily	Squirming, shifting back and forth, tense	Arched, rigid or jerking
Cry	No cry (awake or asleep)	Moans or whimpers, occasional complaint	Crying steadily, screams or sobs, frequent complaints
Consolability	Content, relaxed	Reassured by occasional touching, hugging or being talked to, distractable	Difficult to console or comfort

Bibliography

1. Malviya S, Voepel-Lewis T, Burke C, Merkel S, Tait AR. The revised FLACC observational pain tool: improved reliability and validity for pain assessment in children with cognitive impairment. *Pediatric Anesthesia* 2006, 16(3): 258–265.

2. National Institute for Health and Clinical Excellence. *Analgesia – Mild-to-moderate pain*. London: NICE, 2015. Available from: https://cks.nice.org.uk/analgesia-mild-to-moderate-pain#!scenario.

3. National Institute for Health and Clinical Excellence. *When Using Paracetamol or Ibuprofen in Children with Fever, Do Not Give Both Agents Simultaneously*. London: NICE, 2013. Available from: https://www.nice.org.uk/donotdo/when-using-paracetamol-or-ibuprofen-in-children-with-fever-do-not-give-both-agents-simultaneously.

Patient Confidentiality

1. Introduction

- Health professionals have a duty of confidentiality regarding patient information. They also have a priority, which is to ensure that all relevant information about their patients, their assessments, examinations and advice is recorded clearly and accurately, and passed to other staff whenever it is necessary for provision of ongoing care.

- Sometimes, aspects of legislation relating to these issues appear to conflict with each other. This guideline provides a brief overview of the relevant legislation.

2. Patient Identifiable Information

- Patient identifiable information is any information that may be used to identify a patient directly or indirectly. It may include:
  - Patient's name, address, postcode or date of birth.
  - Any image or audio/digital recording of the patient.
  - Any other data or information that has the potential, however remote, to identify a patient (e.g. rare diseases, drug regimes, statistical analysis of small groups, IP addresses or biometric data).
  - Patients' record numbers.
  - Combinations of any of the items here that may increase the risk of a breach of confidentiality, that include all verbal, written and electronic disclosure, whether formal or incidental.

3. Data Protection Act 2018

- The main principles of the GDPR should be read in conjunction with this guideline. GDPR describes processes for obtaining, recording, holding, using and sharing information, and forms part of the data protection regime in the UK, together with the DPA 2018.
  - Patients must be informed and give explicit consent to any sharing of their personal information.
  - Only the minimum amount of data should be collected and used to achieve the agreed purpose.
  - Information can only be retained for as long as it is needed to achieve its originally intended purpose.
  - Strict rules apply to sharing information and with whom it may be shared.

4. NHS Policy

- All NHS employees must be aware of and respect a patient's right to confidentiality and protect their personal information. A disciplinary offence may have been committed for any behaviour contrary to their organisation's policy or the *NHS Code of Practice: Confidentiality* (in Scotland, the *NHS COP on Protecting Patient Confidentiality*). Ambulance clinicians should be aware of how to gain access to training, support or information, which they may need, and be able to show that they are making every reasonable effort to comply with the relevant standards.

5. Protecting Patient Information

There are five essential steps that all ambulance clinicians should take to ensure that they comply with the relevant standards of confidentiality. They are listed below:

5.1 Record Information Given By, and About, Patients Concisely and Accurately

- Inaccurate clinical records about patients may contain false information that has been created by, for example, omissions, errors, unfounded comments or speculation. This breaches DPA standards. It also brings the professional integrity of ambulance clinicians and their employing organisations into question. Any comments and opinions, whether verbal, written or electronic, must be justifiable and accurate.

5.2 Keep Patient Information Physically Secure

- Ambulance services have particular difficulties in ensuring that information is not shared accidentally with the public. Not only must patients be treated confidentially, but the information gained must not be disclosed to anyone else unless to do so genuinely promotes patient care. (Comments to the public must be guarded.) Information given to other clinicians when handing over patients' care should not be overheard by or shared with people who are not directly involved in each patient's care. Patients' records, either electronic or written, must be protected against unwarranted viewing: thus, patients' clinical records must be shielded from the view of other people, stored securely after case closure and only handed over to staff who are entrusted with ongoing care of particular patients or other authorised personnel who have legitimate reasons for possessing the information. Personal health data must be destroyed in an approved manner and according to each organisation's policies when they have served their function. Discussions of each patient must not disclose personal information unless there is genuine and provable health benefit.

- Leaders of healthcare and health information systems believe that electronic health information systems, which include computer-based patient records, can improve healthcare. Achieving this goal requires systems to be in place that: protect the privacy of individual persons and data about patients; provide appropriate access; and

Patient Confidentiality

use data security measures that are adequate. Sound policies and practices relating to handling confidential information must be in place prior to deploying health information systems. Strong and enforceable policies on the privacy and security of confidential and patient identifiable information must shape the development and implementation of these systems.

5.3 Follow Guidance Before Disclosing Any Patient Information

■ It is not sufficient for ambulance clinicians to understand the basic principles of confidentiality alone. They must also understand and comply with their employing organisations' requirements for information-sharing. Similarly, it is the responsibility of each service to ensure that policies for data-sharing are produced, communicated, monitored, updated and reviewed. Each ambulance service will have a senior advisor available. There must be a Data Protection Officer, Information Governance Manager and/or Caldicott Guardian available to advise ambulance clinicians if they have any doubts about sharing information.

5.4 Conform to Best Practice

■ All grades of ambulance clinicians come into contact with the public and other NHS clinicians. Any temptation for ambulance clinicians to share information unnecessarily with other people who are known to them must be avoided, and the responsibility lies firmly with the holder of the data, both personally and in respect of employing organisations. Commitment to best practice should be applied to all information in any form about patients (e.g. patients' records, electronic data, surface mail, email, faxes, telephone calls, conversations that may be overheard and private comments to friends or colleagues).

■ If, for any reason, ambulance staff discover that personal data has been lost or has the potential for being viewed by anyone not authorised to view it, they have a duty to immediately:
  − take every action possible to recover the data and/or protect them, and
  − to inform immediately an officer in their employing organisation who has responsibility for data (or their immediate supervisor) that such an event has occurred
  − record the event.

5.5 Anonymise Information Where Possible

■ Information about patients is said to be anonymised when items such as those listed in section 2 are removed. It means that patients cannot be identified by any receiver of the information and any possibility of recognition is extremely small.

■ Ambulance clinicians are advised to anonymise confidential data about patients wherever possible and reasonable. If information is recorded, retained or transmitted in any way, it should be anonymised unless to do so would frustrate any genuine reasons for its collection/storage that create identifiable benefits to patients' health.

6. Patients' Rights of Access to Personal Health Records

■ Patients have a right to see, and obtain a copy of, personal health information held about them. This right in law includes any legally appointed representative and those persons who have parental responsibility for children who are patients. Children also have this right provided they have the capability to understand the information. Services have the right to charge for this information; and there are guidelines on the processes that are to be followed.

■ There are exceptions to the rights of patients to see their personal health information. The information is subject to legal restrictions if it could identify someone else and if that information cannot be removed from the record. Also, a request can be refused if there is substantial opinion that access to the information could cause serious harm to a particular patient or to someone else's physical or mental well-being. These instances are extremely rare in ambulance service operations. If there were to be doubt about whether exceptions such as these do exist, staff should consult the Caldicott Guardian, Information Governance Manager or Data Protection Officer and agreement should be reached with each patient's lead-clinician.

■ Notwithstanding the exceptions noted here, clinicians should make every effort to support each patient's right to gain access to their personal health information. It is a requirement that this information should be received by a patient who requests it within 30 days of their request. Services should have clear written procedures in place to deal with these requests.

7. Disclosure to Other Bodies and Organisations

7.1 Police

■ The police have the right of access via ambulance service systems to personal information (name, address, etc.) in their investigation, detection and prevention of any crime. They also have the right of access to confidential health information (type of illness or injury, etc.) in their investigation, detection or prevention of a serious crime (e.g. rape, arson, terrorism, murder, etc.). This information must go

Patient Confidentiality

through an ambulance service system, as per local pathways.

- They have no right to expect to receive information when criminality, crew safety or public safety are not involved. Generalised information regarding attendance at an incident may be passed to the police through locally agreed procedures, when details of the location of an incident and what is involved **may** be disclosed – but passage of personal or confidential health data **may not**.

7.2 Local Authorities

- A local authority officer may require any person holding health, financial or other records relating to a person whom the officer knows or believes to be an adult at risk to give the records, or copies of them, to the officer, for the purposes of enabling or assisting the authority to decide whether it needs to do anything in order to protect an adult at risk from harm.

7.3 Secretary of State (By Proxy)

- The Secretary of State's '**security management functions**' in relation to the health service mean that their powers to take action for the purpose of protecting and improving the security of health service providers (and persons employed by them) includes releasing documents for the purpose of preventing, detecting or investigating fraud, corruption or other unlawful activities.

7.4 Fire Service and Other Emergency Services

- There is no right of access for emergency service personnel other than the police to patients' personal health information. Situations may occur in which ambulance clinicians feel that such disclosure would be in the best interests of a particular patient, or that, by not disclosing it, other emergency workers could be put at risk. Ambulance clinicians should be fully aware of their obligations towards their patients' confidentiality. Avoidable breaches of confidentiality occur when colleagues and authorities (such as the police and persons in a judicial context) ask for information. On these occasions, ambulance clinicians should follow the best practice advice given in the relevant section of the *NHS Code of Practice on Protecting Patient Confidentiality*; otherwise, access to information should be governed by formal documented requests and consideration by the Data Protection Officer, Information Governance Manager and/or Caldicott Guardian.

7.5 The Media

- There is no basis for disclosure of confidential or patient identifiable information to the media. Services may receive requests for information in special circumstances (e.g. requests for updates

on celebrity patients or following large incidents, and when responding to press statements – public interest exemption). In instances such as these, the explicit consent of the persons about whom information is sought should be gained and recorded prior to any disclosure. Occasionally, services or ambulance clinicians can be criticised in the press by patients or by someone else with whom a patient has a relationship. Criticism of this nature may contain inaccurate or misleading details of behaviour, diagnosis or treatment. Services or ambulance clinicians should always seek advice from professional bodies on how to respond (if at all) to press criticism and about any legal redress that may be available. Although these instances may cause frustration or distress, they do not relieve anyone of their duty to respect the confidentiality of any patient.

7.6 For Commercial Purposes

- Ambulance services are not registered to use information for primarily commercial purposes. If such use was permitted, each patient would have to give explicit consent for information given by or about them to be used within the express commercial setting and each patient should be given an opt-out facility. This includes all intended purposes of all parties to the agreement and lists of all persons/groups who would have access to the data. Due to the nature of commercial enterprise, this consent must be explicit (expressly and actively given) as opposed to implied (acceptance without voicing an objection).

8. Research

- All data for research should be anonymised wherever possible. If anonymisation would be contrary to the aims of the research, prior consent must be gained. Formal research guidelines exist for the use of health-related data and they must be adhered to.

9. Consent

- Consent and patients' confidentiality are inextricably linked. In essence, each patient is said to be the owner of their own personal, non-anonymised patient information and/or data. Therefore, each patient should give approval before information provided by or about them is used by other people. There are exceptions to this general rule:
  - There may be legal requirements to disclose data without consent (e.g. due to persons having **notifiable diseases**). Even then, however, each patient must be informed that this situation has arisen.
  - When there is a risk to a patient's well-being by not informing other professionals without consent (e.g. where a child or vulnerable

Patient Confidentiality

adult, an adult without capacity or a patient who is being treated using powers given by the Mental Health Act may be in need of protection) and informing the relevant authorities would appear to be to the patient's wider benefit.

– Inability to consent (e.g. some children, adults who lack capacity or patients who are seriously ill or injured and who could reasonably be expected to give consent if it were otherwise possible to do so). Even in circumstances such as these, information must be used cautiously and anonymised when possible. A proxy, guardian or parent should be consulted if such a person is available.

■ Use of personal information without consent may be justified if it is in the **public interest** to do so. This may occur to prevent or detect a serious crime, for example.

■ In all the instances described here, the advice of the service's Caldicott Guardian, Information Governance Manager and/or Data Protection Officer should be sought prior to using or releasing any personal health information or data. Each service must advise their own ambulance clinicians in relation to consent, and this advice must be studied by ambulance clinicians.

KEY POINTS!

Patient Confidentiality

■ Health professionals have a duty of confidentiality regarding information about or that may identify patients. They also have a priority to ensure that all relevant information is recorded clearly and accurately, and passed to others when this is necessary for providing ongoing care.

■ Inaccurate clinical records may contain false information about patients, which is created by, for example, omissions, errors, unfounded comments or speculation. Any comments or opinions, whether verbal, written or electronic, must be justifiable and accurate.

■ Data Protection Officers, Information Governance Managers and Caldicott Guardians are available to advise and assist ambulance clinicians of the ambulance services.

■ Consent and confidentiality of information that is held about patients are inextricably linked. In essence, patients are the owners of personal, non-anonymised information that is provided by or about them and they, therefore, are required to give approval before it is used by other people.

■ Ensure you are aware of the rules in your service regarding patients' confidentiality and follow them – but remember that ongoing care of patients should never be compromised in their application.

Further Reading

Further important information and evidence in support of this guideline can be found in the Bibliography.[1,2,3,4,5,6,7,8,9,10,11,12,13,14,15,16,17,18,19]

Bibliography

1. Health and Care Professions Council. *Standards of Conduct, Performance and Ethics: Your duties as a registrant.* London: Health Professions Council, 2016. Available from: https://www.hcpc-uk.org/assets/documents/10004EDFStandardsofconduct,performanceandethics.pdf.

2. Gold M, Philip J, McIver S, Komesaroff PA. Between a rock and a hard place: exploring the conflict between respecting the privacy of patients and informing their carers. *Internal Medicine Journal* 2009, 39(9): 582–7.

3. Department of Health. *Confidentiality: NHS Code of Practice.* London: Stationery Office, 2003. Available from: https://www.gov.uk/government/publications/confidentiality-nhs-code-of-practice.

4. NHS Scotland. *NHS Code of Practice on Protecting Patient Confidentiality.* 2010. Available from: https://www2.gov.scot/Publications/2010/04/20142935/0.

5. Department of Health. *Confidentiality: NHS Code of Practice – Supplementary guidance: public interest disclosures.* 2010. Available from: https://www.gov.uk/government/publications/confidentiality-nhs-code-of-practice-supplementary-guidance-public-interest-disclosures.

6. General Medical Council. *Confidentiality: good practice in handling patient information.* London: General Medical Council, 2018. Available from: https://www.gmc-uk.org/ethical-guidance/ethical-guidance-for-doctors/confidentiality.

7. Thomas MG. Team learning: the issue of patient confidentiality. *Work Based Learning in Primary Care* 2004, 2(4): 377–80.

8. Department of Health. *The Caldicott Committee Report on the Review of Patient-Identifiable Information.* London: Stationery Office, 1997.

Patient Confidentiality

Available from: https://webarchive.nationalarchives.gov.uk/20130123204013/http://www.dh.gov.uk/en/Publicationsandstatistics/Publications/PublicationsPolicyAndGuidance/DH_4068403.

9. Woodward B. The computer-based patient record and confidentiality. *The New England Journal of Medicine* 1995, 333(21): 1419–1422.

10. Gostin LO. Health information privacy. *Cornell Law Review* 1995, 80(3): 451–528.

11. Brooks J. Caldicott Guardians: driving the confidentiality agenda. *British Journal of Healthcare Computing and Information Management* 2004, 21(3): 20–21.

12. White C, Hardy J. What do palliative care patients and their relatives think about research in palliative care? A systematic review. *Support Care Cancer* 2010, 18(8): 905–911.

13. Department of Health. *The Data Protection Act 2018*. London: HMSO, 2018. Available from: http://www.legislation.gov.uk/ukpga/2018/12/contents/enacted.

14. Griffith R, Tengnah C. Access to health records: the rights of the patient. *British Journal of Community Nursing* 2010, 15(7): 344–347.

15. Wougare J. Patient rights to privacy and dignity in the NHS. *Nursing Standard* 2005, 19(18): 33–37.

16. Ministry of Justice. *The Mental Capacity Act 2005 Code of Practice 2007.* London: The Stationery Office, 2005. Available from: https://www.gov.uk/government/publications/mental-capacity-act-code-of-practice.

17. British Medical Association. *The Mental Capacity Act 2005: Guidance for Health Professionals.* 2009. Available from: https://egret.psychol.cam.ac.uk/medicine/legal/BMA_MCA_2005_guidance_March2007.pdf.

18. Information Commissioner's Office. *Guide to the General Data Protection Regulation (GDPR).* Cheshire: Information Commissioner's Office. Available from: https://ico.org.uk/for-organisations/guide-to-the-general-data-protection-regulation-gdpr/.

19. NHS Digital. *General Data Protection Regulation (GDPR) guidance*. Leeds: NHS Digital. Available from: https://digital.nhs.uk/data-and-information/looking-after-information/data-security-and-information-governance/information-governance-alliance-iga/general-data-protection-regulation-gdpr-guidance.

Patients with Communication Difficulties

1. Introduction

- This guideline comprises generic guidance intended to be used for any patient interaction where there are communication difficulties, e.g. patients with learning disabilities (LDs), autism, dementia, mental health problems or hearing or speech difficulties. The guidance does not relate directly to any specific patient group or condition. It has been developed without individual direct consultation with specific patient groups, given the number of patient groups that would potentially be involved. This is intentional due to the nature and breadth of out-of-hospital care and the need to ensure all patients receive the most appropriate care in an emergency situation.

2. Background

- A learning disability is a reduced intellectual ability and difficulty with everyday activities, e.g. household tasks, socialising or managing money, that affects someone for their whole life. The level of impairment can vary from mild to severe in all conditions.

- A learning disability is different from a learning difficulty, as a learning difficulty does not affect general intellect.

- There are many different types of learning difficulty. Some of the more well-known are dyslexia, attention deficit-hyperactivity disorder (ADHD), dyspraxia and dyscalculia. A person can have one, or a combination.

- Autism is a lifelong developmental disability that affects how people perceive the world and interact with others.[1] There is a triad of impairment: social interaction, communication and imagination or flexibility of thought.[1]

- People with learning disabilities are likely to die 20 years earlier than people without them. Reasons include increased comorbidities, challenges with accessing healthcare, difficulties in assessment and inappropriate or delayed care.[2,3]

- People with LD are three times more likely to die of something treatable compared to others.[2]

- The top three causes of death in people with LD are pneumonia, sepsis and aspiration pneumonia.[3]

- 2.16% of adults and 2.5% of children have a learning disability.[4]

- People with dementia, frailty needs, mental health problems and other communication needs are also at higher risk of ill health. This is for similar reasons to people with learning disabilities, such as difficulties accessing healthcare, multiple comorbidities, medications and assessment challenges.

- Communication is vital to assessment.

- Be aware of polypharmacy. This needs to be taken into consideration when assessing a patient. Consider drug interactions, potential accidental overdoses or toxicity.

3. Communication

- Help the patient to feel as secure and safe from harm as possible.

- Speak clearly and slowly enough for the patient, and keep instructions short and straightforward.

- Give your patient time to process information and to reply.

- Try and keep background noise to a minimum.

- Consider light level or the intensity of light.

- Eye contact can help communication with some people, although others with autism may find it very uncomfortable.

- Find out how your patient usually communicates. Can someone help you with sign language? Would pointing to equipment help? Can you use symbols or pictures? Would gestures help?

- Makaton sign language is simple and easy. You don't have to sign every word, just key words. Many signs are similar to everyday gestures.

- Watch out for non-verbal communication for both yourself and your patient.

- Your patient may have an individualised care plan such as a hospital or health passport or an All About Me book, which can give you valuable information.

- Communication and understanding are not the same. Some patients can understand but not communicate. Some can communicate but not understand.

- Ensure your patient has as much choice and control over their treatment as possible.

4. Examination

- Explain things as clearly as you can using the previously established method of communication, e.g. via a hospital or health passport, or a family member or care giver.

- You may need to alter the order or structure of your examination — start with less-threatening things and work towards things that are more uncomfortable or scary.

- Your patient may have a sensory processing disorder, where sensations are perceived inappropriately by the body. For example, a light touch may be very painful whilst a firmer touch may be more comfortable. Noises and lights can also present challenges. Find out more from family, carers or the hospital or health passport.

- Your patient may have had very bad experiences of previous healthcare, which can make examining them difficult. Use reassurance and

Patients with Communication Difficulties

explanation, and consider distraction or altering your examination.

- Some patients may be more settled if distracted by family, videos, books, fidget toys, etc. Others may not be distractible at all. Find out more about this.
- You may need to be opportunistic, flexible and resourceful.
- If possible, conduct the examination in a familiar or calming environment, e.g. in a specific room or sensory room.

4.1 Vital Signs and Scoring Systems

- Some patients may always have abnormal vital signs and NEWS2 — find out their baseline score.
- Some patients may be very unwell but have normal vital signs and NEWS2. For example, some patients with neurological conditions may not mount a tachycardia or pyrexia; some may not be able to sustain an increased respiratory rate.
- The Learning Disabilities Mortality Review (LeDeR)[3] found issues with NEWS2 and patients with LD, including the score not being recorded, or being recorded and not acted upon. These both lead to avoidable deaths.
- Many illnesses may not present in a typical way in patients with underlying conditions such as Down/Down's syndrome.
- Pain scores are also difficult to interpret as some patients with autism or other sensory processing conditions may have a very 'high pain threshold'.

4.2 Soft Signs

- These are signs that vary from patient to patient, which may mean someone is unwell. Families and carers are more likely to notice these than healthcare professionals.

- For example, someone might be unwell if they are refusing their favourite food, not interested in their favourite TV programme, more pale than usual or quieter than usual.
- Pay attention to soft signs as they can indicate serious illness in people with normal vital signs or a normal NEWS2 score.

4.3 Diagnostic Overshadowing

- This occurs when someone already has a pre-existing diagnosis and a healthcare professional puts any new symptoms or signs down to this diagnosis, rather than looking for another cause.
- For example, someone with autism or mental health problems presents with agitation. Rather than looking for a cause such as pain or infection, the healthcare professional assumes the agitation is purely due to the autism or mental health condition.
- Be aware of diagnostic overshadowing; make sure you are thorough and consider other causes for symptoms and signs. Finding out what is normal for your patient from sources such as family, carers or a hospital or health passport can help.

5. Reasonable Adjustments

- These are required by law, under the Equality Act 2010.[5]
- In essence, this means doing your best to make things as easy as possible for your patient, whilst still doing a thorough job.
- Consider things such as the environment you assess your patient in, the language you use, whether you need any help from family or carers and how best to communicate with your patient.
- Do what needs to be done now without delay, making appropriate adjustments. Avoid unnecessary interventions or interventions that could wait until the patient reaches hospital.

KEY POINTS!

Patients with Communication Difficulties

- **The TEACH mnemonic may help ambulance clinicians with communication.**
  - **TIME: you may need to spend more time on your assessment.**
  - **ENVIRONMENT: consider the impact of your surroundings on your patient. Are they quiet enough? Too distracting? Too unfamiliar? How can you make things better for your patient?**
  - **ATTITUDE: don't assume anything about quality of life. Be as thorough as you would with anyone else, although you may need to adjust how you work. Admit what you don't know.**
  - **COMMUNICATION: how can you best communicate with your patient? Using symbols or signs? Checking for understanding? Can family or carers help?**
  - **HELP: who or what can help you? Family? Carers? An LD nurse? A hospital or health passport? An individualised care plan?**

SECTION 1 General Guidance

Patients with Communication Difficulties

Bibliography

1. National Autistic Society. *About Autism*. 2020. Available from: https://www.autism.org.uk/about.aspx.

2. HQIP. *Confidential Enquiry into Deaths of People with Learning Disabilities CIPOLD 2013*. 2013. Available from: https://www.hqip.org.uk/resource/confidential-enquiry-into-deaths-of-people-with-learning-disabilities-cipold-2013/#.Xbya1fZ2vlU.

3. University of Bristol. *Learning Disabilities Mortality Review (LeDeR)*. 2020. Available from: http://www.bristol.ac.uk/sps/leder/.

4. Mencap. *How Common Is Learning Disability?* 2020. Available from: https://www.mencap.org.uk/learning-disability-explained/research-and-statistics/how-common-learning-disability.

5. Mencap. *Learning Disability Explained*. 2020. Available from: https://www.mencap.org.uk/learning-disability-explained.

6. Public Health England. *Reasonable Adjustments: A legal duty*. 2016. Available from: https://www.gov.uk/government/publications/reasonable-adjustments-a-legal-duty/reasonable-adjustments-a-legal-duty.

7. Makaton. *Healthcare Cards*. 2020. Available from: https://www.makaton.org/shop/shopping/freeDownloadDetails/Lanyard-cards.

8. PEM Infographics. *Triaging and Treating Kids with Down's Syndrome*. 2019. Available from: https://www.peminfographics.com/infographics/triaging-and-treating-kids-with-down-s-syndrome.

9. Mencap. *Resources for Healthcare Professionals*. 2020. Available from: https://www.mencap.org.uk/learning-disability-explained/resources-healthcare-professionals.

10. RCEM Learning. *Learning Difficulties in the ED*. 2018. Available from: https://www.rcemlearning.co.uk/foamed/learning-difficulties-in-the-ed/.

11. My PECS. *Communicating PECS*. 2020. Available from: http://www.mypecs.com/Search.aspx?catid=30&isParent=true.

12. O'Dwyer M, Peklar J, McCallion P, et al. Factors associated with polypharmacy and excessive polypharmacy in older people with intellectual disability differ from the general population: a cross-sectional observational nationwide study. *BMJ Open* 2016, 6:e010505.

13. St Oswald's Hospice. *Distress and Discomfort Assessment Tool*. 2020. Available from: https://www.stoswaldsuk.org/how-we-help/we-educate/education/resources/disability-distress-assessment-tool-disdat/.

14. Regnard C, Matthews D, Gibson L, Clarke C & Watson B. Difficulties in identifying distress and its causes in people with severe communication problems. *International Journal of Palliative Nursing* 2003, 9: 173–176.

15. Regnard C, Reynolds J, Watson B, Matthews D, Gibson L, Clarke C. Understanding distress in people with severe communication difficulties: developing and assessing the disability distress assessment tool (DisDAT). *Journal of Intellectual Disability Research* 2007, 51: 277–292.

16. Fuchs-Lacelle S et al. Development and preliminary validation of the pain assessment checklist for seniors with limited ability to communicate (PACSLAC). *Pain Management Nursing* 2004, 5(1): 37–49. Available from: https://www.painmanagementnursing.org/article/S1524-9042(03)00122-X/fulltext.

SECTION **1** General Guidance

Safeguarding Adults at Risk

1. Introduction

- Everyone has the right to live their life free from harm. Safeguarding adults at risk from significant harm is reliant on effective joint working and communication between agencies and professionals.

- This guidance is for the management of people aged 18 years and over; for those under 18 years, refer to **Safeguarding Children**.

- Ambulance clinicians are often the first professionals to make contact with an adult at risk and may identify initial concerns regarding abuse. The role of the ambulance service is not to investigate suspicions but to ensure that any suspicion is passed, with the consent of the adult (where no consent, state why), to the appropriate agency (e.g. social care or the police) in line with locally agreed procedures.

- Ambulance clinicians need to be aware of local policies and procedures relating to the abuse of vulnerable adults. The aim of this guideline is to assist ambulance clinicians to recognise and report cases (with consent) of suspected abuse of adults at risk.

- The principles of adult protection differ from those of child protection in that adults have the right to take risks and may choose to live at risk if they have the capacity to make such a decision (refer to **Mental Capacity Act 2005**).

- Anyone can be a victim of abuse.

- An abuser may be anyone, including a friend, family member, carer or professional involved in delivering care to the adult.

The introduction of the Care Act 2014[1] provides a statutory framework to safeguard adults at risk of abuse or neglect. The Care Act puts the wishes and experience of the adult at the centre of safeguarding and is a move away from the previous process-led culture.

2. Making Safeguarding Personal

2.1 'No Decision About Me Without Me'[2]

Under the Care Act 2014 there has been a move away from process-led practice to a person-centred approach that works in partnership with the adult to achieve the outcomes that they need to make them feel safe. In the words of Lord Justice Munby, 'What good is it making someone safer if it merely makes them miserable?'.[3]

2.2 Six Key Principles

There are six key principles underpinning the Care Act guidance that put the patient at the heart of decision making:

1 **Empowerment** 'I am asked what I want as the outcome from the safeguarding process, and this directly informs what happens'.

2 **Prevention** 'I receive clear and simple information about what abuse is, how to recognise the signs and what I can do to seek help'.

3 **Proportionality** 'I am sure that the professionals will work in my interests, as I see them, and they will only get involved as much as needed'.

4 **Protection** 'I get help and support to report abuse and neglect. I get help so that I am able to take part in the safeguarding process to the extent that I want'.

5 **Partnership** 'I know that staff treat any personal and sensitive information in confidence, only sharing what is helpful and necessary. I am confident that professionals will work together and with me to get the best result for me.'.

6 **Accountability** 'I understand the role of everyone involved in my life and so do they'.

The aim of safeguarding is to:

- Stop abuse or neglect wherever possible

- Prevent harm and reduce the risk of abuse or neglect to adults with care and support needs

- Safeguard adults in a way that supports them in making choices and having control about how they want to live

- Promote an approach that concentrates on improving life for the adult concerned.

3. Definition of Adult at Risk

Not every adult will require safeguarding. To meet the criteria set out in the Care Act 2014, the adult must meet the following criteria:

- Demonstrates a need for care and support (whether or not the local authority is meeting any of those needs) **and**

- Is experiencing, or at risk of, abuse or neglect **and**

- As a result of those care and support needs, is unable to protect themselves from either the risk or the experience of abuse or neglect.

An adult's needs meet the eligibility criteria for care and support if:

1 Their needs arise from, or are related to, a physical or mental impairment or illness

2 As a result of the adult's needs, the adult is unable to achieve two or more of the outcomes

3 As a consequence there is, or is likely to be, a significant impact on the adult's well-being.

The specified outcomes are the adult:

1 Managing and maintaining nutrition

2 Maintaining personal hygiene

3 Managing toilet needs

4 Being appropriately clothed

5 Being able to make use of their home safely

6 Maintaining a habitable home environment

Safeguarding Adults at Risk

7 Developing and maintaining family or other personal relationships

8 Accessing and engaging in work, training, education or volunteering

9 Making use of necessary facilities or services in the local community, including public transport, and recreational facilities or services

10 Carrying out any caring responsibilities they have for a child.

TABLE 1.16 – Types and Signs of Abuse	
TYPES OF ABUSE	**SIGNS OF ABUSE**
Physical: hitting, slapping, misuse of medication, restraint.	▪ Multiple bruising ▪ Fractures ▪ Burns ▪ Bed sores ▪ Fear ▪ Depression ▪ Unexplained weight loss ▪ Assault (can be intentional or reckless).
Domestic violence: incidents, or pattern of incidents, of controlling, coercive or threatening behaviour, violence or abuse by someone who is, or has been, an intimate partner or family member, regardless of sex or sexuality.	Includes: psychological, physical, sexual, financial, emotional abuse; so-called 'honour'-based violence; female genital mutilation; forced marriage. Note: The age range extended down to 16 (for the purpose of the safeguarding adult arrangements; safeguarding children arrangements would be applied to a person under 18).
Sexual abuse: rape, indecent exposure, subjection to pornography, not consented or pressured to consent.	▪ Loss of sleep ▪ Unexpected or unexplained change in behaviour ▪ Bruising ▪ Soreness around the genitals ▪ Torn, stained or bloody underwear ▪ Preoccupation with anything sexual ▪ Sexually transmitted diseases ▪ Pregnancy ▪ Rape – e.g. a male member of staff having sex with a mental health client (see Mental Health Act 1983) ▪ Indecent assault.
Psychological abuse: emotional abuse, threat of harm or abandonment, blaming, humiliation, isolation.	▪ Fear ▪ Depression ▪ Confusion ▪ Loss of sleep ▪ Unexpected or unexplained change in behaviour ▪ Deprivation of liberty could be false imprisonment ▪ Aggressive shouting causing fear of violence in a public place may be an offence against the Public Order Act 1986, or harassment under the Protection from Harassment Act 1997.

(continued)

Safeguarding Adults at Risk

TABLE 1.16 – Types and Signs of Abuse *(continued)*	
Financial or material abuse: internet scamming, will issues, inheritance, financial transactions, theft.	▪ Unexplained withdrawals from the bank ▪ Unusual activity in bank accounts ▪ Unpaid bills ▪ Unexplained shortage of money ▪ Reluctance on the part of the person with responsibility for the funds to provide basic food and clothes etc. ▪ Fraud, theft.
Modern slavery: human trafficking, forced labour, domestic servitude, coerce, deceive and force individual into life of abuse.	Modern slavery is an international crime; it can include victims that have been brought from overseas, and vulnerable people in the UK. Slave masters and traffickers will deceive, coerce and force adults into a life of abuse, callous treatment and slavery.
Discriminatory abuse: slurs, issues of race, gender, disability etc.	Abuse can be experienced as harassment, insults or similar actions due to race, religion, gender, gender identity, age, disability or sexual orientation.
Organisational abuse: neglect or poor care within an institution or care setting. Neglect or poor professional practice as a result of policies and processes.	▪ Inflexible and non-negotiable systems and routines ▪ Lack of consideration of dietary requirements. ▪ Name-calling; inappropriate ways of addressing people. ▪ Lack of adequate physical care – an unkempt appearance.
Neglect and acts of omission: ignoring medical, emotional or physical care needs. Failure to provide access to appropriate healthcare.	▪ Malnutrition. ▪ Untreated medical problems. ▪ Bed sores. ▪ Confusion. ▪ Over-sedation. ▪ Deprivation of meals may constitute 'wilful neglect'.
Self-neglect: wide-ranging neglect for one's personal hygiene, health or surroundings; includes behaviour such as hoarding.	This includes various behaviours: disregarding one's personal hygiene, health or surroundings, resulting in a risk that impacts on the adult's wellbeing – this could consist of behaviours such as hoarding.

Incidents can be a one-off or multiple and may affect one person or more.

▪ Bruising in darker skin tones may appear as purple or dark brown discolouration, and it may be more difficult to see very recent bruising on darker skin tones (on lighter skin tones very recent bruising may appear red). It may only become obvious as the colour of the bruising develops into a dark purple, brown or black colour which is then darker than the surrounding skin. Also, the yellow discolouration of older bruises may be more subtle in darker skin tones.

▪ Enquiring about how long the colour change has been there and what might have caused it is important. The colour of the bruising will change over time but it is not possible to reliably date bruising based on appearance alone.

▪ Note that bruising could also be caused by bleeding disorders or medicines.

4. Wellbeing

▪ Ambulance clinicians often come across adults who have an unmet or increasing care need. Whilst these are unlikely to meet the threshold for safeguarding, raising an alert is still possible with the patient's consent. Please follow your local reporting procedures.

5. Consent

▪ Adults at risk should, where possible, be given full information about any concerns for their safety to enable them to give informed consent

Safeguarding Adults at Risk

to the ambulance service raising a safeguarding alert with the local authority or other appropriate agency. Where the adult does not have capacity (refer to **Mental Capacity Act 2005**), or having a discussion may increase the risk to the adult, ambulance clinicians can raise an alert in the patient's best interests.

- If there is a risk to others (i.e. other residents in a care setting or an identified fire or public health risk), ambulance clinicians can share information without consent (refer to **Mental Capacity Act 2005**).

6. Mandatory Reporting of Female Genital Mutilation (FGM)

- From 31 October 2015, the FGM Act introduces a mandatory reporting duty which requires health and social care professionals as well as teachers to report known cases of FGM in those under 18 years of age to the police.

- FGM is child abuse and the current procedure is set out below:
  - **Children and vulnerable adults:** if any child (under 18) or vulnerable adult in your care has symptoms or signs of FGM, or if you have good reason to suspect they are at risk of FGM having considered their family history or other relevant factors, they **must** be referred using existing safeguarding procedures as with all instances of child abuse. This will involve referral to police and social care in the usual way.
  - **Adults:** there is no requirement for automatic referral of adult women with FGM to adult services or the police. Ambulance clinicians should be aware that a disclosure may be the first time that a woman has discussed her FGM with anyone. Referral to police must not be introduced as an automatic response when identifying adult women with FGM, and each case must be individually assessed. Ambulance clinicians should seek to assist women by offering referral to community groups for support, clinical intervention or other services as appropriate, for example through an NHS FGM clinic. The wishes of the woman must be respected at all times. If she is pregnant, the welfare of the unborn child or others in her extended family must be considered at this point as they are potentially at risk, and action taken accordingly.
  - In all cases where staff are unsure of their actions, they should seek the advice of the Trust Safeguarding Service.

7. Prevent

7.1 Introduction

- The NHS, including the ambulance service, has a statutory responsibility to comply and engage with *Prevent*.[1]

- This involves the formulation of policy and procedures, the training of staff and, importantly, having appropriate mechanisms in place to ensure that concerns are noted and shared.

The three key objectives of the national *Prevent* strategy are to:

1 Challenge the **ideology** that supports terrorism and those who promote it.

2 Prevent vulnerable **individuals** from being drawn into terrorism, and ensure that they are given appropriate advice and support.

3 Work with sectors and **institutions** where there are risks of radicalisation.

- It remains clear that while the focus is an imminent threat from Al-Qaida or Islamic State (IS), it should be noted that radicalisation of vulnerable individuals can be undertaken by any extremist group. These forms of terrorism include (but are not limited to):
  - Far-right extremists, e.g. English Defence League
  - Al-Qaida-influenced groups
  - Environmental extremists
  - Animal rights extremists.

7.2 Definitions

- The following examples of vulnerability are included within 'Building Partnerships, Staying Safe' (DoH, 2011).
  - **Identity crisis** Adolescents/vulnerable adults who are exploring issues of identity can feel both distant from their parents/family and cultural and religious heritage, and uncomfortable with their place in the society around them. Radicalisers can exploit this by providing a sense of purpose or feelings of belonging. Where this occurs, it can often manifest itself in a change in a person's behaviour, their circle of friends and the ways in which they interact with others and spend their time.
  - **Personal crisis** This may, for example, include significant tensions within the family, which produce a sense of isolation in the vulnerable individual from the traditional certainties of family life.
  - **Personal circumstances** The experiences of migration, local tensions or events affecting families in countries of origin may contribute

SECTION 1 General Guidance

---

1   Section 26 of the Counter-Terrorism and Security Act 2015 places a duty on certain bodies (including the NHS) in the exercise of their functions to have 'due regard to the need to prevent people from being drawn into terrorism'.

Safeguarding Adults at Risk

to alienation from UK values and a decision to cause harm to symbols of the community or state.

- **Unemployment or under-employment** Individuals may perceive their aspirations for career and lifestyle to be undermined by limited achievements or employment prospects. This can translate into a generalised rejection of civic life and the adoption of violence as a symbolic act.

- **Criminality** In some cases, a vulnerable individual may have been involved in a group that engages in criminal activity or, on occasion, a group that has links to organised crime, and be further drawn to engagement in terrorist-related activity.

▪ An additional vulnerability is around young people moving from childhood into adulthood, and, in particular, those children known to children's services as they transition into adult services.

7.3 Duties/Responsibility

▪ Any member of staff identifying concerns that vulnerable people may be radicalised should report to the safeguarding service, their *Prevent* lead or their line manager in the Trust.

▪ If the incident occurs outside of office hours, staff should contact police for advice.

8. Assessment and Management

▪ Identify an adult(s) at risk.

▪ Report concerns following local guidelines:
- Ascertain the patient's wishes wherever possible.
- Gain consent if it is safe and appropriate to do so.
- Consider the use of the Mental Capacity Act (MCA) if needed.

▪ Ensure concerns are clearly and concisely documented and jargon free.

> **KEY POINTS!**

Safeguarding Adults at Risk

▪ **Stop abuse and neglect wherever possible.**

▪ **Respect the adult's wishes wherever possible.**

▪ **Concerns of suspected abuse must be reported as soon as possible following trust policy and procedures.**

▪ **Ambulance clinicians must document fully the reasons for concern and any action taken.**

▪ **Documentation of consent or the reason it has not been obtained must be clearly recorded.**

▪ **Ambulance clinicians should not investigate concerns, but should identify and report appropriately.**

Further Reading

Further important information and evidence in support of this guideline can be found in the Bibliography.[4,5,6,7,8,9,10,11]

Bibliography

1. Department of Health. *Care Act 2014*. London: HMSO, 2014. Available from: http://www.legislation.gov.uk/ukpga/2014/23/pdfs/ukpga_20140023_en.pdf.

2. Department of Health. *Liberating the NHS: No decision about me without me*. London: HMSO, 2012.

3. Munby J. *Safeguarding Adults: Advice and guidance to directors of adult social services*. 2013. Available from: https://www.adass.org.uk/safeguarding-adults/public-content/advice-and-guidance-to-directors-of-adults-social-services-march-2013.

4. Office of the Public Guardian. *Office of the Public Guardian and Local Authorities: A protocol for working together to safeguard vulnerable adults*. London: HMSO, 2008.

5. Office of the Public Guardian. *Safeguarding Policy: Protecting vulnerable adults*. 2015. Available from: https://www.gov.uk/government/publications/safeguarding-policy-protecting-vulnerable-adults.

6. Lord Chancellor's Department. *Who Decides? Making decisions on behalf of mentally incapacitated adults*. London: HMSO, 1997.

7. Department of Health. *Clinical Governance and Adult Safeguarding: An integrated process*. London: HMSO, 2010. Available from: http://webarchive.nationalarchives.gov.uk/20130107105354/http://www.dh.gov.uk/en/Publicationsandstatistics/Publications/PublicationsPolicyAndGuidance/DH_112361.

8. Department of Health. *Safeguarding Adults: Report on the consultation on the review of No Secrets*. London: HMSO, 2009. Available from: http://webarchive.nationalarchives.gov.uk/20130107105354/http://www.dh.gov.uk/prod_consum_dh/groups/dh_digitalassets/documents/digitalasset/dh_102981.pdf.

Safeguarding Adults at Risk

9. Department of Health. *No Secrets: Guidance on developing and implementing multi-agency policies and procedures to protect vulnerable adults from abuse.* London: HMSO, 2000. Available from: https://www.gov.uk/government/uploads/system/uploads/attachment_data/file/194272/No_secrets__guidance_on_developing_and_implementing_multi-agency_policies_and_procedures_to_protect_vulnerable_adults_from_abuse.pdf.

10. Department of Health. *Safeguarding Adults: The role of health services.* London: HMSO, 2011. Available from: http://www.dh.gov.uk/en/Publicationsandstatistics/Publications/PublicationsPolicyAndGuidance/DH_124882.

11. Biarent D, Bingham R, Eich C, López-Herce J, Maconochie I, Rodriguez-Nunez A, et al. European Resuscitation Council Guidelines for Resuscitation 2010 Section 6: Paediatric life support. *Resuscitation* 2010, 81(10): 1364–1388.

SECTION **1** General Guidance

Safeguarding Children

- Safeguarding is everyone's responsibility and a statutory duty under the Children Act.[1] Ambulance clinicians must be aware of the signs, symptoms and indicators of abuse and neglect that constitute harm. This applies to staff who have direct contact, either face-to-face or on the telephone.

- Throughout this section, reference to a child equates to someone who is not yet 18 years of age.

- Members of staff in an ambulance trust have a **duty of care to report abuse or neglect**. If the abuse is not reported, the victim may be at greater risk. They may also feel discouraged from disclosing again, as they may feel they were not believed. This may put other people at risk.

- All partners who work with children, including local authorities, police, the health service, courts, professionals, the private and voluntary sectors and individual members of local communities, share the responsibility for safeguarding and promoting the welfare of children and young people. It is vital that all partners are aware of, and appreciate, the role that each of them plays in this area.[2]

- Healthcare professionals have a statutory duty to report, while social care and the police have statutory authority to investigate allegations or suspicions of child abuse.

- Ambulance clinicians are often the first professionals on scene and, therefore, may identify initial concerns regarding a child's welfare and alert social care, the police, the GP or another appropriate health professional, in line with locally agreed procedures. Accurate recording of events/actions may be crucial to subsequent enquiries.

- The role of the ambulance service is not to investigate suspicions but to use professional curiosity to identify risk and to ensure that any concern is passed to the appropriate agency (e.g. social care or the police). Ambulance clinicians need to be aware of child abuse issues and the aim of this guideline is to:
  - ensure all staff are aware of, and can recognise, cases of suspected child abuse or children at risk of significant harm, and provide guidance enabling operational and control staff to assess and report cases of suspected child abuse
  - where appropriate, ensure that all staff involved in a case of suspected abuse are aware of the possible outcome and of any subsequent actions.

- Further information on local procedures can be obtained from the safeguarding services within individual ambulance trusts.

- All children have the right:
  - to be protected from harm/ill-treatment
  - to be protected from impairment of their health[1] and development
  - to grow up in circumstances consistent with the provision of safe and effective care.

- The maltreatment of children, physically, emotionally, sexually or through neglect, can have a major impact on their health, well-being and development.

- There are no absolute criteria on which to rely when judging what constitutes significant harm. In some cases, a single traumatic event may constitute significant harm, but more generally it is a compilation of significant events, both acute and longstanding, which interrupt, change or damage the child's physical and psychological development. Considerations include:
  - the degree and extent of physical harm
  - the duration and frequency of abuse and neglect
  - the extent of premeditation
  - the degree of threat, coercion, sadism and bizarre or unusual elements.

- In order to understand and identify significant harm, consider:
  - the nature of harm, in terms of maltreatment or failure to provide adequate care
  - the impact on the child's health and development
  - the child's development within the context of the family and wider environment
  - any special needs, such as a medical condition, communication impairment or disability, that may affect the child's development and care within the family and the capacity of parents/carers to meet adequately the child's needs.

- Take a 'think family' approach to identifying and assessing risk. Consideration is needed towards other siblings and/or vulnerable people living in the household/establishment.

- Abuse and neglect are forms of maltreatment, and children may suffer as a result of a deliberate act or failure on the part of a parent, legal guardian or carer to act to prevent harm (descriptions of abuse and neglect are detailed in Table 1.17).

- Children can be abused in any care or community setting, and abuse can be perpetrated by those known to them or by a stranger.

---

1   Health means physical or mental health.

Safeguarding Children

TABLE 1.17 – Examples of Types of Abuse and Neglect

Emotional abuse

- The persistent emotional maltreatment of a child so as to cause severe and persistent adverse effects on the child's emotional development, which may:
  - involve conveying to the child(ren) that they are worthless or unloved, inadequate or valued only insofar as they meet the needs of another person
  - involve not giving the child opportunities to express their views, deliberately silencing them or 'making fun' of what they say or how they communicate
  - feature age or developmentally inappropriate expectations being imposed on children (e.g. interactions that are beyond the child's developmental capability), as well as overprotection and limitation of exploration and learning, or preventing the child from participating in normal social interaction
  - involve seeing or hearing the ill-treatment of another
  - involve serious bullying (including cyberbullying), causing children frequently to feel frightened or in danger, or the exploitation or corruption of children
  - involve witnessing domestic abuse.
- Some level of emotional abuse is involved in all types of maltreatment of a child, though it may occur alone.
- Emotional abuse alone can be difficult to recognise as the child may be physically well cared-for and the home in good condition. Some common factors that may indicate emotional abuse are:
  - if the child is constantly denigrated/humiliated in front of others
  - if the child is constantly given the impression that the parents are disappointed in them
  - if the child is blamed for things that go wrong or is told they may be unloved/sent away
  - if the parent does not offer any love or attention (e.g. leaves them alone for a long time)
  - if the child is obsessive about cleanliness, tidiness etc.
  - if the parent has unrealistic expectations of the child (e.g. educational achievement/toilet training)
  - if the child is either bullying others or being bullied themselves
  - if there is an atmosphere of domestic abuse, adults or parents with mental health problems or a history of drug or alcohol abuse
  - if there is evidence of self-harm, intentional overdose or the excessive use of alcohol on the part of either the parent(s) or child
  - unusual behaviour of the parents/carers towards the child(ren) in an emergency situation (e.g. are they comforting a distressed child? What is the interaction like between the child and care giver?).

Sexual abuse

- Sexual abuse involves forcing or enticing a child or young person to take part in sexual activities. Both girls and boys of all age groups are at risk.
- The sexual abuse of a child is often planned and chronic. A large proportion of sexually abused children have no physical signs, and it is therefore necessary to be alert to behavioural and emotional factors that may indicate abuse.
- The activities may involve physical contact, including assault by penetration (e.g. rape or oral sex) or non-penetrative acts (e.g. masturbation, kissing, rubbing and touching outside of clothing). They may include non-contact activities, such as involving children in looking at, or in the production of, sexual images, watching sexual activities, encouraging children to behave in sexually inappropriate ways or grooming a child in preparation for abuse (including via the internet).
- Men, women and children perpetrate sexual abuse. However, most abuse is perpetrated by someone known to the child.

(continued)

SECTION 1 General Guidance

Safeguarding Children

TABLE 1.17 – Examples of Types of Abuse and Neglect *(continued)*

Child sexual exploitation/abuse (CSE/CSA)

- Sexual exploitation/abuse of children and young people under 18 can involve gangs or individuals. It is defined when children and young people receive something (such as food, accommodation, drugs, alcohol, cigarettes, affection, gifts or money) as a result of performing, and/or others performing on them, sexual acts. It can occur through direct contact or the use of the internet or mobile phones. Perpetrators have power over the child(ren) because of their age, gender, intellect, physical strength and/or resources. Both girls and boys of all age groups are at risk.

There are four models used to describe CSE:

1 **Peer-on-peer exploitation:** outlines instances when children are sexually exploited by their own peers who could be known to them at school, through mutual friends or in the neighbourhood.

2 **Boyfriend model:** the perpetrator targets children by posing as their boyfriend and showering them with attention, which results in them becoming infatuated. The perpetrator then initiates a sexual relationship with the child, who is then expected to return it as 'proof of their love', or they are told they owe money for the gifts, and sexual activities are a way of paying back.

3 **Party model:** organised by groups who lure young people by offering drinks, drugs and car rides often for free and as an introduction to an exciting environment. This often results in incriminating evidence being obtained at e.g. parties, such as photos or videos of sexual acts, that is then used to exploit through fear.

4 **Exploitation through befriending and grooming:** befriending directly by the perpetrator, either in person or online, or through other children or young people.

- All children can be vulnerable to CSE/CSA but those who are most vulnerable are:
  - missing or runaway children
  - children in care
  - those with experience of sexual abuse or violence in the home
  - neglected children
  - children who are homeless/sofa-surfing
  - children who are misusing substances
  - children with mental health issues
  - those with a learning disability
  - unaccompanied children
  - children not in education, employment or training (NEET).

Physical abuse

- Physical abuse may involve hitting, shaking, throwing, poisoning, burning (including cigarette burns or scalding), suffocating, use of restraint, spitting, force-feeding or otherwise causing physical harm. Physical harm may also be caused when a parent or carer fabricates the symptoms of, or deliberately induces, ill-health; this situation is commonly described as 'fabricated or induced illness' (FII).

Neglect

- Neglect is the persistent failure to meet a child's basic physical and/or psychological needs, and is likely to result in the serious impairment of the child's health or development. Neglect may occur during pregnancy as a result of maternal substance abuse.

- A neglected or abused infant may show signs of poor attachment. They may lack the sense of security to explore, and appear unhappy and whining. There may be little sign of attachment behaviour, and the child may move aimlessly around a room or creep quietly into corners.

- Signs of potential neglect include:
  - poor weight gain
  - failure to use prescribed medication or medication withheld by parent/carer
  - severe nappy rash
  - tooth decay
  - failure to immunise

Safeguarding Children

TABLE 1.17 – Examples of Types of Abuse and Neglect *(continued)*
– poor hygiene and dirty clothes – obesity – poor growth – delayed development – failure to attend appointments – delayed presentation – poor physical condition – child not at school – child not registered with a GP – clothes not consistent with the climate. ▪ Do not rely on this list when assessing risk. Take a holistic approach and use professional curiosity to identify and assess risk. An absence of identifiable risk factors does not mean that a child is always safe.

2.1 Children in Need

▪ Children are defined as being 'in need' when:
- they are unlikely to reach or maintain a satisfactory level of health or development
- their health and development will be significantly impaired without the provision of services (section 17 (10) of the Children Act 1989)[1]
- they have a disability.

▪ Local authorities have a duty to safeguard and promote the welfare of children in need.

3. Recognition of Abuse

▪ Ambulance clinicians may receive information or make observations that suggest that a child has been abused or is at risk of harm, for example:
- the nature of the illness/injury
- observation of hazards in the home (e.g. alcohol or drug paraphernalia, home conditions such as lack of bedding)
- child(ren) has/have been locked in a room
- signs of distress shown by other children in the home
- observations regarding the condition of other children or adults in the household (e.g. an environment where domestic abuse has taken place). In the case of domestic dispute between adults, the presence of children in the household creates a need to notify even if the child(ren) was/were not injured
- parents or carers who seek medical care from a number of sources.

3.1 Non-accidental/Deliberate Injury

▪ When assessing an injury in any child, you should be aware of the possibility of the injury being non-accidental/deliberate and you should consider this possibility in every case, even if you promptly dismiss the idea.

▪ For an injury to be accidental it should have a clear, credible and acceptable history and the findings should be consistent with the history and with the development and abilities of the child.

3.2 Suspicion of Abuse

▪ Suspicions should be raised by:
- any injury in a non-mobile (non-independent) baby
- accidents/injuries in unusual places (e.g. the buttocks, trunk, inner thighs)
- extensive injuries or signs of both recent and old injuries
- small, deep burns in unusual places
- repeated burns and scalds
- 'glove and stocking' burns
- poor state of clothing, cleanliness and/or nutrition
- delayed reporting of the injury
- inappropriate sexual knowledge for the child's age
- overt sexual approaches to other children or adults
- fear of particular people or situations (e.g. bath time or bedtime)
- drug and alcohol abuse
- suicide attempts and self-injury
- running away and fire-setting
- environmental factors and family situations (e.g. domestic abuse, drug or alcohol abuse, learning disabilities that affect parents, carers and/or child).

▪ The following symptoms should give cause for concern and further assessment:
- soreness, discharge or unexplained bleeding in the genital area (including anal area and severe nappy rash)
- chronic vaginal/anal infections

SECTION 1 General Guidance

Safeguarding Children

- bruising, grazes or bites to the genital/anal or breast area
- sexually transmitted infections
- pregnancy, especially when the identity of the father is vague or if it is a concealed or denied pregnancy.

- When assessing an injured child, you should use your clinical knowledge regarding what level of accidental injury would be appropriate for their stage of development. Although stages of development vary (e.g. children may crawl or walk at different ages), injuries can broadly be divided between mobile and non-mobile children.

- Bruising in darker skin tones may appear as purple or dark brown discolouration, and it may be more difficult to see very recent bruising on darker skin tones (on lighter skin tones, very recent bruising may appear red). It may only become obvious as the colour of the bruising develops into a dark purple, brown or black colour which is then darker than the surrounding skin. Also, the yellow discolouration of older bruises may be more subtle in darker skin tones.

- Enquiring about how long the colour change has been there and what might have caused it is important. The colour of the bruising will change over time but it is not possible to reliably date bruising based on appearance alone.

- Note that bruising could also be caused by bleeding disorders or medicines.

- Any non-mobile child with skin discolouration that could be attributed to bruising should be seen by a paediatrician.

3.3 Disguised Compliance

- Disguised compliance involves parents and carers appearing to co-operate with professionals to allay concerns and stop professional engagement. This can mean that social workers and other practitioners may be unaware of what is happening in a child's life and the risks they face may be unknown and unassessed by local authorities. Staff should remain professionally curious when engaging with families and ensure that they share safeguarding concerns with the local authority even if they are led to believe this information is already known to them.

4. Extra-Familial Harm

- As adolescents begin to develop their independence and engage more in their local communities in the absence of their parents, they can be at increased risk of experiencing harm from outside the family environment. Extra-familial harm is the term used when children and young people's experience of harm is beyond their home, family or carers. This can include:
  - sexual abuse/exploitation
  - criminal exploitation

- peer-on-peer pressure
- gang affiliation
- trafficking and modern-day slavery
- serious youth violence
- radicalisation.

- Professionals will need to remain alert and make a safeguarding referral should they suspect a child is at risk of or is experiencing extra-familial harm.

5. Duty to Report to Police

- The Serious Crime Act 2015 enhances the protection of children from cruelty and abuse and adults at risk. Serious and organised crime includes drug trafficking, human trafficking, organised illegal immigration, child sexual exploitation, high-value fraud and other financial crime, counterfeiting, organised acquisitive crime and cybercrime.

- The Act places a duty on healthcare professionals and others to report serious crime, including and not limited to:
  - Serious domestic abuse (Domestic Abuse Act 2021)
  - Female genital mutilation (FGM) risk or actual (children)
  - Mandatory duty to notify the police – The 2015 Act places a duty on practitioners in regulated professions (health, teaching and social work) to notify the police when they identify that an act of FGM appears to have been carried out on a girl under the age of 18. This applies in cases where the victim discloses the offence to the practitioner or where the practitioner has observed physical signs of FGM. Failing to comply with the duty will be dealt with via existing disciplinary measures, which may include referral to the professional regulator
  - Gang-related activity
  - CSE/CSA
  - Cybercrime

- Depending on individual circumstances, you should either request immediate police support or report via 101. Please refer to own trust safeguarding policies.

6. Non-mobile (Non-independent) Babies

- Babies aged under one year are the most vulnerable group of children, as they cannot speak for themselves and are dependent on their parents/carers. Any injury in a non-mobile baby requires review by a clinician. If there is any doubt, the clinician should speak with the on-call paediatrician in the acute trust and/or the child should be conveyed.

Safeguarding Children

- Healthy babies do not bruise or break their bones easily. They do not bruise themselves with their fists or toys, bruise themselves by lying against the bars of a cot or acquire bruises on the legs when they are held for a nappy change. When in an environment, checks can be made for safety equipment, such as stair gates etc.

- Bruising on the ears, face, neck, trunk and buttocks is particularly suspicious. A torn frenulum (behind the upper lip) is rarely accidental in babies, and bleeding from the mouth of a baby should always be regarded as suspicious. Try to avoid using diagnostic terms such as 'bruise' when writing a referral. Use objective language and descriptive terminology instead.

6.1 Fractures

- Fractures may not be obvious on observation and the baby may present only with crying on handling. Often a fracture will not be diagnosed until an X-ray is performed. Fractures in babies are seldom caused by 'rough handling' or putting their legs through the bars of the cot. Babies rarely fracture their skull after a fall from a bed or a chair. Fractures in non-mobile infants should be assessed by an experienced paediatrician to exclude non-accidental injury (refer to Table 1.18 for types of fractures).

- Children's bones tend to bend rather than break and require considerable force to damage them. There are various kinds of fractures (refer to Table 1.18), depending on the direction and strength of the force that caused them.

- Unless there is an obvious bony deformity, bone injuries may not be apparent on initial clinical assessment. A clear history and appreciation of the mechanism of injury are crucial parts of the initial assessment and must be clearly documented.

TABLE 1.18 – Types of Bone Fractures

Greenstick

The bones bend rather than break. This is a very common accidental injury in children.

Transverse

The break goes across the bone and occurs when there is a direct blow or a direct force on the end of the bone (e.g. a fall on the hand may break the forearm bones or the distal humerus).

Spiral or oblique

A fracture line that goes right around the bone or obliquely across it is due to a twisting force, which may be a feature in non-accidental injuries.

Metaphyseal

These fractures occur at the extreme ends of the bone and are usually only confirmed radiologically. These are caused by a strong twisting force.

Skull

These must be consistent with the history and explanation given. Complex (branched), depressed or fractures at the back of the skull are suspect of abuse.

Rib

These do not occur accidentally, except in a severe crushing injury. Any other cause is highly suspicious of non-accidental injury.

6.2 Shaking Injuries

- When small babies are shaken violently, their head and limb movements cannot be controlled, causing brain damage and haemorrhage within the skull. This can also be caused by being thrown.

- Finger bruising on the chest may indicate that a baby has been held tightly and shaken. These babies usually present with collapse or respiratory problems and the diagnosis is only made on further detailed assessment.

7. Mobile Babies and Toddlers

7.1 Bruising

- It is normal for toddlers to have accidental bruises on the shins, elbows and forehead. Bruises in unusual areas such as the back, upper arms and abdomen do not tend to occur accidentally. Defensive wounds commonly occur on the forearm, upper arm, back of the legs, hands or feet. You may see clusters of bruises on the upper arm, outside of the thigh or on the body. You may see bruises with dots

Safeguarding Children

of blood under the skin. A bruised scalp and swollen eyes may suggest that hair has been pulled violently.

- Bruising caused by a hand slap leaves a characteristic pattern of 'stripes' representing the imprint of fingers. Forceful gripping leaves small round bruises corresponding to the position of the fingertips. 'Tramline' bruising is caused by a belt or stick, and shows as lines of bruising with a white patch in between.

7.2 Burns and Scalds

- Burns and scalds can result from hot liquids, hot objects, flames, chemicals or electricity.

- Burns are caused by the application to the skin of dry heat, and the depth of the burn will depend on the temperature of the object and the length of time it is in contact with the skin.

- Abusive burns are frequently small and deep, and may show the outline of the object (e.g. the soleplate of an iron), whereas accidental burns rarely do so because the child will pull away in response to pain.

- Cigarette burns are not common. They are round, deep and have a red flare around a flat brown crust. These burns usually leave a scar.

- Scalds are caused by steam or hot liquids. Accidental scalds may be extensive but show splash marks unlike the sharp edges of damage done when the child is dunked in hot water (although splash marks may also feature in a non-accidental burn, indicating that the child had tried to escape hot water). The glove and stocking pattern of burns on the arms and legs is typical of non-accidental injury. The head, face, neck, shoulders and front of the chest are the areas affected when a child pulls over a kettle accidentally.

7.3 Bite Marks

- Bites result in small bruises forming part or all of a circle. They are usually oval or circular in shape. There may be visible wounds, indentations or bruising from individual teeth.

7.4 Deliberate Poisoning and Attempted Suffocation

- These are very difficult to assess and may need a period of close observation in hospital. Deliberate poisoning, such as might be found in a child in whom illness is fabricated or induced by carers with parenting responsibilities (fictitious or induced illness), may be suspected when a child has repeated puzzling illnesses, usually of sudden onset. The signs include unusual drowsiness, apnoeic attacks, vomiting, diarrhoea and fits. There may be respiratory problems due to suffocation.

8. Older Children and Adolescents

- If the injury is accidental, older children will give a very clear and detailed account of how it happened. The detail will be missing if they have been told what to say.

- Overdosing and other self-harm injuries must be taken seriously in this age group, as they may indicate sexual or other abuse (such as exploitation).

8.1 Parental Factors

- Parental unavailability for whatever reason increases the risk to the child of all forms of abuse, especially neglect and emotional abuse. Specific consideration of the effects of the parent's problem on the children must be made, whatever the circumstances of presentation. Sources of stress within families may have a negative impact on a child's health, development or well-being, either directly or because they affect the capacity of parents to respond to their child's needs. Sources of stress may include social exclusion, domestic abuse, unstable mental illness of a parent or carer or drug and alcohol misuse. Parents who appear overanxious about their child when there is no sign of illness or injury may be signalling their inability to cope.

- Parental factors that might have a negative impact on parenting capacity include:
  - learning difficulties
  - mental health problems
  - substance abuse
  - domestic abuse
  - chronic ill-health
  - physical disability
  - unemployment or poverty
  - homelessness/frequent moves
  - social isolation
  - young, unsupported parents
  - parents with poor role models of their own
  - lack of, or poor, education
  - criminality
  - unwanted or unplanned pregnancy.

9. Special Circumstances

9.1 Individuals Who Pose a Risk to Children

- Once an individual has been sentenced and identified as presenting a risk of harm to children, agencies have a responsibility to work collaboratively to monitor and manage the risk of harm to others.

Safeguarding Children

- Where an offender is given a community sentence, offender managers or youth offending team workers will monitor the individual's risk of harm to others and their behaviour, and liaise with partner agencies as appropriate.

- Multi-Agency Public Protection Arrangements (MAPPAs) should be in place to enable agencies to work together within a statutory framework for managing risk of harm to the public.

- There are certain work forces that are exempt from the Rehabilitation of Offenders Act 1974. Patient-facing roles within the ambulance service are part of this. Safer recruitment checks will be undertaken, including an enhanced DBS (Disclosure and Barring Service).

9.2 Disabled Children

- Abuse may be difficult to separate from symptoms of disability (e.g. increase in seizures in a child with epilepsy if anticonvulsants are withheld). Induced and fabricated illness may be even more difficult to recognise because the child may have coexistent diagnoses.

- Important points to remember about abuse of disabled children are:
  - It may be more common than abuse of non-disabled children, but evidence for this is poor.
  - It may be under-reported.
  - Children may have difficulty communicating their abuse.
  - Abuse may compound pre-existing disability, or be the cause of the disability.
  - All forms of abuse are seen, including neglect and sexual abuse.
  - It is easy to fail to recognise abuse in disabled children by making too many allowances for the disability as a cause of problems.
  - Be aware that professionals can be drawn into collusion with families; this is a term known as 'disguised compliance'.

- These children are at risk of achieving poor outcomes. Ambulance clinicians need to be aware of the role they can play in recognition of these children, identifying their particular needs and preventing significant harm. In the current multicultural society of the United Kingdom, it is important to recognise that there may be children and families in need of skilled interpreters, and that differences may exist in child-rearing practices in minority groups.

9.3 Special Circumstances for Consideration

- **Children and young people living away from home** – many looked-after children and young people that live independently have been abused or neglected prior to going into care. This is a particular group where assessment may be made more difficult because of pre-existing symptoms and behaviour. There should be a low threshold for seeking advice from experienced professionals in these circumstances (e.g. designated/named professional).

- **Asylum-seeking children or refugees, both with families and unaccompanied** – the importance of having skilled interpreters in assessment of these children cannot be over-emphasised. The children's behaviour on entering the country may already have been influenced by previous experience. It is important to remember their general health needs and that families will need help in accessing services. It is also important to refer children who are victims of human trafficking.

- **Children with maladjusted parent(s)/carers** (see also Parental Factors) – these include children of substance-misusing parents/carers, children living with domestic abuse, children whose parents/carers have chronic mental or physical health problems, children whose parents/carers have a learning disability, children with a parent/carer in prison and children living in flexi-families. Effects on the child/ren can be profound and include fearfulness, withdrawal, anxious behaviour, lack of self-confidence and social skills, difficulties in forming relationships, sleep disturbance, non-attendance at school, aggression, bullying, post-traumatic stress disorder and behaviour suggestive of ADHD.

The following children may also have unmet health needs (low immunisation levels, poor dental health and either poor or non-attendance at clinic appointments).

- **Children of Gypsy/Roma/Traveller background** – these children are subjected to the same problems because of frequent moves. They may also suffer from poor health, poor access to primary healthcare and vaccinations, in addition to poor living conditions.

- **Runaway children and exploitation** – many runaway children may already have been the subject of abuse and are at risk of exploitation. They are also at risk of child trafficking for sexual exploitation.

- **Children as young carers** – neglect and emotional abuse may be part of the difficulties of taking on parental responsibilities and a caring role at a young age. Young carers lose out on normal childhood experiences and should be considered at higher risk of abuse, whether intentional or unintentional (e.g. school attendance, peer groups).

Safeguarding Children

- For some pregnant women, complex social factors are likely to impact on their engagement with their maternity care (NICE, 2010). Examples of complex social factors in pregnancy include:
  - Trafficked/modern slavery
  - Mental ill-health
  - Substance/alcohol misuse
  - Recent migrant/refugee/asylum-seeker
  - Language barrier
  - Domestic abuse
  - Sexual assault/rape/sexual exploitation
  - Previous child/ren removed from care
  - Learning disabilities
  - Teenage pregnancy
  - Difficult childhood (ACES)
  - Homelessness/financial difficulties

- Ambulance services are in a very unique position whereby we may be the first point of contact for the pregnant/post-natal woman during her pregnancy.

- Any staff that attend to a woman who has delivered (whether unassisted or attended to by ambulance crew), who presents late in pregnancy and has engaged with little to no antenatal care (whether free-birthing or otherwise) or who has delivered yet declined to convey should undertake a safeguarding risk assessment and use professional curiosity to establish whether there are any safeguarding concerns identified which would warrant further management to protect the unborn/born and mother from harm.

- In the event of a BBA where the mother declines to be conveyed in the absence of a midwife in attendance, or a situation where there are immediate risks of harm to a baby or any other children within the household, staff should contact Children's Social Care and **should not leave the baby/children alone** with the mother until the staff has had a direct discussion with the Duty Social Worker and a plan is put in place. Staff should also consider contacting the police for a PPO (Police Protection Order) **after** a discussion has taken place with the Duty Social Worker, or if the risk of harm is so high, then the police should be contacted immediately.

- For pregnant women who are visiting the UK from abroad, the above recommendations also apply. Staff should be mindful that overseas visitors will not have an NHS number and must be considered as a potential increased risk for absconding, particularly in the event of a BBA.

- If the pregnant woman speaks limited to no English, then appropriate interpretation services must be used. Staff must not rely on family and friends to translate for the woman.

SECTION **1** General Guidance

Safeguarding Children

Maternity Safeguarding Flow Chart

If the woman is a visitor to the UK

- A children's safeguarding risk assessment should be carried out using the child assessment framework and using your professional curiosity, consider; *the gestation the pregnant woman is travelling at, any other siblings and their whereabouts, details of others associated with the pregnant woman such as her partner / family & or friends the woman is visiting in the UK, history of antenatal care (NB it may vary significantly depending on where the woman has travelled from)*
- Encourage the woman to attend the local maternity unit / ED for a full antenatal check – reassure her that treatment will be provided without request for payment up front
- Consider informing the local maternity unit, depending on the gestation and clinical picture
- If she has delivered, follow the process as for women who have delivered and had no antenatal care in the UK
- Remember visitors from overseas will NOT have an NHS number and must be considered as a potential risk for absconding

Claire Sidley-Jenkins, RM, PMA, May 2022

- If ambulance staff are referring women for antenatal care, then establish whether there is an online booking system in multiple languages.

- If the pregnant woman advises that she has transferred her care from another trust but is unable to share her antenatal records/notes with staff, then this should be considered as a safeguarding concern and a children's safeguarding risk assessment should be carried out with consideration for a safeguarding referral.

12. Mandatory Reporting of Female Genital Mutilation (FGM)

- On 31 October 2015, the FGM Act introduced a mandatory reporting duty that requires health and social care professionals as well as teachers to report known cases of FGM in those under 18 years of age to the police.

- FGM is child abuse and the current procedure is set out below:
  - **Children and vulnerable adults** – if any child (under 18) or vulnerable adult has symptoms or signs of FGM, or if there is good reason to suspect they are at risk of FGM on consideration of their family history or other relevant factors, they **must** be referred using existing safeguarding procedures as with all instances of child abuse. This will involve referral to police and social care in the usual way.
  - In all cases where staff are unsure of their actions, they should seek the advice of the Trust Safeguarding Service.

13. Assessment and Management

- If physical, sexual or emotional abuse or neglect is suspected, follow local procedures; information can be obtained from the named professional for safeguarding within individual ambulance trusts. Ambulance clinicians may obtain contact information from ambulance control.

13.1 If the Child Is the Patient

- The first priority is the health and safety of the child. Ambulance clinicians should follow the usual **ABCDE** and **<C>ABCDE** assessment (refer to **Medical Emergencies in Children – Overview** and **Trauma Emergencies in Children – Overview**). Children with significant injury should be transferred to further care without delay.

- Where a child is thought to be at immediate risk, they should be referred to the police as an emergency by contacting ambulance control for a 999 response.

Safeguarding Children

In all circumstances:

- Ensure that no action taken will place the child at further risk of harm.

- Limit questions to those of routine history-taking, asking questions only in relation to the injury or for clarification of what is being said. It is important to stop questioning when suspicions are clarified. Unnecessary questioning or probing may affect the credibility of subsequent evidence.

- Accept the explanations given and do not make any suggestions to the child as to how an injury or incident may have happened.

- Care must be taken not to directly accuse parents or carers of abuse, as this may result in a refusal to transfer to further care and place the child at further risk. Always work in partnership with parents or carers as far as possible, and inform them of concerns and the need to share these with the statutory agencies, unless to do so would put the child or others at greater risk of harm. Professional curiosity and judgement is crucial as to what information should be shared with parents.

- Any allegation of abuse made by a child is an important indicator and should always be taken seriously – it is important to listen to the 'voice of the child' and what they are saying. Do not ask probing questions. Consider what is a 'safe space' for them to talk.

- Adult responses can influence how able a child feels to reveal the full extent of the abuse. Listen and react appropriately to instil confidence. It is important to note that children may only tell a small part of their experience initially.

- It is important to make an accurate record of events and actions. Write down exactly what the child says. Their first language may not be English and care must be taken not to use family members or carers as interpreters in cases of suspected abuse. Take note of any inconsistency in history and any delay in calling for assistance. A child should not be asked to repeat what they have told you to someone else.

- On arrival at hospital, inform the receiving staff and the most senior member of nursing staff on duty of any concerns or suspicions. When reporting suspected abuse, the emphasis must be on shared professional responsibility and immediate communication.

- Complete safeguarding documentation/report as per local procedures; complete in private if possible. Follow local/trust protocols/guidelines.

- Ambulance clinicians must report suspected child abuse to the relevant statutory bodies (e.g. social care and the police), but they do not have a statutory duty to investigate it.

- Where a practitioner feels that their concerns have not been taken up (commonly known as professional challenge), they have a duty to escalate their concerns to a higher level by discussing this with their line manager, a more experienced colleague or named/designated doctor or nurse.

13.2 If the Child Is Not the Patient

- If the circumstances are suspicious, the ambulance clinician(s) should consider the implications of leaving the child.

- If the child is accompanying another person (e.g. a parent/carer) who is being conveyed, the ambulance clinician(s) should inform ED staff of their concerns and remember to report through their own safeguarding services as required.

- If no one is transferred to hospital, follow local/trust protocols/guidelines and inform safeguarding services of the incident/concerns at the earliest opportunity.

- Complete safeguarding documentation/report as per local procedures; complete in private if possible. Follow local/trust protocols/guidelines.

13.3 Allegations Against Ambulance Service Employees and Volunteers

- An allegation made by a child against ambulance service employees and volunteers is no different from an allegation made against any other healthcare professional, and the appropriate procedures should be followed, that is a referral to social care or the police. In other words, a child protection inquiry must follow such allegations.

- No staff, regardless of their position, volunteer, commissioned service or person associated with delivering services on behalf of an NHS Trust must act in any way that constitutes any of the following:
  - Behaviour that harms, or may harm, a child, young person or adult
  - Behaviour that results in a criminal offence against, or related to, a child, young person or adult
  - Behaviour towards a child, young person or adult that indicates they are unsuitable to work in a position of trust.

- The member of staff who is alleged to have abused the child must report the allegation to their line manager/named professional, who should follow employment procedures, that is a possible restriction of practice or suspension while investigations are conducted. There should be close liaison between the police carrying out the investigation and the line manager/named professional, who should be guided by the police as to how much information about the inquiry should be relayed to the member of staff. There will also need to be a support system in place for the member of staff.

Safeguarding Children

Safeguarding Children

- The safety and welfare of the child are paramount.
- There is a duty to report concerns. Staff should not investigate concerns themselves.
- Be aware of any special circumstances that the child is in which may increase the risk of abuse.
- Police should be involved where there may be an immediate risk to the child.
- Staff should document the circumstances giving rise to their concern as soon as possible.

Further Reading

Further important information and evidence in support of this guideline can be found in the Bibliography.

Other useful resources include:

Barnado's – http://www.barnados.org.uk/

Child Exploitation and Online Protection Command – http://www.ceop.gov.uk

Childline – http://www.childline.org.uk/

Children's Legal Centre – http://www.childrenslegalcentre.com

Family Lives – http://www.familylives.org.uk/

Kidscape – http://www.kidscape.org.uk

NSPCC – http://www.nspcc.org.uk

Samaritans – http://www.samaritans.org.uk

Victim Support – http://www.victimsupport.org.uk

NSPCC Learning – Recently published case reviews: https://learning.nspcc.org.uk/case-reviews/recently-published-case-reviews

Bibliography

1. Department of Health. *The Children Act 2004*. London: HMSO, 2004. Available from: https://www.legislation.gov.uk/ukpga/2004/31/content.

2. HM Government. *Working Together to Safeguard Children: A guide to inter-agency working to safeguard and promote the welfare of children*. London: HMSO, 2018. Available from: https://assets.publishing.service.gov.uk/government/uploads/system/uploads/attachment_data/file/942454/Working_together_to_safeguard_children_inter_agency_guidance.pdf.

3. National Institute for Health and Clinical Excellence. *Child Abuse and Neglect (NG76)* London: NICE, 2017. Available from: https://www.nice.org.uk/guidance/ng76.

4. NSPCC Learning. *Guidance on Protecting d/Deaf and Disabled Children and Young People from Abuse*. 2022. Available from: https://learning.nspcc.org.uk/safeguarding-child-protection/deaf-and-disabled-children.

5. HM Government. *Information Sharing: Advice for practitioners providing safeguarding services to children, young people, parents and carers*. 2018. Available from: https://assets.publishing.service.gov.uk/government/uploads/system/uploads/attachment_data/file/1062969/Information_sharing_advice_practitioners_safeguarding_services.pdf.

6. Department of Health. *Responding to Domestic Abuse: A resource for health professionals*. London: HMSO, 2017. Available from: https://assets.publishing.service.gov.uk/government/uploads/system/uploads/attachment_data/file/597435/DometicAbuseGuidance.pdf.

7. Home Office. *Adoption and Children Act 2002*. London: HMSO, 2002. Available from: http://www.legislation.gov.uk/ukpga/2002/38/contents.

8. Home Office. *Female Genital Mutilation Act 2003*. London: HMSO, 2003. Available from: http://www.legislation.gov.uk/ukpga/2003/31/pdfs/ukpga_20030031_en.pdf.

9. Royal College of Nursing. *Safeguarding Children and Young People: Roles and competencies for healthcare staff*. 2019. Available from: https://www.rcn.org.uk/-/media/Royal-College-Of-Nursing/Documents/Publications/2019/January/007-366.pdf.

10. Scottish Parliament. *Prohibition of Female Genital Mutilation (Scotland) Act 2005*. Edinburgh: HMSO, 2005. Available from: https://www.legislation.gov.uk/asp/2005/8/contents.

11. WHO. *Fact Sheet: Female Genital Mutilation*. 2022. Available from: https://www.who.int/news-room/fact-sheets/detail/female-genital-mutilation.

12. NICE. *Pregnancy and Complex Social Factors: A model for service provision for pregnant women with complex social factors*. 2010. Available from: https://www.nice.org.uk/guidance/cg110.

SECTION **1** General Guidance

Sexual Assault

1. Introduction

- Sexual assault is extremely distressing, causing a broad spectrum of psychological, emotional and physical effects on patients. They may be agitated or hysterical, in shock or disbelief or calm and extremely controlled. Clinicians should understand that there is no 'normal' response and have no expectation of the patient exhibiting a prescribed pattern of behaviour.[1]

- It may be appropriate for the patient to be accompanied by another person. The patient may be anxious when left alone with a person of the same sex as the assailant. On the other hand, they may be reassured by the presence of a professional person. The wishes of the patient must be considered and attempts made to reassure them and make them feel safe.

- The patient has just experienced a major psychological and potentially physical trauma, often committed by someone they believed in and trusted. The clinician must not only manage their physical, medical and psychological needs, but must absolutely act as the patient's advocate, facilitating their wishes wherever possible.

- Patients experiencing sexual assault may believe they are responsible for the assault and need reassuring that they are victims and that what has happened was not their fault.[2]

- A sensitive and kind approach by those providing an initial response is known to be beneficial in facilitating recovery and decreasing long-term use of health services post rape. In contrast, health professionals inexperienced in dealing with survivors, who use insensitive language, subscribe to rape myths and stereotypes, who are judgemental, inconsiderate or critical, are known to increase the risk of revictimising the survivor, delaying recovery, sometimes forever.[3]

- Importantly, victims of sexual violence must be treated with respect and dignity irrespective of either the victim's or the clinician's social status, race, religion, culture, sexual orientation, lifestyle, sex or occupation.[1]

- It is not the role of the clinician to determine if the assault has occurred; that is the job of the courts. Instead they must provide a sensitive, non-judgemental, holistic approach that is neither moralistic nor opinionated. Victims who blame themselves, or fear being blamed or doubted, are less likely to report sexual assault. Recovery may also be hampered by the blame or disbelief of others, whether real or perceived. Body language, gestures and facial expressions all contribute to conveying an atmosphere of believing the patient's account, which is known to be critical to recovery.[4]

- The intimate nature of sexual assault, combined with the inevitable feelings of guilt and shame these patients experience, complicates their care. During the assault, they may have seen, experienced and been forced to do things that are outside their normal moral or ethical code. They may believe it to be unspeakable.

- Many victims cite fear of not being believed as a reason for not reporting sexual assault, and recovery may be hindered when others disbelieve or blame the patient for the assault. Validation of the patient's feelings is thus critical to recovery.[3] Body language, gestures and facial expressions all contribute to conveying an atmosphere of believing the patient's account.

2. Disclosure to Police

- Some patients will refuse care or transfer to hospital because they believe police may be informed without their consent and fear perceived catastrophic consequences. Historically, reporting without patient consent has been common practice amongst both control room and operational staff of all levels.

- The decision to report a sexual assault on an adult is entirely the decision of the victim. There is no statutory obligation for victims of sexual violence to report to police, and many victims elect not to report to protect their safety, privacy or both.[5]

- Similarly, no statutory obligation mandates the reporting by healthcare professionals of cases involving rape or sexual assault.[5] Where the patient is an adult with full capacity to consent, and is not classed as 'vulnerable', there is no requirement for clinicians to breach confidentiality and report to police without consent. Control room staff should not routinely inform police and request their attendance unless this is the specific wish of the patient, and no attempt to persuade or coerce the patient to agree to police attendance should be made by anyone involved in their care pathway at any time.[6,7]

- The only exception to this would be where disclosing the information is necessary to prevent a serious crime or serious harm to others. Generally, if the ambulance service is involved, the serious crime has already occurred. Unless there are reasonable grounds to assume there is imminent risk to either the patient or the public, the patient's decision, as an autonomous adult, should be fully respected.[8]

- Where it is perceived there is a clear and present immediate danger to the patient or others if disclosure to police is not made, and that risk is greater than the possible consequences to the patient of disclosure, then it would be appropriate to breach that confidentiality.

Sexual Assault

3. Forensic Requirements

- Where the victim requests police involvement, forensic awareness is essential. Within the limits of any immediate care needs, there is a responsibility to preserve evidence. Where police are on scene and injuries do not require emergent care, the police will normally take responsibility for the patient.[9]

- While awaiting police arrival, patients should be kept within the environment in which they present, unless this is unsafe or increasing the patient's distress; if so, they can be moved to the ambulance, seated on a clean sheet and wherever possible discouraged from any activities that jeopardise collection of evidence. This will include cutting, removing or changing clothing, eating or drinking, passing urine or opening bowels or washing.[9]

- Where the patient cannot be dissuaded from the natural need to clean themselves, they should be encouraged to place any tissues or towels along with any bloodstained clothes into paper (not plastic) bags, which do not destroy biological evidence.[9]

- Where patients are transported to hospital and police action is requested, all blankets, sheets, towels and associated paraphernalia should be passed to police for forensic retrieval.[9]

Additional forensic information:

- Where patients have not presented for immediate care following rape, clinicians should be aware of how long forensic material may be preserved within the patient. The approximate times after contact for which evidentially relevant material has been identified – the 'forensic window' – are detailed in Table 1.19.

- Differences exist between pre- and post-pubescent patients; this is because the vaginal area is hostile to semen in the pre-pubescent patient.

TABLE 1.19 – Preservation of Forensic Material[9]

Type of Incident	Type of Sample	Forensic Window
Digital penetration	Vulval, vaginal, peri-anal and anal swabs	Up to 12 hours
Oral penetration	Mouth swabs and oral rinse	Up to 48 hours – even where the patient has eaten, drunk or brushed their teeth
Anal penetration	Peri-anal, perineal, internal anal and rectal swabs Penile swabs	Up to 72 hours
Vaginal penetration	Vulval, vaginal and endocervical swabs	Pre-pubescent: Up to 72 hours Post-pubescent: Up to 120 hours

4. Care Pathways

As primary caregiver and advocate, clinicians should inform the patient of their options without judgement, bias or coercion. Any physical examination should allow identification of life-threatening injuries and those requiring emergent care only. Genital areas should only be exposed and examined if there is evidence of bleeding requiring immediate treatment.

Allow the patient space and as much choice about options for their treatment as possible. Options for the care of sexual assault victims may be summarised as:

- **Accident and Emergency:**
  - if the victim has injuries requiring emergent care
  - if the level of distress makes it impossible for the patient to consent or coherently express their wishes.

- **Police:**
  - only where the patient gives express and informed consent, as discussed above.

- **Sexual Assault Referral Centres (SARCs):**
  - SARCs provide recent victims of sexual assault with immediate care and crisis support from specialist staff trained to allow patients to make informed decisions. They also provide access to acute physical assessment with testing for STIs and provision of post-infection prophylaxis and emergency contraception.[10]
  - SARCs also facilitate access to the criminal justice system. Forensic retrieval may be undertaken regardless of whether the patient reports to police or not. Where the patient decides not to report, forensic samples may be stored, allowing patients time to consider their options until after the immediate 'crisis period'.[10]

Sexual Assault

- SARCs provide direct access to Independent Sexual Violence Advisers (ISVAs) who provide advice, support and access to follow-up services addressing the patient's medical, safeguarding, psychosocial and ongoing needs.
- ISVAs will also support patients through the judicial process; importantly, patients supported by ISVAs are more likely to go through the full course of criminal justice proceedings, which highlights the importance of encouraging patients to access SARCs wherever possible.[11]

4.1. Access to SARCs

- **Self-referral** – patients may self-refer to SARCs by telephone; clinicians may also call on the patient's behalf. Patients have a brief conversation with a crisis worker who helps them decide on an immediate plan and makes an appointment for them to attend. Where this appointment is immediate, subject to time constraints and local protocols, ambulance crews may transport the patient directly to the SARC or alternatively make certain the patient will be able to be taken safely by a third party.
- Local SARC contact details should be held centrally by ambulance control rooms; they are also available on NHS Choices.
- **Police referral** – the patient reports to police, who contact the SARC and arrange for the patient to be transferred.

4.2. Refusal of Care

- Patients refusing referral to support services place a duty of care on clinicians to ensure their immediate safety. Encouraging patients to call a friend or relative for support is a priority. In these cases, patients should be given details of their nearest GUM clinic and rape crisis services. These conversations require tact and sensitivity, as patients may not have considered the risk of STIs or pregnancy, and this alone may create another crisis.
- In cases of sexual assault in vulnerable adults and children, refer to **Safeguarding Adults at Risk** and **Safeguarding Children**.

5. Incidence

- Approximately 11 adults are raped every hour in England and Wales. That amounts to 85,000 women and 12,000 men becoming victims of rape every year, while nearly half a million adults are sexually assaulted.
- Of these, 90% know the perpetrator prior to the offence, and only around 15% of these will choose to report to police.[12]
- In 2012–13, 23,663 sexual offences against children were reported to police in England and Wales, including 6,296 rapes, with 80% of these involving girls.[13]
- Given this incidence, as a profession, paramedics should be well versed in the care of this most vulnerable group and have a comprehensive understanding of the care pathways and services available to them.

6. Severity and Outcome

- The severity of the assault can vary from sexual touching to sustaining life-threatening injuries. The outcome of the assault can lead to long-term psychological and physical effects.

7. Pathophysiology

The Sexual Offences Act (2003) defines four offences:[14]

- Rape – penetration of the vagina, anus or mouth with a penis without consent.
- Assault by penetration – non-consensual, intentional insertion of an object (other than a penis) into the vagina or anus.
- Sexual assault – non-consensual violation of the victim's sexual anatomy, e.g. touching another person in a sexual way without consent.
- Causing a person to engage in sexual activity without consent.

8. Assessment and Management

For the assessment and management of sexual assault, refer to Table 1.20.

TABLE 1.20 – ASSESSMENT and MANAGEMENT of: Sexual Assault
Assess <C>ABCD
If any **TIME-CRITICAL** features present major ABCD problems:
▪ Start correcting <C>ABCD problems.
▪ Undertake a TIME-CRITICAL transfer to nearest receiving hospital.
▪ Continue patient management en-route.
▪ Provide an ATMIST information call.

Sexual Assault

TABLE 1.20 – ASSESSMENT and MANAGEMENT of: Sexual Assault *(continued)*

Assess

- Limit questions to those identifying the need for medical treatment, but allow the patient to talk and document what is said. **NB** It is not appropriate to probe for details of the assault and could affect the outcome of criminal investigations.

- Manage according to condition:
  - Acute injury – refer to **Trauma Emergencies in Adults – Overview** and **Trauma Emergencies in Children – Overview**.
  - Acute illness – refer to **Trauma Emergencies in Adults – Overview** and **Trauma Emergencies in Children – Overview**.

- It may be appropriate to delay assessment for non-urgent injuries until transfer to a Sexual Assault Referral Centre to avoid further distress and disturbing the evidence.

Approach

- Rape is about power and control, not the sexual act. Listen to the patient with a sensitive and respectful manner and return control to them.

- Establish the patient's safety.

- Let the patient know you believe them.

- If possible, ensure privacy.

- Consider cultural/religious issues.

- Where possible accommodate patient's requests.

- Where possible avoid disturbing the scene.

- Where possible avoid being alone with the patient.

- Patients are not required by law to report sexual violence to police.

- Healthcare professionals are not required by law to report cases of sexual violence to police unless:
  - the patient does not have capacity to consent
  - the patient is classed as 'vulnerable'
  - there is a clear and present danger of immediate risk to the patient or public.

- No attempt should be made to persuade the patient to agree to police attendance; decision making should be facilitated by presenting available options.

- Where this is requested, police should be called promptly so the scene may be secured.

- Where patients decline any support or referral, they should be encouraged to obtain community support ensuring their ongoing safety is secured. These patients should be encouraged with tact and care to contact their nearest GUM clinic or local rape crisis services.

Forensic Examination

- Forensic examination will focus specifically on the areas affected, including wounds, mouth, anus and vagina and other areas where the patient has been kissed, licked or bitten, as these areas may well be contaminated with the assailant's DNA.

- Clinicians should be aware of forensic windows, and where this is relevant patients should be encouraged not to:
  - wash (shower/bathe) or brush their teeth
  - change, throw away or destroy clothes
  - urinate – the police will want to collect early evidence samples including a urine sample to screen for the presence of drugs, as some drugs have a very short half-life
  - smoke, eat or drink – a mouth swab and mouth wash may also be requested by the police
  - defecate.

- If a blanket is required for modesty or warmth, a single-use blanket should be used and kept with the patient – the blanket needs to be retained in order to analyse cross-contamination.

- If the patient is not wrapped in a single-use blanket, place a sterile sheet or single-use blanket under the patient where they sit or lie and retain for forensic examination.

(continued)

SECTION 1 General Guidance

Sexual Assault

TABLE 1.20 – ASSESSMENT and MANAGEMENT of: Sexual Assault *(continued)*

- Avoid cleaning any wounds unless clinically absolutely necessary – if possible, keep 'washings'.
- If required, lightly apply dry dressings – retain any used dressing and swabs for forensic examination; also keep the sterile packets in which they were contained in order to examine for cross-contamination.

NB All of these recommendations are vital to conserve evidence for a successful prosecution of the offender; BUT the need for this approach must be conveyed with great sensitivity to the patient, who may well want to wash and change.

Care Pathways

Accident and Emergency is appropriate:

- if the patient has injuries requiring emergency care
- if the level of distress makes it impossible for them to consent or coherently express their wishes.

Sexual Assault Referral Centres can provide:

- immediate care and crisis support
- acute physical assessment
- testing for STIs
- post-infection prophylaxis
- emergency contraception
- access to the criminal justice system
- forensic retrieval with storage where police involvement is declined
- access to ISVA services
- access to follow-up services addressing medical, safeguarding, psychosocial and ongoing needs.

Access to SARCs, where the patient consents, is either by:

- **Self referral** – the patient telephones the SARC themselves (this can easily be initiated by the ambulance crew), who give them an appointment normally within a few hours unless they are busy. There is no reason why ambulance crews – subject to local protocols and time restraints, should not transport the patient directly to the SARC or alternatively make certain the patient will be able to be taken safely by a third party.
- **Police referral** – the patient reports to police, who make contact with the SARC and arrange for the patient to be transferred.

Sexual Health Clinics provide treatment for:

- sexually transmitted infections
- emergency contraception
- post-exposure prophylaxis.

Rape Crisis Centres provide:

- confidential telephone helpline and support
- face-to-face counselling for survivors of rape or sexual assault
- ISVA services
- handover to an appropriate member of staff and not in a public area.

Where a patient is competent and refuses hospital treatment, advise them to seek further medical attention. They may need post-exposure prophylaxis, vaccination and/or contraception, all of which can be provided confidentially.

Documentation

- Complete the clinical record in great detail contemporaneously and document:
  - only facts, not personal opinion
  - what the patient says
  - clinical findings with relevant timings
  - the ambulance identification number.
- A police statement may be required later.

Sexual Assault

Figure 1.7 – Assessment and management of sexual assault.

KEY POINTS!

Sexual Assault

- Sexual assault may be concurrent with other injuries that will need treating.
- Treatment should avoid disturbing evidence where possible.
- The patient's rights to autonomy should be respected unless they do not have capacity to consent or are 'vulnerable'.
- Leave the investigation to the police.
- Accommodate the patient's wishes where possible.
- Police may have special facilities for managing patients.

Further Reading

Further important information and evidence in support of this guideline can be found in the Bibliography.[15,16,17,18,19,20,21,22,23]

Bibliography

1. World Health Organization. *Guidelines for Medico-legal Care for Victims of Sexual Violence*. Geneva: WHO, 2003. Available from: http://apps.who.int/iris/bitstream/10665/42788/1/924154628X.pdf.

2. Beckmann CR, Groetzinger LL. Treating sexual assault victims. A protocol for health professionals. *Female Patient* 1989, 14(5): 78–83.

3. Ranibar V, Speer SA. Revictimization and recovery from sexual assault: implications for health professionals. *Violence and Victims* 2013, 28(2): 274–287.

4. Dunn S, Gilchrist V. Sexual assault. *Primary Care* 1993, 20: 359–373.

5. Department of Health. *Public Health Functions to be exercised by NHS England – Service Specification No 30, Sexual Assault Services*. London: HMSO, 2013. Available from: https://www.gov.uk/government/uploads/system/uploads/attachment_data/file/256501/30_sexual_assault_services.pdf.

6. British Association for Sexual Health and HIV. *UK National Guidelines on the Management of Adult and Adolescent Complainants of Sexual Assault 2011*. Macclesfield: BASHH, 2011. Available from: http://www.nordhaven.co.uk/BASHH.PDF.

7. Department of Health. *Confidentiality: NHS Code of Practice*. London: HMSO, 2003.

8. Department of Health. *Confidentiality: NHS Code of Practice Supplementary Guidance on Public Interest Disclosures*. London: HMSO, 2010.

Sexual Assault

9. Crown Prosecution Service. *Prosecution Policy and Guidance; Legal Guidance; Rape and sexual offences: forensic, scientific and medical evidence.* Available from: https://www.cps.gov.uk/legal-guidance/rape-and-sexual-offences-chapter-9-forensic-scientific-and-medical-evidence.

10. Department of Health, Home Office, Association of Chief Police Officers. *Revised National Service Guide – A resource for developing Sexual Assault Referral Centres.* London: HMSO, 2009. Available from: https://www.sericc.org.uk/pdfs/4313_sacentres.pdf.

11. Robinson AL. *Independent Sexual Violence Advisers: A process evaluation.* University of Cardiff funded by the Home Office, 2009. Available from: http://library.college.police.uk/docs/horr/horr20.pdf.

12. Ministry of Justice, Home Office and Office of National Statistics. *An Overview of Sexual Offending in England and Wales.* London: HMSO, 2013. Available from: https://www.gov.uk/government/statistics/an-overview-of-sexual-offending-in-england-and-wales.

13. Jutte S. et al. *How Safe Are Our Children?* London: NSPCC, 2014.

14. Legislation.gov.uk. Sexual Offences Act (2003). Available from: http://www.legislation.gov.uk/ukpga/2003/42/part/1.

15. Avegno J, Mills TJ, Mills LD. Sexual assault victims in the emergency department: analysis by demographic and event characteristics. *Journal of Emergency Medicine* 2009, 37(3): 328–334.

16. Dalton M. *Forensic Gynaecology: Towards better care of the female victim of sexual assault.* London: Royal College of Obstetricians and Gynaecologists Press, 2004.

17. Department of Health. *Improving Services for Women and Child Victims of Violence: The Department of Health Action Plan.* 2010. Available from: http://www.dh.gov.uk/prod_consum_dh/groups/dh_digitalassets/@dh/@en/@ps/documents/digitalasset/dh_122094.pdf.

18. Du Mont J, White D, McGregor MJ. Investigating the medical forensic examination from the perspectives of sexually assaulted women. *Social Science and Medicine* 2009, 68(4): 774–780.

19. Martin EK, Taft CT, Resick PA. A review of marital rape. *Aggression and Violent Behavior* 2007, 12(3): 329–347.

20. Mein JK, Palmer CM, Shand MC, Templeton DJ, Parekh V, Mobbs M et al. Management of acute adult sexual assault. *Medical Journal of Australia* 2003, 178(5): 226–230.

21. Pesola GR, Westfal RE, Kuffner CA. Emergency department characteristics of male sexual assault. *Academic Emergency Medicine* 1999, 6(8): 792–798.

22. Regan L, Lovett J, Kelly L. *Forensic Nursing: An option for improving responses to reported rape and sexual assault.* London: Home Office, 2004.

23. Taskforce on the Health Aspects of Violence Against Women and Children Improving Safety. *Responding to Violence Against Women and Children – The role of the NHS.* 2010. Available from: http://www.fflm.ac.uk/wp-content/uploads/documentstore/1268669895.pdf.

Staff Health and Wellbeing

1. Introduction

- The importance of good mental health and wellbeing cannot be underestimated. The World Health Organization defines good mental health as: 'a state of wellbeing in which every individual realizes his or her own potential, can cope with the normal stresses of life, can work productively and fruitfully and is able to make a contribution to her or his community'.[1]

- However, there is evidence to suggest that, for those who work in the emergency services, the risk of experiencing a mental health issue is greater than average.[2] The number and type of significant tragedies and events in the UK in recent years combined with the ever-increasing workload placed upon emergency services has highlighted the difficulties often experienced by staff. As a result, the subject has been looked at from a fresh perspective, with many new and useful resources becoming available.

- The blue light scoping survey undertaken by Mind – the mental health charity – suggested that there are a number of areas that are directly attributable to a change in the mental wellbeing of ambulance service workers.[3] Similarly, it highlighted some worrying trends:
  - Emergency service staff are twice as likely to identify work as the cause of their mental health issue, with over 85% of staff experiencing stress, low mood, anxiety or depression at some point in their career.
  - Over 50% of staff are unaware of services they can access to help them with their mental health needs.
  - Despite the Equality Act (2010) offering protection, only 12% would approach a line manager for help and almost 80% said they would never speak to their HR departments.

- But this need not be the case and there is a wealth of resources at hand. The most common issues around ambulance staff mental wellbeing are centred upon several key themes.[3]

2. Anxiety

- Anxiety is a perfectly normal reaction to a stressful situation and is linked closely to the fight-or-flight response. Anxiety disorders can take several different forms, the most common of which is generalised anxiety disorder and is widely experienced.

- The most commonly experienced symptoms are very much in line with those of PTSD:[3,4]
  - palpitations
  - shortness of breath
  - diarrhoea
  - nausea.

- Once the trigger for the symptoms of anxiety stop, you would expect the anxiety to reduce.

However, if the anxiety starts to influence our lives too greatly, we must look for ways to deal with it effectively.

3. Post-traumatic Stress Disorder (PTSD)

- Post-traumatic stress disorder (PTSD) can affect anyone and is closely associated with very intense situations in which someone experiences life-threatening or life-changing events, especially those that involve witnessing death and dying.[5]

- These types of situation are not uncommon for ambulance clinicians, and recognising that you may have been negatively influenced by a single event or accumulation of events should never be considered a weakness. Research points towards the severity, intensity and number of exposures to stressful experiences as being the key reason someone may suffer from PTSD and not because of an individual's personality traits.[6]

- Common symptoms include:
  - flashbacks or reliving traumatic incidents
  - nightmares
  - feeling constantly on edge
  - a numbing of emotions
  - an unwillingness to talk about or visit memories and reminders of an event.

- Other symptoms can include:
  - pain
  - nausea
  - diarrhoea
  - choosing to withdraw and becoming socially isolated
  - increased drug and alcohol use
  - depression
  - low mood
  - anxiety
  - a strong sense of guilt.[7]

4. Low Mood and Depression

- It is estimated one in five people in the UK suffer from depression at some point throughout their lives, making depression amongst the most common of disorders.[8]

- A sense of hopelessness, sadness, loss and reduced interest in your normal life and activities is felt over an extended period. It can affect appetite, sleep, concentration, self-worth and relationships. At its worst it can lead to feelings and thoughts of self-harm and suicide.[9]

- There are a range of services such as talking therapies, self-help and medication which are available to anyone experiencing symptoms and these can be accessed quickly and easily.

Staff Health and Wellbeing

5. Spotting the Signs

- The potential for reduced mental wellness is greater throughout the emergency services in all roles. As clinicians, we often assist the people we encounter by finding the most appropriate source of help for their current situation. Recognising a need in yourself or a colleague is difficult, but research suggests that ambulance personnel are far more likely to confide in each other rather than their own GP.[3]

- Even when we do recognise the need for help, fear of discrimination and stigma still presents a significant concern for many, despite the protection afforded by the 2010 Equality Act.

- Anyone can experience any number of mental health issues at any point in their lives regardless of their history or circumstance. The cause and nature of any individual's issues can be as unique as the individual and can be cumulative in nature, building over time and for any number and combination of reasons.

- It is not unusual in today's workplace for individuals to see concentrating upon work and careers as vital to maintaining professionalism; however, achieving a healthy work–life balance can have a very positive influence upon the stress and productivity experienced by any individual.[10]

- There is a wealth of independent, confidential and high-quality sources of help. Accessing help in a timely manner can have a significant impact upon the speed and quality of an individual's recovery. The benefits of spending time on relationships outside of work, family, hobbies and interests, volunteering, exercising and continued learning all have a role to play in maintaining and improving wellbeing. This in turn can have benefits not only to ourselves, but also to the many people we encounter in our roles.

6. Sources of Help and Signposting

- Ambulance Hub on NHS Employers website – Head First tool. Available from: https://www.nhsemployers.org/headfirst

- HR/work-related sources

- College of paramedics. Available from: https://www.collegeofparamedics.co.uk

- MIND Blue light. Available from: https://www.mind.org.uk/news-campaigns/campaigns/bluelight/

- TASC. Available from: http://www.theasc.org.uk/

- Samaritans. Available from: https://www.samaritans.org/

- CALM. Available from: https://www.calm.com/

- Step change. Available from: https://www.stepchange.org/

- Alcoholics Anonymous (AA). Available from: https://www.alcoholics-anonymous.org.uk/

- TRiM. Available from http://www.marchonstress.com/page/p/trim

Bibliography

1. World Health Organization. *Mental Health: a state of wellbeing.* 2014. Available from: https://www.who.int/features/factfiles/mental_health/en/.

2. Fjeldheim CB, Nöthling J, Pretorius K, Basson M, Ganasen K, Heneke R, Cloete KJ, Seedat S. Trauma exposure, post-traumatic stress disorder and the effect of explanatory variables in paramedic trainees. *BMC Emergency Medicine* 2014, 14: 11. Available from: https://www.ncbi.nlm.nih.gov/pubmed/24755358.

3. Mind. *Blue Light Scoping Survey.* 2015. Available from: https://www.mind.org.uk/media/4627950/scoping-survey.pdf.

4. Rethink Mental Illness. *What Are Anxiety Disorders.* 2018. Available from: https://www.mind.org.uk/media/4627950/scoping-survey.pdf.

5. Royal College of Psychiatrists. *Post-traumatic Stress Disorder.* 2015. Available from: https://www.rcpsych.ac.uk/healthadvice/problemsanddisorders/posttraumaticstressdisorder.aspx.

6. Javidi H and Yadollahie M. Post-traumatic stress disorder. *International Journal of Occupational and Environmental Medicine*, 2012, 3(1). Available from: http://theijoem.com/ijoem/index.php/ijoem/article/view/127/247.

7. National Health Service. *Post-traumatic Stress Disorder (PTSD).* 2015. Available from: https://www.nhs.uk/conditions/post-traumatic-stress-disorder-ptsd/symptoms/.

8. Royal College of Psychiatrists. *Depression: Key facts.* 2014. Available from: https://www.rcpsych.ac.uk/healthadvice/problemsanddisorders/depressionkeyfacts.aspx.

9. World Health Organization. *Depression: Let's talk.* 2018. Available from: https://www.who.int/mental_health/management/depression/en/.

10. Burn SM. *How's Your Work-Life Balance? The importance of work-life balance and how to achieve it.* 2015. Available from: https://www.psychologytoday.com/us/blog/presence-mind/201509/hows-your-work-life-balance.

SECTION **1** General Guidance

2

Resuscitation

Out-of-Hospital Cardiac Arrest: Overview

Every five years, the International Liaison Committee on Resuscitation (ILCOR) reviews current resuscitation science from which the European Resuscitation Council (ERC) then draws up evidence-based guidelines. These guidelines then form the basis from which the Resuscitation Council (UK) provides national, NICE-accredited guidelines for both hospital and pre-hospital UK practice.

JRCALC guidelines are based directly on these RC UK guidelines, currently the 2021 iteration (https://www.resus.org.uk/resuscitation-guidelines).

1. Incidence of Cardiac Arrest and Epidemiology

- 2020 NHS England data indicate that ambulance services respond to approximately 94,000 cardiac arrest calls and attempt to resuscitate approximately 32,000 people from out-of-hospital cardiac arrest (OHCA) each year. (https://warwick.ac.uk/fac/sci/med/research/ctu/trials/ohcao/publications/epidemiologyreports/ohca_epidemiological_report_2020_-_england_overview.pdf). This is in addition to the annual 3,200 resuscitation attempts reported by Scotland (https://www.gov.scot/publications/scottish-out-hospital-cardiac-arrest-data-linkage-project-2018-19-results/), 2,800 cardiac arrests reported by Wales and 1,400 resuscitation attempts reported by Northern Ireland.

- Table 2.1 shows the rate of return of spontaneous circulation (ROSC) on arrival at hospital and survival to hospital discharge when resuscitation is attempted.

- The Utstein group is defined as those with witnessed cardiac arrests where the initial rhythm is found to be ventricular fibrillation (VF).

- 2% of cases were children; of the remainder, one third were less than 64 years of age.

TABLE 2.1 – Current Resuscitation Outcomes (2020)

	ROSC on arrival at hospital	Survival to Discharge
All patients	26%	8%
Utstein patients	48%	25%

- The incidence of bystander cardiopulmonary resuscitation (CPR) rates before ambulance arrival is approximately 70%.

- The initial rhythm is VF in approximately 23% and asystole in 51% of cases. The remainder present in pulseless electrical activity (PEA).

- Unless in a specialist role, most paramedics attend cardiac arrests relatively infrequently.

- Anyone involved in the resuscitation of patients in cardiac arrest (including those involved in the training) should have annual competency assessments and regular face-to-face training to include high-quality CPR and associated skills, such as airway management, aligned to their scope of practice. This should include adult and paediatric resuscitation.

- This guideline refers to enhanced care. This includes specialist and advanced practice roles above the paramedic skillset. Refer to local procedures and definitions.

2. Chain of Survival

The Chain of Survival, Figure 2.1, links the critical actions required to treat cardiac arrest, recognising that all links need to be intact and functioning to achieve neurologically intact survival. The links are:

1 Early recognition and call for help.

2 Early CPR to support circulation to the heart and brain until normal heart activity is restored.

3 Early defibrillation to treat cardiac arrest caused by shockable rhythms.

4 Post-resuscitation care to improve survival rates.

The earlier links contribute far more to survival than the later links, because rapid recognition and good-quality basic life support (BLS) with defibrillation are the key factors influencing a good outcome.

3. Human Factors in Out-of-Hospital Cardiac Arrest: Team Resource Management

- A coordinated, well-rehearsed resuscitation attempt, with a team leader and all team members effectively delivering specific roles, will improve the effectiveness of CPR and the overall resuscitation.

- Four people with a minimum skillset of basic life support and defibrillation should attend patients in cardiac arrest where possible. This should include at least one registered healthcare professional with ALS competencies. One person with clinical decision making and leadership skills should form part of the team. Some members of the team may be non-ambulance staff, for example a Community First Responder (CFR) or other emergency service personnel trained in BLS.

- An effective resuscitation attempt requires a series of actions, skills and decisions to be delivered quickly and efficiently, including:
  - scene management
  - clear roles and responsibilities

Out-of-Hospital Cardiac Arrest: Overview

The Chain of Survival

Figure 2.1 – The chain of survival.

- — clinical assessment
- — effective delivery of interventions
- — teamwork
- — communication.
- These often-simultaneous tasks can have a cumulative effect on workload and potentially compromise the overall effectiveness of the resuscitation attempt.

4. Pathophysiology of Cardiac Arrest and Resuscitation

- The pathophysiology of cardiac arrest, due to a primary cardiac cause resulting in ventricular fibrillation, consists of three phases:

1 **Electrical phase** Constitutes the initial 4–5 minutes during which tissue metabolism is relatively normal and restoration of a perfusing rhythm can lead to a good chance of neurologically intact survival. Early defibrillation in the electrical phase can achieve survival rates in excess of 50%.

2 **Circulatory phase** From 4–5 minutes to approximately 10–15 minutes after cardiac arrest. Worsening tissue hypoxia and accumulating metabolites reduce the likelihood of successful defibrillation. The most important treatment is to initiate high-quality CPR to optimise tissue oxygenation and to deliver defibrillation. Restoration of a spontaneous circulation requires a coronary perfusion pressure (CPP) >15–20 mmHg, which may require the administration of adrenaline.

3 **Metabolic phase** Extends beyond approximately 10–15 minutes after cardiac arrest. Survival becomes less likely due to myocardial and cerebral ischaemia. Reperfusion injury is more likely to occur if ROSC is achieved. Defibrillation and drug therapy become less effective in this phase.

- CPR aims to circulate adequate amounts of oxygen to vital organs (particularly the heart and brain) to maintain tissue viability until ROSC is achieved. In the immediate few minutes after cardiac arrest, reserves in the arterial circulation can provide adequate tissue oxygenation through compression-only CPR, although they are rapidly depleted and rescue breaths are then needed to oxygenate the blood.

5. Mechanisms of Forward Blood Flow

- There are three main mechanisms thought to generate forward blood flow:

  - **Cardiac pump theory** Direct compression of the cardiac chambers between the sternum and vertebral column increases intracardiac pressure. This ejects blood from the heart into the pulmonary artery and aorta. Recoil of the sternum generates a negative pressure, which contributes to the passive filling of the ventricles before the subsequent compression.

  - **Thoracic pump theory** Chest compressions increase the pressure in the thorax which raises the pressure in the great vessels. The thinner-walled veins tend to collapse, while the arteries remain patent, and blood flows from the arterial to venous circulation due to the resulting pressure gradient.

  - **Lung pump theory** It has been suggested that neither the heart compression nor thoracic pump hypotheses fully explain blood flow resulting from cardiac compressions. The 'lung pump' model suggests that chest compressions cause a cyclical rise in intrathoracic pressure, which acts to compress the pulmonary vasculature and eject blood from the lungs with each compression (like wringing a sponge).

- Chest compressions must generate a coronary perfusion pressure of >15–20 mmHg to create

Out-of-Hospital Cardiac Arrest: Overview

sufficient coronary blood flow for the heart to be re-oxygenated and start contracting. Achieving this coronary perfusion pressure requires high-quality chest compressions. When chest compressions are interrupted, coronary perfusion pressure drops very quickly but takes some time to increase again after compressions are restarted – this may contribute to worse survival and hence the importance of minimising interruptions to chest compressions.

- Adequate cerebral blood flow is also dependent on high-quality chest compressions.

6. Rate and Depth of Chest Compressions

- Chest compressions hold the key to survival. Even when chest compressions are performed optimally, cardiac output is no more than 25–40% of pre-arrest values.

- Every effort must be made to ensure that compressions are carried out correctly and effectively. Rescuer fatigue is well described, with an onset time between 1 and 3 minutes. Ideally no one should perform chest compressions for greater than 2 minutes, wherever practicable.

- Interruptions to CPR are associated with a reduced chance of survival and must be avoided wherever possible.

- Too slow a compression rate fails to generate sufficient circulatory pressure, resulting in inadequate coronary blood flows. An excessive rate reduces the time for passive ventricular filling between compressions and also reduces coronary blood flow.

- Inadequate compression depth fails to generate adequate circulatory pressures, but excessive depth does not increase cardiac ejection and may risk myocardial and other organ damage.

- Allowing complete recoil of the sternum between each chest compression optimises the negative pressures generated inside the thorax during passive chest recoil and draws some blood back into the heart. This assists the passive refilling of the heart and increases the amount of blood ejected with the subsequent compression. Inadvertent leaning on the chest, preventing it from fully recoiling after each compression, reduces the above mechanisms.

- Where a patient presents in a shockable rhythm, chest compressions and defibrillation are the most effective treatment. Do not allow any advanced life support intervention to compromise delivery of high-quality BLS and defibrillation in these patients.

- For the solo responder, over-the-head CPR may be considered until other help arrives.

- Delivering good chest compression means:
  - Interruptions are minimised.
  - Proper depth is ensured (5–6 cm).
  - Full recoil is ensured between compressions.
  - Appropriate rate is maintained (100–120 per minute); metronome or feedback device use is recommended.
  - CPR compressions provider is swapped every 2 minutes.
  - When changing the compressions provider, work as a team, communicate with each other and plan to minimise the time spent with hands off the chest.
  - Be ready to charge the defibrillator after the rhythm check and deliver a shock with no more than a 5-second interruption to CPR. (Charging the defibrillator 5 seconds before rhythm check, and either delivering the shock or dumping the charge as required, is an acceptable alternative.)
  - Recommencing CPR as soon as rhythm check/shock is complete.
  - Minimal interruptions to CPR for airway manoeuvres.
  - No interruptions for IV/IO placement.

7. Ventilation

- Ventilation aims not only to deliver oxygen but also to remove CO_2 from the blood.

- Each positive pressure breath inflates the lungs, enabling oxygenation of pulmonary blood and CO_2 excretion. The ventilation tidal volume should be approximately 6–7 ml/kg (about 600 ml for most adults), delivered as either two breaths after 30 compressions or at a rate of 10/min as asynchronous breaths. Inadequate ventilation rates and/or tidal volumes will not provide sufficient blood oxygenation/CO_2 removal.

- Positive pressure breaths increase intrathoracic pressure, which has the adverse effect of reducing venous return to the heart and therefore reducing cardiac filling. Too much ventilation (excessive rates and/or tidal volumes) has a significant adverse impact on cardiac output.

- Each positive pressure breath also increases intracranial pressure (ICP), thus reducing cerebral blood flow. Optimising cerebral and myocardial oxygen delivery therefore requires no more than gentle ventilation that is sufficient to inflate the lungs and remove CO_2.

7.1 Gasping

- Gasping occurs in about 40% of patients in the first few minutes after cardiac arrest and may also be seen during CPR that is sufficiently effective to oxygenate the brainstem. Gasping during CPR creates negative intrathoracic pressure. This causes inhalation of air, increases

Out-of-Hospital Cardiac Arrest: Overview

venous return to the heart and decreases ICP, facilitating increased cerebral and coronary perfusion. It is this mechanism that is thought to be responsible for the more favourable outcomes that result in patients who have been gasping.

- Do not mistake gasping (slow, deep, irregular breaths) for normal breathing. An unresponsive patient who is gasping requires CPR.

8. Drug Therapy

- **Adrenaline:** Adrenaline acts to stimulate beta-adrenergic receptors to increase the force and rate of contraction and stimulate alpha-adrenergic receptors to cause vasoconstriction.

- Following the publication of the PARAMEDIC-2 trial, the use of adrenaline in cardiac arrest continues unchanged.

- **Amiodarone:** Ischaemic myocardial cells may spontaneously depolarise as they lose the ability to control their internal metabolism. Cumulatively, this may result in wave fronts of depolarisation that spread across the myocardium to cause ventricular ectopic beats, ventricular tachycardia or ventricular fibrillation.

- Antiarrhythmic medicines, primarily amiodarone, are used to:
  - decrease conduction velocity
  - reduce myocyte excitability
  - suppress abnormal automaticity

  which assists in terminating shockable rhythms in conjunction with defibrillation and maintaining a perfusing rhythm.

- **Atropine:** Vagal (parasympathetic) stimulation is not thought to be the cause of cardiac arrest in sustained asystole. That is why atropine is not recommended in the mangament of asystolic cardiac arrest. However, it may be a mechanism that causes peri-arrest bradycardia by slowing the sinoatrial node. Vagal tone may be blocked by atropine in patients where bradycardia is contributing to hypotension.

8.1 Acid–base Balance

- The acid–base balance of the body is carefully regulated to optimise cellular metabolism. During cardiac arrest, the build-up of metabolites and CO_2 may cause an acidosis, which acts to reduce oxygen delivery to cells, reduce myocardial contractility and cause myocardial irritability. This makes ROSC more difficult to achieve. The longer the duration of cardiac arrest, the more severe the acidosis.

- CO_2 build-up that causes respiratory acidosis can be limited by ventilating with the correct rate and tidal volume. The use of sodium bicarbonate is not routinely indicated unless blood gas measurements are available on scene.

9. Ambulance Services Response to Out-of-Hospital Cardiac Arrest

9.1 Checklist Use in Resuscitation

- Cardiac arrest checklists should be used by all responders.

- The out-of-hospital paramedic does not usually function as an individual – they are part of a team, and members usually have varying levels of expertise.

- The checklist may help compensate to some degree for this.

- The purpose of a checklist is to help ensure efficient and effective treatment delivery by individuals and teams, to minimise the risk of elements of care and avoid treatment being omitted, delayed or delivered inappropriately in a stressful situation, as a result of human factors.

- The ERC states that the use of checklists may improve adherence to guidelines as long as they do not cause delays in starting CPR.

9.2 Cardiac Arrest Downloads

- Data downloads should be used to review each cardiac arrest to understand the quality of care and chest compressions for future and real-time improvement.

- Auditing and reviewing data downloads will help determine how quickly shocks are being delivered. Decisions can be made based on local data as to whether to recommend using AED mode for the first shock in order to minimise shock delays. Local audit data can help inform the decision making process.

- Hot debriefs after cardiac arrest incidents should be undertaken wherever possible. There is evidence to suggest that where these downloads are reviewed and an appropriate debriefing session is held, rescuer performance improves.

- Where download summaries are available, paramedics should take advantage of this opportunity to reflect on the resuscitation attempt, critically analysing their performance and planning how they could improve on their next attempt.

9.3 Use of CPR Feedback Devices

- The use of CPR feedback and coaching devices is strongly recommended on all occasions where resuscitation is taking place.

- A number of studies have shown that the quality of CPR during training and in clinical practice is often suboptimal, with inadequate compression depth, interruptions in chest compression, prolonged pre- and post-shock pauses and hyperventilation occurring frequently.

Out-of-Hospital Cardiac Arrest: Overview

- CPR feedback and prompt devices (e.g. voice prompts, metronomes, visual dials, numerical displays, waveforms, verbal prompts and visual alarms) aim to improve the performance of resuscitation skills.

- These devices enable the CPR provider to receive real-time objective feedback on the quality of CPR, and have been evaluated in several clinical studies that support their use to improve the quality of CPR delivered.

- Devices on the market give prompts (i.e. signal to perform an action, e.g. metronome for compression rate or voice feedback), give feedback (i.e. after-event information based on the effect of an action, such as a visual display of compression depth) or give a combination of prompts and feedback.

9.4 Clinical Handover

- Clinical handover begins with a pre-alert. Concise and appropriate information should be passed to the emergency department using the ATMIST format (or a format as per local protocol).

- The clinical handover with the patient can be challenging to deliver succinctly. Standardised tools such as ATMIST should be used as per locally agreed protocols (refer to Table 2.2).

- Useful information includes the time of collapse, whether bystander CPR was being performed, the time of arrival of the first crew, the initial rhythm and the patient's pre-arrest co-morbidities.

- Try to speak loudly and clearly, be concise and use the template headings before communicating the information for each heading.

TABLE 2.2 – ATMIST

A	Age
T	Time of incident
M	Mechanism of injury
I	Injuries
S	Signs and symptoms
T	Treatment given and immediate needs

Bibliography

1. Resuscitation Council (UK). *Resuscitation Guidelines 2021*. London: Resuscitation Council (UK), 2021. Available from: https://www.resus.org.uk/resuscitation-guidelines.

2. NHS England. *Resuscitation to Recovery: A national framework to improve care of people with out-of-hospital cardiac arrest (OHCA) in England*. London: NHS England, 2015. Available from: https://aace.org.uk/wp-content/uploads/2017/03/FINAL_Resuscitation-to-Recovery_A-National-Framework-to-Improve-Care-of-People-with-Out-of-Hospital-Cardiac-Arrest-in-England_March-2017.pdf.

3. Scottish Government. *Scottish Out-of-Hospital Cardiac Arrest Data Linkage Project: 2018–2019*. Edinburgh: Scottish Government, 2020. Available from: https://www.gov.scot/publications/scottish-out-hospital-cardiac-arrest-data-linkage-project-2018-19-results/.

4. Perkins GD, Brace-McDonnell SJ. The UK Out of Hospital Cardiac Arrest Outcome (OHCAO) project. *BMJ Open* 2015, 5: e008736. Available from: https://bmjopen.bmj.com/content/5/10/e008736.

5. Weisfeldt ML, Becker LB. Resuscitation after cardiac arrest: a 3-phase time-sensitive model. *JAMA* 2002, 288: 3035–3038. Available from: https://www.researchgate.net/publication/10992588_Resuscitation_after_cardiac_arrest_A_3-phase_time-sensitive_model.

6. Georgiou M, Papathanassoglou E, Xanthos T. Systematic review of the mechanisms driving effective blood flow during adult CPR. *Resuscitation* 2014, 85: 1586–1593. Available from: https://www.sciencedirect.com/science/article/abs/pii/S0300957214007400.

7. Lurie KG, Nemergut EC, Yannopoulos D, Sweeney M. The physiology of cardiopulmonary resuscitation. *Anesthesia & Analgesia* 2016, 122(3): 767–783. Available from: http://umanitoba.ca/faculties/health_sciences/medicine/units/anesthesia/media/The_Physiology_of_Cardiopulmonary_Resuscitation.pdf.

8. Perkins GD, Ji C, Deakin CD et al. on behalf of PARAMEDIC2 collaborators. A randomized trial of epinephrine in out-of-hospital cardiac arrest. *New England Journal of Medicine* 2018, 379: 711–721. Available from: https://www.nejm.org/doi/full/10.1056/NEJMoa1806842.

9. Soar J, Berg B, Andersen L et al. Adult advanced life support 2020 international consensus on cardiopulmonary resuscitation and emergency cardiovascular care science with treatment recommendations. *Resuscitation* 2020, 156: A80–119. Available from: https://www.resuscitationjournal.com/article/S0300-9572(20)30460-3/pdf.

10. Olasveengen T, Mancini M, Perkins GD et al. Adult basic life support: international consensus on cardiopulmonary resuscitation and emergency cardiovascular care science with treatment recommendations. *Resuscitation* 2020, 156: A35–79. Available from: https://www.resuscitationjournal.com/article/S0300-9572(20)30458-5/fulltext.

Advanced Life Support

1. Advanced Life Support Overview

1.1 Introduction

- Advanced life support (ALS) may be defined as the use of resuscitation drugs and interventions above and beyond basic life support and AED use. However, if a trained ALS provider attends as a solo responder, they are limited to basic life support (BLS) and defibrillation until other responders arrive.

- The availability of ALS must not affect the provision of high-quality basic life support and appropriate defibrillation.

- Out-of-hospital cardiac arrest (OHCA) management follows similar principles for ALS as in-hospital treatment. It is recognised, however, that the environment, equipment, resources, access to the patient, extrication and transportation of the patient play a pivotal part in the overall clinical management decisions.

- A team approach should be adopted as early as possible and a team leader appointed (resources allowing), who can use cardiac arrest checklists for the overall management of the cardiac arrest and for specific clinical skills, e.g. intubation checklists.

1.2 Stages of Assessment and Management

- The assessment and management of an out-of-hospital medical cardiac arrest includes:
  - Confirmation of the cardiac arrest.
  - Immediate implementation and continuation of effective BLS and defibrillation.
  - The addition of ALS, including IV/IO access, the administration of medicines, advanced airway management and clinical decision making, where appropriate.
  - Early identification and management of reversible causes.
  - Early decision making on:
    - the appropriateness of the resuscitation attempt (ReSPECT, recognition of life extinct, futility and best interests).
    - an early transportation plan if a reversible cause is identified that cannot be treated on scene or if admission to a cath lab is considered appropriate (according to local protocols).
    - requesting enhanced care resources to attend the scene to help with clinical decision making, enhanced assessments (e.g. ultra-sound) and interventions (e.g. blood products)
    - seeking senior remote advice where available through a structured and governed system.

2. Advanced Life Support in Adults

Refer to ALS algorithm, Figure 2.2.

Additional Information

- Once adrenaline has been administered, further doses should be given every 3–5 minutes, irrespective of rhythm, while the patient remains in cardiac arrest.

- Peripheral IV access should be established as soon as possible. However, paramedics should attempt intraosseous access if two cannulation attempts have failed (or initially if IV cannulation is unlikely to succeed). External jugular vein access is also acceptable as an alternative for those appropriately trained.

- If a patient who is being **monitored** has a **witnessed** arrest:
  - Confirm cardiac arrest.
  - Request further resources if appropriate.
  - A precordial thump is no longer recommended for initial treatment of shockable rhythms even if a defibrillator is not immediately available.
  - If the rhythm is VF/pVT and a defibrillator is immediately available, give a shock first and immediately commence CPR; treat any recurrence of VF/pVT following the shockable rhythm algorithm.
  - Where the arrest is witnessed but unmonitored, defibrillation pads must be applied immediately.
  - Three stacked shocks may be considered as per local protocols in a witnessed and monitored cardiac arrest, only when the patient is already connected to a manual defibrillator. For the purposes of medicine administration, these three shocks should be treated as the first shock in the ALS algorithm.
  - If VF persists, refer to **Defibrillation**.

ADULT ALS – SUMMARY

- During ALS, the priority remains to deliver high-quality chest compressions and effective ventilations with high-flow (100%) oxygen.

- When indicated, defibrillate and resume chest compressions for two minutes without re-assessing the rhythm or feeling for a pulse.

- Defibrillation energy levels should be at least 150 J for the first shock. Consider escalating energy for subsequent shocks.

- Give amiodarone 300 mg IV/IO after three shocks for VF/pVT, irrespective of whether these are sequential or intermittent shockable rhythms.

- A further 150 mg may be administered after a total of 5 shocks (check dose/volume if using a pre-filled syringe).

- Promptly identify and treat reversible causes (4Hs and 4Ts).

Advanced Life Support

Adult advanced life support

Maintain personal safety

Unresponsive and not breathing normally

CPR 30:2
Attach defibrillator/monitor

Assess rhythm

SHOCKABLE
(VF/Pulseless VT)

1 shock

Immediately resume CPR for 2 min

Return of spontaneous circulation (ROSC)

NON-SHOCKABLE
(PEA/Asystole)

Immediately resume CPR for 2 min

Give high-quality chest compressions, and:
- Give oxygen
- Use waveform capnography
- Continuous compressions if advanced airway
- Minimise interruptions to compressions
- Intravenous or intraosseous access
- Give adrenaline every 3–5 min
- Give amiodarone after 3 shocks
- Identify and treat reversible causes
- Glucose control

Identify and treat reversible causes
- Hypoxia
- Hypovolaemia
- Hypo-/hyperkalaemia/metabolic
- Hypo/hyperthermia
- Thrombosis – coronary or pulmonary
- Tension pneumothorax
- Tamponade – cardiac
- Toxins

Consider ultrasound imaging to identify reversible causes

Consider
- Coronary angiography/percutaneous coronary intervention
- Mechanical chest compressions to facilitate transfer/treatment

After ROSC
- Use an ABCDE approach
- Aim for SpO_2 of 94–98% and normal $PaCO_2$
- 12-lead ECG
- Identify and treat cause
- Targeted temperature management

Figure 2.2 – Advanced life support in adults algorithm. Reproduced with permission from the Resuscitation Council (UK) Guidelines 2021 algorithm (www.resus.org.uk).

Advanced Life Support

In most patients where ROSC is not achieved on scene, despite appropriate ALS and treatment of any reversible causes, there is little to be gained from transferring these patients to hospital. The exceptions are:

- Children – aim for minimum scene time.
- Refractory/recurrent VF (or pVT) – consider early departure from scene for PPCI, according to local protocols.
- Cardiac arrest in pregnancy – make plans to undertake a time-critical transfer to hospital – this should be commenced within 5 minutes of arrival at the cardiac arrest (seek senior advice early).
- Penetrating traumatic cardiac arrest – make plans to undertake a time-critical transfer to hospital – this should be commenced within 5 minutes of arrival at the cardiac arrest. These patients are absolutely time-critical if they are to survive.
- Possible electrolyte disturbances (e.g. renal dialysis patients, anorexic patients, dehydration, excessive fluid intake, chronic diarrhoea and vomiting etc.).
- Hypothermia as a contributory factor.

In cases of **persistent** and **continuous** asystole for 30 minutes in adults, despite ALS and where all reversible causes have been identified and treated, the chances of survival are so unlikely that resuscitation can be ceased.

3. Advanced Life Support in Children

3.1 Introduction

Paediatric ALS resuscitation broadly follows adult protocols.
Differences between adult and paediatric resuscitation largely reflect a differing aetiology; paediatric cardiac arrest is most commonly due to hypoxia, whereas adult cardiac arrest is usually due to myocardial disease.
The definition of a child is between 1 year and 18 years of age. A clinician should use judgement and information from relatives/bystanders to estimate the age and weight of the child. If the rescuer believes the victim to be a child, they should use the paediatric guidelines. If a misjudgement is made, and the victim turns out to be a young adult, little harm will result.

This guideline covers:

- infants (defined as under 1 year old)
- children (defined as between 1 year and 18 years of age).

In this guideline, the term 'child' includes infants, unless specified otherwise.

Newborn life support is not covered in this guideline. For newborn babies, refer to **Newborn Life Support**.

ALS procedures (e.g. establishing vascular access) must not delay the transfer of the child to hospital – start and continue good-quality BLS on scene as the priority. Attempt ALS procedures en-route, if practical; oxygenation, ventilation and chest compressions remain the priority.

Paediatric defibrillation (4 J/kg) should be carried out using paediatric defibrillation pads. However, if these are not available, use adult defibrillation pads. Ensure that the defibrillation pads are not in contact with each other; usually a front-to-back (anterior–posterior) pad placement ensures adequate pad separation.

PAEDIATRIC ALS – SUMMARY

During ALS, the priority remains the delivery of high-quality chest compressions and effective ventilations with high-flow oxygen. Particular focus should be to ensure reversal of any hypoxia.

Supraglottic airways (SGAs) may be considered if BVM ventilation is ineffective.

Intubation is rarely indicated and should only be undertaken by those with appropriate skills, according to local protocols and only when waveform capnography is available.

Defibrillation should be delivered at 4 J/kg, rounded up to the energy level the defibrillator can deliver.

As with adults, give amiodarone IV/IO after three shocks and a further dose after five shocks. Refer to **Amiodarone Hydrochloride**, **Page for Age** for children.

Do not delay on scene to deliver ALS interventions. Early extrication and transport to hospital is mandatory; aim to deliver ALS en-route.

In children where hypovolaemia is thought to be a contributory factor, give a fluid bolus of 10 ml/kg (N.saline (0.9%) or Hartmann's solution), repeated once if indicated. Seek appropriate medical opinion if further boluses are thought to be indicated.

4. Defibrillation

4.1 Principles of Defibrillation

The purpose of defibrillation is to terminate VF/pVT by passing an electrical current across the heart to depolarise a critical mass of myocardial cells.

Defibrillation is more likely to be successful if:

- Time from collapse to shock is minimised.
- The collapse has been witnessed and the patient has received bystander CPR.
- BLS is of good quality (correct rate and depth, complete chest recoil, minimal interruptions and maximal chest compression fraction).

Advanced Life Support

Paediatric advanced life support

Recognise cardiac arrest

Commence/continue CPR
(5 initial breaths then CV ratio 15:2)
Attach defibrillator/monitor
Minimise interruptions

Assess rhythm

SHOCKABLE
VF/Pulseless VT

1 shock 4 J kg⁻¹

Immediately resume CPR
for 2 min
Minimise interruptions

After 3 shocks give:
- Adrenaline IV/IO 10 mcg kg⁻¹ (and every alternate cycle thereafter) **AND**
- Amiodarone IV/IO 5 mg kg⁻¹ (and repeat 5 mg kg⁻¹ once more only after 5th shock)

Return of spontaneous circulation (ROSC)

Post cardiac arrest care:
- Use an ABCDE approach
- Aim for SpO₂ of 94–98% and normal PaCO₂
- Avoid hypotension
- Targeted temp management
- Glucose control

NON-SHOCKABLE
PEA/asystole/brady < 60 min⁻¹

Immediately resume CPR
for 2 min
Minimise interruptions

Give adrenaline IV/IO
10 mcg kg⁻¹
as soon as possible
and then every 3–5 min

During CPR
- **Ensure high quality chest compressions are delivered:**
  – Correct rate, depth and full recoil
- Provide BMV with 100% oxygen (2 person approach)
- Provide continuous chest compressions when a tracheal tube is in place.
- Competent providers can consider an advanced airway and capnography, and ventilate at a rate (breaths minute⁻¹) of:

Infants: 25	1–8 years: 20	8–12 years: 15	> 12 years: 10–12

- Vascular access IV/IO
- Once started, give Adrenaline every 3–5 min
- Maximum single dose Adrenaline 1 mg
- Maximum single dose Amiodarone 300 mg
- Glucose control

Identify and treat reversible causes
- Hypoxia
- Hypovolaemia
- Hyperkalaemia, hypercalcaemia, hypermagnesemia, hypoglycaemia
- Hypo-/hyperthermia
- Thrombosis – coronary or pulmonary
- Tension pneumothorax
- Tamponade – cardiac
- Toxic agents

Adjust algorithm in specific settings (e.g. special circumstances)

Figure 2.3 – Advanced life support in children algorithm. Reproduced with permission from the Resuscitation Council (UK) Guidelines 2021 (www.resus.org.uk).

- The pre-shock pause is as short as possible (< 5 secs).
- The defibrillation pads are placed correctly (refer to Figure 2.4).

- Minimise pre-shock pauses, by resuming chest compressions immediately after the rhythm check while the defibrillator charges. It is also acceptable to charge the defibrillator as the end of the 2 minutes of CPR approaches while continuing chest compressions. All team members should stand clear for the rhythm check so that the shock can be delivered without delay if appropriate, before immediately resuming CPR.

SECTION **2** Resuscitation

Advanced Life Support

- Current guidelines for biphasic waveforms recommend commencing with an initial shock of at least 150 J if using a manual defibrillator. Consider increasing the energy for second and subsequent shocks if using a manual defibrillator.

- A range of defibrillation energy levels have been recommended by manufacturers and previous guidelines, ranging from 120–360 J. In the absence of any clear evidence for the optimal initial and subsequent energy levels, any energy level within this range is acceptable for the initial shock, followed by a fixed or escalating strategy up to maximum output of the defibrillator. We suggest a starting energy of at least 150 J, escalating to maximum output for refractory rhythms.

- Paediatric defibrillation should be delivered at 4 J/kg, rounded up to the nearest energy level the defibrillator can deliver. (NB Defibrillators that deliver a maximum output of 200 J at least match the current delivered by defibrillators with a 360 J output).

- When using a monitor that filters out ECG movement artefact and the underlying rhythm can be clearly seen without having to pause for a rhythm check, charge the defibrillator with ongoing CPR. If using manual chest compressions, stand clear to then deliver the shock. If using mechanical chest compression, there is no need to stop this when the shock is delivered. Note that the mechanical chest compression device may move when the shock is delivered, therefore it is important to ensure the device remains correctly positioned.

4.2 Priorities in Delivery of Defibrillation

- Delivering the first shock as soon as possible is the priority. Therefore, when attending as a solo responder equipped with a defibrillator, immediate assessment of the rhythm and defibrillation (when indicated) should take precedence over airway or breathing interventions. If possible, use a bystander to start and continue chest compressions while the defibrillator is attached. Although defibrillation is an initial priority, it is important to minimise delays and interruptions in delivering chest compressions.

4.3 Fine VF

- Immediate defibrillation should always be performed in patients where a shockable rhythm is identified on the ECG, irrespective of the amplitude. Automated defibrillators use a low threshold for the recognition of fine VF.

4.4 AED vs Manual Modes

- Most manual defibrillators carried in ambulances can also be used in an AED mode where they analyse the ECG and recommend delivery of a shock when appropriate. There are advantages and disadvantages of each mode. Although AED mode may improve the time to first shock, manual mode may reduce pre-shock pauses and increase chest compression fraction, which is associated with increased ROSC. Therefore, although manual defibrillation should be the preferred option for appropriately trained paramedics, it should be recognised that solo responders are potentially in a stressful environment and are attempting to manage multiple complex factors. Therefore, the initial use of the AED function is acceptable in these situations until additional help arrives.

4.5 Defibrillator Pads

- It is important to ensure correct pad positioning so that adequate current traverses the myocardium in order to optimise defibrillation success. In the conventional sternal–apical position the right (sternal) pad is placed to the right of the sternum, below the clavicle. The apical pad is placed in the left mid-axillary line, approximately level with the V6 ECG electrode (i.e. just below the armpit). This pad must be placed sufficiently laterally, as shown in Figure 2.4.

- Other acceptable pad positions include:
  - Anterior–posterior – one pad anteriorly, over the left precordium, and the other pad posteriorly to the heart just inferior to the left scapula and spine.
  - Bi-axillary – one pad placed just below each axilla, in the mid-axillary line (for example in patients with burns, or where a subcutaneous pacing box may preclude standard pad placement).

Figure 2.4 – Correct placement of defibrillation pads in the antero–lateral position. Note the relatively high and lateral positioning of the lateral pad (just below the armpit). © Charles D. Deakin. Reproduced with permission.

Advanced Life Support

- When paediatric defibrillation pads are not available, adult pads can be used as an alternative for children. Ensure that the pads are not in contact with each other; usually a front to back (anterior–posterior) pad placement ensures adequate pad separation.

- Self-adhesive defibrillation pads have a water/electrolyte-based matrix to improve conductivity with the skin. Defibrillation pads do not need to be changed during a resuscitation attempt unless visibly damaged, although they may be replaced if the pads need to be moved for an alternative position.

- Quickly shaving the chest prior to defibrillation not only ensures better electrical contact (and therefore defibrillation success) but is likely to reduce the risk of electrical arcing between pads, which may trigger a fire.

4.6 Hands-on Defibrillation

- Delivering continuous chest compressions during defibrillation can minimise pre-shock pause and prevent interruption of chest compressions. However, the benefits of hands-on defibrillation are not proven, and further studies are required to assess the safety and efficacy of this technique. Standard clinical examination gloves (or bare hands) do not provide a safe level of electrical insulation.

4.7 Recurrent and Refractory VF

- Recurrent VF refers to VF that is cardioverted following each shock but returns before the next rhythm check. Recurrence of VF after a successful shock is common.

- Refractory VF refers to VF that persists despite several defibrillation attempts. In the out-of-hospital environment, it may be difficult to determine whether persistent VF is recurrent or refractory, as CPR is resumed immediately post-shock.

- Administer 300 mg amiodarone IV after the third shock and give a further 150 mg IV dose after the fifth shock.

- Optimise oxygenation and ventilation and ensure high-quality CPR.

- Ensure that the defibrillation pads are placed correctly and that electrical contact is not impaired by moisture or a hairy chest. If using antero–lateral defibrillation pad placement, ensure that the lateral pad is placed sufficiently laterally, as shown in Figure 2.4.

- Consider early transport to a primary percutaneous coronary intervention (PPCI) centre. Consider requesting enhanced care support.

4.8 Dual Sequential Defibrillation (DSD)

- DSD involves the use of two separate manual defibrillators, delivering shocks at the same time or in rapid succession.

- This is not recommended practice and it is not licensed or recommended by the defibrillator manufacturers.

- Delivering twice as much defibrillation energy carries with it the risk of myocardial stunning and conversion to asystole rather than a perfusing rhythm.

- No cohort studies or meta-analysis have demonstrated any benefits over conventional defibrillation. Until further studies are concluded, the true benefit (or harm) of DSD remains unknown.

4.9 Pacemakers and External Pacing

External pacing is not recommended as a core paramedic competency. If the patient is bradycardic, consider requesting enhanced care teams or clinical advice as per local procedures.

- Pacemakers (and internal defibrillators) are generally positioned below the left clavicle, although on occasion they may be placed on the right side. They appear as a subcutaneous firm mass, approximately 5 x 5 cm, over which is a scar from the insertion. Check the patient for a MedicAlert bracelet.

- In relation to resuscitation, pacemakers may have several different functions:
  - **Pacing only** – to keep the heart rate above a set level (may be ventricular pacing only, but may be set to deliver both atrial and ventricular pacing).
  - **Defibrillation only** (implantable cardioverter-defibrillator – ICD) – to monitor the heart continually and deliver a shock when a shockable arrhythmia is detected. They give no warning when firing and are programmed to give repeated shocks if indicated.
  - **Pacing and defibrillation** – a combination of both functions.

- These devices may be damaged during defibrillation if current is discharged through pads placed directly over the device.

- Place the pad away from the device (at least 8 cm) or use an alternative pad position (anterior–lateral, anterior–posterior, bi-axillary).

- Pacemakers will continue to discharge even in a patient who is deceased. This appears as very narrow pacing spikes on the ECG and the monitor may even display a heart rate. However, an ECG showing pacing spikes not followed by any ventricular (or atrial) complex is effectively an asystolic trace.

- Placing a magnet over a pacing device will generally result in it pacing at a fixed (asynchronous mode) rate of 50–100/min and does not stop pacemaker function.

- Placing a magnet over an ICD will result in disabling of the defibrillation function and shocks will not be delivered. This may be necessary in

Advanced Life Support

some cases of fast atrial arrhythmias, or if the pacing (sensing) lead is faulty, when the ICD may repeatedly discharge erroneously, which is distressing for the patient.

4.10 Safe Use of Oxygen

- Use oxygen safely during defibrillation by:
  - removing any oxygen mask or nasal cannulae and placing them at least 1 m away from the patient's chest during defibrillation
  - leaving the ventilation bag connected to the tracheal tube or SGA.
- Oxygen-powered LUCAS devices discharge large amounts of oxygen over and around the defibrillation pads which may be a significant hazard, particularly in a closed environment (e.g. the back of an ambulance).

5. Airway and Breathing Management

5.1 Introduction

- The Airways2 trial found that the initial approach to airway management is bag-mask ventilation (BVM) for approximately half of all cardiac arrest patients, with the remainder managed with a supraglottic airway (SGA) (20%) or tracheal intubation (25%).
- The most common reason cited by paramedics for changing from BVM was to carry out ALS, followed by regurgitation and inadequate ventilation.
- Inadequate ventilation was the most common reason cited for removing an SGA.
- A stepwise approach to airway management is recommended. This should include a strategy on how and when to progress from one airway technique to another.
- It should be noted that the stepwise approach is not one way. If a technique is failing, then it is sometimes more appropriate to move to a less advanced technique than to attempt techniques that are more advanced.
- However, in the context of out-of-hospital cardiac arrest, it might also be appropriate to move directly to more advanced techniques, depending on the circumstances. For example, the early application of an SGA may be beneficial, rather than attempting oropharyngeal or nasopharyngeal airways. Tracheal intubation as the initial airway is not recommended; use of a BVM or SGA should proceed any attempt at tracheal intubation.
- Laryngoscopy remains an important skill for visually inspecting the oropharynx in choking, and should be part of ongoing competency assessments.

- Staff attending the arrest will need to be trained to provide support to the clinician that is performing the intubation, such as preparing and passing the equipment.

Spinal precautions must be started at the same time as airway management, but these do not take priority. Refer to **Spinal Injury and Spinal Cord Injury**.

5.2 Bag-mask Ventilation (BVM)

- The initial approach to airway management should usually be BVM. An oropharyngeal airway (OPA) or nasopharyngeal airway (NPA) may be used to improve the efficacy of ventilations via the BVM.
- A complication of ventilation with a BVM is gastric inflation, resulting in impaired ventilation and regurgitation, especially where forceful ventilations are delivered. This risk is reduced where gentle ventilations are delivered over 1 second or where an SGA is used. As such, it is reasonable to place a suitable SGA as part of BLS, when trained in its use.

5.3 Airway Sizes

- Table 2.3 provides a guide for airway sizes in children and adults.

5.4 Supraglottic Airways

- There are several SGAs (e.g. iGel and laryngeal mask airway); all sit above the larynx, and are simpler and quicker to insert than a tracheal tube. They can be inserted with minimal interruption to chest compressions.
- A number of case reports exist describing patients who have been found to have foreign bodies deep within their oropharynx. It is therefore recommended that if there is a high degree of suspicion of foreign body airway obstruction, inspection of the oropharynx should be undertaken with a laryngoscope before inserting any SGA.
- Once an SGA has been placed, continuous chest compressions with 10 ventilations per minute are preferred. However, 30 compressions to two ventilations are acceptable if ventilation is inadequate when delivering continuous compressions.
- Waveform capnography should always be used when using a supraglottic device and BVM.
- Air leaks from around the SGA are common. If the chest wall can be seen to be moving, ventilation is generally adequate. However, repositioning or replacement of the airway with a more suitable size may be necessary if the air leak is of sufficient magnitude to prevent the chest rising and falling with each breath.

2 **Resuscitation**

SECTIONSECTION

2022

Advanced Life Support

89

Advanced Life Support

5.5 Tracheal Intubation

- The tracheal tube is a challenging airway device to insert successfully and requires both adequate initial training and ongoing practice. Paramedics must ensure that they have appropriate competence to undertake it safely and that this skill has been regularly updated and evidenced through maintaining an airway skills log.

- There is no evidence that patient outcome is any better following tracheal intubation compared with any other type of airway.

- When tracheal intubation is undertaken, the availability of a bougie and use of waveform capnography is mandatory.

- Where, as a paramedic, the governance system you work within allows you to intubate, you should only do so if you have maintained your skills and have evidence of self-audit with a success rate of greater than 95% success rate within two attempts.

- Visualisation of the tube entering the trachea, auscultation over both axillae and epigastrium, and observation of chest wall movement should all aid confirmation but are not in themselves 100% diagnostic of correct tube placement. This can only be achieved by using waveform capnography.

- If the capnography trace is flat (or only shows minimal baseline fluctuation), then it must be assumed that the tracheal tube is sited incorrectly and must be removed.

- Once a tracheal tube is in place, continue continuous chest compressions with 10 gentle ventilations per minute. Avoid hyperventilation and high airway pressures during manual ventilation which adversely affect outcome.

- It is important to remember the following for tracheal intubation:
  - Ensure 360° access around the patient where possible. (This may involve rapidly moving the patient to give better access.)
  - Prepare a kit dump of all the necessary equipment close to the patient before starting the process of intubation. This must include suction, a bougie and immediate access to capnography monitoring and any additional airway equipment necessary for a failed intubation.
  - Do not routinely use cricoid pressure for tracheal intubation during CPR.
  - If during laryngoscopy the paramedic needs a better view, use external laryngeal manipulation. Pressure directed to move the trachea backwards, upwards and to the right (BURP manoeuvre) may improve visualisation of the vocal cords.
  - Secure the tracheal tube immediately after insertion, noting length at incisors. This is approximately:
    - adult males: 22–24 cm
    - adult females: 21–23 cm.
  - Listen to any team member who suggests that the attempt has become a 'Can't intubate, can't ventilate scenario', irrespective of clinical grade.
  - Avoid hypoxaemia during intubation: pre-oxygenate the lungs before and between intubation attempts.
  - Where possible, use two team members to attempt intubation, and ensure a failed intubation plan has been communicated to all the team.

5.6 Capnography

- Capnography (measurement of exhaled (end-tidal) carbon dioxide – $EtCO_2$) assists in confirmation and continuous monitoring of tracheal tube placement, can provide feedback on the quality of CPR and can provide an early ROSC.

- Waveform capnography is a real-time waveform display of $EtCO_2$ and is more accurate and reliable than a paper indicator.

- The use of waveform capnography is mandatory in paramedic intubation. Tracheal intubation and subsequent monitoring must only be performed with the assistance of waveform capnography monitoring. Recorded values must be documented on the patient record at 5-minute intervals. In the absence of waveform capnography, an alternative airway technique or device should be employed.

A-B: Baseline

B-C: Expiratory upstroke

C-D: Expiratory plateau

D: $EtCO_2$

D-E: Inspiration

Figure 2.5 – Capnography.

Advanced Life Support

■ Any decision to terminate resuscitation should not be based on either the presence or absence of EtCO$_2$ alone.

■ Waveform capnography is recommended where an SGA has been placed, as it is useful in providing positive feedback on the quality of CPR.

TABLE 2.3 – Airway Sizes by Type

Age	Airway Size by Device Type		
	Oropharyngeal	SGA	Tracheal tube Internal diameter Length at the lips
Birth	000	1.0	Diameter: 3.0 mm Length: 10 cm
1 month	00	1.0	Diameter: 3.0 mm Length: 10 cm
3 months	00	1.5	Diameter: 3.5 mm Length: 11 cm
6 months	00	1.5	Diameter: 4.0 mm Length: 12 cm
9 months	00	1.5	Diameter: 4.0 mm Length: 12 cm
12 months	00 OR 0	1.5 OR 2.0	Diameter: 4.5 mm Length: 13 cm
18 months	00 OR 0	1.5 OR 2.0	Diameter: 4.5 mm Length: 13 cm
2 years	0 OR 1	1.5 OR 2.0	Diameter: 5.0 mm Length: 14 cm
3 years	1	2.0	Diameter: 5.0 mm Length: 14 cm
4 years	1	2.0	Diameter: 5.0 mm Length: 15 cm
5 years	1	2.0	Diameter: 5.5 mm Length: 15 cm
6 years	1	2.0	Diameter: 6.0 mm Length: 16 cm
7 years	1 OR 2	2.0	Diameter: 6.0 mm Length: 16 cm
8 years	1 OR 2	2.5	Diameter: 6.5 mm Length: 17 cm
9 years	1 OR 2	2.5	Diameter: 6.5 mm Length: 17 cm
10 years	2 OR 3	2.5 OR 3.0	Diameter: 7.0 mm Length: 18 cm
11 years	2 OR 3	2.5 OR 3.0	Diameter: 7.0 mm Length: 18 cm
Adult >70 kg	4 OR 5	4.0 OR 5.0	Female diameter: 7.0–8.0 mm Length: 21–23 cm Male diameter: 8.0–9.0 mm Length: 22–24 cm

Advanced Life Support

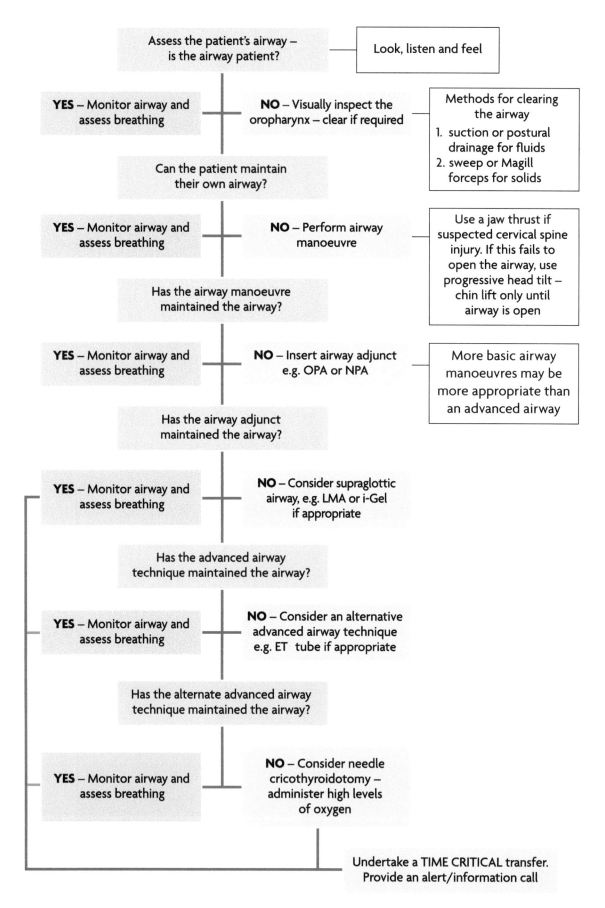

Figure 2.6 – Breathing assessment and management overview.

Advanced Life Support

6. Mechanical Chest Compression Devices (mCPR)

- Mechanical chest compression (mCPR) devices are designed to provide consistent high-quality chest compressions to the required depth and frequency for prolonged periods of time.

- mCPR can act as an additional rescuer, enabling uninterrupted chest compressions while attention is focused on delivering other aspects of ALS.

- Delivery of manual chest compressions is often inconsistent and subject to fatigue, particularly when wearing PPE, during prolonged resuscitation. mCPR can be of particular benefit during extrication and transport in a moving vehicle to ensure continuous chest compressions and ensure rescuer safety.

- In patients presenting with a shockable rhythm, mechanical devices should not be used prior to the first shock.

- However, large randomised controlled trials of the routine use of mCPR in the out-of-hospital setting have found no evidence of improved patient outcome compared with manual CPR. Routine use of mCPR is therefore not indicated.

- In particular mCPR should be considered during the extrication and transportation of a patient in cardiac arrest, when prolonged CPR is indicated (e.g. ECMO, hypothermia, refractory VF etc.) or for patients being taken to the cath lab for PCI where manual chest compression during the procedure is not possible.

- mCPR should be deployed by dedicated teams that are regularly drilled, practised and signed off in its deployment to ensure effective use and minimal interruption to CPR during its placement.

6.1 Impedance Threshold Valve

- In the same way that gasping generates negative intrathoracic pressure, mechanical devices that enhance negative intrathoracic pressure during CPR may also increase venous return and enhance forward blood flow.

- Some, but not all, studies have shown that impedance threshold devices (ITDs) may improve outcome; but where they are effective, they appear to be so only in the context of CPR that delivers correct compression rate and depth.

- Further studies are required to understand the possible benefits of this device.

7. Head-up CPR

- A head-up position improves cerebral venous return by facilitating cerebral venous drainage. It also lowers intracranial pressure, which together results in an increase in cerebral perfusion pressure.

- Animal and human cadaver studies have suggested that gradual head and thorax elevation to an angle of 30° while performing CPR, **when combined with** an ITD and active compression–decompression CPR, improves cerebral perfusion pressures.

- In the absence of any clinical studies, the use of head-up CPR must only be undertaken in the context of a closely monitored trial or evaluation, with regular review of neurological outcome in survivors.

8. Extra-Corporeal Membrane Oxygenation (ECMO) and Possible Out-of-Hospital Applications

- One area of growing interest is the use of ECMO in refractory cardiac arrest, where survival is poor.

- Conventional cardiopulmonary resuscitation involves chest compressions, which produce a 'low-flow' cardiac output. The longer the period of chest compressions, the greater the likelihood of irreversible organ damage, and the less the chance of an ROSC.

- Because ECMO can match a normal native cardiac output (5.0 litres/min), it is very effective in perfusing the heart and the brain, and preventing on going damage despite a patient being in cardiac arrest.

- When used in this way, it is referred to as extracorporeal cardiopulmonary resuscitation (ECPR). It is normally achieved by placing a large cannula in the femoral vein to drain venous blood, and pumping oxygenated blood back through another large cannula placed in the femoral artery.

- Some ambulance services in Europe and North America have begun trials of pre-hospital ECPR for out-of-hospital cardiac arrest. Trials are shortly planned for the UK.

9. CPR-induced Consciousness

- In some patients, the application of CPR, particularly when using mCPR, may produce sufficient cerebral perfusion for signs of consciousness in the absence of ROSC.

9.1 Characteristics

- Patients may display a variety of signs, including:
  - eye opening
  - increased jaw tone
  - incomprehensible sounds
  - recognisable words or speech

Advanced Life Support

- limb movement
- purposeful movements, e.g. localising to pain
- combative movements, e.g. pushing rescuers away.

9.2 Key Points for CPR-induced Consciousness

- Even if a patient is displaying any of these features, ad hoc rhythm checks are not recommended and paramedics should limit rhythm checks to once every 2 minutes, as per conventional guidance.

- CPR-induced consciousness (CPR-IC) should be recognised at the earliest opportunity. Signs that may help paramedics distinguish CPR-IC from ROSC may include:
  - an absence of palpable pulses
  - a rapid deterioration in consciousness when chest compressions are stopped
  - a cardiac rhythm considered incompatible with life.

- In patients with symptoms that create difficulty in delivering high-quality CPR, or when the patient may be distressed, paramedics may wish to consider requesting enhanced care support or advice as per local procedures/pathways or rapid conveyance to hospital to facilitate ongoing treatment.

10. Reversible Causes and Specialist Circumstances in Cardiac Arrest (4Hs and 4Ts)

10.1 Hypoxia

- All patients in cardiac arrest should be ventilated with high-concentration (100%) oxygen to minimise the risk of hypoxia. Ensure regular checks of the oxygen cylinder and replace it if needed before the cylinder runs empty.

10.2 Hypovolaemia

- Most patients who suffer a cardiac arrest due to a cardiac cause are not hypovolaemic. IV fluids are not indicated in these patients during CPR because excess intravascular filling may worsen coronary perfusion. However, in patients who suffer a cardiac arrest due to blood loss or a depleted intravascular volume (e.g. sepsis or severe dehydration), hypovolaemia may require treatment. Prioritise management of hypovolaemia by controlling any catastrophic haemorrhage. Where hypovolaemia is suspected, intravascular volume should be restored rapidly with IV (or IO) fluid. Up to 2 litres of normal saline should be rapidly infused.

Early transportation of these patients should be considered

10.3 Hypo/hyperkalaemia (and Hypoglycaemia)

- Diagnosing this in the pre-hospital setting is challenging. The patient's medical history or identification of a dialysis fistula may give an indication of dialysis history and potential hyperkalaemia. Patients with a history of diabetic ketoacidosis (DKA) will often also have a high serum potassium. Patients living with frailty, or patients with eating disorders, who have a recent history of gastric disease, may have low serum potassium. On suspicion or identification of any potential reversible metabolic disorder, a time-critical transfer to hospital should be considered.

- Blood sugar should remain an important consideration during cardiac arrest and should be undertaken as soon as practical, commencing during the actual cardiac arrest itself. Hypoglycaemia can cause significant brain injury, and this will occur if the patient is hypoglycaemic during the actual cardiac arrest itself. Blood sugar should therefore be monitored both during the arrest and in the post-ROSC period. Hypoglycaemia is rarely, if ever, a primary cause of cardiac arrest; hypoglycaemia is usually a result of cardiac arrest itself. However, identification and treatment of hypoglycaemia is important, in order to optimise the chances of neurologically intact survival. When measuring blood sugar during a cardiac arrest, a venous sample should be used where possible (a capillary sample may be less accurate but is acceptable if it is not possible to obtain a venous sample). Blood glucose monitors are not calibrated for venous samples (although they are likely to still be accurate). If hypoglycaemia is identified, IV glucose should be administered as appropriate (refer to **Glycaemic Emergencies in Adults and Children**), and the blood sugar rechecked at regular intervals until normal levels are obtained.

10.4 Hypothermia

- Accidental hypothermia is often under-diagnosed in temperate climates. Generally, hypothermia can develop during exposure to cold environments and in people who have been immobilised or immersed in cold water. In the older/frail person and the very young, where thermoregulation is impaired, hypothermia can follow a very mild insult. The risk of hypothermia is also increased by exhaustion, illness, injury, neglect, reduced

Advanced Life Support

level of consciousness or when drugs or alcohol have been ingested.

- Severe hypothermia is associated with the depression of cerebral blood flow and oxygen requirement, reduced cardiac output and decreased arterial pressure. Patients can appear to be clinically dead because of significant depression of brain and cardiovascular function, but the threshold for full resuscitation should remain low, as recovery with intact neurology is possible.

- The patient's peripheral pulses and respiratory effort may be difficult to detect. Therefore, resuscitation should not be withheld based on clinical presentation. Consider whether on the basis of history, hypothermia is believed to be the primary cause of the cardiac arrest. If hypothermia is believed to be the primary cause, follow the guidance below.

- Pre-hospital core temperature measurement can be inaccurate and so should not always be relied upon to confirm hypothermia. In a hypothermic patient, resuscitation should not be withheld unless the cause of the cardiac arrest is clearly attributable to fatal illness, prolonged asphyxia, lethal injury or if the chest is incompressible.

- Because hypothermia itself may produce a very slow, small-volume, irregular pulse and unrecordable blood pressure, signs of life may be so minimal that it is easy to overlook them. Palpate a major artery, obtain an ECG and look for signs of life (pulse, chest rise, breathing efforts, movements, eye opening or shockable rhythm) for up to 1 minute before concluding that there is no cardiac output. Hypothermia can cause stiffness of the chest wall, making chest compressions and ventilations difficult; however, if the patient is pulseless, start chest compressions and ventilations at the same rate as for normothermic patients.

- It is important to prevent further heat loss from the patient's body core, by removing wet garments (providing this does not result in additional exposure) and protecting against heat loss and wind chill by using blankets/ heated blankets, head coverings and insulating equipment.

- The hypothermic heart may be unresponsive to cardioactive drugs and defibrillation; therefore, when the temperature is 30–35°C, double intervals between medicines should be used, e.g. adrenaline every 6–10 minutes.

- Where the core temperature is <30°C, no drugs should be administered until the temperature reaches 30°C, at which point double intervals should be used. A maximum of three shocks should be delivered to a patient in a shockable rhythm below 30°C. **NB:** Consideration should be given where Trusts do not have equipment to differentiate between <35°C and <30°C. In these cases, double intervals between medicines should be used.

- Consider hospital bypass to a centre that can provide extracorporeal rewarming and phone ahead to discuss the case, as per local procedures.

10.5 Hyperthermia

- Hyperthermia occurs when the body's ability to thermoregulate fails and core temperature exceeds that normally maintained by homeostatic mechanisms. Either the body's metabolic heat production or environmental heat load exceeds the body's normal heat loss capacity, or heat loss is impaired.

- In addition to heat stroke, patients with acute behavioural disorder (ABD) often present with hyperthermia. Both groups are at risk of hyperthermia, contributing to metabolic disturbance and an ensuing cardiac arrest.

- When managing the hyperthermic patient in cardiac arrest, follow standard procedures for basic and advanced life support and cool the patient by removing excess clothing and adjusting the surrounding environmental temperature if possible.

- Prognosis is poor when compared to normothermic cardiac arrests. High body temperature is capable of producing irreversible brain damage and the risk of unfavourable neurological outcome increases for each degree of body temperature above 37°C.

10.6 Toxins

- Patients who may have ingested a deliberate or accidental amount of toxin before their cardiac arrest should be transported to the ED, with effective resuscitation delivered en-route. Consider mechanical CPR if resuscitation attempts are likely to be prolonged. If possible, communication regarding the suspected ingestion substance should be made with the ED as early as possible. Crew safety regarding cross-contamination must always be a high priority in these situations.

- Where there is suspicion of poisoning of unknown origin (e.g. snake or animal bites), the antidote is required rapidly and will rarely be available in the pre-hospital setting. Paramedics should therefore aim for rapid conveyance with pre-alert.

- Refer to **Overdose and Poisoning in Adults and Children**.

Advanced Life Support

10.7 Tension Pneumothorax

■ The diagnosis of a tension pneumothorax in the pre-hospital environment can be challenging. If there is suspicion of tension pneumothorax, supported by clinical findings, the chest should be decompressed using needle thoracentesis. This procedure may not always relieve the tension and even in patients where it does, a tension pneumothorax may recur as the cannula becomes blocked or dislodged. A high index of suspicion should be applied to any re-occurrence of tension pneumothorax.

■ Consider enhanced care for insertion of a more definitive thoracostomy incision.

10.8 Thrombosis – Coronary or Pulmonary

■ **Coronary** Where the rhythm is shockable, this should be managed as outlined in the ALS algorithm.

■ **Pulmonary** This will be challenging to diagnose in the cardiac arrest situation. If available, the patient's history before cardiac arrest may give some indication. If pulmonary thrombosis is suspected, a time-critical transfer to hospital is indicated. In situations where thrombolysis is administered, CPR for as long as 90 mins may be required to break up the clot. In these circumstances, consider mechanical CPR.

Intra-arrest thrombolysis can be considered if available: follow local pathways but do not delay conveyance to hospital.

10.9 Cardiac Tamponade

■ Diagnosis of this in the pre-hospital environment is challenging due to its occult nature. Cardiac tamponade compresses the heart, prevents adequate filling and ejection and leads to cardiac arrest; it requires urgent decompression. Therefore, if suspected, a time-critical transfer to hospital is indicated. Consider enhanced care support where available.

■ In patients presenting in pulseless electrical activity (PEA), evaluation of the ECG waveform may assist in identifying any reversible causes. Figure 2.7 shows a classification of PEA according to the reversible cause.

11. Special Considerations in Cardiac Arrest

Use of Ultrasound

Ultrasound can be a useful tool in supporting and guiding resuscitation practice to help determine the cause of the arrest. It should not be used as the sole determinant to terminate resuscitation. Staff must have had appropriate additional training in order to use it and this is unlikely to be available for core paramedics.

11.1 Pregnancy

■ Refer to **Maternal Resuscitation**.

■ Establishing effective resuscitation, focusing on delivering ALS to the mother, is the first priority. Specific modifications include:

– The hand position for chest compressions may need to be slightly higher on the sternum for patients in the third trimester.

– Hypoxia and hypovolaemia are common causes of maternal cardiac arrest and should be considered early.

– Tracheal intubation may be considerably more difficult. A tracheal tube may need to be 0.5–1.0 mm smaller than that for a non-pregnant woman of the same size.

– Manually displace the uterus to the left to ensure that there is adequate venous return to the heart. Add left lateral tilt (ideally 15–30° but even a small amount of tilt may be better than no tilt).

– Make plans to undertake a time-critical transfer to hospital – this should be commenced within 5 minutes of arrival at the cardiac arrest.

■ Advanced life support intervention can be carried out en-route. Emphasise the pregnancy at the earliest opportunity during pre-alert to allow for further specialist hospital staff to be available to perform a peri-mortem caesarean section on arrival to resus if indicated.

11.2 Drowning

■ Drowning is defined as a process resulting in primary respiratory impairment from submersion/immersion in a liquid medium and is the third leading cause of accidental death in Europe.

■ Patients who have been submerged for less than 10 minutes have a very high chance of a good outcome, whereas those submerged for more than 25 minutes are likely to have a poor outcome. Rescue efforts of up to 90 minutes may be appropriate for children or those submerged in icy cold water (see Figure 2.6).

■ Ensure personal safety and the safety of other rescuers. Establish whether the patient was alone or if there may be other patients. Ensure additional resources, including enhanced or specialist units, are requested as required.

■ Hypoxia is the most common cause of arrest in drowning, but hypothermia or arrhythmia should also be considered. In those recovered from shallow water; consider cervical spine injury.

■ Resuscitative efforts should be made where there is a possibility of an air pocket from which the patient could breathe while under water or where the patient's airway has only been intermittently

PEA – EVALUATION

QRS NARROW MECHANICAL (RV) PROBLEM	QRS WIDE METABOLIC (LV) PROBLEM
• Cardiac tamponade • Tension PTX • Mechanical hyperinflation • Pulmonary embolism	• Severe hyperkalemia • Sodium-channel blocker toxicity
	AGONAL RHYTHM
ACUTE MI **Myocardial rupture**	**ACUTE MI** **Pump failure**

Figure 2.7 – Classification of PEA based on its initial electrocardiographic manifestation. LV = Left ventricular; PTX = pneumothorax; RV = right ventricular. Source: Littmann L et al. Med Princ Pract 2014. Simplified and Structured Teaching Tool for the Evaluation and Management of Pulseless Electrical Activity. Republished with permission.

submerged (e.g. wearing a life jacket), provided there are no signs unequivocally associated with death.

- Palpation of the pulse as the sole indicator to confirm the presence or absence of cardiac arrest is unreliable. Use an ECG and waveform capnography (EtCO$_2$) monitoring to confirm cardiac arrest.

- There is no difference in the management of salt and fresh water drowning.

- Regurgitation of stomach contents and large amounts of foam can be common during resuscitation from drowning. Efforts to remove the foam may be futile; therefore, early intubation may assist airway management and ventilation. In most drowning incidents, patients will aspirate small amounts of water, and this is absorbed into the central circulation. Where contaminants prevent ventilation, the patient can be turned on their side or direct suction can be used to remove the regurgitated material as best as possible.

- Administer IV fluids to correct hypovolaemia if indicated.

- If submersion occurs in cold water (<5°C), hypothermia may develop rapidly and provides some protection against hypoxia. If hypothermia is considered to be the primary cause of the cardiac arrest, manage as per hypothermia section.

Management

- Give five initial rescue breaths while administering high-flow oxygen, then follow standard ALS protocols.

- Consider head and neck injuries, which may be present if the patient dived into shallow water;

these are present in <0.5% of all cases and rescue should take precedence over c-spine protection.

- The patient's heart may be extremely slow and external cardiac chest compressions may be required.

- Consider early tracheal intubation, as high ventilation pressure may be required because of poor compliance resulting from pulmonary oedema.

11.3 Asthma

- Cardiac arrest in the asthmatic patient is often a terminal event after a period of hypoxaemia and respiratory exhaustion, and is associated with:
  - Severe bronchospasm and mucous plugging leading to asphyxia.
  - Cardiac arrhythmias due to hypoxia, stimulant drug or electrolyte abnormalities.
  - Dynamic hyperinflation where a gradual build-up of pressure occurs which reduces venous return and blood pressure.
  - Tension pneumothorax (sometimes bilateral).

- Consideration of reversible causes (the 4Hs and 4Ts) will help identify these causes of cardiac arrest. Management of cardiac arrest in asthma patients should follow standard ALS guidelines while incorporating the following recommendations:
  - Ventilation may be difficult because of increased airway resistance; a two-person technique may assist.
  - If dynamic hyperinflation is suspected during CPR, manual compression of the chest wall and/or a period of planned apnoea achieved

Advanced Life Support

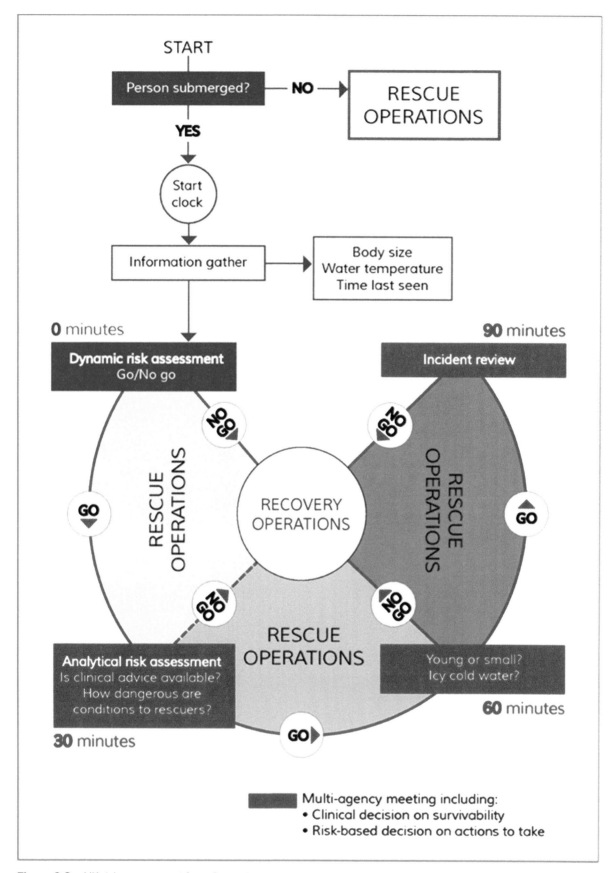

Figure 2.8 – UK risk assessment for submersion.

by disconnecting the BVM from the tracheal tube may reduce gas trapping.

- There is a significant risk of gastric inflation and hypoventilation of the lungs when ventilating a severely asthmatic patient; therefore, consider early tracheal intubation where required.
- Regularly check for evidence of reversible causes, specifically tension pneumothorax.

- Decompress suspected pneumothoraces and consider enhanced/critical care support to perform a thoracostomy. **NB:** Bilateral needle decompression will not make the situation worse and may reverse the cause of the cardiac arrest.

11.4 Opiate Overdose

- Cardiac arrest following opiate overdose (OD) is usually secondary to a respiratory arrest. If cardiac arrest occurs, follow standard resuscitation guidelines while incorporating the following modifications:
  - Administering naloxone is unlikely to cause harm; it can be given where opiate OD is likely. The usual adult dose is 400 microgram IV/IO, which should be titrated to affect every 60 seconds, with the subsequent doses being 800 microgram IV/IO. Administer incrementally until the patient is breathing adequately and is able to protect their airway.
  - If no response is observed after a total of 10 mg IV/IO naloxone, consider a non-opioid-related drug or other cause.
  - The administration of Naloxone should not compromise the provision of quality CPR, early defibrillation and adequate airway management and effective ventilation.
  - Prolonged resuscitation may be appropriate in this cohort of patients, as good neurological outcome is possible. Cessation of resuscitation should be in consultation with a senior clinician.

11.5 Rhythm-affecting Drugs

- Consider the effect that rhythm-affecting drugs (e.g. beta blockers, tricyclic anti-depressants, cocaine etc.) and non-opiate recreational drugs may have on cardiac output before terminating a resuscitation attempt. Follow normal ALS guidance for these patient groups.

11.6 Bariatric Patients

- While normal ALS guidance and shock protocols should be followed in the resuscitation of bariatric patients, it is recognised that delivery of effective CPR may be challenging. Chest compressions will be difficult to perform in many patients, simply because of suboptimal positioning of

rescuers. A step or platform may be required, or compressions can be performed from the patient's head end.

- Additional rescuers may be required to assist due to rescuer fatigue, particularly in relation to the delivery of chest compressions. It may be necessary to change the CPR provider more frequently and mechanical devices may not accommodate this patient group. Although chest compressions are most effective when performed with the patient lying on a firm surface, where it is unsafe to attempt to move the patient they may remain on a mattress, as the heavier torso compresses the surface, leaving less potential for displacement during chest compressions.

- Higher inspiration pressure is needed for positive pressure ventilation due to increased intra-abdominal pressure. In all patients with extreme obesity, difficult intubation must be anticipated, with a clear failed intubation drill if necessary.

- It is important to request additional resources to assist with moving the patient, with consideration for specially adapted vehicles. Weight limits of equipment must be checked before use. Underestimation of the technical aspects of rescue operations may cause trauma or prohibit safe transfer of bariatric patients.

12. Chemical, Biological, Radiological and Nuclear (CBRN) Incidents

- The key priority of the first medical personnel on arrival at a chemical, biological, radiological and nuclear (CBRN) incident is to ensure all emergency service control centres are alerted and specialist resources are summoned early.

- If there is one casualty, rescuers may approach as usual. If there are two casualties, only approach with caution, considering all options. If there are three or more casualties, one should not approach. Instead withdraw, contain the scene, report the situation, self-isolate and await specialist resources.

- A patient in cardiac arrest as a result of a CBRN incident should only be approached and treated once the risk to rescuers is known. A chemical incident may initially present with patients in a peri or actual cardiac arrest. Proper scene management of chemical incidents is crucial for preventing further exposure and incident escalation. Early pattern recognition of chemical agent syndromes is vital, and paramedics should be aware of the constant threat of this type of

Advanced Life Support

incident. These can result from terrorist action, or industrial and chemical incidents, as well as isolated cases of toxic exposure.

■ The signs of a CBRN incident can often be subtle or delayed, and emergency medical personnel should always be vigilant for abnormal situational or patient factors that raise suspicion of a CBRN incident. Exposure to a CBRN agent can occur through direct contact, inhalation, injection, ingestion or irradiation.

12.1 Personal Protection

■ Rescuers must not approach potential casualties unless adequate PPE is worn.

■ Personal protection is paramount if a CBRN incident is suspected. If in doubt, the rescuer should withdraw to a place of safety until the CBRN threat can be accurately identified and the necessary PPE brought to the scene.

■ Entering a CBRN scene without adequate PPE puts the rescuer at risk of harm and also risks spread of contamination. A CBRN patient will need decontamination before being able to receive advanced medical care.

■ There are also an increasing number of individual chemical exposure incidents in the UK, this may occur as a result of suicide or agricultural accidents, for example. There are a number of different agents commonly used, which include:
 – hydrogen sulphide (made by mixing a combination of household chemicals)
 – aluminium phosphide (from rat poison)
 – cyanide salts
 – helium gas
 – nitrogen gas
 – carbon monoxide (e.g. from a disposable BBQ or car exhaust).

13. Trauma

■ Establishing the cause of cardiac arrest may not be straightforward. A primary medical arrest can occur before a patient suffers a secondary traumatic insult. Primary medical cardiac arrests

resulting in falls from height or while driving are examples that can typically result in rescuers suspecting cardiac arrest of traumatic origin.

■ Pay close attention to a witness history and perform an accurate scene assessment to establish the course of events and mechanism of injury. If there is a possibility that the patient has had a primary medical cardiac arrest, follow standard BLS and ALS guidelines. Where trauma is considered to be the primary cause of the arrest, consider early enhanced care support and follow the traumatic cardiac arrest algorithm in Figure 2.5.

■ Patients who are in cardiac arrest following drowning, hanging or asphyxiation should not automatically be conveyed to a major trauma centre (MTC) (unless there is significant mechanism to trigger TU bypass). However, all patients for whom ROSC has been achieved following traumatic cardiac arrest should be conveyed to an MTC unless airway and/or catastrophic haemorrhage cannot be safely managed, when a pit stop at the nearest Emergency Department is indicated.

■ Consider termination of the resuscitative effort if the patient presents in asystole and has not responded to 30 minutes of ALS **with likely reversible causes treated successfully (rapid MTC conveyance is indicated where reversible causes cannot be corrected, or for patients with penetrating trauma)**. The exceptions to termination at 30 minutes are for pregnancy, children and where hypothermia may be a contributory factor. Consider senior advice when appropriate.

13.1 Blunt Trauma

■ In the pre-hospital setting, advanced life support and exclusion of reversible causes using the 4Hs and 4Ts or the HOT approach should take priority. The commonest causes of traumatic cardiac arrest are **h**ypovolaemia, **o**xygenation (hypoxia) and **t**ension pneumothorax, which form the mnemonic 'HOT' – a helpful short checklist of reversible causes for the management of these patients.

Hypovolaemia	• Control external haemorrhage • Splint pelvis / fractures • IV/IO fluid bolus • Early administration of TXA (IV/IO/IM)
Oxygenation (hypoxia)	• Basic/advanced airway management • Maximise oxygenation
Tension pneumothorax	• Decompress chest

Advanced Life Support

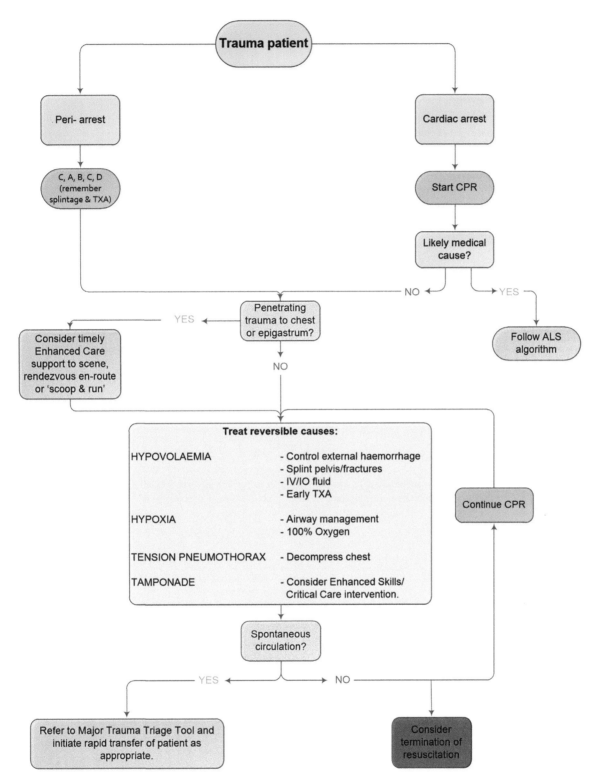

Figure 2.9 – Traumatic cardiac arrest algorithm. Source: Resuscitation Council (UK), 2015.

- Rapid treatment of reversible causes should take priority over chest compressions and ALS drug administration. However, high-quality chest compressions are important and may generate some forward flow, even in cases of severe hypovolaemia or cardiac tamponade; it is therefore important to continue chest compressions as soon as sufficient personnel are available to allocate someone to this task.

- Undertake only essential lifesaving interventions on scene. If the patient has signs of life (pulse, chest rise, breathing efforts, movements, eye opening or shockable rhythm), rapidly transfer to hospital or arrange rendezvous with enhanced/critical care support. Do not delay for spinal immobilisation.

- Effective airway management using a stepwise approach is essential to maintain oxygenation

Advanced Life Support

of the severely compromised trauma patient. In low cardiac output conditions, positive pressure ventilation may cause further circulatory depression or even cardiac arrest by impeding venous return to the heart. Monitor ventilation with continuous waveform capnography and adjust rate to achieve normocarbia.

- Consider performing all further interventions en-route and administer tranexamic acid early. Refer to **Tranexamic Acid**, **Page for Age** for children.

- Hypovolaemia due to blood loss that is sufficient in volume to cause cardiac arrest is difficult to treat. Gain large bore IV access. Although IV normal saline may restore blood volume (often requiring 2–3 litres), excessive crystalloid causes coagulopathy, acidosis and hypothermia, which in itself worsens outcome. Request enhanced care, particularly if it enables blood and blood products to be brought to scene without delay. Once ROSC is achieved, only give IV fluids to achieve a systolic BP no higher than 80 mmHg.

- Consider whether the patient can be conveyed for early blood or blood product intervention, or whether this can be brought to the scene or to a rendezvous point in a timely manner by enhanced care assets.

- In blunt trauma cases, where ALS (including attempts to address reversible causes) is being delivered, clinical judgement may be applied as to whether enhanced care assets may be accessed, or the patient can be conveyed to an MTC (or TU if necessary) in a timely manner. If likely reversible causes of traumatic cardiac arrest have been treated and there has been no ROSC after 30 minutes of ALS, resuscitation may stop.

13.2 Penetrating Trauma

- In penetrating traumatic cardiac arrest, patients should be transferred rapidly to hospital because surgical intervention is often needed to treat the cause of the arrest. A rapid transport approach is appropriate to the nearest MTU (or TU if necessary), but crew safety should be a consideration where there are prolonged journey times in a moving vehicle.

- Enhanced care assets should be requested early for attendance at the scene (but do not delay departure from scene while waiting for these assets) and/or during conveyance.

- Rapidly address immediate issues:
  - catastrophic haemorrhage (splinting, trauma dressings, tourniquet etc.)
  - airway and breathing (consider tension pneumothorax, sucking chest wound etc.)
  - defibrillation, if indicated.

- Consider performing all further interventions en-route and administer tranexamic acid early.

- The principles for volume resuscitation for penetrating trauma are similar to those for blunt trauma. However, the priority for rapid conveyance to hospital often precludes any significant pre-hospital volume being administered. Do not delay on scene to obtain IV access. If IV fluids are administered, a systolic BP no greater than 80 mmHg is adequate. Surgical intervention is often the only intervention that will save the patient's life, and rapid conveyance to hospital is vital to achieve this.

Bibliography

1. Resuscitation Council (UK). *Resuscitation Council Guidelines 2021: Adult advanced life support.* London: Resuscitation Council, 2021. Available from: https://www.resus.org.uk/resuscitation-guidelines/adult-advanced-life-support.

2. Resuscitation Council (UK). *Resuscitation Council Guidelines 2021: Paediatric advanced life support.* London: Resuscitation Council, 2021. Available from: https://www.resus.org.uk/resuscitation-guidelines/paediatric-advanced-life-support.

3. Resuscitation Council (UK). *Resuscitation Council Guidelines 2021: Peri-arrest arrhythmias.* London: Resuscitation Council UK, 2021. Available from: https://www.resus.org.uk/resuscitation-guidelines/peri-arrest-arrhythmias.

4. Resuscitation Council (UK). *Resuscitation Council Guidelines 2021: Prehospital Resuscitation.* London: Resuscitation Council UK, 2021. Available from: https://www.resus.org.uk/resuscitation-guidelines/prehospital-resuscitation/.

5. Soar J, Nolan JP, Bottiger BW et al. European Resuscitation Council Guidelines for Resuscitation 2015: Section 3. Adult advanced life support. *Resuscitation* 2015, 95: 100–147. Available from: https://www.resuscitationjournal.com/article/S0300-9572(15)00328-7/fulltext.

6. Truhlar A, Deakin CD, Soar J et al. European Resuscitation Council Guidelines for Resuscitation 2015: Section 4. Cardiac arrest in special circumstances. *Resuscitation* 2015, 95: 148–201. Available from: https://www.resuscitationjournal.com/article/S0300-9572(15)00329-9/fulltext.

7. Maconochie I, Bingham R, Eich C, López-Herce J, Rodriguez-Nunez A, Rajka T, Van de Voorde P, Zideman D, Biarent D. European Resuscitation Council Guidelines for Resuscitation 2015 Section 6: Paediatric life support. *Resuscitation* 2015, 95: 223–248. Available from: https://www.resuscitationjournal.com/article/S0300-9572(15)00340-8/fulltext.

8. Deakin CD, Soar J, Morley P, Drennan I. Double sequential defibrillation for refractory ventricular fibrillation cardiac arrest: a systematic review. Resuscitation 2020, 155: 24–31. Available from: https://doi.org/10.1016/j.resuscitation.2020.06.008.

9. Finn J, Jacobs I, Williams TA et al. Adrenaline and vasopressin for cardiac arrest. *Cochrane Database of*

Advanced Life Support

Systematic Reviews 2019, 327(15): 1051. Available from: http://doi.org/10.1002/14651858.CD003179.

10. Soar J, Perkin G, Maconochie I et al. European Resuscitation Council Guidelines for Resuscitation: 2018 update – antiarrhythmic drugs for cardiac arrest. *Resuscitation* 2019, 134: 99–103. Available from: https://www.sciencedirect.com/science/article/pii/S0300957218310967/pdfft?md5=22f72cc33ecab8b1e38130bfb18dc680&pid=1-s2.0-S0300957218310967-main.pdf.

11. Perkins GD, Ji C, Deakin CD et al, on behalf of PARAMEDIC2 collaborators. A randomized trial of epinephrine in out-of-hospital cardiac arrest. *New England Journal of Medicine* 2018, 379: 711–721. Available from: https://www.nejm.org/doi/full/10.1056/NEJMoa1806842.

12. Holmberg MJ, Geri G, Wiberg S et al. Extracorporeal cardiopulmonary resuscitation for cardiac arrest: a systematic review. *Resuscitation* 2018, 131: 91–100. Available from: https://www.resuscitationjournal.com/article/S0300-9572(18)30373-3/pdf.

13. Benger J, Kirby K, Black S et al. Effect of a strategy of a supraglottic airway device vs tracheal intubation during out-of-hospital cardiac arrest on functional outcome: the AIRWAYS-2 randomized clinical trial. *JAMA* 2018, 320: 779–791. Available from: https://www.ncbi.nlm.nih.gov/pmc/articles/PMC6142999/.

14. Poole K, Couper K, Smyth MA et al. Mechanical CPR: Who? When? How? *Critical Care* 2018, 22: 140. Available from: https://ccforum.biomedcentral.com/track/pdf/10.1186/s13054-018-2059-0.

15. Dee R et al. The effect of alternative methods of cardiopulmonary resuscitation – cough CPR, percussion pacing or precordial thump – on outcomes following cardiac arrest. A systematic review. *Resuscitation* 2021, 162: 73–81.

Basic Life Support in Adults

1. Introduction

- When there is only one person on scene, resuscitation is limited to providing basic life support (BLS) and defibrillation.
- When available, the first priority is to attach defibrillation pads to reduce the time to first shock and then begin BLS with minimal delay.
- If a bystander is willing and able to provide good-quality chest compressions, utilise their skills until further trained assistance arrives. This is particularly helpful in ensuring that immediate uninterrupted chest compressions are delivered while the defibrillator is attached.
- Once other providers are in attendance, BLS and defibrillation should continue, while advanced life support (ALS) interventions are provided.

2. Assessment and Management

- The assessment and management of a collapsed patient is detailed in Table 2.4. The adult BLS sequence is detailed in Figure 2.10.

TABLE 2.4 – ASSESSMENT and MANAGEMENT of: Basic Life Support in Adults

This sequence is for a single ambulance paramedic; however, when more than one person is present, tasks can be shared and undertaken simultaneously.

Assess Safety

- Ensure that you are safe.

Check Responsiveness

- Check the responsiveness of the patient.
- If there are no signs of life (and the patient is not breathing normally) and it is in the best interests of the patient, begin CPR.
- A pulse check is often inaccurate and may lead to an erroneous diagnosis, delaying CPR.
- Agonal breathing (occasional irregular gasps; slow, laboured, noisy breathing) is common in the early stages of cardiac arrest and should not be confused with signs of life/circulation.

Next Steps

- As a solo responder, the first priority is to attach defibrillation pads to reduce the time to first shock, but commence BLS as quickly as possible with minimal delay. (With two or more responders, chest compressions/ventilations should be commenced immediately while the defibrillator is applied by the second responder).
- Ensure further/enhanced resources are en-route.
- BLS should be commenced while obtaining details to inform a best interests decision.
- Every effort should be made to gain 360° access to the patient.
- Start chest compressions at a rate of 100–120 per minute.
- Compression depth should be 5–6 cm.
- Allow the chest to recoil completely after each compression.
- Take approximately the same amount of time for each compression and recoil.
- Use of a CPR feedback device allows optimisation of BLS delivery and assessment of performance.
- Minimise interruptions to chest compressions.
- A palpable pulse (carotid, femoral or radial) during CPR is not a gauge of effective blood flow.

Combine Chest Compressions with Ventilations

Refer to **Airway and Breathing Management**.

- Maintain patency of the airway during CPR:
  - Consider the use of a laryngoscope and forceps if foreign body airway obstruction (FBAO) is suspected. Refer to **Foreign Body Airway Obstruction**.
  - Establishing a patent airway takes priority over concerns about a potential spinal injury.
- After 30 compressions:
  - Open and inspect the airway.
  - Provide two ventilations with the most appropriate equipment available.
  - Use an inspiratory time of 1 second with adequate volume to produce a visual rise of the chest.

Basic Life Support in Adults

- Resume chest compressions without delay.
- Add high-flow oxygen as soon as possible; refer to **Oxygen**.
- Continue chest compressions and ventilation in a ratio of 30:2.
- Stop to recheck only if the patient starts breathing normally; otherwise do not interrupt chest compressions and ventilation.
- Performing chest compressions is tiring; try to change the person doing chest compressions every 2 minutes; ensure the minimum of delay during the changeover.
- Ventilate gently 10 times per minute. Hyperventilation and hyperinflation must be avoided. Refer to **Airway and Breathing Management**.
- Do not attempt more than two breaths each time before returning to chest compressions.

Adult basic life support in community settings

Unresponsive and not breathing normally?

30 chest compressions

2 rescue breaths

Continue CPR 30:2

As soon as Defibrillator arrives, switch it on and follow instructions

Figure 2.10 – Adult basic life support sequence. Reproduced with permission from the Resuscitation Council (UK) Guidelines 2021 (www.resus.org.uk).

KEY POINTS!

Basic Life Support in Adults

- **High-quality basic life support is a key determinant of survival from OHCA. Begin and maintain chest compressions and ventilations without interruption.**
- **Chest compressions should be provided at a rate of 100–120 per minute and a depth of 5–6 cm using a ratio of 30:2 compressions to ventilations.**
- **Attach defibrillator pads as soon as available, to identify and treat shockable rhythms.**
- **Agonal breathing is common in the early stages of cardiac arrest and should not be confused as a sign of life or spontaneous circulation.**

Basic Life Support in Adults

Bibliography

1. Olasveengen TM, Semeraro F, Ristagno G et al. European Resuscitation Council Guidelines for Resuscitation 2021: basic life support. *Resuscitation* 2015, 95: 81–99. Available from: https://cprguidelines.eu/assets/guidelines/European-Resuscitation-Council-Guidelines-2021-Ba.pdf.

2. Perkins GD, Colquhoun M, Deakin CD et al. Resuscitation Council (UK). *Adult Basic Life Support Guidelines 2021*. London: Resuscitation Council (UK), 2021. Available from: https://www.resus.org.uk/library/2021-resuscitation-guidelines/adult-basic-life-support-guidelines.

Basic Life Support in Children

1. Introduction

- Cardiac arrest in children is different from that of the adult patient in its aetiology and early pathophysiology, with the vast majority of cases being caused by hypoxia.

- It is a rare phenomenon, with an incidence of 9 per 100,000 children. Paramedics are less likely to encounter a paediatric than adult cardiac arrest.

- Proactive dispatch of enhanced care, where available, should be considered. Most calls coded as paediatric cardiac arrest are subsequently found to be post-ictal; unresponsive children with abnormal breathing may also appear blue.

- Due to the prevalence of hypoxia as a cause of paediatric cardiac arrest, paediatric resuscitation focuses primarily on ensuring a patent airway and adequate oxygenation/ventilation.

- A small number of paediatric patients will experience cardiac arrest without warning, often during exertion, and present in a shockable rhythm as a result of an often undiagnosed cardiac abnormality. The possibility of a successful outcome is high if appropriate action is taken promptly in these cases, i.e. rapid defibrillation.

2. Age Definitions

- This guideline covers:
  - infants (defined as under one year old)
  - children (defined as between 1 and 18 years of age).

- In this guideline, the term 'child' includes infants, unless specified otherwise.

- Newborn life support is not covered in this guideline. For newborn babies, refer to **Newborn Life Support**.

3. General Principles

- The priorities should include:
  - effective airway management
  - effective ventilations
  - effective chest compressions
  - early defibrillation, if appropriate.

- Do not delay on scene once these interventions have been attempted.

- Consider conveyance to the most appropriate hospital with early pre-alert.

- In the event of a life-threatening episode for any child, consideration must be given to the need for clinical assessment of other siblings in the property if the cause of illness is unknown.

- In the event of a life-threatening episode for any child, consideration must be given to safeguarding concerns for that child and siblings.

4. Airway Management

- Bag-mask ventilation (BVM) is the recommended first-line method for achieving airway control and ventilation in children.

- Appropriate padding behind the shoulder blades, which also supports the head in children, may aid airway management.

- Gastric insufflation is a complication of paediatric resuscitation, leading to splinting of the diaphragm, vomiting and compression of the vena cava causing diminished venous return. This is best avoided by delivering gentle ventilations over 1 second, just sufficient to cause chest rise.

- Basic airway adjuncts may assist in maintaining an open airway.

- Although bag-mask ventilation remains the recommended first-line method for achieving airway control and ventilation in children, a supraglottic airway is an acceptable airway device for providers trained in its use. It is particularly helpful in airway obstruction caused by upper airway anatomical supraglottic airway abnormalities or if bag-mask ventilation is not possible.

TABLE 2.5 – ASSESSMENT and MANAGEMENT of: Basic Life Support in Children

This sequence is for a solo paramedic; however, when more than one person is present, tasks can be shared and undertaken simultaneously.

Assess Safety

- Ensure that you are safe.

Check Responsiveness

- Check the responsiveness of the patient.

- Agonal breathing (occasional irregular gasps; slow, laboured, noisy breathing) is common in the early stages of cardiac arrest and should not be confused with signs of life/circulation.

- It may be difficult to be certain that there is no pulse. If there is any doubt and it is in the best interest of the patient, begin CPR.

(continued)

Basic Life Support in Children

TABLE 2.5 – ASSESSMENT and MANAGEMENT of: Basic Life Support in Children *(continued)*

Next Steps

- Every effort should be made to gain 360° access to the patient.
- The first priority is to open, inspect and clear the airway and begin effective ventilations using BVM with high-flow oxygen.
- Open the child's airway by tilting the head and lifting the chin:
  - Place your hand on the forehead and gently tilt the head back. Be careful not to hyperextend the neck.
  - At the same time, lift the point of the chin with your fingertip(s). Do not push on the soft tissues under the chin as this may block the airway.
  - If you still have difficulty in opening the airway, try a jaw thrust: place the first two fingers of each hand behind each side of the child's mandible (jawbone) and push the jaw forward.
- Maintain patency of the airway during CPR:
  - Refer to **Airway and Breathing Management**.
- There is a high incidence of choking in children.
  - Consider the use of a laryngoscope and forceps if FBAO is suspected. Refer to **Foreign Body Airway Obstruction**.
  - Establishing a patent airway takes priority over concerns about a potential spinal injury.
- Give five ventilations.

Ventilations – Child

- Ensure head tilt and chin lift.
- Use paediatric BVM (with a mask appropriate to the size of the child) and inflate the chest steadily over 1 second, watching for chest rise.
- Maintaining head tilt and chin lift, watch the chest fall.
- Repeat this sequence 5 times.
- Identify effectiveness by observing the child's chest rise and fall in a similar fashion to the movement produced by a normal breath.

Ventilations – Infant

- Ensure a neutral position of the head and apply a chin lift.
- Use paediatric BVM (with a mask appropriate to the size of the child) and inflate the chest steadily over 1 second, watching for chest rise.
- Maintaining the chin lift, watch the chest fall.
- Repeat this sequence 5 times.
- Identify effectiveness by observing the child's chest rise and fall in a similar fashion to the movement produced by a normal breath.

If There Is Difficulty Achieving an Effective Breath, the Airway May Be Obstructed

- Open the child's mouth and remove any visible obstruction.
- **DO NOT** perform a blind finger sweep.
- Ensure that there is adequate head tilt and chin lift but also that the neck is not over-extended.
- If head tilt and chin lift has not opened the airway, try the jaw thrust method.
- Make up to 5 attempts to achieve effective breaths.
- If still unsuccessful, examine the oropharynx with a laryngoscope and remove any obstruction. If an obstruction is removed, make 5 further attempts at ventilations.
- If still unsuccessful, move on to chest compressions.

Assess the Child's Circulation

- Look for signs of life. This includes checking for a pulse, any movement, coughing or normal breathing (not agonal gasps – these are infrequent, irregular breaths).

NB If you are not sure if there is a pulse, assume there is no pulse.

Basic Life Support in Children

TABLE 2.5 – ASSESSMENT and MANAGEMENT of: Basic Life Support in Children *(continued)*

Pulse Check – Child

■ Feel for the carotid pulse in the neck.

Pulse Check – Infant

■ Feel for the brachial pulse on the inner aspect of the upper arm.

⚑ **Remember that pulse checks may be unreliable and are prone to errors. The detection of circulation therefore should also include other intra-arrest parameters such as EtCO$_2$, blood pressure and SpO$_2$.**

Where a Pulse Is Present and Breaths Are Absent:

■ Continue ventilating, until the child starts breathing effectively on their own.

■ Re-asssess the child frequently.

If There Are No Signs of Circulation – OR There Is Any Doubt:

■ Start chest compressions.

■ Combine ventilations and chest compressions.

NB – For paediatric patients in a collapsed state, with no signs of life and a heart rate <60 beats per minute, compressions must be commenced.

For all children, compress the lower half of the sternum.

■ Avoid compressing the upper abdomen, by locating the xiphisternum (i.e. find the angle where the lowest ribs join in the midline) and compressing the sternum one finger's breadth above this point.

■ Compressions should be sufficient to depress the sternum by at least one-third of the depth of the chest (approximately 4 cm for an infant and 5 cm for a child).

■ Release the pressure, and repeat at a rate of 100–120 per minute.

■ After 15 compressions, give two ventilations.

■ Continue compressions and ventilations in a ratio of 15:2.

■ Solo rescuers may use a ratio of 30:2, particularly if they are having difficulty with the transition between compressions and ventilations.

■ The best method for compression varies slightly between infants and children (see below).

Compressions – Child

■ Place the heel of one hand over the lower half of the sternum (as above).

■ Lift the fingers to ensure that pressure is not applied over the child's ribs.

■ Position yourself vertically above the child's chest and, with your arm straight, compress the sternum to depress it by approximately 5 cm.

■ In larger children or for small rescuers, this may be achieved most easily by using both hands with the fingers interlocked.

■ Ensure complete recoil following each compression.

Compressions – Infant

■ The solo rescuer should compress the sternum with the tips of two fingers.

■ If there are two or more rescuers, an alternative method would be to use the encircling technique:
  – Place both thumbs flat, side by side on the lower half of the sternum (as above) with the tips pointing towards the infant's head.
  – Spread the rest of both hands with the fingers together to encircle the lower part of the infant's rib cage with the tips of the fingers supporting the infant's back.
  – Press down on the lower sternum with the two thumbs to depress it by approximately 4 cm.

■ Ensure complete recoil following each compression.

Basic Life Support in Children

Paediatric basic life support

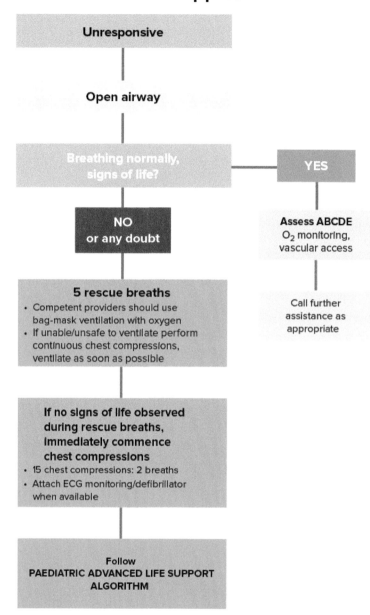

Figure 2.11 – Child basic life support sequence algorithm (modified). Reproduced with permission from the Resuscitation Council (UK) Guidelines 2021 algorithm (www.resus.org.uk).

KEY POINTS!

Basic Life Support in Children

- Hypoxia is the most common cause of cardiac arrest.
- Some children may present in a shockable rhythm as a result of an often undiagnosed cardiac abnormality.
- Treatment should focus on rapidly correcting the cause where possible.
- If the child is not breathing, carefully remove any obvious airway obstruction but DO NOT perform blind finger sweeps.
- Give five initial ventilations using a BVM, watching for chest rise.
- Adopt a high index of suspicion of airway obstruction and treat accordingly.
- The duration of ventilations is about 1 second (comparable with adult practice).

Basic Life Support in Children

- If there are:
  - no signs of life
  - or an absent or slow pulse (<60 bpm with poor perfusion)
  - or you are not sure

  start chest compressions at a rate of 100–120 per minute.
- Continue alternating compressions and breaths at a ratio of 15:2.

Bibliography

1. Van de Voorde P, Turner NM, Djakow J et al. European Resuscitation Council Guidelines 2021: paediatric life support. *Resuscitation* 2021, 161: 327–387. Available from: https://doi.org/10.1016/j.resuscitation.2021.02.015.

2. Skellett S, Maconochie I, Bingham B et al. *Resuscitation Council (UK). Paediatric Basic Life Support Guidelines 2021.* London: Resuscitation Council (UK), 2021. Available from: https://www.resus.org.uk/library/2021-resuscitation-guidelines/paediatric-basic-life-support-guidelines.

SECTION 2 Resuscitation

Emergency Tracheostomy and Laryngectomy Pre-Hospital Management

1. Introduction

'A patient with a tracheostomy or laryngectomy is at risk of death or harm if inappropriate or inadequate care is provided. This patient group requires airway devices to be safely inserted, securely positioned and appropriately cared for, in order to continue to provide the patient with a patent airway. Failure to do so may lead to a displaced or blocked tube, which, if not dealt with immediately, may be fatal within minutes'.[1]

An increasing number of patients with long-term tracheostomies and laryngectomies are now being managed in the community. Approximately 12,000 tracheostomy procedures are performed each year in the UK.[2] Patients are discharged from hospital once the tracheostomy is stable and the patient or carer is competent with self-care along with support from community nurses.

2. Incidence

- All trusts can expect to see more patients requiring emergency care due to the increase in head and neck cancers. These are the fifth leading cause of cancer and the sixth leading cause of cancer mortality.[3]

- Approximately 34 people receive a diagnosis every day in the UK[4] and this is the most common cause of a laryngectomy.[5]

- There are approximately 15,000–20,000 tracheostomies performed annually throughout the NHS.[6]

3. Severity and Outcome

- Commonly, patients are discharged with all the necessary equipment to manage most emergencies. The majority of patients are also discharged with a hospital passport or digital care plan that provides vital details in relation to the specifics of the patient, their airway management and the history of their condition.

- The most common tracheostomy airway emergencies are displacement, accidental de-cannulation and obstruction.[1]

- Obstruction of the tube is the third most common cause of death in patients with tracheostomies.[4] Maintaining a patent airway is the priority. Clinicians must be able to recognise a blocked tube in the presence of severe difficulty in breathing or apnoea. Tubes can become blocked with plugs of mucous, blood and crusts, and the clinician must be competent and trained in suction techniques. They should also be aware of the different types of tracheostomy tubes in use in order to clear the tube safely and effectively.

4. Physiology

4.1 Laryngectomy

- Laryngectomy is the total removal of the larynx and the separation of the airway from the nose, mouth and oesophagus. In a total laryngectomy, the laryngectomee breathes through an opening in the neck. This becomes the patient's primary airway. Total laryngectomy results in permanent changes to the airway anatomy; the trachea is pulled forward during surgery and stitched to the anterior neck skin, forming a new stoma (Figure 2.12).

- It is vital to recognise that following a laryngectomy, the patient's airway does not communicate with their nose or mouth at all.

4.2 Tracheostomy

- A tracheostomy is an opening in the trachea performed via a surgical incision or a percutaneous technique. A tracheostomy tube is passed into the trachea between the second and third tracheal rings, and a stoma is formed 3–5 days post surgery. The airway is then secured. Tracheostomies can be permanent or temporary (Figure 2.13).

Figure 2.12 – Airway anatomy before and after laryngectomy.

Emergency Tracheostomy and Laryngectomy Pre-Hospital Management

Tracheostomy tube – this is sometimes referred to as the outer tube, or outer cannula. This is the main tube which secures the airway through the stoma. It may or may not be cuffed, and it may or may not be fenestrated dependent on need and manufacturer.

Inner cannula – this may or may not be present, dependent on the manufacturer of the tracheostomy tube. It is sometimes known as the inner tube. It is the part of the equipment which can be removed and replaced. Its purpose is secretion management. It should lock into the outer tube by either clicking or twisting into place, to prevent accidental removal.

NB: A fenestrated tube has small holes in the tube shaft.

There will be a code on the flange that will state:

- Fen: Fenestrated
- Non-Fen: Non-fenestrated. Some tubes will allow our equipment such as BVM or EtCO$_2$ to be connected to the main tube, though some makes will only allow connection to the inner cannula.

5. Assessment and Management

For the assessment and management of tracheostomy and laryngectomy, refer to Table 2.6 and Figures 2.13 to 2.15.

TABLE 2.6 – ASSESSMENT and MANAGEMENT of: Suction and Oxygen
ENSURE PPE INCLUDING FACE MASK PROTECTION. REMOVE FENESTRATED TUBES BEFORE SUCTIONING. REMEMBER SUCTION IS A HYPOXIC PROCESS.
Indications for Suction Found on Assessment: - Excessive secretions not cleared by coughing - Increase in pulse, BP or respiratory rate - Decrease in O$_2$ saturations, prolonged capillary refill - Difficulty in mechanically ventilating the patient - Assess the need for oxygen based on reliable saturation readings.
Aims of Suction and Oxygenation: - Prevent respiratory distress. - Maintain a patent airway. - Clear excessive secretions. - Reassurance. - Pre-oxygenate* the patient before the suction procedure; aim for 94–98% SpO$_2$ (88–92% SpO$_2$ for COPD patients). Explain your actions to the patient. - Remove the inner cannula and clean it if blocked. Replace and assess for improvement. - When suctioning, replace a fenestrated inner cannula with a non-fenestrated one; this will reduce the chance of the suction catheter damaging the tracheal wall through the fenestrations. - Set suction at 150–200 mmHg. - When using a soft catheter, go no further than 2 cm beyond the tube length; suction on the way out. (Remove the inner cannula from the tube to measure against the suction catheter to get an idea of length). - Remember to re-oxygenate* the patient after suctioning. - If you are unable to pass suction beyond the length of the tube, refer to the conscious patient algorithm.
*High-flow oxygen 15 l/min, tracheostomy O$_2$ mask at the neck, non-rebreather mask over the nose and mouth.

Emergency Tracheostomy and Laryngectomy Pre-Hospital Management

Figure 2.13 – Tracheostomy.

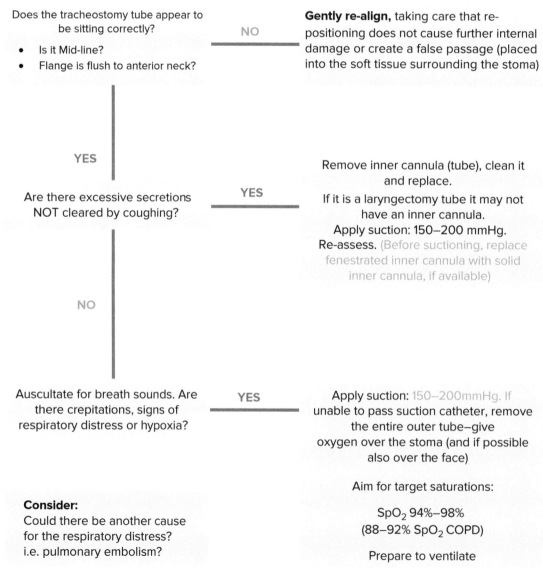

Does the tracheostomy tube appear to be sitting correctly?

- Is it Mid-line?
- Flange is flush to anterior neck?

NO → **Gently re-align,** taking care that re-positioning does not cause further internal damage or create a false passage (placed into the soft tissue surrounding the stoma)

YES

Are there excessive secretions NOT cleared by coughing?

YES → Remove inner cannula (tube), clean it and replace.

If it is a laryngectomy tube it may not have an inner cannula.

Apply suction: 150–200 mmHg.

Re-assess. (Before suctioning, replace fenestrated inner cannula with solid inner cannula, if available)

NO

Auscultate for breath sounds. Are there crepitations, signs of respiratory distress or hypoxia?

YES → Apply suction: 150–200mmHg. If unable to pass suction catheter, remove the entire outer tube–give oxygen over the stoma (and if possible also over the face)

Aim for target saturations:

SpO_2 94%–98%
(88–92% SpO_2 COPD)

Prepare to ventilate

Consider:
Could there be another cause for the respiratory distress? i.e. pulmonary embolism?

Figure 2.14 – Steps for confirming tracheostomy patency on the conscious patient.

Emergency Tracheostomy and Laryngectomy Pre-Hospital Management

Is the patient presenting with respiratory distress or dyspnoea? — NO → **Assess as appropriate to presenting complaint**

yes

Consider requesting support (Enhanced Care)

Assess breathing at MOUTH and NECK
Attach EtCO$_2$ to inner cannula – a positive reading indicates a patent, or partially patent, airway.

Commence CPR if no signs of life ← NO — **Is the patient breathing?** — YES → **Hi-flow O$_2$ to face and neck (15 1/min)**

Assess tracheostomy/stoma patency.
Remove the stoma cover, speaking valve or cap (if present).
Remove inner tube and clear blockage – may need to be replaced with non-fenestrated inner tube.
If it's a laryngectomy tube it may not have an inner-cannula – move on to the next step.
DO NOT remove tracheoesophageal puncture (TEP) prosthesis.

Can you pass a suction catheter? — YES → **Tracheostomy tube/stoma is patent;** Perform tracheal suction (150–200mmHg). Ventilate via tracheostomy if not breathing. Continue ABCDE assessment. **Remain alert as there may be a partial obstruction.**

NO

Deflate the cuff (if present).

If the patent breathing adequately? — YES → **Tracheostomy tube/stoma partially obstructed or displaced:** Continue ABCDE assessment.

NO

Remove the whole tube (if present).
Assess breathing at mouth and neck.

Is the patient breathing? — YES → **Continue ABCDE assessment.**

NO

Commence CPR if no signs of life.

TRACHEOSTOMY | **LARYNGECTOMY or uncertain**

STEPWISE APPROACH

Cover the stoma (swabs/hand).
Attempt to ventilate via MOUTH–LOOK FOR CHEST RISE

Ventilate the STOMA with a paediatric face mask or adult SGA or I gel attached to an adult bag and valve, occlude the mouth and nose.

Do not move to next step if this is successful | Do not move to next step if this is successful

Attempt inserting tube into STOMA: open the stoma with a finger if it has closed, gently insert a bougie and carefully railroad a size 6 ET tube up to the first black line and inflate cuff.

Last resort: If all else fails and airway remains closed you could try inserting a spare tracheostomy tube, attempt to fashion a bougie from a soft suction catheter to allow an ET tube to be placed over or insert finger to open stoma and use as a guide to slide the ET or tracheostomy tube in next to it). Always remember to attach EtCO2.

Be mindful that this is a last resort and will be dependent on what equipment is available to you at the time, i.e. the soft suction catheter will have to be cut off at the top to allow an ET tube to be railroaded meaning you will need another soft catheter to continue suctioning.

Figure 2.15 – Emergency tracheostomy and laryngectomy management.

Emergency Tracheostomy and Laryngectomy Pre-Hospital Management

TABLE 2.7 – Glossary of Commonly used Tracheostomy/Laryngectomy Terms	
Tracheotomy/tracheostomy	Technically, the suffix -otomy means 'to cut into'. The suffix -ostomy means 'opening into'. So a tracheotomy is the surgical procedure to create an opening into the trachea to enable a tracheostomy.
Inner and outer cannula	The inner part of the tracheostomy tube can be removed, cleaned or replaced. The outer part of the tube stays in place.
Cuff Republished with permission of Fuji Systems.	The balloon at the end of the tracheostomy tube that can be inflated, similar to that of inflatable cuffs on ET tubes.
De-cannulation	Removal or accidental removal of the whole tracheostomy tube.
Fenestrated tracheostomy tube Republished with permission of Kapitex.	The word fenestration comes from the French word fenêtre, meaning window. A fenestration is an opening in the shaft of the tube allowing air to pass through. This allows people to speak when it is correctly fitted. **NB** A fenestrated inner cannula must be removed and replaced with a non-fenestrated inner cannula before suctioning.
Flange Republished with permission of Kapitex.	The part of the tracheostomy tube that fits against the anterior neck and around the stoma. It also carries written information about the tube. The flange provides anchoring for securing straps and stops the tube from slipping into the stoma.
Laryngectomee	A person who has had a laryngectomy.
Laryngectomy	The surgical removal of the larynx.

SECTION 2 Resuscitation

TABLE 2.7 – Glossary of Commonly used Tracheostomy/Laryngectomy Terms *(continued)*

Mucus plug	An accumulation of mucus that can obstruct the lumen of the tracheostomy tube.
Speaking valve Republished with permission of Kapitex.	Usually a one-way valve that fits on the tracheostomy tube. It allows air to pass into the tracheostomy, but closes with exhalation, forcing air into the mouth and nose which allows speech. Used only on cuffless tubes or in 'cuff down' mode. This is more commonly known as a 'Passey Muir valve' by patients, family and carers.
Stoma	Translates as 'mouth' in Greek. It refers to the skin around the opening.
Suctioning	Removal of tracheal secretions or blood in the airway.
Heat moisture exchanger (HME) Republished with permssion of Intersurgical.	A device that fits on the tracheostomy tube. It collects exhaled water vapour, allowing it to be inhaled, which aids humidification. Patient or family may know this as a 'Swedish nose'.
Laryngectomy tube Republished with permission of Kapitex.	This appears very similar to the tracheostomy tubes but with no inner cannula. It is for use in laryngectomies and is placed to support the stoma.

(continued)

Emergency Tracheostomy and Laryngectomy
Pre-Hospital Management

TABLE 2.7 – Glossary of Commonly used Tracheostomy/Laryngectomy Terms *(continued)*

Buchanan bibs	Buchanan DeltaNex® is a three-layer system with a hydrolox foam core and a breathable soft cotton outer mesh. It is designed specifically for airway protection, to filter fine particles and allow moisture transfer. It is a bib of plastic foam covered with knitted fabric of honeycomb pattern. The neck band includes Velcro strips for fastening onto the strip on the bib and around the neck.
Republished with permission of Kapitex.	
Phonation	Using the voice.

TABLE 2.8 – Stepwise Approach to Airway Management

A tracheostomy tube in situ with a dressing, neck tie, cuffed tube and a heat moisture exchanger (HME). 1. Any attachment that covers the tube must be removed if the patient is experiencing difficulty in breathing. Ensure that the tube is in neutral alignment.	
2. Dependant on the manufacturer, the inner part of the tracheostomy tube can be removed either by twisting and gently extracting or by directly pulling out, dependent on the manufacturer. It can then be cleaned or replaced. The outer part of the tube stays in place. The BVM and catheter mount will fit to the inner cannula. They may also fit to some tracheostomy tubes once the inner cannula has been removed, though this is not universally the case and depends on the manufacturer.	

Emergency Tracheostomy and Laryngectomy Pre-Hospital Management

TABLE 2.8 – Stepwise Approach to Airway Management *(continued)*

3. If there are **no airway problems** and the **airway is patent,** you can use a **CUFFED** tube with the inner tube in place as an advanced airway. The cuff must be inflated to achieve positive pressure ventilations. $EtCO_2$ must be recorded to confirm advance airway. **Look for equal bilateral chest rise.**	
4. If the tube is blocked, it must be removed. As a last resort open the stoma with a finger if it has closed, gently insert a bougie and carefully railroad a size 6 ET tube up to the first black line. Inflate the cuff. This is a two-person procedure; be gentle in your technique and remember the delicate nature of tracheal tissue. Be careful not to create a false passage by inserting the tube into the subcutaneous tissue rather than the stoma.	
5. Once the cuff is inflated, attach the catheter mount, filter, $EtCO_2$ line and BVM. **Do not let go of the tube, and do not use a Thomas™ tube holder.** Best practice is to appoint someone to hold the tube and monitor the airway constantly. This is a two-person technique. **Look for equal bilateral chest rise.** If there is no chest rise and surgical emphysema develops in the neck, a false passage has been created and the ET tube should be removed.	
6. If the tracheostomy tube is blocked, it must be removed. The nose and mouth must be occluded to prevent any air escape. Use a small paediatric mask attached to an adult bag and valve, seal over the stoma and ventilate the patient, you can also use an i-Gel to cover the stoma if required. This is best carried out as a two-person technique. **Look for equal bilateral chest rise.**	

Images republished with kind permission of Dorothy Antrim, London Ambulance Service.

Emergency Tracheostomy and Laryngectomy Pre-Hospital Management

KEY POINTS!

Emergency Tracheostomy and Laryngectomy Pre-Hospital Management

- A third of deaths associated with tracheostomy and laryngectomy patients are due to hypoxia caused by a blocked tube.
- Early recognition of a blocked tube is vital.
- Inability to pass suction catheters beyond the tube indicates a blockage.
- Accidental removal of the whole tracheostomy tube (de-cannulation) is a TIME-CRITICAL emergency.
- Try to remember to take the patient's emergency box to hospital; it contains their appropriately sized tubes.
- NEVER reintroduce a tracheostomy tube.
- Emphasis must be on oxygenation to reverse the hypoxia together with reassurance.
- Always be prepared to ventilate airway-compromised patients.

Acknowledgements

Acknowledgements to Jacqueline Mitchell, CNS Tracheostomy Specialist at Guy's and St Thomas' NHS Foundation Trust; Lewis Etherington at London Ambulance Service; and Dr Lucy Bates at the National Tracheostomy Safety Project.

Bibliography

1. McGrath BA. Executive summary key recommendations. In BA McGrath, *Comprehensive Tracheostomy Care*. Chichester: John Wiley & Sons Ltd, 2014: xix.

2. Wilkinson KA, Freeth H, Kelly K. On the right trach. A review of care received by patients who underwent a tracheostomy. *British Journal of Hospital Medicine* 2014, 76(3): 163–165.

3. Goon PKC, Stanley MA, Ebmeyer J, Steinsträsser L, Upile T et al. HPV and head and neck cancer: a descriptive update. *Head and Neck Oncology* 2009, 1: 36.

4. Feber T. Tracheostomy care for community nurses: basic principles. *British Journal of Community Nursing* 2016, 11(5): 186–193.

5. Heathline. *Laryngectomy: Purpose, Procedure, and Recovery*. Available from: https://www.healthline.com/health/laryngectomy.

6. McGrath et al. Improving tracheostomy care in the United Kingdom: results of a guided quality improvement programme in 20 diverse hospitals. *British Journal of Anaesthesia* 2020, 125(1): e119–112.

SECTION
2
Resuscitation

Foreign Body Airway Obstruction

1. Introduction

- Foreign body airway obstruction (FBAO) is an uncommon but potentially treatable cause of accidental death.

- Most cases occur when eating or playing (in children) and are consequently witnessed. Therefore, interventions are usually initiated when the patient is conscious.

- The signs and symptoms vary, depending on the degree of airway obstruction (refer to Table 2.9).

- FBAO is characterised by the sudden onset of respiratory distress associated with coughing, gagging or stridor.

- Similar signs and symptoms may also be associated with other causes of airway obstruction such as laryngitis or epiglottitis, which tend to be of slower onset and require different management.

- This guideline covers:
  - infants (defined as under one year old)
  - children (defined as between one year and 18 years of age)
  - adults (aged >18 years of age).

- In this guideline, the term 'child' includes infants, unless specified otherwise.

2. General Management Principles

- When a foreign body enters the airway, the patient will usually react immediately by coughing in an attempt to expel it.

- A spontaneous cough is likely to be more effective and safer than any manoeuvre a rescuer might perform.

- If coughing is absent or ineffective and the object completely obstructs the airway, the patient will rapidly become asphyxiated.

- Active interventions to remove FBAO are only required when coughing becomes ineffective; but when required, these should be commenced confidently and rapidly.

- A high index of suspicion of airway obstruction must be maintained where airway compromise is noted, and paramedics should examine the oropharynx with a laryngoscope at an early stage if chest rise is not witnessed.

- Finger sweeps are not recommended, particularly when paramedics have the benefit of McGill forceps and suction, as they may drive any foreign body deeper into the airway. If an obstruction is seen and it can be grasped easily, make an attempt to remove it with forceps and/or suction.

- There will be occasions when a patient who has a DNACPR form may have a cardiac arrest that is considered unnatural and not in the envisaged circumstances and has a potentially reversible cause such as choking. All reversible causes should be considered (refer to Section 10, ALS Reversible Causes). In these circumstances, resuscitation and rapid conveyance to hospital should be considered, as the cause of the arrest is unrelated to their main clinical problem(s) and could be reversible.

TABLE 2.9 – General Signs of Foreign Body Airway Obstruction	
Mild airway obstruction	**Severe airway obstruction**

- The patient is able to:
  - speak
  - cough
  - breathe.
	- The patient is unable to:
	  - speak
	  - breathe.
	- Attempts at coughing are silent.
	- The patient may be unconscious.

Other indicators

- The episode was witnessed.
- The patient may clutch their neck.
- The patient may appear panicked or anxious.
- Coughing or choking may be present:
  - Cough may be ineffective, silent, quiet or loud.
- A stridor or wheeze may be present.
- Onset is sudden.
- There is recent history of playing with, or eating, small objects.
- The patient is cyanosed.
- The patient has a decreasing level of consciousness.
- The patient was able to breathe before coughing.

Foreign Body Airway Obstruction

3. Assessment and Management

For the assessment and management of foreign body airway obstruction, refer to Table 2.10.

TABLE 2.10 – Foreign Body Airway Obstruction (FBAO)
Assess for Severity of Obstruction
Adult, Child > 1 year and Infant < 1 year
▪ Consider enhanced care.
▪ Determine the patient's level of consciousness.
▪ Refer to Table 2.9.
▪ Consider severe allergic reaction which can cause airway obstruction (refer to **Allergic Reactions including Anaphylaxis**).
Mild Airway Obstruction
Adult and Child > 1 year
▪ Encourage the patient to cough but do nothing else.
▪ Monitor carefully and re-assess frequently.
▪ Rapid transport to hospital.
Infant < 1 year
▪ Monitor carefully and re-assess frequently.
▪ Rapid transport to hospital.
Severe Airway Obstruction – Conscious Patient
Adult and Child > 1 year
▪ Give up to 5 back blows – after each back blow, check to see if the obstruction has been relieved.
▪ If 5 back blows do not relieve the airway obstruction, give up to 5 abdominal thrusts.
▪ These manoeuvres increase intrathoracic pressure and may dislodge the foreign body.
▪ Alternate these until the obstruction is relieved or the patient loses consciousness.
Infant < 1 year
▪ Give up to 5 back blows – after each back blow, check to see if the obstruction has been relieved.
▪ If 5 back blows do not relieve the airway obstruction, give up to 5 **CHEST** thrusts.
▪ These manoeuvres increase intrathoracic pressure and may dislodge the foreign body.
▪ Alternate these until the obstruction is relieved or the infant loses consciousness.
Severe Airway Obstruction – Unconscious Patient
Adult, Child > 1 year and Infant < 1 year
▪ Open the mouth and look for any obvious obstruction.
▪ Attempt to visualise the vocal cords with a laryngoscope.
▪ If an obstruction is seen and it can be grasped easily, make an attempt to remove it with forceps, or suction.
▪ **DO NOT** attempt finger sweeps – these can cause injury and force the object more deeply into the pharynx.
▪ If the patient is unconscious or becomes unconscious, begin basic life support (refer to **Basic Life Support in Adults** and **Basic Life Support in Children**).
▪ If all other measures fail and airway remains obstructed, also consider cricothyroidotomy or surgical airway (<u>not</u> infants) where trained and authorised.
▪ During CPR, the patient's mouth should be checked for any foreign body that has been partly expelled each time the airway is opened.

Foreign Body Airway Obstruction

TABLE 2.10 – Foreign Body Airway Obstruction (FBAO) *(continued)*

Additional Information

Adult, Child and Infant

- Chest thrusts/compressions generate a higher airway pressure than back blows.
- Following successful treatment for FBAO, foreign material may remain in the upper or lower respiratory tract and cause complications later.
- Patients with a persistent cough, difficulty swallowing or the sensation of an object being stuck in the throat must be assessed further.
- Abdominal thrusts can cause serious internal injuries and all patients who receive them must be assessed for injury in hospital.
- Infants (< 1 year of age): 5 back blows, alternating with 5 chest thrusts. Child (> 1 year of age): 5 back blows, alternating with 5 abdominal thrusts.

Back Blows

Child > 1 year

- Back blows are more effective if the child is positioned head down.
- A small child may be placed across the rescuer's lap.
- If this is not possible, support the child in a forward-leaning position and deliver the back blows from behind.

Infant < 1 year

- Support the infant in a head-down, prone position, to allow gravity to assist the removal of the foreign body.
- Support the infant's head by placing the thumb of one hand at the angle of the lower jaw, with one or two fingers from the same hand at the same point on the other side of the jaw.
- Do not compress the soft tissues under the infant's jaw, as this will exacerbate the airway obstruction.
- Deliver up to 5 sharp back blows with the heel of one hand in the middle of the back between the shoulder blades, aiming to relieve the obstruction with each blow.

Chest/Abdominal Thrusts

Abdominal thrusts – children

- Stand or kneel behind the child. Place your arms under the child's arms and encircle their torso.
- Clench your fist and place it between the umbilicus and the xiphisternum. Grasp this hand with the other hand and pull sharply inwards and upwards.
- Repeat up to 5 times (if required).
- Ensure that pressure is not applied to xiphoid process or lower rib cage (as this may result in abdominal trauma).

Chest thrusts – infants

- Turn the infant into a head-down, supine position (this can be safely achieved by placing the paramedic's arm along the infant's back and encircling the occiput with the hand). Rest this arm against a solid surface or the paramedic's thigh.
- Identify the landmark for chest compression (lower sternum, approximately a finger's breadth above the xiphisternum).
- Deliver 5 chest thrusts (if required).
- These are similar to external chest compressions but sharper in nature and delivered at a slower rate.

Foreign Body Airway Obstruction

Adult choking

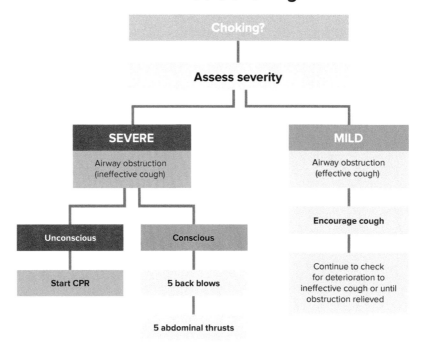

Figure 2.16 – Foreign body airway obstruction in adults. Reproduced with permission from the Resuscitation Council (UK) Guidelines 2021 algorithm (www.resus.org.uk).

Paediatric foreign body airway obstruction

Figure 2.17 – Foreign body airway obstruction in children (modified). Reproduced with permission from the Resuscitation Council (UK) Guidelines 2021 algorithm (www.resus.org.uk).

Foreign Body Airway Obstruction

Foreign Body Airway Obstruction

- FBAO is a potentially treatable cause of death that often occurs while playing or eating. It is more common in children.

- It is characterised by the sudden onset of respiratory distress.

- If the patient is coughing effectively, encourage them to cough.

- If coughing is ineffective, back blows should initially be given.

- If the patient becomes unconscious, use chest thrusts in infants and abdominal thrusts in children and adults.

- Avoid finger sweeps; use suction and/or McGill forceps.

- Check after each manoeuvre to see if the obstruction is removed.

- If the object is expelled successfully, assess the patient's clinical condition. It is possible that part of the object may remain in the respiratory tract and cause complications.

- Abdominal thrusts may cause internal injury – patients who have received abdominal thrusts require further hospital assessment.

Bibliography

1. Perkins GD, Handley AJ, Koster RW, Castrén M, Smyth MA, Olasveengen T et al. European Resuscitation Council Guidelines for Resuscitation 2015: Section 2. Adult basic life support. *Resuscitation* 2015, 95: 81–99. Available from: https://cprguidelines.eu/sites/573c777f5e61585a053d7ba5/content_entry573c77e35e61585a053d7baf/573c781e5e61585a053d7bd1/files/S0300-9572_15_00327-5_main.pdf.

2. Maconochie I, Bingham R, Eich C, López-Herce J, Rodriguez-Nunez A, Rajka T, Van de Voorde P, Zideman D, Biarent D. European Resuscitation Council Guidelines for Resuscitation 2015: Section 6. Paediatric life support. *Resuscitation* 2015, 95: 223–248. Available from: https://www.resuscitationjournal.com/article/S0300-9572(15)00340-8/fulltext.

3. Resuscitation Council (UK). *Adult Basic Life Support and Automated External Defibrillation 2021*. London: Resuscitation Council (UK), 2021. Available from: https://www.resus.org.uk/resuscitation-guidelines/adult-basic-life-support-and-automated-external-defibrillation.

4. Resuscitation Council (UK). *Paediatric Resuscitation Guidelines 2021*. London: Resuscitation Council (UK), 2021. Available from: https://www.resus.org.uk/resuscitation-guidelines/paediatric-basic-life-support/.

Return of Spontaneous Circulation

1. Introduction

- Gaining return of spontaneous circulation (ROSC) is the initial step towards recovery from out-of-hospital cardiac arrest (OHCA). As such, it is important that paramedics are aware of the critical nature of the post-ROSC patient. A large proportion of patients who have achieved ROSC will re-arrest, the chances of which are minimised by appropriate and timely post-ROSC care.

- Undertake an accurate and complete patient assessment and rapidly provide all interventions to ensure that the patient's condition has been optimised before transfer to hospital, except where an intervention only available in hospital is required or it is unsafe to remain on scene.

- Be prepared for re-arrest; the recurrence rate of a shockable rhythm is at its highest during this period.

- Following ROSC, patients may present with a varying degree of post-cardiac arrest syndrome. Post-cardiac arrest syndrome comprises four key elements:

  – **Brain injury** – coma, seizures, myoclonus, varying degrees of neurocognitive dysfunction and brain death; this may be exacerbated by microcirculatory failure, impaired autoregulation, hypercarbia, hyperoxia, pyrexia, hyper/hypoglycaemia and ongoing seizures.
  – **Myocardial dysfunction** – this is common after cardiac arrest, but usually improves in the following weeks.
  – **Systemic ischemia/reperfusion response** – the whole-body ischaemia/reperfusion that occurs with resuscitation from cardiac arrest activates immunological and coagulation pathways contributing to a systemic inflammatory response syndrome (SIRS).
  – **Persistence of the precipitating pathology.**

- The management of post-cardiac arrest syndrome requires ambulance paramedics to assimilate their clinical assessment and findings, with a view to targeting therapy to the patient's needs.

2. Assessment and Management

TABLE 2.11 – ASSESSMENT and MANAGEMENT of: Return of Spontaneous Circulation
Return of Spontaneous Circulation
▪ Early recurrence of VF is common; ensure appropriate ongoing monitoring through defibrillator pads.
▪ Undertake a structured <C>ABCD assessment that enables appropriate treatment to be applied, as described in the immediate management below. Consider and continue to treat any reversible cause of the initial cardiac arrest. Refer to **Medical Emergencies in Adults – Overview** and **Medical Emergencies in Children – Overview**.
▪ Measure and record a full set of observations and repeat these at regular intervals.
▪ Early optimisation of airway, breathing and circulatory support will assist in the heart and brain recovery.
▪ Forward planning – ensure appropriate resources are on scene or requested to the scene; this may include enhanced care.
▪ Consider the extrication plan and facilitate preparations for extrication and onward transfer.
▪ Transfer the patient directly to the nearest appropriate hospital in accordance with local pathways for primary percutaneous coronary intervention (PPCI) or ECMO (where available).
▪ Provide an ATMIST pre-alert call to the receiving facility.
Airway and Breathing
▪ Ensure an effective airway; consider enhanced care support for advanced airway insertion or maintenance.
▪ Maintain oxygen saturations of 94–98%; titrate oxygen to prevent hypoxia or hyperoxia. Refer to **Oxygen**.
▪ Assist ventilations where required.
▪ Use of a mechanical ventilator (if available) is preferable to manual ventilation; ensure the settings are appropriate for age, weight and rate (generally a tidal volume of 6–7 ml/kg with a rate of 10/min).
▪ Monitor waveform capnography.
▪ Ventilate lungs to normocarbia (4.6–6.0 kPa); consider the reason for readings that fall outside normocarbia, i.e. is this a perfusion, ventilation or metabolic issue?

Return of Spontaneous Circulation

TABLE 2.11 – ASSESSMENT and MANAGEMENT of: Return of Spontaneous Circulation *(continued)*

Circulation

- Perform a 12-lead ECG.

NB Post-ROSC ECGs frequently demonstrate a 'recovering heart'; therefore, ECGs should be obtained at regular intervals.

- Ensure adequate vascular access.

- Following ROSC, patients are often haemodynamically unstable, arrhythmogenic and hypotensive. Aim for a systolic blood pressure (SBP) >100 mmHg. In patients with an adequate heart rate, attempt to achieve this with IV (or IO) fluids, together with IV (or IO) adrenaline (see below for the management of **bradycardia**).

- Most patients who suffer a cardiac arrest due to a cardiac cause are not hypovolaemic, but vasodilation may result in the circulation being relatively underfilled. Administer a 250 ml IV/IO bolus of 0.9% saline, repeated as necessary to a maximum of 500 ml. Patients with sepsis, anaphylaxis, respiratory conditions and dehydration may benefit from larger volumes; seek medical advice in these cases.

- Although 250–500 ml of IV (or IO) fluid may support the circulation, it may take several minutes to administer. If hypotension is present during or after this fluid administration, provide additional circulatory support using careful administration of an adrenaline bolus, repeated as required, every 3–5 mins to maintain the systolic BP >100 mmHg.
  - Initial dose: 50 mcg (0.05 mg) IV/IO. (0.5 ml from a 1:10,000 pre-filled 10 ml adrenaline syringe).
  - Subsequent doses: 50–100 mcg (0.05–0.10 mg). (0.5–1.0 ml from a 1:10,000 pre-filled 10 ml adrenaline syringe).

- Follow each adrenaline bolus with a flush of 20 ml 0.9% normal saline.

- In the event of symptomatic bradycardia in adults (HR <60/min), atropine should be administered.

- In the event of symptomatic bradycardia in children/infants, first ensure that hypoxia has been reversed (the commonest cause of bradycardia). Refer to **Atropine Sulfate**, **Page for Age** for children.

- If bradycardia persists, external pacing should be considered.

Control Temperature

- There is no evidence that cooling patients post-ROSC is of benefit, but extremes of temperature are harmful. Some patients post ROSC will have a mild hypothermia. Use no more clothing/blankets than is necessary. Vehicle heating is only required to provide a comfortable ambient temperature.

- Aim for a core temperature no higher than 37.5°C.

Blood Glucose Level

- Measure and record blood glucose for hypo/hyperglycaemia (refer to **Glycaemic Emergencies in Adults and Children**).

- Accuracy of blood glucose measurements immediately following ROSC may be impaired by capillary blood stasis. Venous blood glucose is preferred to capillary samples and should be measured and repeated 10 minutes following ROSC.

Combative Patient

- Following ROSC, patients may be cerebrally irritated, agitated or combative, which can make oxygenation difficult.

- Exclude hypoglycaemia and hypoxaemia.

- Try to establish why the patient may be agitated, such as in pain, need for oxygenation or airway device removal.

- If available, request additional support from enhanced care teams to consider the need for anaesthetic management or sedation, as per local procedures.

- This should only be provided by defined teams or individuals in line with robust governance and scope of practice.

(continued)

SECTION **2**

Return of Spontaneous Circulation

TABLE 2.11 – ASSESSMENT and MANAGEMENT of: Return of Spontaneous Circulation *(continued)*
Pain Relief
▪ CPR is a painful procedure, therefore the patient is likely to be in pain.
▪ Consider the provision of analgesia (IV paracetamol, supplemented with small dose of opiates) following resuscitation efforts.
▪ Observe and manage respiratory function after opiate administration.
Seizure Control
▪ Seizures that do not self-terminate within 5 minutes may be treated with a benzodiazepine (refer to **Diazepam, Page for Age** for children).
▪ The administration of diazepam or midazolam (where available) should be carried out in line with clinical practice guidelines or PGD (in the context of midazolam).

3. Disposition

▪ Acute coronary syndrome (ACS) is a frequent cause of OHCA. Adult patients with a cardiac arrest of presumed primary cardiac aetiology should be transported directly to a hospital with 24/7 coronary angiography capability (this includes both STEMI and non-STEMI patients).

▪ Adult patients with non-traumatic OHCA should be considered for transport to a recognised centre of care for appropriate specialist treatment, according to local protocols. There is no evidence for a preference for a policy of primarily transporting via ambulance (using bypass protocols) or one of secondary inter-hospital transfer.

▪ Patients who obtain ROSC following traumatic cardiac arrest should be conveyed in line with the local major trauma pathways, normally to a major trauma centre, assuming criteria for trauma unit bypass are met.

Bibliography

1. Nolan JP, Sandroni C, Bottiger B et al. European Resuscitation Council and European Society of Intensive Care Medicine Guidelines 2021. Post-resuscitation care. *Intensive Care Med* 2021, 47: 369–421. Available from: https://link.springer.com/content/pdf/10.1007/s00134-021-06368-4.pdf.

2. Nolan JP, Neumar RW, Adrie C et al. Post-cardiac arrest syndrome: epidemiology, pathophysiology, treatment, and prognostication: A Scientific Statement from the International Liaison Committee on Resuscitation; the American Heart Association Emergency Cardiovascular Care Committee; the Council on Cardiovascular Surgery and Anesthesia; the Council on Cardiopulmonary, Perioperative, and Critical Care; the Council on Clinical Cardiology; the Council on Stroke. *Resuscitation* 2008, 79: 350–379. Available from: https://www.ilcor.org/data/Post-cardiac_arrest_syndrome.pdf.

3. Dankiewicz J, Cronberg T, Lilja J et al. Hypothermia versus normothermia after out-of-hospital cardiac arrest. *N Engl J Med* 2021, 384: 2283–2294. Available from: https://www.nejm.org/doi/pdf/10.1056/NEJMoa2100591?articleTools=true.

Return of Spontaneous Circulation

Prepare for Transfer

a. Early recurrence of VF is common; ensure appropriate ongoing monitoring through defibrillator pads.

b. Transfer the patient directly to the nearest appropriate hospital in accordance with local pathways.

c. Provide an ATMIST pre-alert call to the receiving facility.

Airway & Breathing

a. Ensure an effective airway; consider enhanced support

b. Record and maintain oxygen saturations of 94–98%, refer to Oxygen.

c. Monitor waveform capnography.

d. Ventilate lungs to normocarbia (4.6–6.0 kPa)

Circulation

a. Record Blood Pressure and aim for SBP > 100 mmHg.

b. First: Fluid (crystalloid) - restore normovolaemia. Refer to Intravascular Fluid in Adults and Intravascular Fluid in Children.

c. Second: Consider small doses of adrenaline to support the circulation if unresponsive to fluid resuscitation – refer to Adrenaline.

d. In the event of symptomatic bradycardia, atropine should be administered, refer to Atropine.

ECG

Perform a 12-lead ECG

Temperature

a. Measure temperature.

b. Patients post-ROSC should be allowed to cool passively.

BM

Measure and record blood glucose for hypo/hyperglycaemia, refer to Glycaemic Emergencies in Adults and Children.

Other

a. Consider the provision of analgesia (small dose opiates or IV Paracetamol) for the management of pain

b. Seizures that do not self-terminate within five minutes may be treated with a benzodiazepine, refer to Diazepam.

c. Combative patients may benefit from anaesthetic management or sedation. Consider enhanced care.

Figure 2.18 – Assessment and management of return of spontaneous circulation (ROSC).

Termination of Resuscitation and Verification of Death in Adults

1. Introduction

Clinical management aims to differentiate between those for whom cardiac arrest is their natural end of life event and for whom resuscitation is not indicated, and those where there is a chance to restore life to a quality acceptable to the patient and in accordance with their wishes, through provision of optimum pre-hospital care.

- Where no explicit decision about CPR has been considered and recorded in advance, there should be an initial presumption in favour of CPR.

- However, in some circumstances where there is no recorded explicit decision regarding CPR, but death is imminent and unavoidable and CPR would not be successful (for example, a person in the advanced stages of an irreversible illness), a decision not to commence CPR should be considered in order to allow a natural death to occur. For patients in whom there is no chance of survival, CPR is not supported; for example:
  - where resuscitation would be both futile and distressing for the patient, relatives, friends and healthcare personnel
  - where time and resources would be ineffective undertaking such measures.

- Every effort should be made to identify patients with a DNACPR decision, Recommended Summary Plan for Emergency Care and Treatment (ReSPECT) form, treatment escalation plan or Advance Decision to Refuse Treatment (ADRT).

- The views of the patient's general practitioner (GP) or relevant third party should be considered. Ask if the patient has a care plan or ADRT in place. Family members may be able to provide verbal information about the patient's wishes, although this is not legally binding in this format.

- CPR should not be attempted, or it should be abandoned if already started by the general public or volunteer responders, if the ambulance clinician is as certain as they can be that a person is dying as an inevitable result of underlying disease (it is therefore their natural end of life event) and CPR would not restart the heart and breathing for a sustained period.

- Where there is uncertainty, it is acceptable to commence basic life support (BLS) while further information is rapidly gathered to enable the decision to be made about whether resuscitation can be stopped.

- On rare occasions, it may be appropriate to continue CPR until patient privacy and dignity can be assured, before stopping the resuscitation attempt.

- Refer to local policies and procedures regarding the clinical grade of ambulance clinician that is permitted to undertake verification of death.

2. Conditions Unequivocally Associated with Death in Adults

The following conditions are unequivocally associated with death in adults (for children, refer to **Termination of Resuscitation and Verification of Death in Children**), and can be used by ambulance clinicians to verify death:

- **Decapitation**.

- **Massive cranial and cerebral destruction**.

- **Hemicorporectomy** or similar massive injury.

- **Decomposition/putrefaction** – where tissue damage indicates that the patient has been dead for some hours, days or longer.

- **Incineration** – the presence of full-thickness burns with charring of greater than 95% of the body surface.

- **Hypostasis** – the pooling of blood in congested vessels in the dependent part of the body in the position in which it lies after death. Initially, hypostatic staining may appear as small round patches looking rather like bruises but later these will combine to merge as the familiar pattern. Above the hypostatic engorgement, there is obvious pallor of the skin.

  The presence of hypostasis is diagnostic of death – the appearance is not present in a live patient. In extremely cold conditions, hypostasis may be bright red in colour, and in carbon monoxide poisoning it is characteristically 'cherry red' in appearance.

- **Rigor mortis** – the stiffness occurring after death from the post-mortem breakdown of enzymes in the muscle fibres.
  - Rigor mortis occurs first in the small muscles of the face, next in the arms, then in the legs, with these changes taking between 30 minutes and 3 hours. The recognition of rigor mortis can be made difficult where, rarely, death has occurred from tetanus or strychnine poisoning.
  - In some, rigidity never develops (infants, cachectic individuals and the aged), while in others it may become apparent more rapidly, i.e. in conditions in which muscle glycogen is depleted, e.g. exertion (which includes struggling), strychnine poisoning and local heat (e.g. from a fire, hot room or direct sunlight).
  - Rigor should not be confused with cadaveric spasm (sometimes referred to as instant rigor mortis), which develops immediately after death without preceding flaccidity following intense physical and/or emotional activity. Examples include death by drowning or a fall from a height. In contrast with true rigor mortis, only one group of muscles is affected and **not** the whole body. Rigor mortis will develop subsequently.

Termination of Resuscitation and Verification of Death in Adults

— Rigor is also distinct from trismus (spasm of the muscles around the jaw which may occur in those with a reduced level of consciousness). Rigor mortis is not isolated to jaw muscles alone.

Note:

In cases that do not meet these criteria, where it is thought that CPR is futile or inappropriate, do not withhold or terminate resuscitation until senior clinical advice has been sought.

If access to the patient is restricted and it is believed that one of the conditions above may exist, then a multi-agency decision (Fire, Police, Coast Guard etc.) should be made on whether ongoing rescue should continue or whether the incident becomes that of body recovery. The JESIP principles should be followed and include factors such as risks posed to the rescue teams.

3. Other Conditions Where Resuscitation May Be Withheld or Discontinued

- In addition to the conditions above, there are other criteria which can be used to confirm death, and which indicate that resuscitation should not be attempted, or may be discontinued:

A) The presence of a DNACPR (do not attempt cardiopulmonary resuscitation) decision or ReSPECT form that advises resuscitation is not to be attempted.

B) A valid Advance Decision to Refuse Treatment (ADRT), which refuses cardiopulmonary resuscitation, or a Lasting Power of Attorney (LPA) for Health and Welfare that includes decisions related to life-sustaining treatments and where CPR is refused by the attorney.

C) If a person is known to be in the final stages of an advanced, irreversible condition, in which attempted CPR would be both inappropriate and unsuccessful, CPR should not be started or can be stopped if already commenced. Even in the absence of a recorded DNACPR decision, ambulance clinicians may be able to recognise this situation and make an appropriate decision, based on clear evidence that they should document. Examples of clear evidence include the presence of anticipatory medications, hospice or palliative care notes and advance care plans, but always refer to local guidance. While seeking evidence or where there is doubt, it is appropriate to start BLS and seek senior clinical advice. The relatives/carers should be included in the decision making process.

> **NB: An advanced and irreversible condition** is an illness or injury that can no longer be cured and care is refocused to promote quality of life, comfort and symptom control. Examples of conditions are not confined to cancer, but also include organ failure (e.g. heart, respiratory, renal and liver), neurological illness (e.g. motor neurone disease, Parkinson's, Dementia) and advanced frailty in older people.

When identifying patients near end of life, it is useful to utilise available screening tools, such as the Gold Standards Framework (GSF) or the Supportive and Palliative Care Indicators Tool (SPICT). They offer insight into a patient's pattern of deterioration and an overall impression of their stage of illness. Further information to support this can also be gleaned from the patient's history, medical notes and any completed advance personalised care plan.

D) Submersion for longer than 90 minutes (refer to **Immersion and Drowning**).

E) There is no realistic chance that CPR would be successful if **ALL** the following exist together:

- >15 minutes has elapsed since the onset of cardiac arrest.
- No evidence of bystander CPR in the 15 minutes before the arrival of the ambulance.
- Exclusion factors are absent (drowning, hypothermia, poisoning/overdose, pregnancy, child/neonate).
- Asystole for >30 seconds on the ECG monitor screen. CPR should only be paused for a 30-second asystole check if all other criteria are met.

- Whenever possible, a confirmatory ECG demonstrating asystole should be documented as evidence of death. In this situation, a 3- or 4-electrode system using limbs alone will cause minimum disturbance to the deceased. If a paper ECG trace cannot be taken, it is permissible to make a diagnosis of asystole from the screen alone (**NB** due caution must be applied in respect of electrode contact, gain and, where possible, using more than one ECG lead).

- It is important that in order to confirm death, the rhythm is unequivocally persistent and continuous asystole. If CPR is stopped when any other rhythm is present (i.e. agonal rhythm or PEA), it is important to wait until all cardiac electrical activity has ceased and the ECG shows asystole. Only at this stage should the patient be declared life extinct and the family/relatives informed that this is the case. This is because there have been well-documented cases where spontaneous ROSC has occurred following termination of resuscitation.

Termination of Resuscitation and Verification of Death in Adults

4. Advance Care Planning

- Advance care planning is a voluntary process involving a person-centred discussion that helps an individual in understanding choices and sharing their preferences and priorities for future care.

- The aim of advance care planning is to ensure that individuals receive medical care that is appropriate and consistent with their values, goals and preferences, when they no longer have the mental capacity to make such decisions.

- The outcome of advance care planning discussions may include an ADRT, or context-specific recommendations such as emergency care plans or treatment escalation plans. A trusted person/s may also be nominated as an LPA with legal power to make medical treatment decisions, including life-sustaining treatment.

- A DNACPR decision is a part of advance care planning but differs as it is clinician led, in discussion with the patient and their family members wherever possible. The decision is based on a clinical assessment that the person is dying as an inevitable result of an advanced, irreversible disease and that CPR would not be successful and should not be attempted.

- Ambulance clinicians should be familiar with these documents and their legal standing; they are critical elements of resuscitation decision making.

4.1 Advance Decision to Refuse Treatment (ADRT)

- An ADRT enables a person over 18 years of age to refuse specified medical treatment in advance of a time where they are unable to consent or refuse treatment following the loss of mental capacity. **It is legally binding.**

  An ADRT in Scotland is known as an Advance Directive; they do not have the same legal recognition as in England and Wales but are widely recognised under common law and by healthcare professionals. In Northern Ireland, they are not legally recognised. Refer to local policies regarding use of these documents.

- ADRTs are defined within the Mental Capacity Act 2005 (MCA). Providing ADRTs meet all the requirements of the MCA, they are legally binding for health and social care professionals. This makes ADRTs quite distinct from other aspects of advance care planning.

- An ADRT must be valid and applicable to current circumstances. If it is, it has the same effect as a decision that is made by a person with capacity: healthcare professionals (including ambulance clinicians) must follow the decision.

- ADRTs are only valid if the patient is unconscious or lacks capacity. If the patient has capacity, their decision and wishes should be followed.

- Paramedics will be protected from liability if they:
  - stop or withhold treatment because they reasonably believe that an ADRT exists, and that it is valid and applicable
  - treat a person because, having taken all practical and appropriate steps to find out if the person has made an ADRT, they do not know or are not satisfied that a valid and applicable ADRT exists.

- There is no official form for recording an ADRT, although there are several well-known versions for completion. It can be informal, e.g. a hand-written paper copy; the important issue is that it fulfils the criteria for validity.

- If the advance decision refuses life-sustaining treatment, it **must**:
  - be in writing (if the patient cannot write it themselves, it is acceptable to have someone else write it but this must be signed and witnessed by an independent person)
  - be signed by the patient or another in their presence if they are unable to sign it themselves
  - specify the exact treatment being refused; this can be written in layperson's terms
  - specifically acknowledge an intention to refuse treatment even if this puts the patient's life at risk, and must include a statement to this effect
  - be witnessed and dated (there are no legal requirements on who should be a witness, except being over 18 years of age) and it is not necessary to involve a solicitor in this process.

- To establish whether an advance decision is valid and applicable, ambulance clinicians must take reasonable steps to find out if the person:
  - has done anything that clearly goes against their advance decision
  - has withdrawn their decision
  - has subsequently conferred the power to make that decision on an LPA
  - would have changed their decision if they had known more about the current circumstances.

- If any of these apply, then the ADRT is not considered to be valid or applicable. The ADRT would additionally not apply in cases of attempted suicide or suicide. In these cases, seeking urgent senior clinical support is advised.

- If there is any genuine doubt about the validity of an ADRT, ambulance clinicians must act in the patient's best interests. When an advance decision is not followed, the reasons must be clearly documented.

- In Scotland and Northern Ireland, ADRTs are not covered by statute but it is likely that they are

Termination of Resuscitation and Verification of Death in Adults

binding under common law. Although no cases have been taken to court in Scotland or Northern Ireland, it is likely that the principles that emerged from consideration of cases by the English courts (before the MCA) would also guide decision making in these jurisdictions.

- An advance refusal of CPR is likely to be legally binding in Scotland and Northern Ireland if:
  - the person was an adult at the time the decision was made (16 years old in Scotland and 18 in Northern Ireland)
  - the person had capacity when the decision was made
  - the circumstances that have arisen are those that were envisaged by the person
  - the person was not subjected to undue influence in making the decision.

- If an ADRT does not meet these criteria but appears to set out a clear indication of the person's wishes, it will not be legally binding but should be taken into consideration in determining the person's best interests.

4.2 Lasting Power of Attorney (LPA)

- An LPA is a **legally binding** document which allows someone to nominate another person (or persons) to make decisions on their behalf after they lose mental capacity. The document is completed in advance of that person losing capacity, during which time the person continues to make their own decisions.

- The document must be registered with the Office of the Public Guardian (England and Wales) or the Public Guardian (Scotland) and include their official stamp or crest. The original document or a certified copy must be viewed physically or digitally; in England and Wales, an LPA can be viewed online using an access code at www.gov. uk. In Northern Ireland, the Health and Welfare Power of Attorney does not exist.

- In England and Wales, there are two types of LPA: property and financial affairs and health and welfare. Only a health and welfare LPA allows healthcare decisions to be made on the person's behalf when they lack capacity. In Scotland, a Welfare Power of Attorney or Combined Power of Attorney allows an attorney to make decisions related to the person's health.

- An LPA can include decisions relating to life-sustaining treatment. If the donor wishes the attorney to be able to consent to or refuse life-sustaining treatment, it will be clearly included in the document. An attorney cannot insist on any treatment which is inappropriate, including resuscitation.

- The document should be viewed before basing a decision on information provided by the named individual.

- Where both an ADRT and LPA exist for a patient; if the ADRT is dated after the LPA, and is valid, then the ADRT should be followed. If the ADRT is dated prior to the LPA, then the decision of the attorney should be followed if the LPA applies in the specific situation and is in the patient's best interests.

- If there is any genuine doubt about the validity of an LPA, ambulance clinicians must act in the patient's best interests.

4.3 Do Not Attempt Cardiopulmonary Resuscitation (DNACPR) Decision

- A DNACPR decision is an advance clinical assessment, recorded to guide immediate decision making in the event of a cardiac arrest. DNACPR decisions are made when a person is near the end stage of an advanced, irreversible condition (or on some occasions sooner), to ensure that the individual is not exposed to the trauma and indignity of CPR, which has no realistic prospect of benefit.

- A DNACPR decision is **not legally binding** but is one of a number of elements to inform decision making regarding CPR. The final decision regarding whether or not attempting CPR is clinically appropriate lies with the healthcare professional who is responsible for their care at the time.

- The majority of DNACPR decisions are made for adults. Children with advanced irreversible conditions may have recorded within their care plan text stating that, following discussions with family and the child's healthcare team, CPR is not considered appropriate. (Refer to **Termination of Resuscitation and Verification of Death in Children**.)

- DNACPR decisions are only made for advanced, irreversible physical health conditions. Learning disabilities and/or autism are not physical health conditions and should never be used as rationale for a DNACPR decision.

- A DNACPR decision applies solely to cardiopulmonary resuscitation. All other treatment and care that a patient requires is not precluded or influenced by a DNACPR decision.

- DNACPR documents should, ideally, move with patients as they are transferred from one setting to another – particularly when death is expected (e.g. an end of life patient being discharged home to die). It is anticipated that the senior clinician responsible for the patient in each setting (e.g. the GP after patient discharge from hospital) will review the patient at the earliest opportunity. This may not always be possible and although processes can vary by locality, in principle the DNACPR decision remains valid.

Termination of Resuscitation and Verification of Death in Adults

4.4 Resuscitation Decision Making and DNACPR Decisions

- DNACPR recommendations and similar decisions are often recorded on a form approved by the organisation providing the care for the patient. The design and content of these forms can vary significantly.

- Care-planning documents can often contain DNACPR sections, or the decision may be documented in a letter, hospital discharge summary or as an entry in the patient's health records. Formal letters can also be used to communicate resuscitation instructions to other professionals. These are often communicated to ambulance control and logged against the patient's address, or the decision is available to access via an electronic care record database.

- It is important to note that all of the above are acceptable methods for recording and communicating resuscitation decisions. Documentation of the decision includes:
  - Patient identification (e.g. name, DOB, NHS number)
  - The decision, including the date it was made.
  - Rationale for making the decision
  - Name and position of the clinician making the decision
  - Information of any discussions about the decision with the patient and/or those close to them.

- If a review date is specified, expiry of that date DOES NOT invalidate the DNACPR. Many DNACPR forms/records will not have a review date; this is acceptable and indicates that the patient's condition is not expected to improve. A decision must be made and recorded by the ambulance clinician (with senior clinical advice if appropriate) as to whether the document is still considered valid.

- In the absence of the original copy, a photocopy can be considered valid. Refer to local policy as to whether additional verification is required, for example seeking confirmation that the photocopy is the most up-to-date version of the decision.

- Where a DNACPR exists, ambulance clinicians should support dying patients, provide appropriate comfort measures and support relatives and carers. Contact should be made with the patient's GP, district nursing team or specialist team, to arrange the provision of ongoing care and effective symptom control and to ensure the death is managed appropriately.

- Ambulance staff will be protected from liability if they stop or withhold resuscitation because they reasonably believe that a DNACPR exists, and that it is valid and applicable.

- Where there are concerns regarding the validity of the DNACPR decision and its authenticity cannot be confirmed, any evidence obtained should be taken into consideration in determining the person's best interests. This may require paramedics to provide BLS while they seek senior clinical advice.

- There will be occasions when a patient who has a DNACPR decision may have a cardiac arrest that is considered unnatural and not in the envisaged circumstances and has a potentially easily reversible cause (e.g. patient has taken an overdose, is choking or has anaphylaxis). All reversible causes should be considered (refer to Section 10 of **Advanced Life Support**). In these circumstances, resuscitation and rapid conveyance to hospital should be considered, as the cause of the arrest is unrelated to the patient's main clinical problem(s) and could be reversible. In these potentially reversible situations, it is vital to seek urgent senior clinical advice as per local policy. Documented DNACPR decisions are not valid in cases of suicide.

4.5 Recommended Summary Plan for Emergency Care and Treatment (ReSPECT)

- A ReSPECT form summarises treatments to be considered and those that would not be wanted or would not work for the patient in an emergency. It might include recommendations of when transfer to hospital would be desirable or not.

- ReSPECT is a summary of recommendations to help the ambulance clinician make immediate decisions about the patient's care and treatment. It contains recommendations about whether CPR should be attempted.

- A ReSPECT form contains more than a CPR decision: it is not just a replacement for a DNACPR form. It is to promote recording an emergency care plan by many people, and may recommend active treatment, including attempted CPR if it should be needed.

- Like a DNACPR form, it is **not legally binding**; clinical judgement must still be applied and ambulance clinicians may decide not to follow the recommendations on a ReSPECT form. However, paramedics should be prepared to justify valid reasons for overriding the recommendations on a ReSPECT form, remembering that the information contained reflects the patient's wishes and preferences. An example of such a decision would be treating an immediately reversible emergency such as choking if it was believed that this was not the circumstance envisaged when the decision was made for resuscitation not to be attempted.

- The ReSPECT form should be with the person and be readily available; in some areas it may be accessed electronically.

4.6 Best Interests Decision Making

- Ambulance clinicians must consider any evidence as an expression of previous wishes when

Termination of Resuscitation and Verification of Death in Adults

establishing the person's best interests. This may involve the provision of clinical treatment, including resuscitation.

■ It is the most senior member of the ambulance team in charge of a patient's care and treatment who must decide what is in the patient's best interests. However, joint decision making by the entire team is considered best practice.

■ Ambulance clinicians should be guided by advice from those close to a patient regarding the patient's previously expressed wishes and beliefs, even though the patient's spouse, family, friends or colleagues may not be entitled to give or withhold consent to treatment on the patient's behalf.

■ Decisions must not be based on assumptions made solely on factors such as the person's age, disability or a professional's subjective view of a person's quality of life.

■ Refer to the Mental Capacity Act Code of Practice (2007) for guidance on making best interests, decisions. In a resuscitation situation where there is uncertainty about what is in the patient's best interests, gather information rapidly and seek senior clinical support and/or advice from the patient's care team/GP.

5. Termination of Resuscitation

■ If there is a realistic chance that CPR could be successful, then resuscitation should continue to establish the patient's response to ALS interventions (ALS is defined in **Advanced Life Support**).

■ If, following ALS interventions, the patient has been **persistently and continuously** asystolic for 30 minutes and all reversible causes have been

identified and corrected, resuscitation may be discontinued, except in the following cases:

– pregnancy
– hypothermic patients (where hypothermia is the primary cause of the cardiac arrest)
– suspected drugs overdose/poisoning
– infants, children and adolescents (i.e. all those <18 years of age). (Refer to **Termination of Resuscitation and Verification of Death in Children**.)

■ These patients should be transported to the nearest facility with on going resuscitation, unless the circumstances would make transport futile.

5.1 Pulseless Electrical Activity

■ Pulseless electrical activity (PEA) is a scenario that presents challenges to decision making about cardiac arrest management.

■ Although there is ongoing myocardial electrical activity, the outcome is often poor.

■ An early decision around the need for rapid removal to hospital should be considered.

■ The use of cardiac ultrasound, if available, may enable more guided therapy or decision making.

■ Senior clinicians may be asked to advise on situations where the patient remains in PEA following 30 minutes of resuscitation, and where paramedics on scene believe continuing the resuscitation is futile. Refer to local senior clinician guidance.

■ There is limited evidence to support when one should terminate a PEA cardiac arrest; however, the following factors are important to consider when making this decision:

– the interval of time in arrest without life support

Figure 2.19 – Relationship between the duration of cardiopulmonary resuscitation and favourable neurological outcomes after out-of-hospital cardiac arrest.[13] Extending the duration of resuscitation from 20 to 30 minutes will result in a small but significant number of additional survivors.

Termination of Resuscitation and Verification of Death in Adults

- the absence of reversible causes
- the presence of comorbidities
- the rate/width of the QRS complexes
- the trend and absolute value of EtCO$_2$.

- Some patients undergoing prolonged CPR can survive with good outcome.

- Young age, myocardial infarction and potentially reversible causes of cardiac arrest, such as hypothermia and pulmonary emboli, are associated with a better outcome, especially when the arrest is witnessed and followed by prompt and effective resuscitative efforts.

5.2 Refractory ventricular fibrillation (VF)

- A significant number of patients may present in ventricular fibrillation (VF) that is unresponsive to repeated defibrillation shocks and amiodarone.

- Many cases of VF are secondary to myocardial ischaemia as a result of myocardial infarction, which is potentially reversible with primary percutaneous coronary intervention (PPCI). Resuscitation should not therefore be stopped in cases of refractory or persistent VF.

- Where practical, transport patients with persistent/refractory VF or pulseless VT to a cardiac arrest centre with ongoing CPR, because further in-hospital treatment may occasionally be successful.

5.3 Agonal Rhythm

- As resuscitation progresses, organised QRS complexes often deteriorate to wide, low-amplitude, irregular complexes, known as an idioventricular or agonal rhythm. This is typically at a rate <10 bpm and is not associated with effective cardiac output.

- This rhythm is usually a prelude to asystole.

- A persistent agonal rhythm can be treated as asystole and resuscitation can be terminated if it has **persisted continuously** for more than 30 minutes.

6. Deaths During a Major Incident

- In a major incident scenario, deceased patients **MUST** have a mass casualty assessment/triage card attached to them with the following details recorded:
  - That the patient is identified as dead.
  - The time the patient was identified as dead.
  - The identity of the paramedic making the decision.

- Deceased patients should only be moved if they are obstructing an evacuation route for other casualties, as the location is to be treated as a crime scene. Follow major incident protocols.

7. Action to Be Taken after Death Has Been Established

- Following termination of a resuscitation attempt and verification of death, repositioning of the body and removal of advanced airways and/or indwelling cannulae should be in accordance with local protocol.

- Complete documentation, including the factors that influenced resuscitation decision making and those relating to DNACPR decisions/ADRTs/LPAs/ReSPECT forms.

- Actions taken after verification of death by ambulance clinicians will depend on whether the death was believed to be expected or unexpected.
  - **Expected death** This occurs where a death was anticipated, expected and predicted and there are no unusual circumstances, and the person has been assessed by a doctor or healthcare professional either remotely or in person during their last illness and within the last 28 days of life (currently, under the Coronavirus Act). In the majority of cases, the patient's GP will certify the death and issue a Medical Certificate of Cause of Death (MCCD).
  - **Unexpected death** This is where a death is not clinically expected or has occurred in suspicious, unnatural, violent or otherwise unexpected circumstances. These deaths will be referred to HM Coroner's office.

- It is not necessary for a medical practitioner to attend to confirm the fact of death. Subsequent actions to be taken by ambulance clinicians will vary by location; refer to local policies and procedures.

- Services should be encouraged, in conjunction with their Coroner's service (or Procurator Fiscal in Scotland), to develop a local procedure for handling the body once death has been verified by ambulance personnel.

- A locally approved leaflet should be adopted for handing to bereaved relatives.

- Any consideration for organ donation should not influence resuscitation attempt decision making:
  - If there is no ROSC, it is unlikely organ donation will occur.
  - If there is ROSC but the patient is not suitable for critical care, they are unlikely to be admitted solely for donation purposes.
  - A long downtime usually makes organs unsuitable for donation.
  - Tissue donation occurs the next day in the mortuary, not in the hospital, so transport to hospital does not change the chance of tissue donation.

Termination of Resuscitation and Verification of Death in Adults

8. Supporting Bystanders Witnessing Cardiac Arrest

- In many cases of out-of-hospital cardiac arrest (OHCA), a close relative or friend may have performed CPR before ambulance service help arrives; it is important to provide reassurance about the actions they have taken and their resuscitation efforts.

- Relatives may find it more distressing to be separated from their family member during the resuscitation attempt, and there may be advantages to them being present.

- However, it is also important to acknowledge that these are distressing events, and so there can be disadvantages to the relative being present.

- There are a number of key principles, actions and safeguards that ambulance clinicians should be aware of, and adopt, to support relatives through the witnessing of a resuscitation attempt and its termination when appropriate:
  - Always acknowledge the difficulty of the situation.
  - When possible, try to ensure that one member of the team is with the relative at all times. This can be challenging to achieve with limited numbers of people on scene, but will ensure the relative is supported as much as possible during the event.
  - Ensure the bystander understands they have a choice of whether or not to be present.
  - Ensure that introductions are made and names known.
  - Give clear, simple and honest explanations of what is happening.
  - Ask the relative, in a sensitive manner, not to interfere with the resuscitation process, but allow them to touch the patient when it is safe to do so should they so wish (assuming that there are no issues in relation to a possible crime scene).
  - Answer what questions they have and explain the procedures in simple terms.
  - When it becomes clear that the resuscitation attempt is unlikely to have a successful outcome, take time to prepare relatives by keeping them updated, using sensitive warnings. Examples include, 'despite all we are doing there has been no change', 'it is unlikely their heart is going to restart' or 'they are not responding to the drugs we are giving'.
  - When the decision has been made to terminate the resuscitation attempt, explain that you will be stopping CPR and ask if the relative would like to be present when this happens.
  - When the patient has died, explain that there will be a period where actions will need to be taken, for example that equipment will need to be removed. Depending on the situation, explain that some medical devices will need to be left in situ.
  - Allow relatives time to say goodbye; advise that it is ok to talk to the deceased or to touch them if they wish and this is appropriate to the situation.

- Best attempts should be made to ensure that any member of the public who has delivered CPR is supported at the scene and given welfare advice. Bystanders should be signposted to their GP in the first instance.

8.1 Breaking Bad News

- Breaking bad news is best done with a well-prepared, honest and simple approach.

- Relatives will often not remember the details of what was said, but they will remember how they were made to feel.

- Ambulance clinicians should try to:
  - Take time to prepare personal appearance; check and tidy uniform/clothing, remove gloves and, if necessary, wash hands.
  - Confirm the name of the deceased before speaking to the relatives, establish their relationship and confirm the correct relatives where there are multiple patients.
  - Adopt a position at the same level as the relative.
  - Use simple language and avoid medical jargon.
  - Avoid long preamble such as asking about the patient's pre-morbid health.
  - Ensure the word 'dead' or 'died' is introduced early in the conversation.
  - Allow periods of silence to enable the relatives to absorb and process what they are being told.
  - Check if they have understood what you have told them: you may need to repeat the information

- Remember to anticipate the types of reaction or emotional response to the bad news and be ready to support the relatives as much as possible.

8.2 Children and Young People Witnessing Cardiac Arrest

- Children and young people that witness and are present at a cardiac arrest, particularly of a close relative, may need additional support.

- They may have questions about what they have witnessed. Always talk to them with a family member or someone who knows them. Try to ascertain their understanding; their awareness of death and reaction will depend on their age and stage of development. Follow the child's lead, be open and honest, use simple terms and avoid long explanations which may cause confusion.

Termination of Resuscitation and Verification of Death in Adults

- Before leaving the scene, consider making a referral to their GP.

- Consider signposting parents/carers to organisations that provide specific support for bereaved children, as per local procedures.

Termination of Resuscitation and Verification of Death in Adults

- **Paramedics are increasingly being called upon to diagnose death and initiate the appropriate clinical response.**

- **After cardiac arrest, resuscitation efforts including ALS must be made whenever there is a chance of survival, unless the person has made an ADRT refusing CPR in these circumstances.**

- **Some conditions are incompatible with recovery and, in these cases, resuscitation should not be attempted.**

- **In some situations, once the facts of the patient and situation are known, resuscitation efforts can be discontinued.**

- **Patients can and do make anticipatory decisions NOT to be resuscitated. An ADRT must be respected and a DNACPR recommendation should be used to guide decision making on whether or not to attempt CPR.**

- **These guidelines should be read in conjunction with local policies and procedures.**

Bibliography

1. Soar J, Bottiger BW, Carli P, Couper K, Deakin CD, Djavf T, Lott C, Olasveengen T, Paal P, Pellis T, D. Perkins GD, Sandroni C, Nolan JP. European Resuscitation Council Guidelines 2021: adult advanced life support. *Resuscitation* 2021, 161: 115–151. Available from: https://www.resuscitationjournal.com/article/S0300-9572(15)00328-7/pdf.

2. Resuscitation Council (UK). Resuscitation Guidelines 2021. *Prevention of Cardiac Arrest and Decisions about CPR*. 2021. Available from: https://resus.org.uk/resuscitation-guidelines/prevention-of-cardiac-arrest-and-decisions-about-cpr/.

3. British Medical Association, Resuscitation Council (UK), Royal College of Nursing. *Decisions Relating to Cardiopulmonary Resuscitation*. 3rd edn. 2016. Available from: https://resus.org.uk/EasySiteWeb/GatewayLink.aspx?alId=16643.

4. Ambitions Partnership. *Universal Principles for Advance Care Planning (ACP). NHS England and NHS Improvement*. 2022. Available from: https://www.england.nhs.uk/publication/universal-principles-for-advance-care-planning/.

5. British Medical Association. *2020/21 General Medical Services (GMS) Contract Quality and Outcomes Framework (QOF)*. London: NHS England and NHS Improvement, 2021. Available from: https://www.england.nhs.uk/coronavirus/wp-content/uploads/sites/52/2020/03/C0713-202021-General-Medical-Services-GMS-contract-Quality-and-Outcomes-Framework-QOF-Guidance.pdf.

6. UK Government Office of the Public Guardian. *Mental Capacity Act 2005 Code of Practice*. London: The Stationary Office Ltd, 2007. Available from: https://assets.publishing.service.gov.uk/government/uploads/system/uploads/attachment_data/file/921428/Mental-capacity-act-code-of-practice.pdf.

7. Mentzelopoulos, SD et al. European Resuscitation Council Guidelines 2021: ethics of resuscitation and end of life decisions. *Resuscitation* 2021, 161: 408–432. Available from: https://www.resuscitationjournal.com/article/S0300-9572(21)00070-8/pdf

8. Department of Health (NI). *Review of the Law Relating to Advance Decisions to Refuse Treatment Mental Capacity Act (NI) 2016 section 284*. 2019. Available from: Mental Capacity Act (NI) 2016 Advance Decision to Refuse Treatment and Mental Health Paper – Review (health-ni.gov.uk).

9. Hospice UK. *Special Edition of Care After Death: Registered Nurse Verification of Expected Adult Death (RNVoEAD) Guidance*. 2020. Available from: https://professionals.hospiceuk.org/docs/default-source/What-We-Offer/Care-Support-Programmes/Care-after-death/rnvoead-special-covid-19-edition-final_2.pdf?sfvrsn=2H.

10. Resuscitation Council (UK). *ReSPECT Recommended Summary Plan for Emergency Care and Treatment*. 2017. Available from: https://www.resus.org.uk/respect/.

11. Ridley D. *Regulation 28 Report to Prevent Future Deaths. Mary Johnson*. 2020. Available from: Mary Johnson, Courts and Tribunals Judiciary.

12. Scottish Government. *Adults with Incapacity (Scotland) Act 2000. Proposals for Reform*. 2018. Available from: Adults with Incapacity (Scotland) Act 2000: Proposals for Reform (www.gov.scot).

13. Yoshikazu G. Relationship between the duration of cardiopulmonary resuscitation and favorable neurological outcomes after out-of-hospital cardiac arrest: a prospective, nationwide, population-based cohort study. *Journal of the American Heart Association* 2016, 5(3). DOI: 10.1161/JAHA.115.002819.

Termination of Resuscitation and Verification of Death in Children

1. Introduction

- Being called to a death of an infant, child or adolescent is one of the most difficult experiences to encounter. Paramedics are usually the first professionals to arrive at the scene, and, at the same time as making difficult judgements about resuscitation, they have to deal with the devastating initial shock of the parents/carers.

- Despite the recent fall in incidence, sudden unexpected death in infancy (SUDI) remains the largest single cause of death in infants aged 1 month to 1 year. SUDI can also occasionally occur in children older than one year of age. The 1991 national 'Reduce the Risk' campaign advocating that infants sleep on their backs produced a dramatic reduction (70%) in sudden infant deaths.

- In 50% of SUDIs, a specific cause for the death is found. The vast majority of SUDIs occur from natural causes. SUDIs can result from child prompting a joint paediatric and police investigation. When informed of a SUDI, ambulance control should immediately notify the police to initiate this process.

- This section draws on national experience and follows the Kennedy Report's (2016) recommendations.

2. Considerations for Paediatric Cardiac Arrest/Death

Resuscitation should always be attempted unless there is a condition unequivocally associated with death or the child has an advanced and irreversible condition and their Advance Care Plan recommends that CPR is not appropriate.

- The immediate consideration(s) when called to a paediatric cardiac arrest/child death include:

  1) **Resuscitation** This must be attempted in **ALL** cases, unless there is a condition unequivocally associated with death or the child has a life-limiting condition AND the child has an Advance Care Plan that states that CPR is not appropriate (refer to **Basic Life Support in Children** and **Advanced Life Support**).

  2) **Verification of death and termination of resuscitation** As in adult practice, asystole should be confirmed by ECG when determining death. (Pulse checks are particularly unreliable in sick children. Similarly, sick infants may demonstrate marked peripheral cyanosis and cold extremities prior to death (refer to **Medical Emergencies in Children – Overview** and **Trauma Emergencies in Children – Overview**).

- Unlike for adults, resuscitation of children should almost always be undertaken and continued (unless an Advance Care Plan recommends otherwise) while rapidly conveying the child to the nearest suitable Emergency Department, continuing resuscitation en-route (even in circumstances where resuscitation appears futile and death inevitable).

- Parents/carers need to be assured that resuscitation was attempted (even if unsuccessful), rather than forever questioning whether their child was denied potentially life-saving treatment(s).

- An initial presumption in favour of performing CPR should be made when a child does not have an Advance Care Plan and there is no documented advance decision about attempting resuscitation.

- Every effort should be made to identify children with an Advance Care Plan, Recommended Summary Plan for Emergency Care and Treatment (ReSPECT) form or Treatment Escalation Plan that includes recommendations for resuscitation.

- On rare occasions, it may be appropriate to continue CPR when a child has a condition unequivocally associated with death until patient privacy and dignity can be assured before stopping the resuscitation attempt.

2.1 Conditions Unequivocally Associated with Death in Children

- **Decapitation**.

- **Massive cranial and cerebral destruction**.

- **Hemicorporectomy** (or similar massive injury).

- **Decomposition/putrefaction** – where tissue damage indicates that the patient has been dead for some hours, days or longer.

- **Incineration** – full-thickness burns and charring of greater than 95% of the body surface.

- **Hypostasis** – pooling of blood in congested vessels in the dependent parts of the body, in the position in which it lies after death. In very sick children, mottling of the skin may mimic hypostasis so hypostasis alone should not be used as the only factor to withhold paediatric resuscitation.

- **Rigor mortis** – stiffness occurring after death as a result of the enzymic muscle fibres breakdown. This can occur rapidly in children but sometimes does not occur at all, so resuscitation should be attempted unless there is another condition unequivocally associated with death.

- **Foetal maceration in a newborn** – children delivered with severe abnormalities incompatible with life. A stillborn child that died more than a day before birth may have skin loosening and sloughing off when touched.

Termination of Resuscitation and Verification of Death in Children

Note:
Do not withhold or terminate resuscitation:

(i) where these criteria have not been met or

(ii) where CPR appears futile or inappropriate, until senior clinical advice has been sought.

If access to the patient is restricted and it is believed that one of the conditions above may exist, then a multi-agency decision (Fire, Police, Coastguard etc.) should be made on whether ongoing rescue should continue or the incident becomes that of body recovery, applying JESIP principles and considering the risks posed to the rescue team.

Other conditions where resuscitation may be withheld or discontinued

In addition to the conditions above, other criteria can be applied to confirm death, and can be used when considering whether resuscitation need not be attempted or should be discontinued:

a. The child has a life-limiting condition, an Advance Care Plan, a ReSPECT form or Treatment Escalation Plan that advises resuscitation is not attempted.

b. Submersion for longer than 90 minutes (refer to **Immersion and Drowning**).

Care Plans for Children and Young People

- Children and young people with complex illnesses are likely to have a detailed Advance Care Plan in place.

- This is likely to be documented within the nationally recognised Child and Young Persons Advance Care Plan (CYPACP), although localised forms may also be used.

- The CYPACP may or may not include a ReSPECT form.

- Children and young people who have reached an age where they have an understanding and competence should be involved in decision making around their care. Parents should also be involved in this joint decision making process.

- For additional support and guidance when using a care plan for children and young people, their specialist care team should be contacted.

2.2 Expected Deaths

- It is uncommon for ambulance paramedics to be called to attend to an expected death of a child.

- When a child has a life-threatening or life-limiting condition and is nearing death, the child's clinical team will have made plans, in conjunction with the child's parents (and the child if appropriate). These can include discussions about care after death, and written Advance Care Planning documentation will be prepared to guide ambulance paramedics.

- It is important to remember that even though the family may have been caring for the child for many years and anticipated their death, when the death occurs they are likely to experience overwhelming grief at their loss.

- Parents may have made decisions in advance about their child's care but can change their mind; be guided by them and contact the child's clinical team for advice and support.

- Following verification of death, family members may want time alone with the child but may be reassured by and benefit from your continuing presence; be guided by their needs. If transporting the child, ask if they have a favourite blanket or toy to take with them and pre-alert the receiving hospital so they can prepare for the child's arrival.

- Remember the needs of wider family members who may be with the child (particularly siblings), who will need support and sensitive communication.

3. Care of the Family

- Families are profoundly affected by the initial response and care that professionals offer their child in these circumstances. Not only is your role essential for immediate practical reasons but it also has a great influence on how the family deals with the death in the future.

- Communication and empathy are essential, and the family must be treated with compassion and sensitivity throughout. The Foundation for the Study of Infant Deaths found that parents/carers regard the actions and attitudes of those who tend to them as extremely important and typically speak very highly of the way both themselves and their child were treated.

- Explain what you are doing at every stage.

- Parents/carers exhibit a variety of reactions (e.g. overwhelming grief, anger, confusion, disbelief or guilt). Be prepared to deal with any of these feelings with empathy and sensitivity, remembering some reactions may be directed towards the attending ambulance paramedics as a manifestation of their distress.

- Avoid any criticism of the parents/carers, either direct or implied.

Termination of Resuscitation and Verification of Death in Children

- Think before you speak. Chance remarks may cause offence and may be remembered indefinitely (e.g. 'I'm sorry; he looks so awful').
- Ask the child's name and use it when referring to them (do not refer to the child as 'it').
- Allow the parents/carers to hold the child if they so wish (unless there are obvious indications of trauma or obvious suspicious circumstances that result in the police declaring a crime scene), as long as it does not interfere with clinical care.
- If possible, do not put children in body bags. It is known that relatives do not perceive very traumatic events in the way that unrelated onlookers might, and it is important they can see, touch and hold their loved one.
- Ensure the family is aware of where you are taking their infant/child. The parents/carers may wish to accompany you when you take the child to hospital. If appropriate, offer to take one or both in the ambulance. Alternatively, ensure that they have other means of transport, and that they know where to go.
- If they have no telephone, offer to help in contacting a relative or friend who can give immediate support, such as looking after other children or making sure the premises are secure.
- Explain sensitively that it is routine practice to involve both the coroner and the police in unexpected child deaths and that they may wish to attend the scene and/or speak to the carers.

4. Document

- Collect information pertaining to:
  - The situation in which you find the child (e.g. position in cot, bedding, proximity to others, room temperature etc.).
  - A history of the last 24–48 hours' events, including a brief description from the parents/carers of the events that led up to them finding the deceased child (e.g. when last seen alive, health at that time, position when found etc.). The police and the paediatrician will go through these events in greater detail, but the parent/carer's initial statement to you may be particularly valuable in the investigation.
  - Any significant past medical history.
- Write all this information down as soon as you have the opportunity, recording times and other details as accurately as possible.

5. Multi-agency Approach

The Kennedy Report requires a multi-agency approach to the management of SUDI, in which all the professionals involved keep each other informed and collaborate. Follow agreed protocols with regards to inter-agency communication and informing the police.

5.1 Communication with Other Agencies

- After you have arrived at the house and confirmed that the infant is deceased, the police Child Abuse Investigation Team (CAIT) must be informed (refer to locally agreed procedure). In unexpected deaths, the police will attend the scene and they can offer further advice regarding the Coroner's Officer's investigation.
- Share the information you have collected with the police and with relevant health professionals.

6. Transferring the Child

- The child should be taken to the nearest appropriate emergency department, not direct to a mortuary, even when the child has clearly been dead for some time and a death has been medically confirmed at home (there will be occasions where it is necessary to remind a doctor that taking the child to a hospital is now the preferred procedure, as recommended by Kennedy).
- Pre-alert the emergency department of your arrival, asking them to be ready to take over resuscitation if this is ongoing. Inform them if the parent(s)/carer(s) are accompanying the child.
- In hospital, an immediate examination will be made by a paediatrician, bodily samples (blood, urine, CSF) can be taken for analysis, parents/carers can talk with the paediatricians and support services can be contacted.

7. Support

- A child death is one of the most emotionally traumatic and challenging events to encounter and is very distressing for all involved.
- Opportunities for debriefing or counselling for ambulance staff should be available.
- Follow local procedures for post-critical incident debriefing local guidelines/processes.
- Some people will feel ongoing distress. This is normal and should be recognised: other forms of therapy, from informal support from colleagues to formal counselling, may be required.
- As part of the ambulance service safeguarding processes, information from local paediatricians and ambulance service safeguarding leads will be available if required for further discussion.
- Unsuccessful attempts at resuscitating children weigh heavily on individuals despite recognised poor outcomes following paediatric out-of-hospital cardiac arrest (OHCA). The vast majority of children having a cardiac arrest outside of hospital die, irrespective of response times, personnel or intervention/availability of advanced life support – less than 10% of paediatric OHCAs survive, despite those attempting resuscitation having done everything possible to help that child.

Termination of Resuscitation and Verification of Death in Children

Arrive at scene

- Unexpected child death-questionable crime scene
  - Viable resuscitation
    - YES → Commence resuscitation → Transport child and parents to ED; inform ambulance control to direct police to hospital
    - NO
      - No obvious cause of death → Ask ambulance control to contact police and await attendance or telephone advice of a child death DI* and follow instruction → Advised by child death DI to take child and parents to ED
      - Obvious cause of death → Ask ambulance control to contact police and await attendance or telephone advice of a child death DI* and follow instruction → Crime scene declared; leave child at scene; inform ambulance control

- Unexpected child death-obvious crime scene
  - Condition unequivocally associated with death
    - YES
    - NO → Commence resuscitation → Ask ambulance control to contact police

Pre-alert and take to appropriate ED that is prepared to accept sudden deaths in children

*Child Death Detective Inspector (child death DI) – A Detective Inspector who is trained in the management of child death; oversees the multiagency investigation and collection of evidence.

Figure 2.20 – Death of a child, including sudden unexpected death in infancy, children and adolescents (SUDICA).

Termination of Resuscitation and Verification of Death in Children

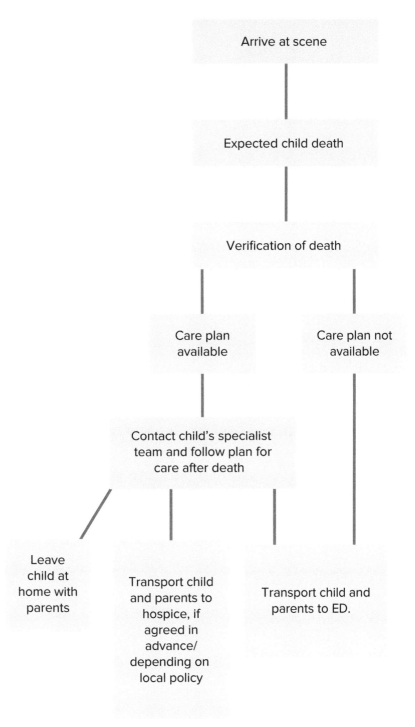

Figure 2.21 – Expected child death.

Termination of Resuscitation and Verification of Death in Children

KEY POINTS!

Termination of Resuscitation and Verification of Death in Children

- A child death is one of the most emotionally traumatic and challenging events to encounter.

- Resuscitation should always be attempted unless there is a condition unequivocally associated with death or a valid advance decision.

- Communication and empathy are essential, and the family must be treated with compassion and sensitivity throughout. Parents/carers regard the actions and attitudes of those who tend to them as extremely important and speak very highly of the way both they and their child were treated.

- Your role is not only essential for immediate practical reasons but also has a great influence on how the family deals with the death, long after the initial crisis is over.

- Ensure the family is aware of where you are taking their infant/child.

- Collect information pertaining to the situation in which you find the child, a history of events and any significant past medical history.

- Follow agreed protocols with regards to inter-agency communication and informing the police.

- In unexpected deaths, explain to the family that the death will be reported to the Coroner and that they will be interviewed by the Coroner's Officer and the police in due course.

Bibliography

1. Resuscitation Council (UK). *Resuscitation Guidelines 2015. Prevention of Cardiac Arrest and Decisions About CPR*. London: Resuscitation Council, 2015. Available from: https://resus.org.uk/resuscitation-guidelines/prevention-of-cardiac-arrest-and-decisions-about-cpr/.

2. British Medical Association, Resuscitation Council (UK), Royal College of Nursing. *Decisions Relating to Cardiopulmonary Resuscitation*. 3rd edn. London: British Medical Association, 2016. Available from: https://resus.org.uk/EasySiteWeb/GatewayLink.aspx?alId=16643.

3. Kennedy H. Royal College of Pathologists, Royal College of Paediatrics. *Sudden Unexpected Death in Infancy and Childhood*. London: Royal College of Pathologists, 2016. Available from: https://www.rcpath.org/uploads/assets/uploaded/af879a1b-1974-4692-9e002c20f09dc14c.pdf.

4. Together for Shorter Lives. *Caring for a Child at End of Life*. 2nd edn. Together for Shorter Lives, 2019. Available from: https://www.togetherforshortlives.org.uk/app/uploads/2019/11/TfSL-Caring-for-a-child-at-end-of-life-Professionals.pdf.

3

Medical Emergencies

Medical Emergencies in Adults – Overview

1. Introduction

Although the care of a wide range of medical conditions will be quite specific to the presenting condition, there are general principles of care that apply to most medical cases, regardless of underlying condition(s).

2. Patient Assessment

- In order to gather as much relevant information as possible, without delaying care, the accepted format of history-taking is as follows:
  - Presenting complaint – why the patient or carer called for help at this time
  - The history of presenting complaint – details of when the problem started, exacerbating factors and previous similar episodes. **NB** The patient history can provide valuable insight into the cause of the current condition
  - Direct questioning about associated symptoms, by system. Ask about all appropriate systems. Refer to Table 3.1
  - Past medical history, including current medication
  - Family history
  - Social history.

- Combined with a good physical examination (primary and secondary survey), this format of history-taking should ensure that you correctly identify those patients who are time-critical, urgent or routine. The history taken must be fully documented. In many cases, a well-taken history will point to the diagnosis.

- The presence of MedicAlert®-type jewellery (bracelets or necklets), or emergency card (steroids, oxygen), can provide information on the patient's pre-existing health risk (e.g. diabetes, anaphylaxis, Addison's disease, COPD etc.)

that may be relevant to the current medical emergency.

- Consider scoring a patient's level of frailty.[2]
  - The Rockwood Clinical Frailty Scale (CFS) is a judgement-based frailty assessment tool. It is not validated for people under the age of 65 years or those with long-term disabilities. Frailty must be sensed, described and measured: not guessed. If the patient you are assessing is acutely unwell and over 65 years, consider using the CFS, as per local pathways.
  - The score is based on the patient's baseline, so use the tool to score how the patient was 2 weeks ago (prior to deterioration) or their usual level of functioning when well, rather than how they present today. If possible, cross-reference what the patient describes to you with a description from relatives/carers.
  - Do NOT compare the patient to the pictures (e.g. person using walking aids) alone to make a judgement on the level of frailty.

2.1 Primary Survey

- The primary survey should take 60–90 seconds for assessment and follow the approach set out in Table 3.1. This rapid assessment should quickly identify patients with actual or potential life-threatening conditions or symptoms.

- Assessment and management should proceed in a 'stepwise' manner and abnormalities should be managed as they are encountered; that is, do not move onto breathing and circulation until the airway is managed. Every time an intervention has been carried out, re-assess the patient.

- If haemorrhage cannot be controlled or airway and breathing cannot be corrected, evacuate immediately, continuing resuscitation as appropriate en-route.

TABLE 3.1 – ASSESSMENT and MANAGEMENT of: Medical Emergencies

Assess <C>ABCD

All stages should be considered, but some more detailed elements may be omitted if not considered appropriate.

At each stage, consider the need for **early senior clinical support**.

- Start correcting any **<C>ABCD** problems as below.
- Undertake a **TIME-CRITICAL** transfer to nearest appropriate receiving hospital.
- Provide an ATMIST information call.

Catastrophic Haemorrhage

- Look for evidence of external catastrophic haemorrhage.
- Consider whether occult catastrophic haemorrhage could be occurring, for example following trauma or as a result of an aneurysm rupture.

Stem external bleeding.

- Apply a tourniquet and/or apply direct pressure to the site.

Medical Emergencies in Adults – Overview

TABLE 3.1 – ASSESSMENT and MANAGEMENT of: Medical Emergencies *(continued)*

- Dress the site with appropriate haemorrhage/trauma dressing.
- Elevate the site if possible.

Airway

- Assess the airway (refer to **Airway and Breathing Management**).
- **Look for** obvious obstructions, e.g. teeth/dentures, foreign bodies, vomit, blood (refer to **Foreign Body Airway Obstruction**).
- **Listen for** noisy airflow, e.g. snoring, gurgling or no airflow (refer to **Dyspnoea**).
- **Feel for** air movement.
- Airway constriction is a life-threatening condition and can result from an immune response to an allergen (refer to Allergic Reactions including **Anaphylaxis**).
- Correct any airway problems immediately by:
  - Positioning – head tilt, chin lift, jaw thrust.
  - Suction (if available and appropriate).
  - Oropharyngeal airway.
  - Nasopharyngeal airway.
  - Supraglottic mask airway (SGA) (if appropriate).
  - Endotracheal intubation (if appropriate, appropriately trained and only if waveform capnography is available).
  - Needle cricothyroidotomy.

Breathing

- Expose the chest and assess (refer to **Airway and Breathing Management**).

Inspect:

- Respiratory rate (<10 or >30).
- Adequacy and depth of chest movements.
- Symmetry of chest movement.
- Effectiveness of ventilation.
- Cyanosis (which may appear pale grey/blue), anaemia or pallor is more difficult to detect in people with darker skin tones. Look for central cyanosis around the lips, inside the mouth and in the oral mucous membranes (buccal or sublingual). Peripheral cyanosis is usually seen in the hands or feet, and may occur with or without central cyanosis.

Figure 3.1 – Conjuctival pallor in a patient with severe anaemia. Reproduced with permission. Available from: https://www.hst.org.za/publications/NonHST%20Publications/malaria_36.pdf.

(continued)

TABLE 3.1 – ASSESSMENT and MANAGEMENT of: Medical Emergencies *(continued)*

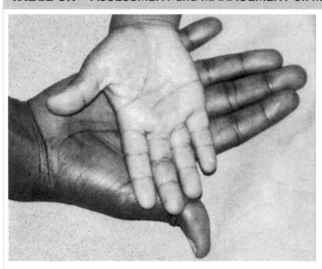

Figure 3.2 – Pallor of a child's palm, with the mother's for comparison. Republished with permission. Available from: https://pubmed.ncbi.nlm.nih.gov/20417858/.

- In anaemia the conjunctiva may appear to be pale pink or white, regardless of the patient's skin tone. In patients with darker skin tones there may be reduced darkness in the palmar creases, although this sign cannot be used on its own. The patient's palms can be compared to that of a family member with the same skin tone.

- Position of trachea in suprasternal notch.

Palpate:

- Any instability of chest wall and note any areas of tenderness.

- Note depth and equality of chest movement.

Percuss for:

- Dullness or hyperresonance.

Auscultate:

- Altered breathing patterns with a stethoscope – ask the patient to take deep breaths in and out briskly through their mouth if possible – listen on both sides of the chest:
  - above the nipples in the mid-clavicular line
  - laterally in the mid-axillary line
  - below the shoulder blade (front and back).

- Auscultate to assess air entry and compare sides. Equality of air entry.

- Crepitations at the rear of the chest (crackles, heard low down in the lung fields at the rear – may indicate fluid in the lung in heart failure).

- Wheezing, noisy respiration on inspiration or expiration.

- Stridor (higher-pitched noise on inspiration), suggestive of upper respiratory obstruction.

Additional crackles and wheeze on inspiration may be associated with inhalation of blood or vomit.

- Correct any breathing problems immediately.

- Consider patient positioning (e.g. sitting upright for respiratory problems).

- If breathing is absent, refer to appropriate **Resuscitation** guidelines.

- If the breathing is inadequate, refer to **Airway and Breathing Management**.

- Treat underlying cause of unilateral chest movement if tension pneumothorax.

Monitor the patient's SpO_2; administer oxygen to achieve saturations of >94% if the patient presents as hypoxaemic on air; refer to **Oxygen**.

NB This is except for patients with COPD or other risk factors for hypercapnia (refer to **Oxygen**).

In patients with a decreased level of consciousness (Glasgow Coma Scale (GCS) <15), administer the initial supplemental oxygen dose until the vital signs are normal, then reduce the oxygen dose and aim for a target saturation (SpO_2) of >94%. Refer to **Altered Level of Consciousness**.

Medical Emergencies in Adults – Overview

TABLE 3.1 – ASSESSMENT and MANAGEMENT of: Medical Emergencies *(continued)*

In patients with sickle cell crisis, administer supplemental oxygen via an appropriate mask/nasal cannula until a reliable SpO$_2$ measurement is available; then adjust the oxygen flow to aim for target saturation within the range of 94–98%. Refer to **Sickle Cell Disease**.

Consider assisted ventilation at a rate of 12–20 respirations per minute if any of the following are present:

- Oxygen saturation (SpO$_2$) <90% on levels of supplemental oxygen.
- Respiratory rate <10 or >30 bpm.
- Inadequate chest expansion.

NB Restraint (positional) asphyxia – If the patient is required to be physically restrained (e.g. by police officers) in order to prevent them injuring themselves or others, or for the purpose of being detained under the Mental Health Act, then it is paramount that the method of restraint allows both for a patent airway and adequate respiratory volume.

- **Under these circumstances, it is essential to ensure that the patient's airway and breathing are adequate at all times.**

Circulation

- Assess for evidence of external haemorrhage (e.g. epistaxis, haemoptysis, haematemesis, melaena). For suspected gastrointestinal bleeding, refer to **Gastrointestinal Bleeding**.
- Assess skin colour and temperature.
- Palpate for a radial pulse – if absent, feel for a carotid pulse. **NB** The estimation of blood pressure by pulse is inaccurate and unreliable; however, the presence of a radial pulse suggests adequate perfusion of major organs. The presence of a femoral pulse suggests perfusion of the kidneys, while a carotid pulse and coherent mental state suggests adequate perfusion of the brain.
- Assess pulse rate, volume and rhythm.
- Check capillary refill time centrally (forehead or sternum – normal <2 seconds).
- Arrest external haemorrhage.
- In cases of internal or uncontrolled haemorrhage, undertake a **TIME-CRITICAL** transfer to further care; provide an alert/information call.
- Patients with acute adrenal insufficiency (adrenal crisis) and/or sepsis will usually benefit from early fluid therapy and an appropriate hospital alert/information call. Adrenal insufficiency patients with hypotension and hypovolaemia must be given IV fluids and injected hydrocortisone prior to transportation to minimise the risk of circulatory collapse. See **Steroid-dependent Patients** and **Sepsis**.

Consider hypovolaemic shock and be aware of its early signs:

- Pallor.
- Cool peripheries.
- Anxiety, abnormal behaviour.
- Increased respiratory rate.
- Tachycardia.

Recognition of Shock

Shock is difficult to diagnose. In certain groups of patients, the signs of shock may appear late (e.g. patients with acute adrenal insufficiency (adrenal crisis), pregnant women, patients on medication such as beta-blockers and the physically fit).

Blood loss of 750–1000 ml will produce little evidence of shock; blood loss of 1000–1500 ml is required before more classical signs of shock appear. **NB** This loss is from the circulation and is NOT necessarily visible externally.

Fluid Therapy

- If fluid replacement is indicated, refer to **Intravascular Fluid Therapy in Adults**.

Rapid fluid replacement into the vascular compartment can overload the cardiovascular system, particularly where there is pre-existing cardiovascular disease and in older people. Gradual rehydration over many hours rather than minutes may be indicated for rehydration. **NB** Monitor fluid replacement closely in these cases.

(continued)

Medical Emergencies in Adults – Overview

TABLE 3.1 – ASSESSMENT and MANAGEMENT of: Medical Emergencies *(continued)*

Disability

- Note the initial level of responsiveness on the AVPU scale and the time of assessment.
- **A** – Alert.
- **V** – Responds to voice.
- **P** – Responds to painful stimulus.
- **U** – Unresponsive.
- Detail how to check pain.
- Assess and note pupil size, equality and response to light.
- **NB** In patients with fixed pinpoint pupils, suspect opiate use.
- Check for purposeful movement in all four limbs.
- Check sensory function.
- Assess blood glucose levels in all patients with diabetes, impaired consciousness, convulsions, collapse, alcohol consumption or a history of Addison's disease or another form of adrenal insufficiency.
- Check blood glucose level to rule out hypo/hyperglycaemia as the cause (refer to **Glycaemic Emergencies in Adults and Children**).
- Also check blood glucose levels in all patients with a history of diabetes, impaired consciousness, seizures, collapse or alcohol/drug consumption.
- Consider adrenal crisis as a cause and provide drug therapy as required; refer to appropriate drug guidelines. In adrenal crisis, refer to **Hydrocortisone** and **Steroid-dependent Patients**.
- If the level of consciousness deteriorates or respiratory depression develops in cases where an overdose with opiate-type drugs may be a possibility, consider administering naloxone; refer to **Naloxone Hydrochloride**.
- For patients with decreased consciousness and active seizure, refer to **Convulsions in Adults**.

Vital Signs and NEWS2

NB Complete a full set of observations for all patients; repeat after intervention or when any value is outside normal parameters.

Respiratory Rate

- Measure and record respiratory rate.

Pulse

- Measure and record pulse.

Oxygen Saturation

- Monitor the patient's SpO_2; administer oxygen to achieve saturations of >94% if the patient presents as hypoxaemic on air; refer to **Oxygen**.

Blood Pressure and Fluids

- Measure and record blood pressure. If required, administer fluids; refer to **Intravascular Fluid Therapy in Adults**.

Blood Glucose

- If appropriate, measure and record blood glucose for hypo/hyperglycaemia; refer to **Glycaemic Emergencies in Adults and Children**.

Temperature

- Measure and record temperature.

NEWS2

For cancer patients, consider UKONS Tool (see **End of Life Care**, 3. Management – Patients Who Are Not Expected to Die Within 72 Hours).

These observations will enable you to calculate a NEWS2 score.

Medical Emergencies in Adults – Overview

TABLE 3.1 – ASSESSMENT and MANAGEMENT of: Medical Emergencies *(continued)*
ECG
▪ If required, monitor and record 12-lead ECG. Assess for abnormality; refer to **Cardiac Rhythm Disturbance**.
Assess the Patient's Pain
▪ Where present, assess the SOCRATES of pain and record initial and subsequent pain scores.
▪ Consider analgesia if appropriate (refer to **Pain Managment in Adults**).
Documentation
▪ Complete documentation to include all clinical findings, advice from other clinicians, onward referral and worsening advice given.

2.2 Secondary Survey

▪ A secondary survey should only commence after the primary survey has been completed and an assessment of the patient's critical status has been made.

▪ The secondary survey is a more thorough 'head-to-toe' assessment of the patient, including their past medical history (refer to Table 3.2). It is important to monitor the patient's vital signs during the survey.

▪ A complete and thorough secondary survey may not be possible in some patients with **TIME-CRITICAL** conditions.

▪ Follow additional medical guidelines as indicated by the patient's condition (e.g. cardiac rhythm disturbance).

TABLE 3.2 – Clinical Assessment
▪ Continually re-assess <C>ABCD throughout clinical assessment.
▪ Assess all patients holistically, considering the implications of any of the following:
– Congenital defects/malformations – kyphosis/scoliosis – causing compression.
– Dentition – this may indicate level of nutrition.
– Jugular vein distension – cardiac history.
– Oedema (ankles/orbital) – failure or kidney disease.
– Central cyanosis.
– Finger clubbing/splinter haemorrhage – respiratory or cardiac history.
– Bruising – injury (consider non-accidental injury in vulnerable patient groups).
– Surgical scars – previous procedures.
Respiratory
▪ Inspect, palpate, percuss and auscultate the chest, examining for signs which could indicate a respiratory cause for the presenting condition:
– Accessory muscles/recession/nasal flaring.
– Chest shape and symmetry.
– Palpate for tactile fremitus which may indicate mucus plug or pneumonia.
– Central trachea.
▪ Assess for pneumothorax – in small pneumothorax no clinical signs may be detected. A pneumothorax causes breathlessness, reduced air entry and chest movement on the affected side. If this is a tension pneumothorax, then the patient will have increasing respiratory distress; distended neck veins and tracheal deviation (late sign) away from affected side may also be present.
Cardiac
▪ Auscultate and palpate, examining for signs which could indicate a cardiac cause for the presenting condition.
▪ Assess skin colour and temperature.
▪ Record pulse oximeter reading, including heart rate.
▪ Assess heart sounds and bruits.
▪ Palpate bilateral pulses for equality.

(continued)

SECTION **3** Medical Emergencies

TABLE 3.2 – Clinical Assessment *(continued)*

- Obtain a blood pressure reading using a sphygmomanometer; consider bilateral and standing and sitting blood pressures – consider postural drop.

Neurological

- Establish GCS (refer to **Altered Level of Consciousness**).

- Assess cranial nerves.

- Consider gait.

- Asses tone, strength and sensation to separate limbs and dermatomes.

- Consider assessing reflexes.

- **NB** Patients on long-term steroids or who have adrenal insufficiency may deteriorate rapidly because of steroid insufficiency. If significantly unwell, the patient should be given hydrocortisone and fluids if required (refer to **Steroid-dependent Patients**).

- Some patients, especially those with spinal cord injury above T6, are particularly susceptible to the potentially life-threatening condition autonomic dysreflexia, which is characterised by a rapid rise in blood pressure, bradycardia, tachycardia, arrhythmia, headache or sweating due to unregulated sympathetic hyperactivity. This can cause cerebral haemorrhage and death.

- A small number of patients who have had a severe stroke or who have severe forms of Parkinson's disease, multiple sclerosis, cerebral palsy or spina bifida may also be susceptible to autonomic dysreflexia.
  - Patients with spinal cord injury or neurological conditions may have neurogenic bowel dysfunction. They may depend on routine interventional bowel care, including manual removal of faeces. Autonomic dysreflexia can be caused by non-adherence to a patient's usual bowel routine or during or following interventional bowel care.

- Patients that present to ambulance services may have difficulty when their normal bowel routine does not occur, for example due to illness or injury. The condition autonomic dysreflexia should always be considered.

Gastrointestinal

- Auscultate, percuss and palpate, examining for signs which could indicate a gastrointestinal cause for the presenting condition.

- Auscultate for bowel sounds and bruits.

Percuss for hypo/hyper resonance (e.g. dull = solid, high pitch = gas, shifting dullness = fluid)

- Feel for tenderness and guarding in all four quadrants.

Musculoskeletal/Skin

- Check for MSC in four limbs:
  - Test for movement and power.
  - Apply light touch to evaluate sensation.
  - Assess pulse and skin temperature.

- Assess for rashes, localised inflammation, bruising, swelling, erythema or other abnormalities.

- Assess for jaundice.

ADDITIONAL INFORMATION

The following may assist in determining the diagnosis:

- Relatives, carers or friends with knowledge of the patient's history.

- Packets or containers of medication (including domiciliary oxygen) or evidence of administration devices (e.g. nebuliser machines).

- Warning stickers, often placed by the front door or the telephone, directing the health professional to a source of detailed information (one current scheme involves storing the patient details in a container in the fridge, as this is relatively easy to find in the house).

- Patient-held warning cards denoting previous thrombolysis, at-risk COPD patients or those taking monoamine oxidase inhibitor (MAOI) medication.

- Patients' individualised treatment plans.

Medical Emergencies in Adults – Overview

TABLE 3.3 – Glasgow Coma Scale		
Item	**Element**	**Score**
Eyes Opening:		
	Spontaneously	4
	To speech	3
	To pain	2
	None	1
Verbal Response:		
	Orientated	5
	Confused	4
	Inappropriate words	3
	Incomprehensible sounds	2
	No verbal response	1
Motor Response:		
	Obeys commands	6
	Localised pain	5
	Withdraws from pain	4
	Abnormal flexion	3
	Extensor response	2
	No response to pain	1

KEY POINTS!

Medical Emergencies in Adults – Overview

- Detect **TIME-CRITICAL** problems early.
- Minimise time on scene.
- Continuously re-assess **<C>ABCD**.
- Initiate treatments en-route if the patient is deteriorating.
- Provide an **ATMIST** information call for **TIME-CRITICAL** patients.

Bibliography

1. Sharif H, Hou S. Autonomic dysreflexia: a cardiovascular disorder following spinal cord injury. *Neural Regen Res* 2017, 12(9): 1390–1400.

2. Rockwood, K et al. A global clinical measure of fitness and frailty in elderly people. *Canadian Medical Association Journal* 2005, 173(5): 489–495. Available from: https://pubmed.ncbi.nlm.nih.gov/16129869/.

Medical Emergencies in Children – Overview

1. Introduction

- A problem-based approach to paediatric emergencies is to be encouraged. Identifying the features of possible serious illnesses (and addressing them) is more important than identifying the child's underlying diagnosis.

- Assessment priorities include the detection of respiratory distress, circulatory impairment or decreased consciousness.

- Good patient assessment will allow potentially life-threatening illnesses or injuries to be recognised sooner. This should allow treatments and interventions to be given at the earliest opportunity, including rapid hospital transfer for urgent assessment and further treatments when needed.

2. History

- In most cases, a well-taken history will point to the diagnosis. When combined with the findings of your physical examination, this format of history-taking should allow **TIME-CRITICAL** patients, urgent patients and routine patients to be correctly identified.

- History-taking should adhere to the following format and be fully documented:
  - **Presenting complaint** — why did the patient or carer call for help?
  - The **history** of the presenting complaint — details of when the problem started, exacerbating factors and previous similar episodes.
  - Direct questioning about associated **symptoms**, by system. Ask about all appropriate systems.
  - **Past medical history**, including current medication.
  - **Family history**.
  - **Social history**.

- The following should also be considered:
  - **Previous** treatment/contact with healthcare services or episodes of a similar nature.
  - **Feeding and appetite** — note how the child is typically fed: bottle/breast/solids. Button battery ingestion may need to be considered (refer to **Overdose and Poisoning in Adults and Children**).
  - **Activity/Apathy** — does the child act and respond appropriately?
  - **Urine and Faeces** — is this more or less than usual? Wet/dry nappies can be used as a measure of hydration/dehydration.
  - **Growth** — is the child's growth following expected and previously measured centiles?
  - **Sleeping** — is this normal for the child?
  - **Pregnancy** — maternal illness or drug ingestion during pregnancy may have affected the child.
  - **Birth** — antenatal complications, premature labour and birth complications may impact a child's weight and development.
  - **Immunisation and Health Screening**.
  - **Development** — is the child meeting their expected developmental milestones, e.g. hearing, speech or motor ability? Have there been any backward steps/developmental regression? The child's *Red Book* or other documentation may provide useful supporting information.

- Remember that the history of the child and parent provides invaluable insights into the cause of the current condition.

- In making an assessment, make use of the following sources of additional information:
  - Relatives, carers or friends
  - Packets or containers of medication
  - Administration devices, e.g. inhalers, spacers etc.
  - MedicAlert®-type jewellery, e.g. bracelets, or emergency cards (steroids, oxygen), detailing underlying health issues (diabetes, anaphylaxis, drug allergy etc.), as well as a 24-hour telephone number to obtain a more detailed patient history
  - Child protection concerns may become apparent during the initial medical assessment and should be appropriately dealt with (refer to **Safeguarding Children**).

- Having called the emergency services, it is also important to address parental ideas, concerns and expectations regarding their child's current health.

3. Assessment and Management

TABLE 3.4 – ASSESSMENT and MANAGEMENT of: Medical Emergencies in Children
Assess <C>ABCDE
All stages should be considered but some more detailed elements may be omitted when not clinically appropriate.
■ At each stage, consider the need for early senior clinical support.
■ Start correcting any **<C> ABCDE** problems.
■ Undertake a **TIME-CRITICAL** transfer to nearest appropriate receiving hospital.

Medical Emergencies in Children – Overview

- Continue patient management en-route.
- Provide an ATMIST information call.

Catastrophic Haemorrhage

- Look for evidence of significant external haemorrhage.
- Consider occult sources of internal bleeding, especially following trauma.

Arrest external bleeding

- Apply a tourniquet and/or apply direct pressure to the site.
- Dress the site with an appropriate haemorrhage or trauma dressing.
- Elevate the site if possible.

Airway

Assess the airway (refer to Airway and Breathing Management).

- Manage the child's airway in a stepwise manner.
- Exercise extreme caution when managing epiglottitis (refer to **Respiratory Illness in Children**).

Position the head to open the airway.

Abnormal upper airway sounds

- **Look for** physical obstructions, e.g. teeth, foreign bodies, vomit or blood (refer to **Foreign Body Airway Obstruction**).
- **Listen for** noisy airflow, e.g. snoring, gurgling or no airflow (refer to **Dyspnoea**).
  - Inspiratory noises (stridor) suggest an airway obstruction near the larynx.
  - A snoring noise (stertorous breathing) may be present when there is obstruction in the pharynx, e.g. enlarged tonsils.
- **Feel for** air movement:
  - Airway constriction is a life-threatening condition and can result from an immune response to an allergen (refer to **Allergic Reactions including Anaphylaxis**).

Manual extension manoeuvres, head tilt, chin lift or jaw thrust

- The younger the child, the less neck extension will be required. A newborn's head should be placed in the neutral position, while an older child should be extended into a 'sniffing the morning air' position.
- Do not place pressure on the soft tissues under the chin or in front of the neck – this can obstruct the airway.

Aspiration, foreign body removal

- Blind finger sweeps must be avoided as they may push material further down the airway or damage the soft palate.
- Refer to **Foreign Body Airway Obstruction**.

Oropharyngeal airway (OPA)

- Ensure the OPA is of the appropriate size (refer to **Page for Age**) and inserted using the correct technique. Discontinue insertion or remove if the child gags (refer to **Paediatric Resuscitation**).

Nasopharyngeal airway

- Correct sizing is essential (refer to **Page for Age**).
- In small children, a size smaller than estimated may be required.
- Care should be taken not to damage tonsillar or adenoidal tissues.

Endotracheal intubation

- The hazards associated with intubation in children are considerable and usually outweigh the advantages. It should only be attempted where other more basic methods of ventilation have failed and only when capnography is available (ETT sizes are listed on **Page for Age**).
- Only attempt paediatric intubation if authorised to do so and follow local protocols.

(continued)

SECTION 3 Medical Emergencies

Medical Emergencies in Children – Overview

Needle cricothyroidotomy

- Needle cricothyroidotomy is considered a method of last resort.
- Surgical airways should not be performed on children under the age of 12 years.
- The initial oxygen (O_2) flow rate in litres per minute should be set to equal the child's age in years and gradually increased (in 1 litre min^{-1} increments) until adequate chest wall movements are seen.
- Allow ~4 sec for exhalation.

Breathing

Assessment and recognition of potential respiratory impairment

Measure the respiratory rate (see **Page for Age**).

- Tachypnoea, a rapid respiratory rate, in a child at rest indicates a need for increased ventilation and suggests:
  - an airway problem
  - a lung problem
  - a circulatory problem or
  - a metabolic problem.

Recession (indrawing, retraction)

- Intercostal recession (indrawing of the space between the ribs) and subcostal recession (along the costal margins at the point of diaphragmatic attachment) are seen when respiratory effort is high, due to the pliable nature of children's rib cages. In infants, the sternum itself may even be drawn in (sternal recession), but as children get older the rib cage becomes less pliable and other signs of accessory muscle use (other than recession) are seen (see below). If recession is seen in older children, it suggests severe respiratory difficulty.

Accessory muscle use

- As in adult life, when the work of breathing is increased, the sternocleidomastoid muscle may be used as an accessory respiratory muscle. This can cause head-bobbing (the head bobs up and down with each breath) in infants.

Flaring of the nostrils

- This is a subtle sign that is easily missed. It indicates significant respiratory distress.

Inspiratory or expiratory noises

- Wheezing indicates lower airway narrowing and is most commonly heard on expiration. The volume of the wheeze is **NOT** an indicator of severity – it may diminish with increasing respiratory distress because less air is being moved.

Inspiratory noises (stridor)

- This suggests an imminent danger to the airway due to reduction in airway circumference to approximately 10% of normal. Again, the volume of stridor does **NOT** reflect severity and may also diminish with increasing respiratory distress as less air is moved.

Grunting

- This is produced by exhalation against a partially closed laryngeal opening (glottis). This is more likely to be seen in infants and is a sign of severe respiratory distress.

Effectiveness of breathing — chest expansion and breath sounds

- Note the degree of expansion on both sides of the chest and whether it is equal.

Auscultate the chest with a stethoscope

- A silent chest is a pre-terminal sign, as it indicates that very little air is moving in or out of the chest.

Pulse oximetry

- This can be used at all ages to measure oxygen saturation (readings are less reliable in the presence of shock, hypothermia and other conditions such as carbon monoxide poisoning and severe anaemia).
- For additional signs of breathing compromise, refer to Table 3.5.

SECTION 3 Medical Emergencies

Medical Emergencies in Children – Overview

- All sick children require adequate oxygenation.
- Administer high levels of supplemental oxygen (O_2) via a non-rebreathing mask.
- If the child finds the face mask distressing, ask the parent to help by holding the mask as close to the child's face as possible. If this still produces distress, wafting O_2 across the face directly from the tubing, with the face mask detached from the tubing, is better than nothing.
- In children with sickle cell disease or cardiac disease, high levels of O_2 should be administered routinely, whatever their oxygen saturation.
- Consider assisted ventilation at a rate equivalent to the normal respiratory rate for the age of the child (refer to paediatric resuscitation charts for normal values) if:
  - The child is hypoxic (SpO_2 <90%) and remains so after being placed on high flows and concentration O_2.
  - Respiratory rate is slower (3 times normal) than normal.
  - Expansion is inadequate.
- Use an appropriately sized mask to ensure a good seal.
- Try to avoid hyperventilation to minimise the risks of gastric insufflation or barotrauma. The bag-valve-mask should have a pressure release valve as an added safety measure. If this is not available, extreme care must be taken not to over-expand the lungs. No bag smaller than 500 ml volume should be used for bag-valve-mask ventilation unless the child is <2.5 kg, i.e. preterm baby size.

Wheezing

- The management of asthma is discussed elsewhere (refer to **Asthma in Adults and Children**).
- See **Respiratory Illness in Children** for further guidance on childhood respiratory illnesses.

Circulation

Assessment and recognition of potential circulatory failure (shock)

- Circulatory assessments in children are difficult, as each physical sign may have a number of confounding variables.
- When assessing whether a child is shocked, it is important to assess and evaluate each of the signs below:

Heart rate: (see **Page for Age**)

- **Tachycardia** results from loss of circulatory volume. Heart rates, particularly in infants, can be very high (up to 220 beats per minute). (Heart rates greater than 220 bpm are seen in supraventricular tachycardia).
- An abnormally slow pulse, or **bradycardia**, is defined as less than 60 bpm or a rapidly falling heart rate associated with poor systemic circulation. Bradycardia is a pre-terminal sign and becomes apparent before cardiac arrest (see above).

Pulse volume

- Peripheral pulses become weak and then absent as shock advances.
- Children peripherally vasoconstrict their extremities as shock progresses, initially cooling skin distally and then more proximally as shock advances.
- There is no validated relationship between the presence of certain peripheral pulses and the systemic blood pressure in children.

Capillary refill

- This should be measured on the forehead or sternum.
- A capillary refill time of >2 seconds indicates poor perfusion, although this is influenced by a number of factors, including cold and poor lighting conditions.

Blood pressure:

- Varies with age
- Is difficult to reliably measure, increasing on-scene times, and therefore is not routinely measured in pre-hospital practice
- Hypotension is a very late (and pre-terminal sign) in shocked children and so other signs of circulatory inadequacy will manifest (and should have been recognised) long before hypotension occurs.
- For other signs of circulatory compromise, refer to Table 3.6.

(continued)

SECTION **3** Medical Emergencies

Medical Emergencies in Children – Overview

Arrest external haemorrhage

- Do not attempt to gain intravenous (IV) or intraosseous (IO) access at the scene. Obtain access en-route unless delay is unavoidable.

Cannulation

- Attempt cannulation with the widest bore cannula that can be confidently placed. The vehicle can be stopped briefly to allow for venepuncture and disposal of the sharp, with transport being recommended before applying the IV dressing.

- The IO route may be required where venous access has failed on two occasions or no suitable vein is apparent within a reasonable timeframe. The IO route is the preferred route for vascular access in all cases of cardiac arrest in young children.

- Blood glucose level should be measured in (i) all children in whom vascular access is being obtained and (ii) any child with decreased conscious level (refer to **Altered Level of Consciousness**).

Fluid administration

- Use sodium chloride 0.9% to treat shock.

- Fluids should be measured in millilitres and documented as volume administered — not as the volume of fluid chosen.

- Fluids should be administered as boluses rather than 'run in'.

- Handover at the receiving unit must include details of volume and type of fluid administered.

Fluid volumes

- 20 ml/kg boluses of 0.9% Sodium Chloride are used to resuscitate medically ill children with shock from circulatory failure, to restore vital signs to normal.

- No more than two boluses should be given except on medical advice (refer to **Intravascular Fluid Therapy in Children** and **Sodium Chloride 0.9%**).

Exceptions

- In diabetic ketoacidosis, fluids are administered more cautiously to reduce the risk of cerebral oedema (refer to **Glycaemic Emergencies in Adults and Children**).

- In diabetic ketoacidosis, fluid should be withheld unless severe shock is present, in which case 10 ml/kg should be administered over 10–15 minutes (refer to **Glycaemic Emergencies in Adults and Children**).

- If a child has heart failure or renal failure, give a 10 ml/kg bolus but stop if the patient deteriorates. Transfer to hospital as a priority.

- Seek medical advice when exceptional circumstances are present, such as a long transfer time.

Disability

Recognition of potential neurological failure

- Note the initial level of responsiveness on the AVPU scale, and time of assessment:
  - **A** — Alert.
  - **V** — Responds to voice.
  - **P** — Responds to painful stimulus.
  - **U** — Unresponsive.

Response to a painful stimulus

- Pinch a digit or pull frontal hair. A child who is unconscious or who only responds to pain has a significant degree of coma (refer to Glasgow Coma Scale — Appendix 1. **NB** the 'adult' GCS should be used in children over 4 years of age).

Posture: observe the child's posture

- Children may:
  - be floppy (hypotonic) – recent floppiness in a child suggests a serious illness
  - be stiff (hypertonic) or
  - have back arching (opisthotonus).

- New onset stiffness suggests severe cerebral disturbance.

- Decerebrate or decorticate postures suggest a serious underlying cerebral abnormality.

Medical Emergencies in Children – Overview

Pupils

- Test pupil size and reaction.

- Pupils should be equal, of normal size and react briskly to light.

- Any abnormality or change in pupil size or reaction may be significant.

- For additional signs of neurological compromise, refer to Table 3.7.

- **NB** The whole assessment should take less than 2 minutes unless intervention is required.

- Re-assessment of <C>ABCD is necessary to assess the response to treatment or to detect deterioration. (Blood glucose levels should be measured in any seriously ill child.)

- The aim of management of any child with a cerebral insult is to minimise further insult by optimising their circumstances. This usually concerns management strategies designed to:
  - prevent hypoxia (see above)
  - normalise circulation without causing fluid overload
  - identify and treat hypoglycaemia (refer to **Glycaemic Emergencies in Adults and Children**).

- Other conditions that can be treated out of hospital and are discussed elsewhere include:
  - convulsions (refer to **Convulsions in Children**)
  - opiate poisoning (refer to **Overdose and Poisoning in Adults and Children**)
  - meningococcal septicaemia (refer to **Meningococcal Meningitis and Septicaemia**).

Vital Signs

NB Complete a full set of observations for all patients, and repeat after intervention or when any value is outside normal parameters.

Respiratory rate

- Measure and record respiratory rate.

Pulse

- Measure and record pulse.

Oxygen saturation

- Monitor the patient's SpO_2; administer oxygen to achieve saturations of >94% if the patient is hypoxic in air (refer to **Oxygen**).

Blood pressure

- Measure and record blood pressure.

- **NB** This is difficult to reliably measure, increasing on-scene times, and as a result is not routinely measured in out-of-hospital practice.

Fluids

- If required, administer fluids (refer to **Intravascular Fluid Therapy in Children**).

Neurology

- Assess AVPU, GCS, pupils and posture.

Blood glucose

If appropriate, measure and record blood glucose for hypo/hyperglycaemia (refer to **Glycaemic Emergencies in Adults and Children**).

Temperature

- Measure and record temperature.

Traffic lights

- Refer to specific guidelines to perform a NICE (National Institute for Health and Care Excellence) '**traffic light**' assessment, prioritising children into three groups according to the presence of certain symptoms and signs:
  - '**Green**' – low risk.
  - '**Amber**' – intermediate risk.
  - '**Red**' – high risk.

- Refer to **Febrile Illness in Children**, Table 3.47.

(continued)

SECTION **3** Medical Emergencies

Medical Emergencies in Children – Overview

TABLE 3.4 – ASSESSMENT and MANAGEMENT of: Medical Emergencies in Children *(continued)*

ECG

- If required, monitor and record 12-lead ECG. Assess for abnormality (refer to **Cardiac Rhythm Disturbance**).

Pain assessment

- Use the **SOCRATES** pain mnemonic and record initial (and subsequent) pain scores.
- Offer analgesia where appropriate (refer to **Pain Management in Children**).

Documentation

- Complete documentation to include all clinical findings, advice from other clinicians, onward referral and worsening advice given.

TABLE 3.5 – Additional Signs of Compromised Breathing

Heart rate

- Tachycardia, or eventually bradycardia, may result from hypoxia and acidosis.
- Bradycardia in a sick child is a pre-terminal sign.

Skin colour

- Flushing of the skin (vasodilation) is seen in early respiratory distress due to elevated carbon dioxide levels.
- Hypoxia causes vasoconstriction and skin pallor.
- Cyanosis is a pre-terminal sign of hypoxia.

Mental status

- Hypoxia makes children agitated and drowsy.
- Agitation may be difficult to recognise due to the child's distress. Use parents to help make this assessment.
- Drowsiness gradually progresses, leading to unconsciousness.

TABLE 3.6 – Additional Signs of Circulatory Compromise

Respiratory rate

- The combination of both rapid respiratory rate and no recession may indicate circulatory insufficiency.
- Tachypnoea occurs as the body tries to correct metabolic derangements.

Skin

- Mottled, cold, pale skin reflects poor perfusion.

Mental status

- Agitation is seen in early shock, progressing to drowsiness as shock advances.
- Poor cerebral perfusion may ultimately result in loss of consciousness.

TABLE 3.7 – Additional Signs of Neurological Compromise

Respiratory system

- Brain insults produce abnormal breathing patterns, e.g. hyperventilation, Cheyne–Stokes breathing or apnoea.

Circulatory system

- Bradycardia may be a result of dangerously raised intracranial pressure.

Medical Emergencies in Children – Overview

Summary

- The primary assessment of the child should establish whether they are seriously ill.
- Immediate correction of any problems must be undertaken without delay at the scene.
- Continually monitor and reassess the child en-route to hospital.
- Children who are found to be seriously ill must be considered to have a **TIME-CRITICAL** condition and be taken to the nearest suitable receiving hospital without delay.
- A hospital **ATMIST** call should be made whenever a seriously ill child is transported.
- Paediatric drug dosages are calculated as 'mg per kilogram' (refer to **Page for Age** and specific medicine guidelines for dosages and information).
- Drug doses **MUST** be checked before **ANY** drug administration, no matter how confident the practitioner may be.

Appendix

TABLE 3.8 – Modified Glasgow Coma Scale for Children Under 4-Years of Age		
Item	**Element**	**Score**
Eyes Opening:		
	Spontaneously	4
	To speech	3
	To pain	2
	None	1
Verbal Response:		
	Orientated (appropriate words or social smiles, and fixes on and follows objects)	5
	Confused (cries, but is consolable)	4
	Inappropriate words (persistently irritable)	3
	Incomprehensible sounds (restless, agitated)	2
	No verbal response (silent)	1
Motor Response:		
	Obeys commands	6
	Localised pain	5
	Withdraws from pain	4
	Abnormal flexion	3
	Extensor response	2
	No response to pain	1

Medical Emergencies in Children – Overview

Medical Emergencies in Children – Overview

- The child and parent's history will provide a valuable insight into the cause of the child's current condition.

- Hypoxia and hypovolaemia need urgent correction.

- Emergency airway management rarely requires intubation.

- Check the blood glucose in all seriously ill children and those with a decreased level of consciousness.

- <C>ABCDE problems should be corrected and managed en-route to further care. Do not delay on scene.

- It is important to address ideas, concerns and expectations, especially of the parents who are often concerned, hence the call to emergency services.

Further Resources

1. Spotting the Sick Child. Available from:
    https://spottingthesickchild.com/.
    SSC is an interactive tool commissioned by the
    Department of Health and Health Education England to
    support health professionals in the assessment of the
    acutely sick child.

SECTION

3

Medical Emergencies

Abdominal Pain

1. Introduction

- Abdominal pain is a common presenting symptom to ambulance services. The specific cause can be difficult to identify in pre-hospital care and a definitive diagnosis may require in-hospital investigations.

- The nature, location and pattern of the pain, together with associated symptoms, may indicate a possible cause (refer to Table 3.9). Many of the causes for abdominal pain can be self-limiting. However, it is important to recognise the risk associated with those conditions that need further input, as well as those that need more urgent life saving interventions.

- The elderly, those with alcohol dependence and immunosuppressed patients may have atypical presentations.

- This guideline covers adults, infants and children. In this guideline, the term 'child' includes infants, unless specified otherwise.

- Abdominal pain can arise from both acute and chronic abdominal conditions:
  - **Acute conditions:** e.g. appendicitis, cholecystitis, intestinal obstruction, ureteric colic, gastritis, perforated peptic ulcer, gastroenteritis, pancreatitis, diverticular disease, leaking or ruptured abdominal aortic aneurysms and gynaecological disorders.
  - **Chronic conditions:** e.g. irritable bowel syndrome (IBS), inflammatory bowel syndromes (ulcerative colitis and Crohn's disease), gastric and duodenal ulcers and intra-abdominal malignancy.

TABLE 3.9 – Causes of Abdominal Pain in Adults and Children

CONDITION	CHARACTERISTICS OF PAIN	ASSOCIATED SYMPTOMS
Abdominal migraine	- Presents typically as recurrent bouts of generalised abdominal pain.	- Nausea and vomiting. - No headache, followed by sleep and recovery.
Acute cholecystitis Accounts for approximately 30% of patients attending ED for acute abdominal pain.	- A sharp pain in the right upper quadrant of the abdomen. - May experience right shoulder-tip pain. - The pain is worse when breathing deeply and on palpation of the right upper quadrant.	- Nausea and vomiting. - Increased temperature >38°C. - History of fat intolerance.
Acute pancreatitis Inflammation of the pancreas.	- Constant pain in the upper left quadrant or middle of the abdomen. - The pain may radiate to the patient's back.	- Abdominal tenderness. - Hypotension. - Nausea and vomiting. - Dehydration. - Shock. - History of alcohol abuse or gallstones.
Appendicitis Frequently misdiagnosed. Approximately one-third of women of childbearing age with appendicitis are considered as having pelvic inflammatory disease or urinary tract infection (UTI). Appendicitis accounts for more than 40,000 hospital admissions in England each year (more common in children aged 12–16).	- A constant pain, increasing in intensity, often starting in the peri-umbilical area. - The pain may settle in the right lower quadrant, but the location may vary in the early stages. - Tenderness on percussion, guarding (muscular rigidity). The site of maximal tenderness is often said to be over McBurney's point, which is two-thirds of the way along a line drawn from the umbilicus to the anterior superior iliac spine.	- Nausea. - Vomiting (profuse vomiting may indicate development of peritonitis). - Loss of appetite. - Constipation. - Increased low grade temperature >37.5°C. - Diarrhoea. - Facial flushing, dry tongue, halitosis. - Tachycardia.

(continued)

Abdominal Pain

TABLE 3.9 – Causes of Abdominal Pain in Adults and Children *(continued)*

	<ul><li>There is rebound tenderness in the right iliac fossa and coughing and walking may exacerbate the pain.</li><li>Older patients may present with generalised pain, distension and decreased bowel sounds.</li><li>In children, if asked to hop, the child will refuse as this causes pain.</li><li>Rovsing's sign – palpation of the left lower quadrant increases the pain felt in the right lower quadrant.</li><li>Psoas sign – extending the right thigh with the person in the left lateral position elicits pain in the right lower quadrant.</li><li>Obturator sign – internal rotation of the flexed right thigh elicits pain in the right lower quadrant.</li></ul>	**NB** Assess for potential complications: <ul><li>Tachycardia and sudden relief of pain may be signs of a perforated appendix.</li><li>Palpable abdominal mass and swinging pyrexia may be signs of an appendix abscess.</li><li>High fever (more than 40°C), severe abdominal tenderness and absent bowel sounds may be signs of peritonitis.</li></ul>
Constipation	<ul><li>Abdominal tenderness.</li></ul>	<ul><li>Infrequent bowel activity.</li><li>Foul-smelling wind and stools.</li><li>Excessive flatulence.</li><li>Irregular stool texture.</li><li>Passing occasional enormous stools or frequent small pellets.</li><li>Withholding or straining to stop passage of stools.</li><li>Soiling or overflow.</li><li>Abdominal distension.</li><li>Poor appetite.</li><li>Lack of energy.</li><li>Unhappy, angry or irritable mood and general malaise.</li></ul>
Diverticular disease Inflammation of diverticula in the large intestine.	<ul><li>Abdominal pain in the lower left quadrant.</li></ul>	<ul><li>Nausea and vomiting.</li><li>Altered bowel habit.</li><li>Bloating.</li><li>Increased temperature >38°C.</li></ul>
Ectopic pregnancy Pregnancy not implanted in the uterus. It affects 1 pregnancy in 80 and accounts for 13% of all pregnancy-related deaths.	<ul><li>Pain in the lower abdomen, pelvic area or back.</li><li>**NB** Patients may present atypically but pain is almost always present.</li></ul>	<ul><li>Nausea.</li><li>Missed last menstrual period (though can occur before this).</li><li>History of pelvic inflammatory disease.</li><li>Previous ectopic pregnancy.</li></ul>

Abdominal Pain

TABLE 3.9 – Causes of Abdominal Pain in Adults and Children *(continued)*		
		If the pregnancy ruptures, patients may report: ▪ Severe lower abdominal pain. ▪ Shoulder-tip pain. ▪ Feeling faint/collapse.
Gastritis An inflammation of the gastric lining can be caused by medication (aspirin, non-steroidal anti-inflammatory drugs), alcohol, *Helicobacter pylori* or stress.	▪ Upper abdominal pain. ▪ Lower/central chest pain/ epigastric pain.	▪ Nausea and vomiting. ▪ Loss of appetite. ▪ Haematemesis.
Hepatitis	▪ Abdominal pain.	▪ This is due to liver swelling.
Infective diarrhoea	▪ Intermittent generalised abdominal pain.	▪ Blood mixed with stools – ask about travel history and recent antibiotic therapy.
Inflammatory bowel disease, midgut volvulus		▪ Blood in stools.
Intestinal obstruction A partial or complete obstruction of the small or large intestine. Intussusception (bowel obstruction caused by a segment of intestine sliding inside another part of the intestines). Most commonly found in infants; another peak in incidence occurs at six years of age. Volvulus (a loop of intestine twisting around itself, resulting in obstruction).	▪ Abdominal pain that is cramping in nature. ▪ Intermittent colicky pain associated with bouts of screaming and drawing up legs.	▪ Abdominal distension. ▪ Nausea and vomiting. ▪ Absolute constipation (late stage). ▪ 'Currant jelly stool' – blood and mucus. ▪ Faecal vomiting. ▪ Bile-stained vomiting. ▪ Absence of normal flatus. ▪ Abdominal distension. ▪ Increased bowel sounds. ▪ Visible distended loops of bowel. ▪ Visible peristalsis. ▪ Scars. ▪ Swellings at the site of hernial orifices and of the external genitalia.
Ischaemic bowel Ischaemic bowel is a group of conditions that are associated with reduced blood flow and potential infarction of the intestines. This can occur within both the small intestine and the large intestine. This is a medical emergency, with mortality rates up to 90% in missed recognition or delayed diagnosis and treatment.	▪ Moderate to severe colic type or constant and poorly localised pain. ▪ Severe left iliac fossa pain.	▪ Physical findings and observations that are out of proportion to the degree of pain reported. ▪ Gastrointestinal symptoms such as nausea and vomiting, PR bleeds and bowel problems may also be present.

(continued)

3 SECTION **Medical Emergencies**

Abdominal Pain

TABLE 3.9 – Causes of Abdominal Pain in Adults and Children *(continued)*		
The main contributing cause is a thrombus, and specific risk factors include AF, particularly where patient is not medicated, mitral stenosis, vasopressors and strangulated hernias.		▪ In early presentation, the abdominal examination may not show any significant findings, but later stages may include signs of peritonitis.
Leaking or ruptured abdominal aortic aneurysms (AAAs) Consider AAA in patients >50 years who present with the symptoms listed. Most deaths occur in older people.	▪ Sudden severe abdominal pain or backache. ▪ Renal colic-type pain – a new diagnosis of renal colic in a patient over 50 years of age raises the concern of AAA even in the absence of a palpable mass. ▪ **NB** Given that <25% of all AAA patients present with classic signs and symptoms, there is a risk of misdiagnosis.	▪ Collapse. ▪ Hypotension with bilateral lower limb ischaemia or mottling (a late sign). ▪ History of smoking. ▪ Hypertension and hypercholesterolaemia.
Lower lobe pneumonia (children)	▪ Abdominal pain.	▪ Fever. ▪ Cough. ▪ Tachypnoea. ▪ Desaturation.
Pelvic inflammatory disease A common cause of abdominal pain in females but rarely presents as an acute collapse.	▪ Pain in the lower abdomen, pelvic area or back. ▪ Abdominal tenderness.	▪ Vaginal discharge. ▪ Nausea. ▪ Fever.
Peritonitis	▪ Refusal or inability to walk. ▪ Slow walk or stooped forward. ▪ Pain on coughing or jolting.	▪ Lying motionless. ▪ Decreased/absent abdominal wall movements with respiration. ▪ Abdominal distention. ▪ Abdominal tenderness – localised/generalised. ▪ Abdominal guarding/rigidity. ▪ Percussion tenderness. ▪ Palpable abdominal mass. ▪ Bowel sounds – absent/decreased (peritonitis). ▪ Associated non-specific signs – tachycardia, fever.
Peptic ulcer An erosion of the lining of the stomach or small intestine, forming an ulcer.	▪ Central burning abdominal pain. ▪ Back pain. ▪ Perforation may lead to abrupt onset epigastric pain.	▪ Nausea and vomiting – haematemesis. ▪ Fatigue. ▪ Weight loss.

Abdominal Pain

TABLE 3.9 – Causes of Abdominal Pain in Adults and Children *(continued)*

Torsion of the testis **NB** This is a surgical emergency and if suspected the patient should be admitted to the nearest appropriate ED immediately.	▪ Sudden onset of severe pain in lower abdominal region or in the scrotum.	▪ Acute swelling of the scrotum (swelling is not *always* present). ▪ Nausea and vomiting often occur. **NB** These symptoms indicate torsion of the testis until proven otherwise.
Urinary tract pathology Infection arising from the kidneys, ureters, bladder and/or urethra. Urinary tract obstruction.	▪ Pain in the lower abdomen and/or back. ▪ Cramping.	▪ Pain/burning sensation when urinating. ▪ Needing to urinate frequently. ▪ Urinary frequency and nocturia. ▪ Offensive urine. ▪ Nausea and vomiting. ▪ Cloudy/bloody urine with a malodour. ▪ Lethargy. ▪ Irritability. ▪ Poor feeding. ▪ Jaundice fever. ▪ If the infection involves the kidneys, the patient may have increased temperature >38°C, and fatigue. ▪ Rigors may be present.

TABLE 3.10 – Common Causes of Abdominal Pain in Children

< 2 Years	2 to 12 Years	12 to 16 Years
▪ Gastroenteritis. ▪ Constipation. ▪ Intussusception. ▪ Infantile colic. ▪ UTI. ▪ Incarcerated inguinal hernia. ▪ Trauma. ▪ Pneumonia. ▪ Diabetes.	▪ Gastroenteritis. ▪ Mesenteric adenitis. ▪ Constipation. ▪ UTI. ▪ Onset of menstruation. ▪ Psychogenic. ▪ Trauma. ▪ Pneumonia. ▪ Diabetes.	▪ Mesenteric adenitis. ▪ Acute appendicitis. ▪ Menstruation. ▪ Mittelschmerz. ▪ Ovarian cyst torsion. ▪ UTI. ▪ Pregnancy. ▪ Ectopic pregnancy. ▪ Testicular torsion. ▪ Psychogenic. ▪ Trauma. ▪ Pneumonia. ▪ Diabetes.

SECTION **3** Medical Emergencies

Abdominal Pain

2. Severity and Outcome

- The most common diagnosis of patients presenting to ED with abdominal pain is non-specific abdominal pain, followed by renal colic.

- Many cases are relatively minor in nature (e.g. constipation, UTI); however, 25% of patients contacting the ambulance service with abdominal pain have serious underlying conditions.

- In patients >65 years there is a 6–8 times higher mortality rate due to atypical clinical presentations and the presence of co-morbidities.

3. Pathophysiology

Abdominal pain can be localised and referred, due to overlapping innervations of the organs contained in the abdomen (e.g. small and large intestines).

4. Assessment and Management

For the assessment and management of abdominal pain, refer to Table 3.11.

TABLE 3.11 – ASSESSMENT and MANAGEMENT of: Abdominal Pain

Assess <C>ABCD

- If any of the following **TIME-CRITICAL** features present:
  - major **<C>ABCD** problems (refer to **Medical Emergencies in Adults – Overview** and **Medical Emergencies in Children – Overview**).
  - suspected leaking or ruptured aortic aneurysm
  - torsion of the testis.
- ectopic pregnancy
  - sepsis resulting from perforation
  - traumatic disruption of abdominal organs, e.g. liver, spleen, then:
- Start correcting any **<C>ABCD** problems.
- Undertake a **TIME-CRITICAL** transfer to nearest appropriate receiving hospital – for patients with suspected leaking or ruptured aortic aneurysm, follow local care pathway.
- Continue patient management en-route.
- Provide an ATMIST information call.

Differential Diagnoses

- If no immediately life-threatening signs are identified during the primary survey, then continue to a secondary survey to understand causes of pain and form differential diagnoses. Refer to Table 3.9.

NB For indigestion-type pain, have a high index of suspicion that it may be cardiac in origin.

Examination

- Assess the patient's abdomen, where possible in a supine position. Flexing the knees to 90 degrees relaxes the abdominal wall. The physical abdominal examination should include:
  - auscultating the abdomen for bowel sounds and their frequency
  - palpating for tenderness, rebound tenderness and guarding.

NB Hyperactive bowel sounds in children commonly stem from gastroenteritis; however, consider bowel obstructions or gastro-intestinal (GI) haemorrhage/infection as a risk when completing the assessment.

History

- During history-taking, be aware of bowel obstructions caused by surgical emergencies, such as intussusception (bowel obstruction caused by a segment of intestine sliding inside another part of the intestines) or volvulus (a loop of intestine twisting around itself resulting in obstruction). These presentations are a surgical emergency and need to be conveyed to an ED within an hour of presentation.

NB Bites, stings and poisons: ask about the possibility of bites, stings or ingestion of poisons. Adder envenomation can result in abdominal pain and vomiting

If Patient Is Female and of Childbearing Age, Consider Additional Causes

- Suggest pregnancy test.
- Consider ectopic pregnancy, pelvic inflammatory disease or other STD.
- Other gynaecological problems.

Abdominal Pain

TABLE 3.11 – ASSESSMENT and MANAGEMENT of: Abdominal Pain *(continued)*
■ Mittelschmerz (one-sided lower abdominal pain associated with ovulation).
■ Torsion of the ovary.
■ Pelvic inflammatory disease.
Known Congenital or Pre-existing Condition
■ Previous abdominal surgery (adhesions).
■ Nephrotic syndrome (primary peritonitis).
■ Mediterranean background (familial Mediterranean fever).
■ Hereditary spherocytosis (cholelithiasis).
■ Cystic fibrosis (meconium ileus equivalent).
■ Cystinuria.
■ Porphyria.
■ Current drug treatment if any.
■ Recent travel.
■ Presence of similar symptoms in others.
Associated Symptoms/Conditions
■ Altered bowel habit.
■ Nausea and vomiting – haematemesis/malaena may indicate gastrointestinal pathology – refer to **Gastrointestinal Bleeding**.
■ Vaginal bleeding/pregnancy/previous ectopic pregnancy – refer to relevant **Maternity Care** guidelines.
■ Burning on urination.
■ Menstrual and sexual history in females of childbearing age (is there any possibility of pregnancy?).
NB For details of signs and symptoms of specific conditions, refer to Table 3.9.
Respiratory Rate
■ Measure and record respiratory rate.
Pulse
■ Measure and record pulse.
Oxygen Saturation
■ Monitor the patient's SpO_2, administer oxygen to achieve saturations of >94% if the patient presents as hypoxaemic on air (refer to **Oxygen**).
Blood Pressure and Fluids
■ Measure and record blood pressure. If required, administer fluids (refer to **Intravascular Fluid Therapy in Adults** and **Intravascular Fluid Therapy in Children**).
Blood Glucose
■ If appropriate, measure and record blood glucose for hypo/hyperglycaemia (refer to **Glycasemic Emergencies in Adults and Children**).
Temperature
■ Measure and record temperature.
NEWS2
■ These observations will enable you to calculate a NEWS2 Score (refer to **Sepsis**).
ECG
■ If required, monitor and record 12-lead ECG. Assess for abnormality (refer to **Cardiac Rhyhm Disturbance**).

(continued)

Abdominal Pain

TABLE 3.11 – ASSESSMENT and MANAGEMENT of: Abdominal Pain *(continued)*
Assess the Patient's Pain
▪ Where present, assess the SOCRATES of pain and record initial and subsequent pain scores.
▪ Consider analgesia if appropriate (refer to **Pain Management in Adults** and **Pain Management in Children**).
Documentation
▪ Complete documentation to include all clinical findings, advice from other clinicians, onward referral and worsening advice given.
Transfer to Further Care
▪ Transfer to further care (consider most appropriate centre).
▪ Transfer all children with bile-stained (green) vomit.
▪ A new diagnosis of renal colic in a patient over 50 years of age raises the concern of AAA even in the absence of a palpable mass.

4.1 Community Management

All patients with abdominal pain being left in the community MUST be discussed with another healthcare professional, such as the general practitioner (GP) or out-of-hours GP, due to the complex nature of the presentation and potential implication for missed diagnosis.

Should the patient be discharged on scene, provide the following advice to the patient/parent/carer:

▪ Reassure the patient and encourage them to rest.

▪ If they are not vomiting, advise regular paracetamol for pain relief.

▪ Advise the patient to avoid aspirin.

▪ Encourage the patient to drink plenty of clear fluids (e.g. cooled boiled water).

▪ Do not push the patient to eat if they feel unwell.

▪ If the patient is hungry, encourage them to eat bland food (e.g. crackers, rice, bananas or toast).

▪ Many patients with abdominal pain get better without intervention over a few hours or days. However, if problems persist, encourage them to seek further medical advice.

KEY POINTS!

Abdominal Pain

▪ **The most important diagnoses to consider are those that are life-threatening, as the result of either internal haemorrhage or perforation of a viscus and sepsis.**

▪ **For indigestion-type pain, have a high index of suspicion that it may be cardiac in origin. Obtain a 12-lead ECG for older patients and patients with cardiac risks presenting with upper abdominal pain.**

▪ **If a patient is in pain, adequate analgesia should be given.**

▪ **A precise diagnosis of the cause of abdominal pain is often not possible without access to tests and investigations in hospital or via primary care.**

Acknowledgements

We would like to gratefully acknowledge the contribution of the South Western Ambulance Service to this JRCALC guideline.

SECTION **3** Medical Emergencies

Abdominal Pain

Bibliography

1. Kavanagh S. The acute abdomen: assessment, diagnosis and pitfalls. *UK MPS Casebook* 2004, 12(1): 11–18.

2. Manterola C, Vial M, Moraga J, Astudillo P. Analgesia in patients with acute abdominal pain. *Cochrane Database of Systematic Reviews* 2011, 1. Available from: http://www.mrw.interscience.wiley.com/cochrane/clsysrev/articles/CD005660/frame.html: doi 10.1002/14651858.CD005660.pub3.

3. Agarwal T, Butt MA. Small bowel obstruction. *Emergency Medicine Journal* 2007, 24(5): 368.

4. Amoli HA, Golozar A, Keshavarzi S, Tavakoli H, Yaghoobi A. Morphine analgesia in patients with acute appendicitis: a randomised double-blind clinical trial. *Emergency Medicine Journal* 2008, 25(9): 586–589.

5. Beck J, Jang TB. Short answer question case series: controversies in the diagnosis and management of diverticulitis. *Emergency Medicine Journal* 2012, 29(6): 517–518.

6. Beck J, Jang TB. Short answer question case series: diagnosis of acute cholecystitis. *Emergency Medicine Journal* 2012, 29(5): 430–431.

7. Beckingham IJ, Bornman PC. Acute pancreatitis. *British Medical Journal* 2001, 322(7286): 595–598.

8. Car J. Urinary tract infections in women: diagnosis and management in primary care. *British Medical Journal* 2006, 332(7533): 94–97.

9. Cartwright SL, Knudson MP. Evaluation of acute abdominal pain in adults. *American Family Physician* 2008, 77(7): 971–978.

10. Chan SSW, Ng KC, Lyon DJ, Cheung WL, Cheng AFB, Rainer TH. Acute bacterial gastroenteritis: a study of adult patients with positive stool cultures treated in the emergency department. *Emergency Medicine Journal* 2003, 20(4): 335–338.

11. Chong CF, Wang TL, Chen CC, Ma HP, Chang H. Preconsultation use of analgesics on adults presenting to the emergency department with acute appendicitis. *Emergency Medicine Journal* 2004, 21(1): 41–43.

12. Gray J, Wardrope J, Fothergill DJ. The ABC of community emergency care: 7 Abdominal pain: abdominal pain in women, complications of pregnancy and labour. *Emergency Medicine Journal* 2004, 21(5): 606–613.

13. Hall J, Driscoll P. The ABC of community emergency care: 10 Nausea, vomiting and fever. *Emergency Medicine Journal* 2005, 22(3): 200–204.

14. Humes DJ, Simpson J. Acute appendicitis. *British Medical Journal* 2006, 333(7567): 530–534.

15. Kingsnorth A, O'Reilly D. Acute pancreatitis. *British Medical Journal* 2006, 332(7549): 1072–1076.

16. Lehnert T, Sorge I, Till H, Rolle U. Intussusception in children: clinical presentation, diagnosis and management. *International Journal of Colorectal Disease* 2009, 24(10): 1187–1192.

17. Lewis SRR, Mahony PJ, Simpson J. Appendicitis. *British Medical Journal* 2011, 343: d5976.

18. Little P, Merriman R, Turner S, Rumsby K, Warner G, Lowes JA, et al. Presentation, pattern, and natural course of severe symptoms, and role of antibiotics and antibiotic resistance among patients presenting with suspected uncomplicated urinary tract infection in primary care: observational study. *British Medical Journal* 2010, 340: b5633.

19. Lynch RM. Accuracy of abdominal examination in the diagnosis of non-ruptured abdominal aortic aneurysm. *Accident and Emergency Nursing* 2004, 12(2): 99–107.

20. Metcalfe D, Holt PIE, Thompson MM. The management of abdominal aortic aneurysms. *British Medical Journal* 2011, 342: d1384.

21. Ranji SR, Goldman L, Simel DL, Shojania KG. Do opiates affect the clinical evaluation of patients with acute abdominal pain? *Journal of the American Medical Association* 2006, 296(14): 764–774.

22. Royal College of Obstetricians and Gynaecologists. *Management of Acute Pelvic Inflammatory Disease* (Green-top Guideline 32). London: RCOG, 2008. Available from: https://www.rcog.org.uk/en/guidelines-research-services/guidelines/gtg32/.

23. Sakalihasan N, Limet R, Defawe OD. Abdominal aortic aneurysm. *The Lancet* 2005, 365(9470): 1577–1589.

24. Touzios JG, Dozois EJ. Diverticulosis and acute diverticulitis. *Gastroenterology Clinics of North America* 2009, 38(3): 513–525.

25. Trowbridge RL, Rutkowski NK, Shojania KG. Does this patient have acute cholecystitis? *Journal of the American Medical Association* 2003, 289(1): 80–86.

26. National Collaborating Centre for Women's and Children's Health. *Urinary Tract Infection in Children: Diagnosis, treatment and long-term management* (CG54). London: Royal College of Obstetricians and Gynaecologists, 2007. Available from: http://www.nice.org.uk/nicemedia/pdf/CG54fullguideline.pdf.

27. National Institute for Health and Clinical Excellence. *Diarrhoea and Vomiting in Children: Diarrhoea and vomiting caused by gastroenteritis: diagnosis, assessment and management in children younger than 5 years* (CG84). 2009. Available from: https://www.nice.org.uk/guidance/cg84.

28. Scottish Intercollegiate Guidelines Network. *Management of Acute Upper and Lower Gastrointestinal Bleeding* (Guideline 105). Edinburgh: SIGN, 2008.

29. Gloucestershire Clinical Commissioning Group. 2015. *The Big 6*.

30. Clinical Knowledge Summaries. *Appendicitis*. Available from: https://cks.nice.org.uk/appendicitis, 2016.

31. Bickley, LS., *Bates' Guide to Physical Examination and History Taking*. Philadelphia: Lippincott Williams & Wilkins, 2013.

Acute Behavioural Disturbance (ABD)

1. Introduction

- This guideline covers caring for patients aged 12 years and over with severe agitation and delirium thought to be due to acute behavioural disturbance (ABD), when the level of agitation is posing a risk to the safety of the patient or others.

- Seek clinical advice if the patient is aged less than 12 years.

- Do **NOT** use this guidance if the patient has agitation without delirium or has delirium without agitation.

1.1 Definition

- ABD has been defined as 'a state of extreme mental and physiological excitement, characterised by extreme agitation, delirium, hyperthermia, hostility, exceptional strength and endurance without apparent fatigue' (refer to Figure 3.3).

- To have agitation, a patient must have an abnormal increase in motor activity or restlessness, e.g. trying to climb off the ambulance stretcher, trolley or cot, or actively resisting assessment, treatment or transport, or some combination of these. Anxiety or signs of mental distress or both are not enough by themselves to define the patient as being agitated.

- To have delirium, a patient must have recently (i.e. in the last few hours or days) developed signs of an abnormal state of mind, e.g. confusion, delusions or significantly abnormal behaviour.

- Clinicians must assess the patient's mental capacity to make decisions about their care and treatment. The presence of ABD signs or symptoms does not automatically mean a patient lacks capacity.

1.2 Terminology

- ABD is not a formal diagnosis. It is the 'umbrella' term for the clinical presentation of a number of possible conditions.

- ABD may also be known as:
  - acute behavioural disorder
  - acute severe behavioural disturbance
  - agitated delirium
  - excited delirium
  - excited delirium syndrome (ExD)
  - severe agitated delirium.

- Many of these terms are used interchangeably but they are not interchangeable terms. The term 'acute behavioural disorder' is widely used by the police but it is not a recognised medical condition.

Figure 3.3 – Acute behavioural disturbance. Republished with kind permission of Professor Keith Rix. Available from: https://napicu.org.uk/wp-content/uploads/2019/04/K-Rix-Acute-Behavioural-Disburbance-20-March-14.05-14.30.pdf.

Acute Behavioural Disturbance (ABD)

- Most clinical professionals prefer the term ABD, as it describes behaviour that can have a number of causes without implying a discrete and defined condition.

- 'Excited delirium' is not a generally recognised medical condition, although it has been used in some health guidance, as well as by witnesses in UK Coroners' Courts, and it is a somewhat controversial concept. It is applied to a number of different conditions that have in common some or all of the following:
  - a state of high psychological and mental arousal
  - agitation
  - tactile warmth or 'warm to touch'
  - hyperthermia, which is abnormally elevated temperature, sweating
  - violence, aggression and hostility with insensitivity to pain.

- Regardless of this terminological controversy, the significance of this group of signs and symptoms is that it constitutes a potentially fatal medical emergency.

2. Incidence, Severity and Outcome

- The incidence of life-threatening ABD in the UK is unknown, partly as there are a number of potential causes of similar presenting features, but there have been a number of deaths attributed to this condition. Its presentation has been associated with sudden death in approximately 10% of cases in some countries. The majority of patients who have died have deteriorated within an hour of the first contact with emergency services. However, it is important to realise that the patient may have been experiencing symptoms for some hours prior to first contact. Patients with ABD may come into contact with the police first as they are usually called to attend due to a person's sudden onset of bizarre or violent behaviour. The presenting behaviours can range from mildly erratic to a state of extreme agitation and physical exertion. ABD may be associated with fatality even when appropriately treated, the risk extending for as long as 24–48 hours after treatment, but the likelihood of successful treatment is increased with immediate appropriate clinical interventions.

- Some high-profile deaths of individuals displaying features of ABD have occurred whilst they have been in police custody. This has attracted much media coverage and ABD has become a controversial condition, with significant distress for the families involved. The early recognition, intervention and proactive treatment of ABD, with a collaborative response between the police and NHS Ambulance Services, may improve outcomes.

3. Pathophysiology

- ABD is most commonly associated with the use of illegal recreational drugs.

- ABD may be caused by drugs, infection; metabolic disorders (e.g. hypoglycaemia, hyponatraemia); liver failure; mental health disorders; dementia; drug or alcohol withdrawal.

- The most common cause internationally is recreational drug ingestion, particularly of methamphetamines, cocaine, legal- or illegal-high drugs or synthetic cannabinoids or novel psychoactive substance, as a toxidrome.

- ABD may be associated with serious mental illness, especially if antipsychotic medicine is stopped abruptly.

- The presentation may be also due to a physical illness. It is thought some individuals may have a genetic predisposition to developing ABD. It is essential to consider a range of differential diagnoses.

- The topic of ABD is controversial for a number of reasons, not least because it describes clinical presentations rather than a single disease.

- Patients have physiological signs of autonomic dysfunction, including significant tachycardia, tachypnoea, hyperthermia and sweating – these may be associated with multi-organ failure and death.

- The mechanism of ABD-related pathophysiological changes is unclear and there are a number of different theories. One current theory is that in some patients, ABD may be related to their dopamine levels, dopamine being a neurotransmitter in the brain. This is especially so in those cases involving novel psychoactive substances, particularly cocaine, illegal- and legal-high drugs or similar stimulants, or where patients on antipsychotic mediations have suddenly stopped taking them. Another theory is related to serotonin pathways, particularly when MDMA has been taken. There is also a theory related to genetic susceptibility, particularly in cocaine use, where some patients have fatal outcomes with lower doses of cocaine use than those who survive. Extreme agitation depletes the patient's oxygen and glucose reserves, producing CO_2 and water. CO_2 dissociates into hydrogen ions and bicarbonate, increasing any metabolic lactic acidosis. CO_2 is removed acutely via an increase in respiratory rate; if respiration is restricted or inadequate, the body cannot correct the resultant acidosis, leading to arrythmia risk and further metabolic disturbances. Patients are also at risk of dehydration, rhabdomyolysis producing acute renal failure from myoglobinaemia and hyperkalaemia, which may provoke life-threatening arrhythmias. It is important to try to minimise physical restraint

Acute Behavioural Disturbance (ABD)

to less than 10 minutes and to avoid airway or respiratory compromise.

- Many factors have been proposed as contributory to sudden death in ABD, such as positional asphyxia secondary to restraint, drug toxicity itself or underlying cardiac disease resulting in cardiac arrhythmias.

- Severe metabolic acidosis associated with life-threatening ABD is now thought to be the most significant factor in cardiovascular collapse and sudden death. Ambulance clinicians must be able to recognise that the presenting signs and symptoms of possible ABD represent an **emergency condition**.

4. Assessment

- The identification of life-threatening ABD can be difficult clinically as the spectrum of behaviours and signs (refer to Table 3.12) overlap with many other disease presentations (refer to Table 3.13). There is no definitive diagnostic test for the condition.

- Once potentially life-threatening ABD is suspected, attending ambulance clinicians should consider the need for additional clinical support and request this as per local procedures.

TABLE 3.12 – Possible Signs and Symptoms of ABD
- Acute psychosis with fear of impending doom or paranoia
- Constant or near-constant physical activity without fatigue
- 'Hot to touch' or tactile hyperthermia, profuse sweating or inappropriate state of undress
- Insensitivity to pain, including that caused by irritant sprays
- Extreme aggression or violent behaviour against inanimate objects or people when restraint is attempted
- Excessive strength or continued struggle in restraint to the point of collapse
- Attraction to glass
- Rapid breathing
- Lack of response to or engagement with others
- Lack of fear, e.g. running into the path of a moving vehicle or standing on a roof.

TABLE 3.13 – Differential Diagnoses of ABD
- Common conditions which may have similar presentations:
– sepsis
– hypoxia
– hypoglycaemia
– substance intoxication or withdrawal
– meningitis or encephalitis
– head injury
– seizure, in the post-ictal phase
– subarachnoid haemorrhage
– psychiatric disorder.
- Rare conditions which may have similar presentations:
– heat stroke
– thyrotoxic storm or hyperthyroid crisis
– neuroleptic malignant syndrome, which is a rare, severe, idiosyncratic adverse reaction to antipsychotics
– serotonin syndrome, which is SSRI antidepressant toxicity
– akathisia, which is an adverse effect of antipsychotic drugs, characterised by restlessness and mental unease, both of which can be intense.

- Although trauma is rarely the cause of death in ABD cases, many patients sustain trauma as part of the condition. It is recognised that this is due to:

  – lack of fear or risky behaviour by the patient

  – accidental injury in agitated state, especially where patients exhibit glass attraction

SECTION **3** Medical Emergencies

Acute Behavioural Disturbance (ABD)

- reduced pain perception
- injury during restraint.

- Other potential pitfalls include:
  - assuming a medical cause or drug-related condition without considering the possibility of significant trauma
  - symptoms of trauma may be masked by the signs of ABD
  - misinterpretation of physiological observations.

- ABD may make the clinical assessment of possible major trauma more difficult. Physiological observations will be difficult to take, symptoms may be masked and a full account of the history is unlikely to be available.

- Information from bystanders and the police can be helpful and signs of minor trauma may be significant as they may indicate underlying major trauma.

5. Management

- The Royal College of Emergency Medicine, UK, published an ABD Guideline in 2016 regarding the management of ABD in the Emergency Department. They and others have recommended joint guidelines between all those involved in the management of ABD from scene to hospital.

- This guideline provides the NHS ambulance services with clinical guidance to link the out-of-hospital phase to the emergency department phase for these patients.

5.1 Verbal Calming and De-escalation

- Verbal de-escalation is often under-utilised. Provided there is not an immediate risk to life, verbal de-escalation should be attempted before restraint or pharmacological agents are used.

- The key aspects to successful verbal and non-verbal de-escalation are:
  - Allow sufficient time to attempt verbal de-escalation.
  - Maintain a safe distance between you and the patient.
  - Have only one person verbally engage with the patient.
  - Introduce yourself; state that you are there to help and provide reassurance.
  - Use a calm voice and adopt a non-threatening stance.
  - Use short sentences and keep messages simple. Repetition is essential as the patient will usually have a short attention span.
  - Minimise the number of people in the immediate vicinity to those required for the safety of the patient and staff on scene.
  - Limit unnecessary noise and distractions, e.g. radio noise, blue lights, sirens, etc.

- Minimise any painful stimuli for the patient.
- Actively listen to the patient and try to gain an understanding of their concerns.
- Try to establish rapport and offer choices; if appropriate, allow them to have a drink or a cigarette.
- Avoid provocative statements, e.g. do not say 'If you don't calm down, we will have to sedate you'.
- Once rapport has been established, continue clinical care.

- Patients with ABD are often highly agitated, with altered mental status or lacking mental capacity, making their response to de-escalation techniques unpredictable.

- In close liaison with police and/or other relevant healthcare professionals on scene, attempts at verbal calming by one person and other de-escalation techniques should be considered as the first-line intervention in attempting to manage individuals displaying possible ABD. Consider removal of any causes of the presenting symptoms where appropriate. Where patients present in the context of custodial settings, it is essential to establish if any pharmacological therapy has already been commenced, as this may affect decisions on further clinical care. A mental capacity assessment must also be undertaken in accordance with relevant legislation and their associated codes of practice (refer to **Mental Capacity Act 2005**).

- NICE recommend all health organisations provide their staff with training in de-escalation for:
  - recognising the early signs of agitation, irritation, anger and aggression
  - understanding the likely causes of aggression or violence
  - using techniques for distraction and calming, and ways to encourage relaxation
  - recognising the importance of personal space
  - responding to a patient's anger in an appropriate, measured and reasonable way to avoid provocation.

- Friends, family members or both may be helpful but ask them to desist if they are making the situation worse.

- In a 2-year audit by the London Ambulance Service for cases where appropriately trained critical care paramedics responded to assess ABD, 62% of patients were managed using only verbal de-escalation followed by standard care.

- Where de-escalation interventions are unsuccessful after a short period, attending ambulance clinicians should consider the need for additional clinical or police support or both and request this via the emergency operations centre if not already done.

Acute Behavioural Disturbance (ABD)

5.2 Physical Restraint

- Physical restraint in ABD may be considered as part of patient management and planned by the police in conjunction with ambulance clinicians where possible before being applied.

- Clinicians should request senior support at the earliest opportunity, especially non-registered ambulance clinicians and newly qualified paramedics (NQPs).

- Clinicians on-scene are responsible for the clinical safety of the patient at all times and should immediately inform any other personnel on-scene if they believe the patient's clinical condition is at risk of deteriorating, particularly if there is any restriction to the patient's airway or breathing.

- The first healthcare professional on scene should be specifically responsible for monitoring and treating the patient. Any other healthcare professionals or ambulance staff in attendance should closely liaise with the designated police safety officer.

- Assistance from police should be requested if:
  - There is significant risk of injury to the patient, personnel or bystanders.
  - The patient has agitation causing a severe to immediate life-threatening risk to safety.

- Physical restraint by the police can form part of patient care. It should be kept to a minimum, using a level of force that is justifiable, reasonable and proportional to the individual case, with close monitoring of the patient clinically. During restraint, clinicians should be prepared for a rapid deterioration in the patient's condition, including cardiovascular collapse.

- If any patient needs physical restraint, the ambulance clinician should actively monitor the patient's vital signs where possible and observe for any deterioration in the patient's condition.

- Police officers must be alerted to any concerns regarding the patient's welfare or clinical deterioration during restraint.

- The police have the legal authority to restrain a patient if:
  - There is an immediate need for care and control of the patient in their best interests under the Mental Capacity Act (MCA).
  - It is needed for the protection of the public.
  - It is needed to remove the patient to a place of safety (s136 MHA).
  - The patient is considered to be 'disturbing the peace'.
  - The police have other grounds in relation to their powers as police officers.

- Where legally possible to do so, consideration must be given by the police to using section 136 (s136) under the Mental Health Act (MHA) to detain the patient, to allow for mental health assessment after clinical management of the initial emergency.

- Section 136 can be used by the police in suspected ABD, **unless** the situation occurs in a private dwelling where s136 cannot legally be used. In those cases, if there is thought to be a potentially life-threatening emergency, the police would assist the ambulance clinician by considering the use of the MCA if the patient lacks capacity, and then acting in the best interests of the patient.

- Before ambulance clinicians use physical restraint they must, if the circumstances permit, consider the patient's mental capacity, their care and treatment. That assessment and the reasons for restraint must be documented after its use.

- Prolonged physical restraint must be, wherever practicable, avoided due to the associated risk of injuries to patients, as well as it being a potentially contributing factor in clinical deterioration. Care must be taken to ensure that the patient's airway or respiratory function is not compromised – this is particularly likely if the patient is kept in a prone position with pressure applied on their head, neck, chest or shoulder region. The use of the prone position should be avoided wherever possible or used for a very short period of time only, with the patient placed on their side and hand restraints moved to the patient's front. Handcuffs restraining the arms to the rear of the body are more likely to cause respiratory compromise than arms placed to the front of the body.

- Particular care should be taken where patients are thought to be obese, critically ill or injured, have a disability or are pregnant.

- When considering the use of restraint under the MCA it is necessary to evidence that the intervention is in the best interests of the patient, necessary in order to prevent the patient from coming to harm and proportionate in terms of the likelihood of the harm occurring and the severity of that harm. Clinicians must achieve a fair and reasonable balance between the risks associated with a particular form of restraint and the aim of the restraint. There are well-evidenced risks associated with any form of restraint (physical, mechanical or pharmacological) that must be considered and mitigated against as far as reasonably possible. The clinician must believe that the use of restraint is the least restrictive available to achieve safe and effective patient care. There must be a genuine belief that restraint is necessary.

- A 'proportionate response' means the least intrusive type and minimum amount of restraint to achieve a specific outcome in the best interests of the patient who lacks capacity.

Acute Behavioural Disturbance (ABD)

- On the occasions when the use of force may be necessary, carers and healthcare and social care staff should use the minimum amount of force for the shortest possible time (MCA Code of Practice).

- Clinicians must not place themselves or others in danger. In some rare circumstances, ambulance clinicians may consider it appropriate to restrain a patient because of the risk of harm the patient potentially poses to the public in the absence of police support. Where appropriate, common law, criminal law and mental health law can be relied upon to justify such action, even though it may not be directly in the patient's best interests.

- Significant physiological derangements, such as acidosis, electrolyte abnormalities, rhabdomyolysis, cardiac arrhythmias, etc., can occur due to the underlying condition or as a result of resisting restraint. These may be exacerbated by other clinical factors, e.g. cardiac disease, obesity or taking medications or illicit substances.

- Physiological monitoring and clinical observations must be undertaken as soon as possible; **the patient may have to be clinically monitored from a distance**.

- Attempts must be made to monitor the patient's respiratory rate, level of consciousness and skin colour, e.g. pallor or other change in colour, during restraint. A NEWS2 score should be measured and documented as soon as possible. If there is new confusion, this scores 3 points in NEWS2.

- If there is **any** evidence of possible trauma, complete a primary survey, extricate rapidly, provide an ATMIST pre-alert (refer to **Trauma** guidelines) and be prepared for sudden cardiovascular collapse.

- There is limited research on the effects of Tasers or conducted energy devices (CEDs) in ABD. A risk assessment will be completed and a decision made on the use of a Taser or CED by the police if other methods of de-escalation have failed. In rare circumstances where an immediate threat to life exists, it may be appropriate for a Taser or CED to be used by police, before or after ambulance clinician arrival, to gain initial control, so that restraint and possibly pharmacological agents can be safely used.

- In patients with ABD, the risks of deploying a Taser or CED predominantly relate to the risk of injury associated with the fall.

TABLE 3.14 – ASSESSMENT and MANAGEMENT of: Acute Behavioural Disturbance
Assessment of the Level of Risk to Safety
- The risk to consider is the likelihood of harm occurring and the severity of that harm. The level of risk may range from mild to immediately life-threatening. Determining the level of risk to safety requires clinical judgement that takes into account the risk to the patient, to emergency services and to others on scene.
Mild to Moderate Risk to Safety

- Signs include but are not limited to:
  – verbal aggression
  – actions not involving immediate risk of serious harm to personnel, e.g. pushing or grabbing
  – pulling at equipment
  – trying to climb off the stretcher
  – agitation preventing control of moderate external bleeding.
 	
- Attempt verbal de-escalation and move sequentially through the steps below if the level of agitation continues to pose a risk to safety. Consider calling for police assistance.
 	
- Provide restraint if safe to do so without additional assistance.
 	
- Gain IV access if it is feasible and safe to do so.
 	
- If the patient has a reduced level of consciousness:
  – Position the patient on their side.
  – Provide restraint as required.
  – Administer oxygen and continually monitor the patient's airway, breathing, SpO_2, end-tidal CO_2 and level of consciousness.
  – Monitor heart rate, blood pressure and capillary refill time, particularly in restrained limbs, if possible.

(continued)

SECTION **3** Medical Emergencies

Acute Behavioural Disturbance (ABD)

TABLE 3.14 – ASSESSMENT and MANAGEMENT of: Acute Behavioural Disturbance *(continued)*

Severe to Immediate Life-threatening Risk to Safety

- Signs include but are not limited to:
  - dangerous physical aggression
  - wielding a weapon
  - actions involving immediate risk of serious harm to personnel, e.g. punching or kicking
  - destruction of physical surroundings
  - trying to get out of a moving ambulance
  - agitation preventing control of severe or life-threatening external bleeding.

- Call for urgent police assistance, clinical advice and additional clinical support in line with local procedures.

- Consider moving to create a safe distance between yourself and the patient.

- Attempt verbal de-escalation or provide restraint or both only if it is safe to do so.

- Once patient control has been obtained:
  - Position the patient on their side or allow them to sit up if cooperative and clinically appropriate.
  - Administer oxygen and continually monitor the patient's airway, breathing, SpO_2, end-tidal CO_2 and level of consciousness.
  - Monitor heart rate, blood pressure and capillary refill time, particularly in restrained limbs, if possible.
  - Gain IV access if not already achieved.
  - Consider IV fluids (refer to **Intravascular Fluid Therapy in Adults**).
  - Undertake a TIME-CRITICAL transfer and hospital pre-alert. The police must travel with the patient.

Assess <C>ABCDE

- If any of the following TIME-CRITICAL features are present:
  - Major <C>ABCDE problems (refer to **Medical Emergencies in Adults – Overview**), then:
  - Start correcting any <C>ABCDE problems.
  - Undertake a TIME-CRITICAL transfer to nearest appropriate receiving hospital.
  - Continue patient management en-route.
  - Provide an ATMIST information call.

Respiratory Rate

- Measure and record respiratory rate.

Pulse

- Measure and record pulse.

Oxygen Saturation

- Monitor the patient's SpO_2; administer oxygen to achieve saturations of >94% if the patient presents as hypoxaemic on air (refer to **Oxygen**).

Blood Pressure

- Measure and record blood pressure.

Blood Glucose

- If appropriate, measure and record blood glucose for hypoglycaemia and hyperglycaemia (refer to **Glycaemic Emergencies in Adults and Children**).

Temperature

- Record temperature. If it has increased, allow passive cooling.

NEWS2

- These observations will enable you to calculate a NEWS2 Score (refer to **Sepsis**).

ECG

- Monitor the ECG and if possible and appropriate record a 12-lead ECG (refer to **Cardiac Rhythm Disturbance**).

Acute Behavioural Disturbance (ABD)

TABLE 3.14 – ASSESSMENT and MANAGEMENT of: Acute Behavioural Disturbance (continued)
Assess the Patient's Pain
▪ Where present, assess the SOCRATES of pain and record initial and subsequent pain scores.   ▪ Consider analgesia if appropriate (refer to **Pain Management in Adults** or **Pain Managements in Children**).
Documentation
▪ Complete documentation to include all clinical findings, advice from other clinicians, onward referral and details of the use of any physical restraint or of rapid tranquilisation.

5.3 Rapid Tranquillisation (RT)

▪ Although verbal de-escalation and joint management with the police have been found to be effective in the majority of possible cases of ABD, in a small proportion of cases rapid tranquilisation (RT) may be an option.

▪ In some ABD cases, appropriately qualified clinicians may use medicines parenterally to calm the patient sufficiently to allow clinical care to be provided or the use of out-of-hospital anaesthesia. Clinicians must follow local trust guidelines and the situation must be otherwise unmanageable.

▪ The National Institute for Health and Care Excellence (NICE) uses the term 'rapid tranquillisation' to define using medicines parenterally to reduce the risk of harm and minimise agitation and violence. Ideally, these would have a very rapid onset of action with a high safety profile. No medicines are ideal for use in these extremely physiologically compromised patients; only a few medicines have been used and these should only be administered by advanced clinicians approved by each ambulance trust, as per local guidelines.

▪ There are currently three types of medicines used internationally for rapid out of hospital tranquilisation in ABD: benzodiazepines, antipsychotics and dissociative agents. Currently, there is a lack of high-quality evidence in the medical literature to determine the most suitable single agent or combination of agents.

▪ There are significant risks during and after RT as usually there is limited access to information on the patient's past medical history or medication and drug history, and the environment is much less controlled. This makes this a high-risk clinical intervention given the already potentially seriously compromised physiology of patients with ABD. People with mental health problems are at increased risk of coronary heart disease, cerebrovascular disease, diabetes, epilepsy and respiratory disease, all of which can be exacerbated by the effects of rapid tranquillisation.

▪ The rapid control and calming of a patient displaying the extreme physical exertion associated with ABD may prevent further deterioration of their metabolic status. Ideally, medicines should be administered via the intravenous route; however, this route is unlikely to be immediately available, and the intra-nasal route is likely to present a risk to the clinician, so the intra-muscular route is generally the most suitable.

▪ The aim of RT is to reduce the level of agitation, making the patient calmer or more 'tranquil' **without** reducing their level of consciousness, although the latter may occur inadvertently if the patient is already physiologically seriously compromised.

▪ The clinician providing the RT must be accompanied by an appropriate second clinician who is able to provide clinical management of the patient's respiratory and cardiovascular systems. Clinicians should ensure that appropriate equipment is immediately available to manage a patient's airway, breathing and circulation.

▪ Clinicians must ensure that appropriately trained and equipped personnel accompany the patient during ambulance transfer to the ED. This will normally be the clinician who administers RT.

After Rapid Tranquilisation (RT)

▪ After RT the patient should be quickly and safely moved into a supine, lateral or reclined position where possible, depending on the risk assessment, then moved onto the ambulance and rapidly transferred to an ED. A police presence in the back of the ambulance will provide ongoing support, including altering any restraints such as handcuffs to reposition the patient.

▪ Physiological monitoring **must** be undertaken immediately post-RT and continued until ED clinicians take over care of the patient.

▪ A brief primary survey should be undertaken, looking for any potentially life-threatening injuries or conditions requiring immediate clinical treatment.

Acute Behavioural Disturbance (ABD)

- An **early** pre-alert to include an SBAR summary and an ATMIST, if there may have been trauma, should be passed to the receiving ED.

- As well as having received agents that might depress respiration, many of these patients will be hypoxic or have a high oxygen demand due to their hyper-metabolic state. Oxygen should be given as soon as possible to achieve a target saturation of 94–98%.

- Hypovolaemia is common in ABD, attributable to the excess physical activity or hyperthermia or both. Where possible, patients should receive IV crystalloid. IV fluid will help correct metabolic acidosis and reduce end organ damage; aim to give 1 litre IV crystalloid stat on the way to hospital. Clinicians must monitor the patient's response to fluids and consider additional IV fluids.

- Hyperthermia is common in individuals presenting with ABD. This is due to a combination of the individual's state of constant physical exertion, which itself will generate heat, and hyperthermia due to dopamine dysfunction. 'Hot-to-touch' ABD patients need to be cooled to, but not below, normal body temperature. This can usually be achieved out of hospital with basic cooling methods such as the removal of clothing, where practical, if not already removed.

- After handover at the ED, detailed information regarding the clinical presentation, clinical risk assessments, clinical decision making, clinical findings and clinical care must be documented.

These cases are also likely to be subject to internal and external reviews.

- Episodes of physical restraint must be documented for monitoring purposes; this must be managed in accordance with individual ambulance trust policy.

5.4 ABD in Custody Suites and Police Stations

- In 2019 the Faculty of Forensic and Legal Medicine (FFLM) in the UK issued guidance to healthcare professionals working in and on-call for police custody suites.

- The FFLM advised healthcare professionals (HCPs) covering custody suites, who may or may not have personally assessed the patient, that if anyone exhibits any of the following, they are to call or advise the custody staff that an ambulance should be called to transfer the patient to an ED: tactile hyperthermia or 'hot to touch'; constant or near-constant physical activity; extreme agitation or aggression. They have also advised the police that any individual with any of these presenting features is to be taken to an ED, not to a custody suite.

- The custody suite HCP may have assessed the patient and given pre-rapid tranquillisation (pre-RT) using oral lorazepam (benzodiazepine) up to a maximum of 4 mg in 24 hours. The effect of pre-RT medication must be taken into consideration when assessing any patient clinically.

KEY POINTS!

Acute Behavioural Disturbance (ABD)

- **The majority of acutely disturbed or delirious patients can be managed using de-escalation techniques.**

- **ABD is a clinical emergency – the patient may suffer sudden cardiovascular collapse or cardiac arrest or both with little or no warning.**

- **Once ABD is identified, additional clinical support must be requested.**

- **Dynamic risk assessments and non-clinical management of ABD cases should be conducted jointly with the police.**

- **The clinician must take all reasonable actions to clinically monitor the patient throughout restraint where possible.**

- **Patient restraint time must be kept to an absolute minimum – the degree of restraint used must be justifiable, reasonable and applied for the minimum time necessary and proportional to the situation.**

- **The risks associated with the selected method of restraint must be considered and mitigated against as far as reasonably possible.**

- **Early management of hyperthermia, hypovolaemia and acidosis should be instituted with IV fluids and oxygen.**

- **Undertake a time-critical transfer and hospital pre-alert.**

Acute Behavioural Disturbance (ABD)

Acknowledgements

We gratefully thank the New Zealand Ambulance Service for sharing their guidelines and the many individuals who have provided invaluable advice and comments on this new guideline.

Bibliography

1. American College of Emergency Physicians. *White Paper Report on Excited Delirium Syndrome*, 2009.

2. NICE. *Violence and Aggression: Short-term management in mental health, health and community settings NICE guideline [NG10]*. 2015. Available from: https://www.nice.org.uk/guidance/ng10/chapter/1-Recommendations.

3. Hick JL, Smith S, Lynch MT. Metabolic acidosis in restraint-associated cardiac arrest: a case series. *Academic Emergency Medicine* 1999, 6(3): 239–243.

4. Rt. Hon. Dame Elish Angiolini DBE QC. Report of the Independent Review of Deaths and Serious Incidents in Police Custody. 2017. Available from: https://assets.publishing.service.gov.uk/government/uploads/system/uploads/attachment_data/file/655401/Report_of_Angiolini_Review_ISBN_Accessible.pdf.

5. The Royal College of Emergency Medicine. *Guidelines for the Management of Excited Delirium/Acute Behavioural Disturbance (ABD)*. 2016. Available from: https://www.rcem.ac.uk/docs/College%20Guidelines/5p.%20RCEM%20guidelines%20for%20management%20of%20Acute%20Behavioural%20Disturbance%20(May%202016).pdf.

6. UK Public General Acts. *Mental Health Act*. 1983, c. 20. Available from: http://www.legislation.gov.uk/ukpga/1983/20/contents.

7. UK Public General Acts. *Mental Capacity Act*. Available from: http://www.legislation.gov.uk/ukpga/2005/9/contents, 2005, c. 9.

8. NICE. *Violence and Aggression: Short-term management in mental health, health and community settings NICE guideline [NG10]*. 2015. Available from: https://www.nice.org.uk/guidance/ng10.

9. Green SM, Roback MG, Kennedy RM, Krauss B. Clinical practice guideline for emergency department ketamine dissociative sedation: 2011 update. *Annals of Emergency Medicine* 2011, 57(5): 449–461.

10. FFLM. *ABD 2019 Guidance*. 2019. Available from: https://fflm.ac.uk/resources/publications/guidelines-for-the-management-of-acute-behavioural-disturbance/.

11. Academy of Medical Royal Colleges. *Safe Sedation Practice for Healthcare Procedures*. 2013. Available from: https://www.rcoa.ac.uk/system/files/PUB-SafeSedPrac2013.pdf.

12. Baldwin S, Hall C, Bennell C et al. Distinguishing features of Excited Delirium Syndrome in non-fatal use of force encounters. *Journal of Forensic and Legal Medicine* 2016, 41: 21–27.

13. Wetli CV, Fishbain DA. Cocaine-induced psychosis and sudden death in recreational cocaine users. *Journal of Forensic Sciences* 1985, 30(3), 873–880.

14. Mash D. Excited delirium and sudden death: a syndromal disorder at the extreme end of the neuropsychiatric continuum. *Front Physiol* 2016, 7: 435.

15. Gonin P, Excited delirium: a systematic review. *Acad Emerg Med* 2018, 25(5): 552–565.

16. NICE. *Violent and Aggressive Behaviours in People with Mental Health Problems, Quality standard [QS154]*. 2017. Available from: https://www.nice.org.uk/guidance/qs154.

SECTION **3** **Medical Emergencies**

Acute Coronary Syndrome

1. Introduction

- The National Institute for Health and Care Excellence (NICE) outlines that:

- 'The term "acute coronary syndromes" encompasses a range of conditions including unstable angina, non-ST-segment-elevation myocardial infarction (NSTEMI) and ST-segment-elevation myocardial infarction (STEMI). All are due to a sudden reduction of blood flow to the heart, usually caused by the rupture of an atherosclerotic plaque within the wall of a coronary artery, and may cause the formation of a blood clot.

- The most common symptom of acute coronary syndromes is severe pain in the chest and/or in other areas (for example, the arms, back or jaw), which can last for several hours. Other symptoms include sweating, nausea and vomiting, breathlessness and feeling faint.

- People with acute coronary syndromes may have a poor prognosis without prompt and accurate diagnosis. Treatments are available to help ease the pain, improve the blood flow and to prevent any future complications.

- The highest priority in managing STEMI is to restore an adequate coronary blood flow as quickly as possible using drug treatment and/ or revascularisation. This applies to all people with STEMI, including those who have been resuscitated after cardiac arrest. The time taken to restore coronary blood flow is very important because heart muscle starts to be lost as soon as the coronary artery is blocked.

- In people with NSTEMI and unstable angina, the aim of treatment is to alleviate pain and anxiety and prevent recurrence of ischaemia. For people with unstable angina, treatment also aims to prevent or limit progression to acute myocardial infarction (AMI). The type of treatment is determined by the person's individual risk of future adverse cardiovascular events (heart attack and stroke, repeat treatment or death)'.[1]

2. Incidence

- In 2016/17, the Myocardial Ischaemia National Audit Project (MINAP), which covers England, Wales and Northern Ireland, recorded more than 95,000 'heart attack' (acute coronary syndrome, ACS) patients on the database. This is likely to be an underestimate. Of those with a confirmed diagnosis of myocardial infarction (MI) on the MINAP database, 40% have ST segment elevation myocardial infarction (STEMI) and 60% non-STEMI.

- Over 80% of patients with STEMI present via ambulance services.

- In England, 99% of STEMI patients who receive reperfusion treatment have primary percutaneous coronary intervention (PPCI).

- According to the British Heart Foundation (BHF), an estimated 7 million people in the UK are living with heart and circulatory diseases. With an ageing and growing population, and improved survival rates from heart and circulatory events, these numbers are expected to rise still further. The most recent BHF statistics, published in November 2018, estimate that:

- Heart and circulatory diseases cause a quarter (25%) of all deaths in the UK; over 150,000 deaths each year – an average of 420 people each day or one death every 3 minutes.

- Around 42,000 people under the age of 75 in the UK die from cardiovascular disease each year.

- Around 80% of people with heart and circulatory diseases have at least one other health condition.

- Coronary heart disease (CHD) is the single biggest cause of death in the UK and is a major cause of premature mortality (i.e. death in people aged under 75).

3. Severity and Outcome

- Case fatality rates at 30 days following hospital admission declined between 2002 and 2010 from 18.5% to 12.2% in men and from 20.0% to 12.5% in women, but are determined by factors such as age, co-morbidity, type of AMI and use of treatments (e.g. PPCI, secondary prevention medicines) recommended in NICE and other guidelines. For non-STEMI, unadjusted all-cause mortality at 180 days decreased from 10.8% to 7.6% from 2003 to 2013.

- The risk of cardiac arrest from ventricular fibrillation (VF) or other arrhythmia is highest in the first few hours from symptom onset. VF can occur without warning. For some patients, cardiac arrest is the first presentation of ACS.

4. Assessment and Management

- The diagnosis and management of a patient with suspected ACS requires a detailed clinical assessment and the recording of a 12-lead electrocardiogram. Reperfusion treatments for STEMI are critically time dependent and immediate clinical assessment of all patients with a suspected ACS is essential.

- Clinical risk factors should be considered together when assessing the likelihood of myocardial ischaemia relating to ACS. Such factors include increasing age, sex, family history of CHD, prior history of ischaemic heart disease and peripheral vascular disease, diabetes mellitus and renal impairment. High-risk features include:

    - worsening angina
    - prolonged pain (>20 minutes)
    - pulmonary oedema

Acute Coronary Syndrome

- hypotension
- arrhythmias.

ECG monitoring with defibrillator availability is indicated as soon as possible in all patients with suspected ACS and should continue until handover at hospital.

The 12-lead ECG

- The pre-hospital 12-lead electrocardiogram (PHECG) supports decision making in three components of immediate care: targeted pre-hospital treatment, transport to the appropriate type of receiving hospital and provision of sufficient information required to activate a receiving cardiac catheter laboratory in preparation for the patient, should STEMI be suspected. Research undertaken in the UK has shown that PHECG (compared with no PHECG) was associated with increased short-term mortality benefit following both STEMI and non-STEMI. However, one third of eligible patients did not receive a PHECG. Women, older people and those with co-morbidities were less likely to have PHECG recorded.

- The European Society of Cardiology (ESC) recommends 12-lead ECG recording and interpretation as soon as possible at the point of 'first medical contact', with a maximum target delay of 10 minutes.

- The diagnostic criteria for STEMI set out by the ESC are as follows:

ST-segment elevation (measured at the J-point): at least two contiguous leads with ST-segment elevation:

- 2.5 mm in men aged under 40,
- 2 mm in men aged over 40 and
- 1.5 mm in women

in leads V2 and V3

and/or

- 1 mm in the other leads (in the absence of left ventricular (LV) hypertrophy or left bundle branch block LBBB)).

- The presence of a Q-wave on the ECG should not necessarily change the reperfusion strategy decision.

- ST-segment depression in leads V1–V3 suggests myocardial ischaemia, especially when the terminal T-wave is positive (ST-segment elevation equivalent), and confirmation by concomitant ST-segment elevation > 0.5 mm recorded in leads V7–V9 should be considered as a means to identify posterior MI.

- Use of additional right precordial leads (V3R and V4R) should be considered in patients with inferior MI (ST elevation in leads II, III and aVF) to identify concomitant right ventricular infarction.

- In the presence of LBBB, the ECG diagnosis of AMI is challenging, but marked ST-segment abnormalities may be seen. There are a number of algorithms available to support ECG diagnosis of STEMI in the presence of LBBB but according to the ESC these do not provide diagnostic certainty. Presence of concordant ST-segment elevation (i.e. in leads with positive QRS deflections) may indicate ongoing MI. Patients with a clinical suspicion of ACS and LBBB should be managed in a way similar to STEMI patients, regardless of whether the LBBB is previously known. The presence of a (presumed) new LBBB does not necessarily predict an MI.

- Patients with MI and right bundle branch block (RBBB) have a poor prognosis. The ESC suggests that a PPCI strategy (emergency coronary angiography and PCI if indicated) should be considered when persistent ischaemic symptoms occur in the presence of RBBB. Refer to locally agreed pathways.

TABLE 3.15 – ASSESSMENT and MANAGEMENT of: Acute Coronary Syndrome

Assess <C>ABCDE

- If any of the following TIME-CRITICAL features are present:
  - major <C>ABCD problems (refer to **Medical Emergencies in Adults – Overview**).
  - 12-lead ECG shows STEMI or bundle branch block (BBB) with other clinical features suggestive of ACS
  - suspected ACS with haemodynamic instability, then:
- Start correcting any <C>ABCDE problems.
- Undertake a TIME-CRITICAL TRANSFER to the nearest appropriate receiving hospital.

For patients with STEMI, undertake a direct admission to a PPCI-capable hospital ('Heart Attack Centre') according to local network pathways.

- Continue management en-route:
  - If facilities exist, transmit 12-lead ECG for expert review where possible in cases of uncertainty about interpretation.

(continued)

Acute Coronary Syndrome

TABLE 3.15 – ASSESSMENT and MANAGEMENT of: Acute Coronary Syndrome *(continued)*

– In comparison with placebo, aspirin halves the rate of vascular events (cardiovascular death, non-fatal MI and non-fatal stroke) in patients with unstable angina and reduces it by nearly a third in those with AMI. Administer aspirin as soon as possible (refer to **Asprin**).

– Administer clopidogrel (refer to Clopidogrel) or follow local guidelines for alternative antiplatelet agents.

– Administer glyceryl trinitrate (GTN) for patients with ongoing ischaemic discomfort unless contraindicated (refer to **Glyceryl Trinitrate (GTN)**).

– Provide an ATMIST information call.

Respiratory Rate

– Measure and record respiratory rate.

Pulse

▪ Measure and record pulse.

Blood Pressure

▪ Measure and record blood pressure.

Blood Glucose

▪ If appropriate, measure and record blood glucose for hypo/hyperglycaemia (refer to **Glycaemic Emergencies in Adults and Children**).

Assess Whether the Chest Pain May Be Cardiac

▪ Pain typically comes on over seconds and minutes rather than starting abruptly – 'classical presentation' is detailed in Table 3.16. If truly sudden onset, consider other diagnoses, such as aortic dissection, and seek advice (refer to **Non-Traumatic Chest Pain/Discomfort**).

NB Many patients do not have 'classical presentation' as described above and some people, especially women, older people and those with diabetes, may not experience pain as their chief complaint. This group has a high mortality. Have a low threshold for recording 12-lead ECG.

Assess for Accompanying Features

▪ Nausea and vomiting.

▪ Marked sweating.

▪ Breathlessness.

▪ Pallor.

▪ Combination of chest pain associated with haemodynamic instability.

▪ Feelings of impending doom.

▪ Skin that is clammy and cold to the touch.

NB These may not always be present.

ECG

▪ A normal 12-lead ECG alone must not be used to **exclude ACS**.

▪ Repeat the 12-lead ECG if there is diagnostic uncertainty (e.g. the initial ECG does not show ST elevation) or a change in the clinical status of the patient.

Assess Oxygen Saturation

▪ There is no high-quality evidence that routine use of supplementary oxygen in normoxic patients with AMI is either helpful or harmful, nor that it reduces ischaemic chest pain. There is some evidence suggesting that hyperoxia may be harmful in patients with AMI.

▪ Monitor the patient's SpO_2 but do not administer oxygen unless the patient is hypoxaemic on air (SpO_2 <94%) (refer to **Oxygen**).

Undertake Further Assessment and Management in the Order Appropriate to the Circumstances

▪ Continuous cardiac monitoring is essential to detect arrhythmias.

▪ Obtain intravenous access if clinically indicated.

Acute Coronary Syndrome

TABLE 3.15 – ASSESSMENT and MANAGEMENT of: Acute Coronary Syndrome *(continued)*

- Monitor vital signs.
- Repeat dose of GTN if chest discomfort persists.
- 12-lead ECG (as above).

Assess Patient's Pain

- Where present, assess the **SOCRATES** of pain and record initial and subsequent pain scores.
- Consider analgesia if appropriate (refer to **Pain Management in Adults** and **Pain Management in Children**).

Documentation

- Complete documentation to include all clinical findings, advice from other clinicians and onward referral.

Additional Information

- National and international standards and guidelines for ACS care consistently emphasise the importance of rapid access to defibrillation and reperfusion, and specialist cardiological care.
- Pre-alerting the hospital can speed up appropriate treatment of STEMI patients.
- **MINAP national data suggest 'call-to-balloon' times are increasing in patients receiving PPCI. Make every effort to reduce delay to hospital.**
- Pre-hospital thrombolysis may be an option where PPCI is not available but is rarely given in England, where 99% of reperfusion patients receive PPCI. Patients who receive thrombolytic treatment should subsequently be transferred urgently to a PPCI-capable hospital.
- Patients post ROSC with ST elevation should be taken to a PPCI-capable hospital.
- The role of emergency angiography (and PCI if indicated) in patients resuscitated from cardiac arrest but without ST-segment elevation on the pre-hospital 12-lead ECG is uncertain. Research is ongoing in London (the ARREST trial) to evaluate this strategy. Such patients should be treated according to locally agreed pathways of care. It is important to establish a history of the events prior to the cardiac arrest and whether the patient suffered chest pain.
- The diagnosis of non-STEMI cannot be made pre-hospital as it requires use of biomarkers. Point-of-care (POC) troponin assays are insufficiently sensitive to 'rule out' ACS in the pre-hospital environment and are not recommended at this time. The Pre-hospital Evaluation of Sensitive Troponin (PRESTO) Study led by the University of Manchester is currently evaluating this approach with NHS ambulance services.

TABLE 3.16 – Features of Different Types of Pain

Features that suggest a diagnosis of myocardial ischaemia include:

- Central chest pain.
- Crushing or constricting in nature.
- Persists for >15 minutes.
- Pain may also present:
  - in the shoulders
  - in upper abdomen
  - referred to the neck, jaws and arm.

Features that suggest a diagnosis of stable angina include:

- Pain typically related to exertion and tending to last minutes, but should it persist for >15 minutes, or despite usual treatment, ACS is more likely.

3 Medical Emergencies

Acute Coronary Syndrome

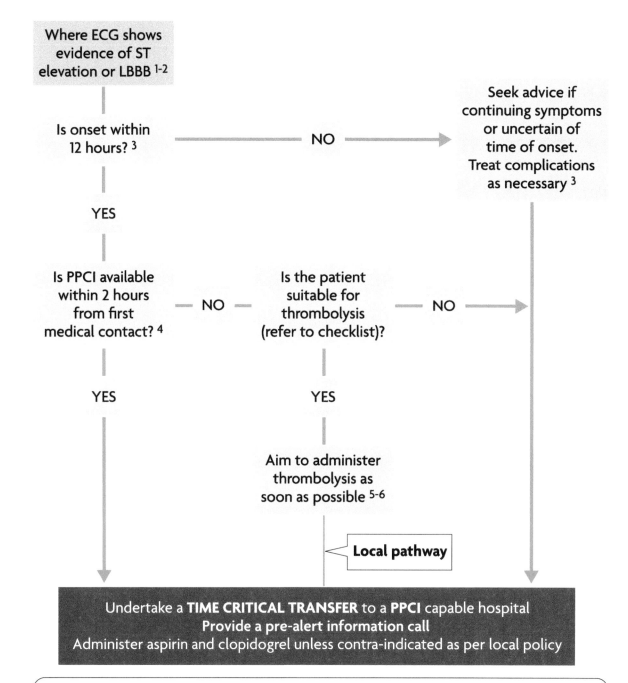

Where ECG shows evidence of ST elevation or LBBB [1-2]

Is onset within 12 hours? [3]

NO → Seek advice if continuing symptoms or uncertain of time of onset. Treat complications as necessary [3]

YES

Is PPCI available within 2 hours from first medical contact? [4]

— NO — Is the patient suitable for thrombolysis (refer to checklist)?

NO →

YES

YES

Aim to administer thrombolysis as soon as possible [5-6]

Local pathway

Undertake a TIME CRITICAL TRANSFER to a PPCI capable hospital
Provide a pre-alert information call
Administer aspirin and clopidogrel unless contra-indicated as per local policy

1. Up to a third of patients with MI will have atypical presentations such as shortness of breath or collapse, without chest pain. This is particularly so in women, patients with diabetes or the elderly. **Have a low threshold for performing a 12-lead ECG in any patient presenting as 'unwell'** Seek advice in 'atypical' patients who have ST elevation or LBBB (see below) as urgent reperfusion may still be indicated.

2. ST-segment elevation (measured at the J-point): at least two contiguous leads with ST-segment elevation 2.5 mm in men aged under 40, 2 mm in men over 40 years, or 1.5 mm in women in leads V2 and V3 and/or 1 mm in the other leads [in the absence of left ventricular (LV) hypertrophy or left bundle branch block LBBB)]

3. If there is uncertainty about the time of symptom onset, or any ongoing chest pain/discomfort or haemodynamic upset beyond 12 hours, seek advice as urgent reperfusion may still be indicated.

4. Refer to local policies for target 'call to balloon' time.

5. Thrombolytic treatment should not be regarded as the end of the emergency care of a STEMI patient. Rapid transfer to an appropriate hospital for timely therapy to prevent re-infarction, and assessment of the need for rescue PPCI, is essential.

6. Refer to tenecteplase guidelines for the checklist to identify eligibility for pre-hospital thrombolysis.

Figure 3.4 – The management of patients presenting with STEMI or LBBB.

Acute Coronary Syndrome

KEY POINTS!

Acute Coronary Syndrome

- Acute coronary syndrome refers to a spectrum of conditions.
- Risk of VF is high in the early stages of ACS. Always take a defibrillator to the patient.
- Patients with ECG evidence of STEMI should be assessed for suitability for reperfusion with PPCI or thrombolysis according to local care pathways. The vast majority of STEMI patients now receive PPCI as their reperfusion treatment.
- Patients with non-STEMI remain at high risk and should be treated as a MEDICAL EMERGENCY.

Bibliography

1. National Institute for Health and Care Excellence. *Acute Coronary Syndromes in Adults*. London: NICE, 2014. Available from: https://www.nice.org.uk/guidance/qs68/chapter/Introduction.

2. National Institute for Health and Care Excellence. *Unstable Angina and NSTEMI: The early management of unstable angina and non-ST-segmentelevation myocardial infarction* (CG94). London: NICE, 2013. Available from: https://www.nice.org.uk/guidance/cg94.

3. Scottish Intercollegiate Guidelines Network (SIGN). *Acute coronary syndrome*. Edinburgh: SIGN, 2016. Available from: https://www.sign.ac.uk/assets/sign148.pdf.

4. Ibanez B, James S, Agewall S, et al. 2017 ESC Guidelines for the management of acute myocardial infarction in patients presenting with ST-segment elevation: The Task Force for the management of acute myocardial infarction in patients presenting with ST-segment elevation of the European Society of Cardiology (ESC). *Eur Heart J* 2018, 29(2): 119–177.

5. British Heart Foundation. *Heart statistics publications*. Birmingham: British Heart Foundation, 2018. Available from: https://www.bhf.org.uk/what-we-do/our-research/heart-statistics/heart-statistics-publications.

6. Sepehrvand N, James S, Stub D, et al. Effects of supplemental oxygen therapy in patients with suspected acute myocardial infarction: a meta-analysis of randomised clinical trials. *Heart* 2018, 104(20): 1691–1698.

7. Sparv D, Hofmann R, Gunnarsson A, et al. DETO2X-SWEDEHEART Investigators. The analgesic effect of oxygen in suspected acute myocardial infarction: a substudy of the DETO2X-AMI trial. *JACC Cardiovasc Interv* 2018, 11(16): 1590–1597.

8. Quinn T, Johnsen S, Gale CP, et al. Myocardial Ischaemia National Audit Project (MINAP) Steering Group. Effects of prehospital 12-lead ECG on processes of care and mortality in acute coronary syndrome: a linked cohort study from the Myocardial Ischaemia National Audit Project. *Heart* 2014, 100(12): 944–950.

9. Manchester University NHS Foundation Trust. *The Pre-hospital Evaluation of Sensitive Troponin (PRESTO) Study*. Washington: U.S. National Library of Medicine, 2019. Available from: https://clinicaltrials.gov/ct2/show/NCT03561051.

Alcohol-use Disorders

1. Introduction

- In 2017 in the UK, 7,697 people died from alcohol-specific conditions. This was equivalent to 12.2 deaths per 100,000 population. The latest figure is the highest rate since 2008, when the rate was recorded as 12.7 alcohol-specific deaths per 100,000.[1] Alcohol-use disorders are a common and increasing reason for a request for an emergency ambulance response.[2]

- Assessment, diagnosis and effective management of patients with alcohol-use disorders improve patient safety by reducing the acute and chronic complications caused by alcohol intoxication and acute withdrawal.[3] Remember that the use of other substances as well as alcohol may enhance the effect of each individual substance.

- Alcohol is associated with an increased chance of avoidable deaths from cancer, trauma and communicable diseases.[3] Whenever the opportunity arises, appropriate advice on consumption should be provided to the patient, and then they should be referred to specialist alcohol liaison services where available or through primary care, in line with Making Every Contact Count (MECC) guidance.

- Co-morbid mental health disorders commonly include depression, anxiety disorders and drug misuse. Physical co-morbidities are common, including gastrointestinal (GI) disorders, in particular liver disease, and GI haemorrhage; neurological and cardiovascular diseases are also common. In some people, these co-morbidities may remit with abstinence or reduced alcohol consumption, but many experience long-term consequences of alcohol-use disorders that may significantly shorten their life expectancy.

- Alcohol-use disorders are also associated with increased safeguarding risks affecting patients, other vulnerable adults around them or children in affected families. There should be a low threshold for safeguarding referrals.

2. Categorisation

2.1 Hazardous Drinking

- Hazardous drinking, or increasing-risk drinking, is categorised by the World Health Organization as 'a pattern of alcohol consumption that increases someone's risk of harm'.[3]

- Consumption, measured as units per week:
  - drinking more than 14 units a week, but less than 35 units a week, for women
  - drinking more than 14 units a week, but less than 50 units, for men.

- Some would limit this definition to the physical or mental health consequences (directly harmful use); others would include the wider social consequences. The term is currently used to describe this pattern of alcohol consumption; it is not a diagnostic term.

2.2 Harmful Drinking

- Harmful drinking (high-risk drinking) is categorised as 'a pattern of alcohol consumption that is causing mental or physical damage'.[3]

- Consumption, measured as units per week:
  - drinking 35 units a week or more for women
  - drinking 50 units a week or more for men.[3]

3. Conditions

3.1 Wernicke-Korsakoff Syndrome

- Wernicke-Korsakoff syndrome is caused by a lack of Vitamin B1 (also known as Thiamine). Thiamine cannot be produced by the body and is absorbed from foods. In chronic alcohol dependency, there is reduced absorption of thiamine as well as impaired utilisation of thiamine by cells, especially those in the cardiac and nervous systems. The condition causes lesions within the brain that disrupt neurological function; this can lead to irreversible neurological changes. Any patient who presents with loss of balance, tremor, confusion, agitation, visual disturbance or loss of muscle control may have an alcohol use disorder and should be considered at high risk of Wernicke-Korsakoff syndrome and be conveyed to hospital.[4]

- Emergency management for this condition may be needed urgently, with an intravenous administration of B vitamins in an Emergency Department.

- People with suspected Wernicke-Korsakoff syndrome are at higher risk if they are malnourished, at risk of malnourishment or have decompensated liver disease.

3.2 Alcohol-related Pancreatitis

- Alcohol-related pancreatitis is a potentially fatal condition, where alcohol even in small amounts may trigger a major inflammatory response. Patients presenting with abdominal pain, nausea and vomiting should be treated and transported to an Emergency Department for further investigation and management. The risk of developing pancreatitis grows with increased acute or chronic consumption of alcohol.

3.3 Delirium

- Alcohol intoxication and withdrawal are frequently associated with delirium. Delirium is an acute, fluctuating change in mental status, with inattention, disorganised thinking and altered levels of consciousness.[5] There is a correlation between recent binge drinking and alcoholic ketoacidosis, which can lead to delirium.

- Delirium Tremens (DTs) is the most severe form of alcohol withdrawal, manifested by altered

Alcohol-use Disorders

mental status (global confusion) and sympathetic overdrive (autonomic hyperactivity), which can progress to cardiovascular collapse.

to a flapping tremor of the limbs and then unconsciousness.

3.4 Gastrointestinal Bleeding

- Patients may have acute or chronic GI haemorrhage; these are a major cause of alcohol-related morbidity and mortality.

- Mallory-Weiss syndrome is a common cause of upper GI haemorrhage in patients with recurrent and active drinking abuse. Alcohol has a reported association with Mallory-Weiss tear in 40% to 80% of patients.[6] Oesophageal or gastric varices (dilated veins) can be a cause of potentially life-threatening upper GI haemorrhage.

3.5 Hepatic Encephalopathy

- This condition can occur in acute or chronic liver failure. Increases in serum ammonia levels cause cerebral oedema. Initially, the signs may be very vague with general malaise, progressing

4. Assessment

- Multiple factors can affect the diagnosis in a patient with chronic alcohol use and there are several differential diagnoses that cannot be formally excluded within the pre-hospital environment.

- Remember that many of these signs (refer to Tables 3.17 and 3.18) can also be present in patients with head injuries, and any history of recent trauma should raise suspicion of an intracranial head injury (refer to **Trauma Emergencies in Adults – Overview** or **Trauma Emergencies in Children – Overview**).

- Consider mixed intentional or unintentional overdose in addition to alcohol use (refer to **Overdose and Poisoning in Adults and Children**).

TABLE 3.17 – Signs and Symptoms of Alcohol Intoxication[4]

- Impairment of tasks requiring skill.
- Increased talkativeness.
- Relaxation.
- Ataxia.
- Hyperreflexia.
- Reduced levels of capacity.
- Lack of coordination.
- Loss of inhibition, change in mood, excitability, aggression.
- Prolonged reaction times.
- Slurred speech.
- Amnesia.
- Diplopia.
- Dysarthria.
- Hypothermia.
- Nausea and vomiting.
- Respiratory depression.
- Reduced consciousness.

TABLE 3.18 – Signs and Symptoms of Acute Alcohol Withdrawal

- Confusion.
- Uncontrollable shaking.
- Nausea or vomiting.
- Paroxysmal sweats.
- Agitation.
- Hallucinations.
- Headaches.

(continued)

Alcohol-use Disorders

TABLE 3.18 – Signs and Symptoms of Acute Alcohol Withdrawal *(continued)*
▪ Convulsions.
▪ Depression.
▪ Tremor.
▪ Anxiety.
▪ Tactile disturbances.
▪ Visual disturbances.
▪ Disorientation.

5. Management

- Refer to Table 3.19 for the assessment and management of alcohol-use disorders.

5.1 Safety

- The management of patients experiencing alcohol-use disorders must always start with an assurance of the safety of the clinicians, the patient and any bystanders. Acute alcohol use can be associated with a sudden change in behaviour that may result in aggressive or violent outbursts.

5.2 Mental Capacity

- Careful assessment of the patient's mental capacity should be undertaken and the least restrictive methods of clinical management used, to ensure patient and clinician safety. Refer to **Safeguarding Adults at Risk** and **Mental Capacity Act 2005**.

5.3 Admission to Hospital

- Patients with signs of acute alcohol withdrawal should attend an Emergency Department or be seen by another healthcare professional. They are at high risk of developing alcohol withdrawal seizures or delirium tremens.

- Have a lower threshold for admission for vulnerable patients. For example, those who are frail or cognitively impaired; those who have multiple co-morbidities, a lack of social support or learning difficulties; and those who are children under 18 years old or pregnant women. These patients often need further physical, psychosocial and safeguarding support.

- Patients without time-critical **<C>ABCDE** issues but with signs of acute alcohol withdrawal **should not** be discouraged from the ingestion of alcohol prior to leaving the scene of the incident.[6]

TABLE 3.19 – ASSESSMENT and MANAGEMENT of: Alcohol-Use Disorders
Assess <C>ABCDE:

▪ If any of the following **TIME-CRITICAL** features are present:
   – major **<C>ABCDE** problems (refer to **Medical Emergencies in Adults – Overview**)
   – convulsions (relatively common in alcohol withdrawal; refer to **Convulsions in Adults** or **Convulsions in Children**).

▪ Start correcting any **<C>ABCDE** problems.
▪ Undertake a **TIME-CRITICAL** transfer to nearest appropriate receiving hospital.
▪ Continue patient management en-route.
▪ Provide an ATMIST information call.
Respiratory Rate
▪ Measure and record respiratory rate.
Pulse
▪ Measure and record pulse
Oxygen Saturation
▪ Measure and record the patient's SpO$_2$, and administer oxygen to achieve saturations of >94% if the patient presents as hypoxaemic on air (refer to **Oxygen**).
Blood Pressure
▪ Measure and record blood pressure.

Alcohol-use Disorders

TABLE 3.19 – ASSESSMENT and MANAGEMENT of: Alcohol-Use Disorders *(continued)*

Blood Glucose

- Measure and record blood glucose for hypo/hyperglycaemia (refer to **Glycaemic Emergencies in Adults and Children**).
- Unless the patient refuses, this assessment should always be undertaken because acute alcohol intoxication and hypoglycaemia share many signs and symptoms.
- Glycogen stores can be very low and rebound hypoglycaemia may occur following pre-hospital glucose administration.
- Have a low threshold for transfer to hospital.

Temperature

- Measure and record temperature.

NEWS2

- Calculate NEWS2 score (refer to **Sepsis**).

ECG

- If required, monitor and record 12-lead ECG. Assess for abnormality (refer to **Cardiac Rhythm Disturbance**).

Assess the Patient's Pain

- Where present, assess the **SOCRATES** of pain, and record initial and subsequent pain scores.
- Consider analgesia if appropriate (refer to **Pain Management in Adults** or **Pain Management in Children**).

Documentation

- Complete documentation to include all clinical findings, advice from other clinicians, onward referral and worsening advice given.
- If the patient is not conveyed to hospital, they must not be advised to suddenly reduce their alcohol intake.
- If convulsions occur, refer to **Convulsions in Adults** or **Convulsions in Children**.

6. Making Every Contact Count

- Ambulance clinicians have a role to play in having conversations with people who are drinking harmful amounts of alcohol. The evidence-based MECC approach can be applied, or other locally agreed methods of ensuring health prevention messages can be given. An MECC interaction takes a matter of minutes and should be part of the clinical conversation with the patient if appropriate.

- Men should drink no more alcohol than 3–4 units each day and women no more than 2–3 units each day, with at least two alcohol-free days every week. A unit is half a pint of (3.5% ABV) beer, cider or lager, a small (125ml) glass of 8% wine or a single (25ml) measure of spirits.

- Most patients express the view that they expect to be asked about lifestyle behaviours by health professionals. Most people want to make changes to their unhealthy behaviours. They do, however, need some support to change. MECC is a great way to deliver consistent lifestyle advice messages.

- Consider referring or signposting the patient to primary care, local pathways or alcohol-use disorder services. Consider leaving an appropriate leaflet with the patient about local services for alcohol-use disorder.

- Discussing conditions associated with long-term alcohol use such as Wernicke-Korsakoff syndrome with patients and relatives helps to warn them about red flag symptoms and their causes.

SECTION **3** Medical Emergencies

2022

Alcohol-use Disorders

191

Alcohol-use Disorders

Alcohol-use Disorders

- Rates of alcohol-use disorders are on the rise.

- Chronic alcohol use is associated with several serious conditions.

- People with chronic alcohol dependency must never be advised to stop drinking without clinically managed withdrawal by a specialist alcohol service.

- There is an increased risk of intracranial haemorrhage with heavy alcohol consumption.

- Paramedics should be aware of the pharmacological interactions that alcohol has, which reduce or increase the effects of some medicines.

Further Reading

Further important information and evidence in support of this guideline can be found in the Bibliography.[7,8,9,10,11,12]

Bibliography

1. ONS. *Alcohol-specific Deaths in the UK*. 2017. Available from: https://www.ons.gov.uk/peoplepopulationand-community/healthandsocialcare/causesofdeath/bulletins/alcoholrelateddeathsintheunitedkingdom/registeredin2017.

2. NAO. *NHS Ambulance Services*. 2017. Available from: https://www.nao.org.uk/wp-content/uploads/2017/01/NHS-Ambulance-Services.pdf.

3. NICE. *Alcohol-use Disorders: Diagnosis and management of physical complications*. 2017. Available from: https://www.nice.org.uk/guidance/cg100/chapter/Recommendations#acute-alcohol-withdrawal.

4. NICE. *Alcohol-use Disorders: Diagnosis, assessment and management of harmful drinking (high-risk drinking) and alcohol dependence*. 2011. Available from: https://www.nice.org.uk/guidance/cg115.

5. Inouye SK, Schlesinger MJ, Lydon TJ. Delirium: a symptom of how hospital care is failing older persons and a window to improve quality of hospital care. *Am J Med* 1999, 106(5): 565–573.

6. Kortas DY, Haas LS, Simpson WG, Nickl NJ, Gates LK. Mallory-Weiss tear: predisposing factors and predictors of a complicated course. *Am. J. Gastroenterol* 2001, 96(10): 2863–2865.

7. Martin RP, Singleton CK, Hiller–Sturmhöfel S. The role of thiamine deficiency in alcoholic brain disease. *Alcohol Research & Health* 2003, 27(2): 134–142. Available from: https://pubs.niaaa.nih.gov/publications/arh27-2/134-142.htm.

8. Vonghia L. Acute alcohol intoxication. 2007. Available from: https://doi.org/10.1016/j.ejim.2007.06.033.

9. Griswold MG, Fullman N, Hawley C, Arian N, Zimsen SR, Tymeson HD, Venkateswaran V, Tapp AD, Forouzanfar MH, Salama JS, Abate KH 2018. Alcohol use and burden for 195 countries and territories, 1990–2016: a systematic analysis for the Global Burden of Disease Study. *The Lancet* 2016, 392(10152): 1015–1035.

10. NICE. *Alcohol-Use Disorders – NICE Pathways*. 2020. Available from: https://pathways.nice.org.uk/pathways/alcohol-use-disorders#path=view%3A/pathways/alcohol-use-disorders/acute-alcohol-withdrawal.xml&content=view-node%3Anodes-information-and-support.

11. NICE. *Alcohol-use Disorders: Diagnosis and management of physical complications*. 2017. Available from: https://www.nice.org.uk/guidance/cg100.

12. Alcohol Change UK. *Unit Calculator*. 2020. Available from: https://alcoholchange.org.uk/alcohol-facts/interactive-tools/unit-calculator.

Allergic Reactions including Anaphylaxis

1. Introduction

- The incidence of allergic reactions continues to rise. It is estimated that allergic reactions affect 30% of adults and 40% of children, while anaphylaxis affects up to 2% of the population.

- The most common triggers are food, drugs/medicines and venom but in 30% of cases the trigger is unknown.

- Anaphylaxis is defined as a severe, life-threatening, generalised or systemic hypersensitivity reaction. This is characterised by rapidly developing life-threatening airway and/or breathing and/or circulation problems, usually associated with skin and mucosal changes.

- Injected allergens can result in cardiovascular compromise, with hypotension and shock predominating. Inhaled and ingested allergens typically cause rashes, vomiting, facial swelling, upper airway swelling and wheeze. Slow release drugs/medicines prolong absorption and exposure to the allergen, meaning the action onset can be delayed.

2. Severity and Outcome

- The severity of symptoms varies from a localised urticaria to life-threatening respiratory and/or cardiovascular compromise – anaphylaxis.

- Some patients relapse after an apparent recovery (biphasic response); therefore, patients who have experienced an anaphylactic reaction should be transferred to hospital for further evaluation. The risk of an individual suffering a recurrent anaphylactic reaction is estimated to be approximately 1:12 per year.

- Patients with other allergic conditions, such as asthma or atopic eczema, are more at risk of developing anaphylaxis, and risk of death is increased in those with pre-existing asthma, particularly if the asthma is poorly controlled.

- Patients who have experienced previous episodes of anaphylaxis may wear a 'Medic Alert' bracelet or necklace and carry an adrenaline auto-injector (e.g. Anapen®, EpiPen®). It is now advised that all patients who have previously experienced an anaphylactic reaction are prescribed two auto-injectors that should be carried at all times.

- The mortality associated with anaphylaxis is estimated to be <1%.

3. Triggers

- Allergic reaction and anaphylaxis can be caused by a broad range of triggers, including food, drugs and insect stings. Food is a common trigger in children, while drugs/medicines are a more common trigger in older people. Virtually any food or class of drug can be implicated, although the classes of foods and drugs responsible for the majority of reactions are well described. For common triggers, refer to Table 3.20.

- The time it takes for the symptoms of anaphylaxis to develop depends on how the trigger enters the body. Death can occur quickly after contact with the trigger or allergen, with approximately 50% of fatalities due to circulatory collapse (shock) and the rest due to respiratory failure (asphyxia).

4. Assessment of Allergic Reactions and Anaphylaxis

- Anaphylaxis is likely when all of the following criteria are met:
  1. Sudden onset and rapid progression of symptoms.
  2. Life-threatening Airway and/or Breathing and/or Circulation problems.
  3. Skin and/or mucosal changes (flushing, urticaria, angioedema).

- The diagnosis is supported if a patient has been exposed to an allergen known to affect them.

TABLE 3.20 – Common Triggers of Allergic Reactions
1 – Foods
Nuts (e.g. peanuts, walnuts, almonds, Brazil nuts and hazel nuts), pulses, sesame seeds, milk, eggs and fish/shellfish.
2 – Venom – insect stings/bites
Insect stings and bites (e.g. wasps and bees). **NB** Bees may leave a venom sac, which should be scraped off (not squeezed).
3 – Drugs
Antibiotics (e.g. penicillin, cephalosporin, ciprofloxacin and vancomycin), non-steroidal anti-inflammatory drugs, angiotensin-converting enzyme inhibitors, gelatins, protamine, vitamin K, amphotericin, etoposide, acetazolamide, pethidine, local anaesthetic, diamorphine and streptokinase.
4 – Other causes
Latex, hair dye, semen and hydatid.

Allergic Reactions including Anaphylaxis

- The skin and/or mucosal changes that occur in allergic reactions and anaphylaxis include:
  - Erythema (superficial reddening of the skin, caused by dilatation of the capillaries)
  - Urticaria (a raised itchy rash (also known as hives), nettle rash, weals or welts)
  - Angioedema (swelling in the dermis, subcutaneous and submucosal tissues).
- Isolated skin or mucosal changes without life-threatening airway, breathing or circulatory problems do not signify an anaphylactic reaction. Skin and mucosal changes can be subtle or absent in up to 20% of anaphylactic patients.
- Angioedema most commonly occurs with urticaria, but may occur in isolation. It can occur anywhere on the body, but most often involves the eye, lips, hands and feet. Less commonly, submucosal swelling affects the airway.

Angioedema may be considered part of the continuum of anaphylaxis, but in isolation, without respiratory difficulty or circulatory collapse, is not anaphylaxis.

- The mechanism for angioedema and anaphylaxis is the same, in that both histamine and bradykinin are involved. However, in anaphylaxis the reaction is more marked, resulting in an increase in vascular permeability and circulatory collapse.
- Anaphylaxis can occur despite a long history of previously safe exposure to a potential trigger. Reactions can be rapid, slow or biphasic.
- For a list of signs and symptoms which may occur during an allergic reaction or anaphylaxis, refer to Table 3.21.
- For the assessment and management of anaphylaxis and allergic reactions, refer to Table 3.22.

TABLE 3.21 – Signs and Symptoms of Allergic Reactions or Anaphylaxis

Airway problems	Throat and tongue swelling (laryngeal/pharyngeal oedema)
	Difficulty in breathing and swallowing
	Hoarse voice
	Stridor (high-pitched inspiratory noise caused by upper airway obstruction).
Breathing problems	Bronchospasm
	Tachypnoea/dyspnoea
	Wheeze/stridor
	Fatigue
	Confusion caused by hypoxia
	Cyanosis (usually a late feature)
	SpO_2 <92%
	Respiratory arrest.
Circulatory problems	Hypotension
	Tachycardia
	Pale and clammy skin
	Dizziness
	Decreased conscious level
	Myocardial ischaemia
	Bradycardia (usually a late feature)
	Cardiac arrest.
Other	Skin/mucosal changes (urticarial/hives)
	Diarrhoea and/or vomiting
	Abdominal pain
	Anxiety.

Allergic Reactions including Anaphylaxis

5. Management of Allergic Reactions and Anaphylaxis

5.1 Immediate Management (Figure 3.5)

- Adrenaline is the first-line treatment for anaphylaxis and immediate administration is a priority. Follow the algorithm for initial treatment of anaphylaxis (Figure 3.5).
  - Give intramuscular (IM) adrenaline early (in the anterolateral thigh) for Airway/Breathing/Circulation problems.
  - A single dose of IM adrenaline is well tolerated and poses minimal risk to an individual having an allergic reaction. If in doubt, give IM adrenaline.
  - Repeat IM adrenaline after 5 minutes if Airway/Breathing/Circulation problems persist.
- Self-administration of IM adrenaline (via an EpiPen® or similar) is not always reliable. Do not assume that any self-administered adrenaline has been delivered effectively.
- Lie the patient flat (elevate legs if hypotensive). A sitting position is acceptable if that makes breathing easier for the patient. If patient is pregnant, lie her on left side. Avoid any sudden change in posture.
- Treat life-threatening features using the Airway, Breathing, Circulation, Disability, Exposure (ABCDE) approach.
- Rapid conveyance to hospital is indicated in patients whose respiratory and/or cardiovascular problems persist despite two doses of IM adrenaline.

5.2 Management of Refractory Anaphylaxis (Figure 3.6)

- Patients who fail to respond to a second IM dose of adrenaline have refractory anaphylaxis. If further treatment is indicated, first ensure that all steps recommended in 'Immediate Management' have been undertaken.
- Continue to administer the appropriate dose of IM adrenaline at 5-minute intervals until the patient begins to improve or is handed over to emergency department (ED) clinicians.
- Histamine release during an anaphylactic reaction leads to increased vascular permeability, causing large volumes of fluid to leak from the patient's circulation. If haemodynamically compromised, refer to **Intravascular Fluid Therapy in Adults** and **Intravascular Fluid Therapy in Children**.
  - Adult: 500–1000 mL per bolus
  - Child: 10 mL/kg per bolus

NB Large volumes may be required (e.g. 3–5 L in adults).

- Consider nebulised Salbutamol for bronchospasm (refer to **Salbutamol**); refer to **Page for Age** for children's doses.

5.3 Management of Cardiac Arrest due to Anaphylaxis

- Start chest compressions early.
- Use IV or IO **Adrenaline 1 milligram in 10 ml (1 in 10,000)** bolus (cardiac arrest protocol).
- Aggressive fluid resuscitation.
- Consider prolonged resuscitation/extracorporeal CPR.

Allergic Reactions including Anaphylaxis

Anaphylaxis?

↓

A = Airway **B** = Breathing **C** = Circulation **D** = Disability **E** = Exposure

↓

Diagnosis – look for:
- Sudden onset of Airway and/or Breathing and/or Circulation problems[1]
- Usually skin changes (e.g. itchy rash)

↓

- Remove trigger if possible (e.g. stop any infusion)
- Lie patient flat (with or without legs elevated)
  - A sitting position may make breathing easier
  - If pregnant, lie on left side

↓

Administer adrenaline[2] ——— **Intramuscular (IM) ONLY**

↓

- Establish airway
- Give high flow oxygen
- Apply monitoring: pulse oximetry, ECG, blood pressure

↓

If no response:
- Repeat IM adrenaline after 5 minutes
- IV fluid bolus[3]

↓

If NO improvement in Breathing or Circulation problems[1] after TWO doses of IM adrenaline:
- Follow REFRACTORY ANAPHYLAXIS ALGORITHM

---

1. Life-threatening problems

Airway
Hoarse voice, stridor

Breathing
↑ work of breathing, wheeze, fatigue, cyanosis, SpO_2 <94%

Circulation
Low blood pressure, signs of shock, reduced consciousness

2. Intramuscular (IM) adrenaline

Use adrenaline at 1 mg/mL (1:1000) concentration

Adult and child >12 years: 500 micrograms IM (0.5 mL)
Child 6–12 years: 300 micrograms IM (0.3 mL)
Child 6 months to 6 years: 150 micrograms IM (0.15 mL)
Child <6 months: 100–150 micrograms IM (0.1–0.15 mL)

The above doses are for IM injection **ONLY**.
Intravenous adrenaline for anaphylaxis to be given **only by experienced specialists** in an appropriate setting.

3. IV fluid challenge

Use crystalloid

Adults: 500–1000 mL
Children: 10 mL/kg

4. Salbutamol

Consider nebulised salbutamol for bronchospasm

Figure 3.5 – Immediate management of anaphylaxis.

Allergic Reactions including Anaphylaxis

Refractory Anaphylaxis
No improvement in respiratory or cardiovascular symptoms despite two appropriate doses of intramuscular (IM) adrenaline

Establish peripheral IV or IO access

Give rapid IV fluid bolus
e.g. 0.9% sodium chloride

Give IM adrenaline every 5 minutes

Give high flow oxygen
Titrate to SpO$_2$ 94–98%

Monitor HR, BP, pulse oximetry and ECG for cardiac arrhythmia

Figure 3.6 – Management of refractory anaphylaxis.

Allergic Reactions including Anaphylaxis

TABLE 3.22 – ASSESSMENT and MANAGEMENT of: Allergic Reactions and Anaphylaxis

Trigger

- Quickly remove the patient from the trigger. Do not delay definitive treatment if this is not possible or where the trigger is unknown.
- Where an insect sting is the trigger, early removal is more important than the method of removal. If the trigger has been ingested, attempts to make the patient vomit are not recommended.

For Anaphylaxis

- Administer Adrenaline **SAFETY NOTE 1:1,000 IM ONLY**. Intramuscular adrenaline is the most important drug for the treatment of anaphylactic reactions (refer to **Adrenaline 1 milligram in 1 ml (1 in 1,000)**; refer to **Page for Age** for children's doses.
- **NB** Drug check **MUST** be completed before administration, including clarification of route to be used **(IM ONLY)**.

Assess <C>ABCD

- If any of the following **TIME-CRITICAL** features are present:
  - Major **<C>ABCD** problems (refer to **Medical Emergencies in Adults – Overview** and **Medical Emergencies in Children – Overview**).
  - Administer high levels of supplementary oxygen to achieve saturations of >94% if the patient presents as hypoxemic on air (refer to **Oxygen**).
- Start correcting any **<C>ABCD** problems.
- Undertake a **TIME-CRITICAL** transfer to nearest appropriate receiving hospital.
- Continue patient management en-route.
- Provide an ATMIST information call.

Mild or Moderate Allergic Reaction

- Consider a mild/moderate allergic reaction if the onset of the presentation has progressed over minutes to hours, and there are skin and/or mucosal changes in the absence of life-threatening features. In this scenario, adrenaline is not appropriate.
  - For mild and moderate allergic reactions, oral antihistamine is the treatment of choice.
  - For a mild reaction, consider the appropriateness of advising the patient to purchase their own over-the-counter antihistamine. If this is not possible, consider referral for oral antihistamine supply.

FOR ALL PATIENTS WITH SYMPTOMS OF ANAPHYLAXIS OR ALLERGY

Respiratory Rate

- Measure and record respiratory rate.

Pulse

- Measure and record pulse.

Oxygen Saturation

- Monitor the patient's SpO_2, administer oxygen to achieve saturations of >94% if the patient presents as hypoxemic on air (refer to **Oxygen**).

Blood Pressure and Fluids

- Measure and record blood pressure; if required, administer fluids (refer to **Intravastcular Fluid Therapy in Adults** and **Intravascular Fluid Therapy in Children**).

Blood Glucose

- If appropriate, measure and record blood glucose for hypo/hyperglycaemia (refer to **Glycaemic Emergencies in Adults and Children**).

Temperature

- Measure and record temperature.

NEWS2

- These observations will enable you to calculate a NEWS2.

Allergic Reactions including Anaphylaxis

TABLE 3.22 – ASSESSMENT and MANAGEMENT of: Allergic Reactions and Anaphylaxis *(continued)*
ECG
■ If required, monitor and record 12-lead ECG. Assess for abnormality (refer to **Cardiac Rhythm Disturbance**).
Assess the Patient's Pain
■ Where present, assess the **SOCRATES** of pain and record initial and subsequent pain scores. ■ Consider analgesia if appropriate (refer to **Pain Management in Adults** and **Pain Management in Children**).
Transfer to Further Care
■ Convey all patients who have experienced an anaphylactic reaction to the Emergency Department as some patients may relapse hours after an apparent recovery from anaphylaxis (biphasic response). ■ Patients who have experienced an allergic reaction and do not require attendance at the Emergency Department should be advised to see their GP for consideration of oral steroids (where not already prescribed) if their symptoms are persistent. For first presentations of an allergic reaction, consider informing the patient's GP.
Documentation
■ Complete documentation to include all clinical findings, advice from other clinicians, onward referral and worsening advice given.

KEY POINTS!

Allergic Reactions including Anaphylaxis

- **Remove from trigger if possible.**
- **Anaphylaxis can occur despite a long history of previously safe exposure to a potential trigger.**
- **Consider anaphylaxis in the presence of acute cutaneous symptoms, bronchospasm or cardiovascular compromise.**
- **Anaphylaxis may be rapid, slow or biphasic.**
- **Immediate administration of adrenaline is key in managing anaphylaxis. Repeat every 5 minutes until symptoms show signs of improving.**
- **Large volumes of intravenous fluids may be needed to support the circulation.**
- **For mild and moderate allergic reactions, oral antihistamine is the treatment of choice.**

Acknowledgements

We would like to gratefully acknowledge the contribution of the Resuscitation Council UK to the JRCALC guideline.

Bibliography

1. Lott C, Truhlar A, Alfonzo A, et al. European Resuscitation Council Guidelines 2021: Cardiac arrest in special circumstances. *Resuscitation* 2021, 161: 152–219.

2. Deakin CD, Soar J, Davies R, et al. (2021) *Resuscitation Guidelines: Special Circumstances Guidelines*. Resuscitation Council UK, 2021. Available from: https://www.resus.org.uk/library/2021-resuscitation-guidelines/special-circumstances-guidelines.

3. National Institute for Health and Clinical Excellence. *Anaphylaxis: Assessment to Confirm an Anaphylactic Episode and the Decision to Refer after Emergency Treatment for a Suspected Anaphylactic Episode (CG134)*. 2011. Last updated 2020. Available from: https://www.nice.org.uk/guidance/cg134.

SECTION 3 Medical Emergencies

Altered Level of Consciousness

1. Introduction

- Pre-hospital presentation of altered level of consciousness (ALoC) can be a major challenge.

- In patients with ALoC it is important to undertake a rapid assessment for **TIME-CRITICAL** conditions.

- It is important to understand, where possible, the cause of altered consciousness which can range from diabetic collapse, to factitious illness (refer to Tables 3.23 and 3.24).

- The patient history may provide valuable insight into the cause of the current condition. Consider the following in formulating your diagnosis. Ask relatives or bystanders if there is:
  - any history of recent illness or pre-existing chronic illness (e.g. diabetes, steroid-dependent adrenal insufficiency or epilepsy)
  - any past history of mental health problems
  - any preceding symptoms such as headache, fits, confusion
  - any history of trauma.

NB Remember, an acute condition may be an exacerbation of a chronic condition or a 'new' illness superimposed on top of a pre-existing problem, such as adrenal crisis triggered by infective gastroenteritis.

- However, often there is little available information – in these circumstances the scene may provide clues to assist in formulating a diagnosis:
  - Environmental factors (e.g. extreme cold, possible carbon monoxide sources).
  - Evidence of tablets, ampoules, pill boxes, syringes, including domiciliary oxygen (O_2), or administration devices (e.g. nebuliser machines).
  - Evidence of alcohol or medication abuse.

TABLE 3.23 – Red Flag Conditions

Condition
Adrenal insufficiency (risk of adrenal crisis with hypoglycaemia) (refer to **Hydrocortisone**).
Epilepsy (refer to **Stroke/Transient Ischaemic Attack**).
Head injury (refer to **Head Injury**).
Hyperglycaemia (refer to **Glycaemic Emergencies in Adults and Children**).
Hypoglycaemia (refer to **Glycaemic Emergencies in Adults and Children**).
Overdose (refer to **Overdose and Poisoning in Adults and Children**).
Stroke/TIA (refer to **Stroke/Transient Ischaemic Attack**).
Subarachnoid haemorrhage (refer to **Headache**).

TABLE 3.24 – Some Conditions That May Result in DLoC (Decreased Level of Consciousness)

Alterations in pO$_2$ (hypoxia) and/or pCO$_2$ (hyper/hypocapnia)
Inadequate airway.
Inadequate ventilation or depressed respiratory drive.
Persistent hyperventilation.
Inadequate perfusion
Cardiac arrhythmias.
Distributive shock.
Hypovolaemia.
Neurogenic shock.
Raised intracranial pressure.
Altered metabolic states
Hypoglycaemia and hyperglycaemia.
Intoxication or poisoning
Alcohol intoxication.
Carbon monoxide poisoning.
Drug overdose.
Medical conditions
Adrenal crisis.
Epilepsy.
Hypo/hyperthermia.
Meningitis.
Stroke.
Subarachnoid haemorrhage.
Head injury

This guideline contains guidance for managing patients with transient loss of consciousness (TLoC) (section 1) and coma (section 2).

2. SECTION 1 – Transient Loss of Consciousness (TLoC)

- Transient loss of consciousness (TLoC) may be defined as spontaneous loss of consciousness with complete recovery, i.e. full recovery of consciousness without any residual neurological deficit.

- An episode of TLoC is often described as a 'blackout' or a 'collapse'. There are various causes of TLoC, including:
  - cardiovascular disorders (which are the most common)
  - neurological conditions such as epilepsy, and psychogenic attacks.

- The diagnosis of the underlying cause of TLoC is often inaccurate and delayed.

Altered Level of Consciousness

2.1 Assessment and Management

For the assessment and management of TLoC, refer to Table 3.25.

TABLE 3.25 – ASSESSMENT and MANAGEMENT of: Transient Loss of Consciousness

Assess <C>ABCD

- If any of the following **TIME-CRITICAL** features are present:
  - major **<C>ABCD** problems
  - unexpected OR persistent loss of consciousness, ECG abnormalities, TLoC during exertion, new, unexplained breathlessness, then:
- Start correcting any **<C>ABCD** problems.
- Undertake a **TIME-CRITICAL** transfer to nearest appropriate receiving hospital.
- Continue patient management en-route.
- Provide an ATMIST information call.

Ascertain from the Patient or Witnesses What Happened Before, During and After the Event

Record details about:

- Circumstances of the event.
- The patient's posture immediately before loss of consciousness.
- Prodromal symptoms (such as sweating or feeling warm/hot).
- Appearance (whether eyes were open or shut) and colour of the patient during the event.
- Presence or absence of movement during the event (limb-jerking and its duration).
- Any tongue-biting (record whether the side or the tip of the tongue was bitten).
- Injury occurring during the event (record site and severity). Refer to relevant guideline.
- Duration of the event (onset to regaining consciousness).
- Presence or absence of confusion during the recovery period.
- Weakness down one side during the recovery period.
- Details of any previous TLoC, including number and frequency.
- The patient medical history and any family history of cardiac disease (personal history of heart disease or family history of sudden cardiac death).
- Current medication that may have contributed to TLoC (diuretics).
- Lying and standing blood pressure if clinically appropriate.
- Other cardiovascular and neurological signs.

ECG

- Monitor and record 12-lead ECG. Assess for abnormality (refer to **Cardiac Rhythm Disturbance**).

If an Underlying Cause Is Suspected

- Undertake relevant examinations and investigations; for example, check blood glucose levels if hypoglycaemia is suspected – refer to relevant guideline.

Assess for Uncomplicated Faint and Situational Syncope

Diagnose uncomplicated faint (uncomplicated vasovagal syncope) on the basis of the initial assessment when:

- There are no features that suggest an alternative diagnosis (**NB** brief seizure activity can occur during uncomplicated faints and is not necessarily diagnostic of epilepsy).

AND

- There are features suggestive of uncomplicated faint (the 3 'P's) such as:
  - **posture** – prolonged standing, or similar episodes that have been prevented by lying down
  - **provoking** factors (such as pain or a medical procedure)
  - **prodromal** symptoms (such as sweating or feeling warm/hot before TLoC).

(continued)

Altered Level of Consciousness

Diagnose situational syncope on the basis of the initial assessment when:

■ There are no features from the initial assessment that suggest an alternative diagnosis.

AND

■ Syncope is clearly and consistently provoked by straining during micturition (usually while standing) or by coughing or swallowing.

Care Pathway

■ Only patients with a GCS 15, with normal blood glucose and responsible adult supervision present may be left at scene. For example, if a diagnosis of uncomplicated faint or situational syncope is made, there is nothing in the initial assessment to raise clinical or social concern and there are no red flags present, the patient may be left at home.

■ **Advise the patient to take a copy of the clinical record and the ECG record to their GP and follow local protocols to safely hand over clinical responsibility.**

■ Take the opportunity, if appropriate, to discuss and record any lifestyle factors which may influence the cause of any TLoC episode.

Red Flags

The presence of any of the following during physical examination should be considered a red flag, resulting in conveyance to the Emergency Department:

■ New ECG abnormalities (listed below).

■ Physical signs of heart failure.

■ TLoC during exertion.

■ Family history of sudden cardiac death in people aged younger than 40 years and/or an inherited cardiac condition.

■ New or unexplained breathlessness.

■ A heart murmur.

Conveyance should be considered for anyone older than 65 years of age who has experienced a TLoC without prodromal symptoms. Where not conveyed, these patients must be discussed directly with a doctor.

The following ECG abnormalities are considered red flags and in these cases the patient must be conveyed to the Emergency Department for assessment:

■ New conduction abnormalities (complete right or left bundle branch block or any degree of heart block).

■ Evidence or prolonged (>440 ms for males or >460 ms for females) or shortened QTc intervals (<350 ms for both).

■ Any ST segment or T-wave abnormalities (e.g. brugada syndrome, abnormal T-wave inversion).

■ Pathological Q waves.

■ Paced rhythm.

■ Inappropriate persistent bradycardia.

■ Ventricular arrhythmia.

■ Ventricular pre-excitation.

■ Sustained atrial arrhythmias.

3. SECTION 2 – Coma

3.1 Introduction

■ Coma is defined as U on the AVPU scale or a Glasgow Coma Score (GCS) (refer to Appendix) of 8 or less; however, any patient presenting with a decreased level of consciousness (GCS <15) mandates further assessment and, possibly, treatment.

■ There are a number of causes of coma; refer to Tables 3.23 and 3.24.

3.2 Assessment and management

For the assessment and management of coma, refer to Table 3.26.

Altered Level of Consciousness

TABLE 3.26 – ASSESSMENT and MANAGEMENT of: Coma (GCS <8)
Assess <C>ABCD
▪ Start correcting any **<C>ABCD** problems.
▪ Undertake a **TIME-CRITICAL** transfer to the nearest appropriate receiving hospital.
▪ Continue patient management en-route.
▪ Provide an ATMIST information call.
Oxygen
▪ Administer high levels of supplementary oxygen and aim for a target saturation within the range of 94–98% (refer to **Oxygen**).
Assess for Hypoxia
▪ Apply pulse oximetry.
▪ Obtain IV access if appropriate.
Assess Heart Rhythm for Arrhythmias
▪ Undertake a 12-lead ECG.
Assess Level of Consciousness
▪ Assess using the AVPU scale or Glasgow Coma Scale (GCS) (refer to Appendix):
A – Alert
V – Responds to voice
P – Responds to painful stimulus
U – Unresponsive.
▪ Assess and note pupil size, equality and response to light.
▪ Check for purposeful movement in all four limbs and note sensory function.
Assess Blood Glucose Level
▪ If hypoglycaemic (<4.0 mmol/l) or suspected, refer to **Glycaemic Emergencies in Adults and Children**.
Blood Pressure
▪ Measure blood pressure.
▪ Correct blood pressure with fluid administration if required (refer to **Sodium Chloride 0.9%**).
Assess for Significant Injury Especially to the Head
▪ If trauma detected or suspected, immobilise spine and refer to **Spinal Injury and Spinal Cord Injury**.
Assess for Other Causes
▪ Breath for ketones, alcohol and solvents.
▪ Evidence of needle tracks/marks.
▪ MedicAlert®-type jewellery (bracelets or necklets), or emergency card (steroids, oxygen), which detail the patient's primary health risk (e.g. diabetes, anaphylaxis, Addison's disease, COPD etc.) – also list a 24-hour telephone number to obtain a more detailed patient history.
▪ Warning stickers, often placed by the front door or the telephone, directing the health professional to a source of detailed information (one current scheme involves storing the patient details in a container in the fridge, as this is relatively easy to find in the house).
▪ Patient-held warning cards, for example for those taking monoamine oxidase inhibitor (MAOI) medication.
▪ **For management, refer to relevant guideline(s).**
Assess for Respiratory Depression
In cases of severe respiratory depressions, refer to **Airway and Breathing Management**.
If the level of consciousness deteriorates or respiratory depression develops in cases where an overdose with opiate-type drugs may be a possibility, consider naloxone (refer to **Naloxone Hydrochloride**).
In a patient with fixed pinpoint pupils, suspect opiate use/overdose.
NB Any patient with a decreased level of consciousness may have a compromised airway.

(continued)

Altered Level of Consciousness

TABLE 3.26 – ASSESSMENT and MANAGEMENT of: Coma (GCS <8) *(continued)*

Re-assess <C>ABCD

- Document any changes/note trends in:
  - GCS
  - altered neurological function
  - base-line observations.

APPENDIX

GLASGOW COMA SCALE

Item	Element	Score
Eyes Opening:		
	Spontaneously	4
	To speech	3
	To pain	2
	None	1
Verbal Response:		
	Orientated	5
	Confused	4
	Inappropriate words	3
	Incomprehensible sounds	2
	No verbal response	1
Motor Response:		
	Obeys commands	6
	Localised pain	5
	Withdraws from pain	4
	Abnormal flexion	3
	Extensor response	2
	No response to pain	1

KEY POINTS!

Altered Level of Consciousness

- **Maintain patent airway.**
- **Support ventilation if required.**
- **Address treatable causes.**
- **History – obtain as much information as possible.**
- **Consider an alert/information call.**

Bibliography

1. National Collaborating Centre for Acute Care. *Head Injury: Triage, assessment, investigation and early management of head injury in infants, children and adults* (CG56). London: National Collaborating Centre for Acute Care at The Royal College of Surgeons of England, 2007. Available from: https://www.nice.org.uk/guidance/cg176.

2. National Institute for Health and Clinical Excellence. *Stroke: The diagnosis and initial management of acute stroke and transient ischaemic attack* (CG68). London: NICE, 2008.

3. National Institute for Health and Clinical Excellence. *The Epilepsies: The diagnosis and management of the epilepsies in adults and children in primary and*

Altered Level of Consciousness

secondary care (CG137). London: NICE, 2012. Available from: https://nice.org.uk/guidance/CG137.

4. National Institute for Health and Clinical Excellence. *Transient Loss of Consciousness in Adults and Young People* (CG109). London: NICE, 2012. Available from: https://www.nice.org.uk/guidance/qs71.

5. Task Force for the Diagnosis and Management of Syncope, European Society of Cardiology, European Heart Rhythm Association, Heart Failure Association, Heart Rhythm Society, Moya A, Sutton R, Ammirati F, Blanc JJ, Brignole M, Dahm JB, et al. Guidelines for the diagnosis and management of syncope (version 2009). *European Heart Journal* 2009, 30(21): 2631–2671.

Asthma in Adults and Children

1. Introduction

- Asthma has varying levels of severity and patients usually present to the ambulance service with one of four presentations: mild/moderate, severe, life-threatening or near fatal (refer to Table 3.27).

- This guideline covers asthma in adults and children. A child is defined as between one year and puberty.

- Typically in patients requiring hospital admission the symptoms will have developed gradually over a number of hours (>6 hours).

- There may be a history of increasing wheeze or breathlessness which is often worse at night or early in the morning. Respiratory infections, allergy, cold weather and physical exertion are common triggers.

- Known asthmatics may be on regular medication, taking inhalers ('preventers' and/or 'relievers') and sometimes oral medications such as Montelukast (Singulair®) or theophyllines.

- Some patients with asthma will have an individualised treatment plan with detailed information regarding their daily symptom control as well as what to do in an acute exacerbation. They may have their own antibiotics and steroids to start when they get an exacerbation.

- **Consider anaphylaxis** where there is a sudden onset or in a patient without a history of asthma that has severe wheezing.

- **Inhaled foreign body:** Consider an inhaled foreign body in a child experiencing their first wheezy episode, or if there is a history of playing with small toys and the wheeze was of sudden onset, particularly if the wheeze is unilateral. These children must be transferred for medical assessment. If they are unwell during transport, bronchodilators may provide some clinical benefit.

- Patients over 50 years of age who are long-term smokers with a history of exertional breathlessness and no other known cause of breathlessness should be treated as having COPD (refer to **Chronic Obstructive Pulmonary Disease**).

2. Incidence

- Asthma is rare in the older population and practitioners should be aware that many people will describe a range of other respiratory conditions as 'asthma', and therefore other causes of breathlessness need to be considered.

- In adults, asthma may often be complicated and mixed in with a degree of bronchitis, especially in smokers. This can make the condition much more difficult to treat, both routinely and in emergencies. The majority of asthmatic patients take regular 'preventer' and 'reliever' inhalers.

- Asthma is rare in very young children (under one year), and other causes of wheeze (such as bronchiolitis or viral induced wheeze) should be considered.

3. Severity and Outcome

- Severe asthma is a **TIME-CRITICAL** emergency – in the UK some 2,000 people a year die as a result of asthma. Patients with severe asthma and one or more risk factor(s) (refer to Table 3.27) are at greater risk of death.

- In patients ≤40 years, asthma deaths peak in the summer (July/August), whereas deaths peak in the winter (December/January) for asthmatics aged >40 years.

TABLE 3.27 – Risk Factors for Developing Near-Fatal Asthma

Medical

- Previous near-fatal asthma (e.g. previous ventilation or respiratory acidosis).
- Previous admission requiring intensive care.
- Previous hospital admission for asthma especially if using three or more classes of asthma medication in the last year.
- Anaphylaxis.
- High β2 agonist requirements, especially with little or no response.
- Repeated asthma-related ED attendances, particularly in the last 12 months.
- Brittle asthma.

Psychological/behavioural

- Non-compliance with treatment or monitoring.
- Failure to attend appointments.
- Fewer GP contacts.
- Frequent home visits.
- Self-discharge from hospital.
- Psychosis, depression, other psychiatric illness or deliberate self-harm.
- Current or recent major tranquilliser use.
- Denial.
- Alcohol or drug abuse.
- Obesity.
- Smoking.
- Learning difficulties.
- Employment problems.
- Income problems.
- Social isolation.
- Childhood abuse.
- Severe domestic, marital or legal stress.

Asthma in Adults and Children

TABLE 3.28 – Features of Severity

Life-threatening asthma

Any one of the following in a patient with severe asthma:

- Altered conscious level.
- Exhaustion.
- Cyanosis.
- Silent chest.
- Poor respiratory effort.
- PEF <33% best or predicted.
- SpO$_2$ <92%.
- Arrhythmia
- Hypotension

Acute severe asthma

Any one of:

- PEF 33–50% best or predicted.
- SpO$_2$ ≥ 92%.
- Inability to complete sentences in one breath.
- Pulse:
  - >110/minute in adults
  - >125/minute in children >5 years
  - > 140/minute in children 1–5 years.
- Respiration:
  - >25/minute in adults
  - >30/minute in children >5 years
  - >40/minute in children 1–5 years.

Moderate asthma exacerbation

- Able to speak in sentences.
- Increasing symptoms.
- PEF >50–75% best or predicted.
- No features of acute severe asthma.
- Heart rate:
  - ≤140/min in children aged 1–5 years
  - ≤125/min in children >5 years.
- Respiratory rate:
  - ≤40/min in children aged 1–5 years
  - ≤30/min in children >5 years.

Mild Asthma

- Below best level of functioning due to wheeze.
- PEFR >75% best or predicted.
- No features of moderate or acute severe asthma.

4. Pathophysiology

- Asthma is caused by inflammation of the bronchi, making them narrower. The muscles around the bronchi become irritated and contract, causing sudden worsening of the symptoms. The inflammation can also cause the mucus glands to produce excessive sputum, which further blocks the air passages.
- Small airway obstruction and narrowing is caused by three factors:
  a bronchial mucosal swelling
  b bronchial muscle spasm and constriction
  c increased bronchial mucus and secretions.
- Since inspiration is an active process involving the muscles of respiration, the obstruction of the airways is overcome on breathing in. Expiration occurs with muscle relaxation and is severely delayed by the narrowing of the airways in asthma, producing the characteristic expiratory wheeze.
- Asthma is managed with a variety of inhaled and tablet medications. Inhalers are divided into two broad categories: preventer and reliever.

1 The preventer inhalers are normally anti-inflammatory drugs and these include steroids and other milder anti-inflammatories and long-acting beta agonists such as salmeterol or formoterol. The common steroid inhalers are beclometasone (Clenil, Qvar), budesonide (Pulmicort), fluticasone (Flixotide) and tiotropium (Spiriva). These drugs act on the lung over a period of time to reduce the inflammatory reaction that causes the asthma. Regular use of these inhalers often eradicates all symptoms of asthma and allows for a normal lifestyle. A combination of maintenance and reliever inhaler therapy (MART) may be given as a single inhaler (AirFluSal, Flutiform, Relvar Ellipta).

2 The short-acting beta agonist reliever inhalers include salbutamol (Ventolin) and terbutaline (Bricanyl); the inhaled muscarinics include ipratropium bromide (Atrovent). These inhalers work rapidly on the lung to relax the smooth muscle spasm when the patient feels wheezy or tight-chested. They are used in conjunction with preventer inhalers. Inhalers are commonly given through a spacer device, such as a Volumatic® or an Aerochamber®, improving drug administration. In mild and moderate asthma attacks, some patients may be treated with high doses of 'relievers' through a spacer device. This has been shown to be as effective as nebulisation.

5. Assessment

- Assess <C>ABCD (refer to **Medical Emergencies in Adults – Overview** and **Medical Emergencies in Children – Overview**), but specifically assess for the severity of the asthma attack (refer to asthma algorithm – Figure 3.8 and Table 3.28).

6. Management

- Refer to the asthma algorithm (Figure 3.8 and Table 3.30) for the management of mild/ moderate, severe, life-threatening and near-fatal.

Asthma in Adults and Children

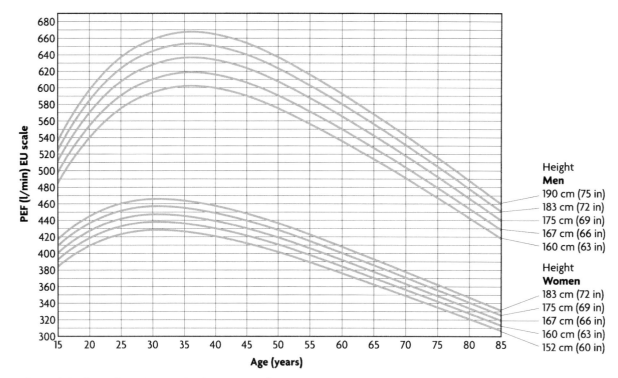

Figure 3.7 – Peak flow charts – Peak expiratory flow rate – normal values. For use with EU/EN13826 scale PEF meters only.

- Always ask if the patient has an individualised asthma treatment plan and follow it, unless clinical circumstances dictate otherwise.

6.1 For less severe attacks

- Where possible, the patient's own β2 agonist should be given (ideally using a spacer) as first-line treatment. Increase the dose by two puffs every 2 minutes according to response, up to ten puffs.

- If symptoms are not controlled by ten puffs, then start nebulised salbutamol whilst transferring to the emergency department (ED).
NB Children aged under two years old who do not appear to be responding to salbutamol (administered with adequate technique) may not be having an asthma attack; alternative diagnosis and treatments should be considered (refer to **Respiratory Illness in Children**).

- Patients (or friends/bystanders) who have previously experienced a severe asthma attack may be more likely to call for help early in the development of an attack, and the symptoms may appear mild on arrival of the ambulance.

- Some patients may be appropriate for alternative care pathways, for example early referral to primary or urgent care. However, apparently minor symptoms should not preclude onward referral, especially where an alternative pathway is not readily accessible. Local care pathways should be followed where patients are considered for non-conveyance. However, caution should be exercised in known severe asthmatics and robust safety-netting of patients must be in place.

- Worsening advice should be given to seek further advice if there is further deterioration, which includes increasing breathlessness, decrease in peak expiratory flow rate (PEFR) and exhaustion.

6.2 Peak expiratory flow rate (PEFR)

- Peak flow is a rapid measurement of the degree of obstruction in the patient's lungs. It measures the maximum flow on breathing out, or expiring, and therefore can reflect the amount of airway obstruction. Whenever possible, peak flow should be performed before and after nebulised treatment. Many patients now have their own meter at home and know what their normal peak flow is. Clearly, when control is good, their peak flow will be equivalent to a normal patient's measurement, but during an attack it may drop markedly (refer to Figure 3.7).

- There is no place for PEFR measurements in pre-school children, as developmentally they do not have the technical ability to reliably perform this task.

- PEFR should be attempted where possible before and after nebulised therapy in mild to moderate asthma. However, care should be taken in severe life-threatening attacks as it could exacerbate the attack and the patient may deteriorate. Predicted PEFR is shown in Figure 3.7.

Adapted by Clement Clarke for use with EN13826/EU scale peak flow meters from Nunn AJ Gregg I, Br Med J 1989:298;1068–70.

Asthma in Adults and Children

TABLE 3.29 – Peak Expiratory Flow Rates

Height (m)	Height (ft)	Predicted EU PEFR (L/min)
1.25	4'1"	192
1.30	4'3"	212
1.35	4'5"	233
1.40	4'7"	254
1.45	4'9"	276
1.50	4'11"	299
1.55	5'1"	323
1.60	5'3"	346
1.65	5'5"	370
1.70	5'7"	393

TABLE 3.30 – ASSESSMENT and MANAGEMENT of: Asthma

Assess <C>ABCD

- If any of the following **TIME-CRITICAL** features present:
  - major <C>ABCD problems (refer to **Medical Emergencies in Adults – Overview** and **Medical Emergencies in Children – Overview**).
  - extreme difficulty in breathing or requirement for assisted ventilations. **NB** Asthma is predominantly a disease of exhalation; therefore care should be taken not to over-ventilate. Adequate expiration must be achieved.
  - exhaustion
  - cyanosis
  - silent chest
  - SpO_2 <92%
  - PEF <33% best or predicted.
- Start correcting any <C>ABCD problems.
- Undertake a TIME-CRITICAL transfer to nearest appropriate receiving hospital.
- Continue patient management en-route.
- Provide an ATMIST information call.

Respiratory Rate

- Measure and record respiratory rate.

Pulse

- Measure and record pulse.

Oxygen Saturation

- Monitor the patient's SpO_2, administer oxygen to achieve saturations of 94–98% if the patient presents as hypoxemic on air (refer to **Oxygen**).

Specifically Assess for the Severity of the Asthma Attack (refer to Figure 3.8 and Table 3.28)

- Move to a calm, quiet environment.
- Encourage use of own inhaler, using a spacer if available. Ensure correct technique is used (refer to Figure 3.8).

NB In children under two who have a poor response to salbutamol, consider an alternative cause (refer to **Respiratory Illness in Children**).

- If unresponsive:
  - Administer high levels of supplementary oxygen.
- Administer nebulised salbutamol (refer to **Salbutamol**; refer to **Page for Age** for children's doses).

(continued)

Asthma in Adults and Children

TABLE 3.30 – ASSESSMENT and MANAGEMENT of: Asthma *(continued)*
Mild Asthma
▪ For cases of mild asthma that respond to treatment, consider alternative care pathway where appropriate. **NB** Exercise caution in known severe asthmatics.
Moderate Asthma
▪ For moderate asthma, administer Prednisolone. Refer to **Prednisolone**.
Severe Asthma
▪ Administer high levels of supplementary oxygen.
▪ Administer nebulised salbutamol (refer to **Salbutamol**; refer to **Page for Age** for children's doses).
▪ If no improvement, administer ipratropium bromide (refer to **Ipratropium Bromide**' refer to **Page for Age** for children's doses).
▪ Administer steroids (refer to **Prednisolone/Hydrocortisone**' refer to **Page for Age** for children's doses).
▪ Continuous salbutamol nebulisation may be administered unless clinically significant side effects occur (refer to **Salbutamol**; refer to **Page for Age** for children's doses).
Life-threatening Asthma
▪ Give early consideration and low threshold to activate enhanced care support.
▪ Continuous salbutamol nebulisation may be administered unless clinically significant side effects occur (refer to **Salbutamol**; refer to **Page for Age** for children's doses).
▪ If there is no improvement, administer ipratropium bromide (refer to **Ipratropium Bromide**; refer to **Page for Age** for children's doses).
▪ If there is no improvement, administer a single dose of intravenous magnesium (refer to **Magnesium Sulfate**; refer to **Page for Age** for children's doses).
▪ If the patient continues to deteriorate, administer adrenaline. **SAFETY NOTE: 1:1000 IM ONLY** (refer to **Adrenaline 1 milligram in 1 ml (1 in 1,000)**; refer to **Page for Age** for children's doses).
NB: Drug check MUST be completed before administration, including clarification of route to be used (IM ONLY).
▪ Administer steroids (refer to **Prednisolone/Hydrocortisone**; refer to **Page for Age** for children's doses).
▪ Assess for bilateral tension pneumothorax.
▪ Transfer rapidly to nearest receiving hospital.
▪ Provide an ATMIST information call.
▪ Continue patient management en-route.
Blood Pressure and Fluids
▪ Measure and record blood pressure; if required administer fluids (refer to **Intravascular Fluid Therapy in Adults** and **Intravascular Fluid Therapy in Children**).
Blood Glucose
▪ If appropriate, measure and record blood glucose for hypo/hyperglycaemia (refer to **Glycaemic Emergencies in Adults and Children**).
Temperature
▪ Measure and record temperature.
NEWS2
▪ These observations will enable you to calculate a NEWS2 Score.
ECG
▪ If required, monitor and record 12-lead ECG. Assess for abnormality (refer to **Cardiac Rhythm Disturbance**).
Documentation
▪ Complete documentation to include all clinical findings, advice from other clinicians, onward referral and worsening advice given.

Asthma in Adults and Children

Figure 3.8 – Asthma assessment and management algorithm.

Asthma in Adults and Children

KEY POINTS!

Asthma in Adults and Children

- Asthma is a common life-threatening condition.
- Its severity is often not recognised.
- Accurate documentation is essential.
- A silent chest is a pre-terminal sign.
- Bronchodilators are the mainstay of treatment.
- Ipatropium bromide should be considered in severe cases.
- Clinical assessment should determine the severity of the asthma attack.
- Consider Magnesium in life-threatening asthma not improving with continuous nebulised Salbutamol.
- Consider adrenaline for life-threatening asthma continuing to deteriorate with continuous nebulised Salbutamol.
- Asthma is rare in very young children (under one year) and other causes of wheeze (such as bronchiolitis or viral-induced wheeze) should be considered.

Bibliography

1. Soar J, Perkins GD, Abbas G, Alfonzo A, Barelli A, Bierens JJLM, et al. European Resuscitation Council Guidelines for Resuscitation 2010 Section 8: Cardiac arrest in special circumstances: electrolyte abnormalities, poisoning, drowning, accidental hypothermia, hyperthermia, asthma, anaphylaxis, cardiac surgery, trauma, pregnancy, electrocution. *Resuscitation* 2010, 81(10): 1400–1433.

2. Health Improvement Scotland, British Thoracic Society, *SIGN 158 British Guideline on the Management of Asthma.* Revised July 2019.

3. Rubin BK, Dhand R, Ruppel GL, Branson RD, Hess DR. Respiratory care year in review 2010. Part 1: asthma, COPD, pulmonary function testing, ventilator-associated pneumonia. *Respiratory Care* 2011, 56(4): 488–502.

4. Nunn AJ, Gregg I. New regression equations for predicting peak expiratory flow in adults. *British Medical Journal* 1989, 298(6680): 1068–1070.

Cardiac Rhythm Disturbance

1. Introduction

- Cardiac arrhythmia is a common complication of acute myocardial ischaemia or infarction and may precede cardiac arrest or complicate the early post-resuscitation period.

- Rhythm disturbance may also present in many other ways and be unrelated to coronary heart disease.

- The management of disorders of cardiac rhythm is a specialised subject, often requiring detailed investigation and management strategies that are not available outside hospital.

- Diagnosis of the precise rhythm disturbance may be complicated and the selection of optimal treatment difficult. Very often, expert advice will be required, yet this expertise is rarely immediately available in the emergency situation.

2. Principles of Treatment

- Management is determined by the condition of the patient as well as the nature of the rhythm. Manage the patient using the standard <C>ABCDE approach.

- In all cases follow the oxygen guideline and aim for a target saturation within the range of 94–98%.

- Gain venous access.

- Always take a defibrillator to any patient with suspected cardiac rhythm disturbance.

- Establish cardiac rhythm monitoring as soon as possible.

- Document the arrhythmia. This should be done with a 12-lead ECG whenever possible. If only a 3-lead ECG is available, lead II provides the best waveform for arrhythmia analysis.

- Provide a printout for the hospital, and, if possible, archive the record electronically so that further copies can be available at a later time if needed. Repeat the recording if the rhythm should change at any time. Record the ECG rhythm during any intervention (vagotonic procedures or the administration of drugs).

- If patients are not acutely ill there may be time to seek appropriate advice.

- The presence of adverse signs or symptoms will dictate the need for urgent treatment. The following adverse factors indicate a patient who is unstable because of the arrhythmia:
  - evidence of low cardiac output: pallor, sweating, cold clammy extremities, impaired consciousness or hypotension (SBP <90 mmHg)
  - excessive tachycardia, defined as a heart rate of >150 bpm
  - excessive bradycardia, defined as a heart rate of <40 bpm
  - heart failure implies the arrhythmia is compromising left ventricular function. This may cause breathlessness, confusion and hypotension or other features of reduced cardiac output
  - ischaemic chest pain implies that the arrhythmia (particularly tachyarrhythmia) is producing myocardial ischaemia. It is particularly important if there is underlying coronary disease or structural heart disease in which ischaemia is likely to lead to life-threatening complications including cardiac arrest.

3. Bradycardia

3.1 Introduction

- A bradycardia is defined as a ventricular rate <60 bpm, but it is important to recognise patients with a relative bradycardia in whom the rate is inappropriately slow for their haemodynamic state.

4. Risk of Asystole

4.1 Assessment and Management

For the assessment and management of bradycardia and risk of asystole, refer to Table 3.31.

TABLE 3.31 – ASSESSMENT and MANAGEMENT of: Bradycardia and Risk of Asystole
Bradycardia: A ventricular rate <60 bpm, but it is important to recognise patients with a relative bradycardia in whom the rate is inappropriately slow for their haemodynamic state.
Assess to Determine If One or More Adverse Signs Are Present
▪ Systolic blood pressure <90 mmHg.
▪ Ventricular rate <40 bpm.
▪ Ventricular arrhythmias compromising BP requiring treatment.
▪ Heart failure.
If one or more signs are present:
▪ Follow oxygen guidelines – aim for target saturation within the range 94–98%.
▪ Gain IV access.

(continued)

SECTION 3 Medical Emergencies

Cardiac Rhythm Disturbance

Cardiac Rhythm Disturbance

TABLE 3.31 – ASSESSMENT and MANAGEMENT of: Bradycardia and Risk of Asystole (continued)

- Administer atropine[1] (refer to **Atropine Sulfate**) and repeat after 3–5 minutes if necessary, or transcutaneous pacing.
- Undertake a 12-lead ECG.
- Transfer to further care.

Risk of asystole: If the patient is initially stable (i.e. no adverse signs are present) or a satisfactory response is achieved with atropine, next determine the risk of asystole.

Assess for Risk of Asystole

- Previous episode of asystole.
- Möbitz II AV block.
- Complete (third-degree) AV block, especially with a broad QRS complex or an initial ventricular rate <40 bpm.
- Ventricular standstill >3 seconds.

If there is a risk of asytole (i.e. one or more signs are present) or the patient shows adverse signs and has not responded satisfactorily to atropine, transvenous pacing is likely to be required. One or more of the following interventions may improve the patient's condition during transport:

- Transcutaneous pacing should be undertaken if available.

If transcutaneous pacing is not available:

- Fist pacing may produce ventricular contraction – give serial rhythmic blows with the closed fist over the lower left sternal edge to pace the heart at a rate of 50–70 bpm.

NOTES:

a **Do not** give atropine to patients with cardiac transplants; their hearts will not respond to vagal blocking by atropine, and paradoxical high-degree AV block or sinus arrest may result.

b Complete heart block with a narrow QRS complex escape rhythm may not require pacing. The ectopic pacemaker (which is situated in the atrioventricular junction) may provide a stable rhythm at an adequate rate.

c Initiate transcutaneous pacing (if equipment is available):
  – if there is no response to atropine
  – if patient is severely symptomatic, particularly when high-degree block (Möbitz type II or third-degree AV block) is present.

NB Transcutaneous pacing may be painful; use analgesia. Verify mechanical capture. Monitor the patient carefully; try to identify the cause of the bradycardia.

5. Tachycardia

5.1 Introduction

- These guidelines are intended for the treatment of patients who maintain a cardiac output in the presence of the tachycardia.
- Pulseless ventricular tachycardia is treated according to the cardiac arrest algorithm for the treatment of pulseless VT/VF.

- Broad complex tachycardia.
- Narrow complex tachycardia.

5.2 Assessment and Management

For the assessment and management of tachycardia broad complex tachycardia and narrow complex tachycardia, refer to Table 3.32.

---

1 Caution – Doses of atropine lower than 500 mcg may paradoxically cause further slowing of the ventricular rate. Use atropine cautiously in acute myocardial ischaemia or infarction; an increased rate may worsen ischaemia.

SECTION 3 Medical Emergencies

Cardiac Rhythm Disturbance

TABLE 3.32 – ASSESSMENT and MANAGEMENT of: Tachycardia, Broad Complex Tachycardia and Narrow Complex Tachycardia

Tachycardia

- These guidelines are intended for the treatment of patients who maintain a cardiac output in the presence of the tachycardia.
- **Pulseless ventricular tachycardia** is treated with immediate attempts at defibrillation following the algorithm for the treatment of pulseless VT/VF.

1 Support the ABCs.

2 Administer high levels of supplemental oxygen – aim for a target saturation of 94–98%.

3 Gain IV access.

4 Establish cardiac rhythm monitoring.

5 Record and monitor BP and SpO$_2$.

6 Record a 12-lead ECG if possible; if not, record a rhythm strip.

7 If the rhythm changes at any time, make a further recording.

8 Make a continuous record of the rhythm during any therapeutic intervention (whether a drug or physical manoeuvre like carotid sinus massage).

9 The response to treatment can provide important additional information about the arrhythmia.

10 Identify and treat reversible causes; give analgesia if indicated.

11 Try to define the cardiac rhythm from the ECG. Determine the QRS duration and determine whether the rhythm is regular or irregular. If the QRS duration is 120 msec or more, the rhythm is a broad complex tachycardia. If less than 120 msec, the rhythm is a narrow complex tachycardia.

Broad Complex Tachycardia

- The rhythm is likely to be ventricular tachycardia, particularly in the context of ischaemic heart disease, in patients showing adverse signs (reduced consciousness, SBP <90 mmHg, chest pain or heart failure) or in the peri-arrest situation.
- In all cases, maintain the supportive measures above and monitor the patient during transport.
- Provide an alert/information call according to local guidelines.
- Atrial fibrillation with aberrant conduction may produce an irregular broad complex tachycardia, but the diagnosis is difficult to make with certainty and often requires expert examination of the ECG. This emphasises the importance of recording the ECG when the arrhythmia is present. Ambulance personnel may greatly assist the subsequent diagnosis and management of patients by obtaining good-quality ECG recordings. It is advantageous if these can also be archived electronically so that additional copies are available in the future.

Narrow Complex Tachycardia

- If the rhythm is narrow complex (QRS <120 msec) **AND REGULAR**, it is likely to be one of the following:
  - sinus tachycardia. This is a physiological response, for example to pain, fever, blood loss or heart failure. Treatment is directed towards the cause. Trying to slow the rate is likely to make the situation worse.
  - supraventricular tachycardia (SVT). This is often seen in patients without other forms of heart disease. There may be a history of previous attacks.
  - atrial flutter with regular AV conduction (often 2:1 and a rate of 150 bpm).
- In cases of SVT, start with vagal manoeuvres. In some cases the patient may be aware of techniques that have terminated previous episodes. The Valsalva manoeuvre (forced expiration against a closed glottis) may be effective and is conveniently achieved (especially in supine patients) by asking the patient to blow into a 10 ml syringe with sufficient force to push back the plunger. If this fails, perform carotid sinus massage provided no carotid bruit is heard on auscultation. A bruit may indicate the presence of atheromatous plaque, rupture of which may cause cerebral embolism and stroke.
- Record the ECG (preferably multi-lead) during each manoeuvre. If the arrhythmia is successfully terminated by vagal procedures, it is very likely to have been SVT. If the rhythm is atrial flutter, slowing of the ventricular rate may occur and allow the identification of flutter waves on the ECG.

(continued)

Cardiac Rhythm Disturbance

> **TABLE 3.32 – ASSESSMENT and MANAGEMENT of: Tachycardia, Broad Complex Tachycardia and Narrow Complex Tachycardia** *(continued)*
>
> - Maintain the supportive measures above and monitor the patient during transport.
> - **AN IRREGULAR** narrow complex rhythm is most commonly atrial fibrillation, less commonly atrial flutter with variable block. Maintain the supportive measures above and monitor the patient during transport.
> - In all cases, ensure the patient is received into a suitable emergency department, maintaining cardiac monitoring throughout. Ensure detailed handover to appropriate staff and that ECGs are safely handed over.

KEY POINTS!

Cardiac Rhythm Disturbance

- **Gain venous access.**
- **Always take a defibrillator to any patient with suspected cardiac rhythm disturbance.**
- **Establish cardiac rhythm monitoring as soon as possible, preferably with a 12-lead ECG.**
- **Record the ECG rhythm during any intervention and archive. Ensure all ECGs are safely handed over to receiving staff, and archive so further copies can be retrieved if necessary.**

Bibliography

1. Deakin CD, Nolan JP, Soar J, Sunde K, Koster RW, Smith GB, et al. European Resuscitation Council Guidelines for Resuscitation 2010 Section 4: adult advanced life support. *Resuscitation* 2010, 81(10): 1305–1352.

2. Soar J, Perkins GD, Abbas G, Alfonzo A, Barelli A, Bierens JJLM, et al. European Resuscitation Council Guidelines for Resuscitation 2010 Section 8: cardiac arrest in special circumstances: electrolyte abnormalities, poisoning, drowning, accidental hypothermia, hyperthermia, asthma, anaphylaxis, cardiac surgery, trauma, pregnancy, electrocution. *Resuscitation* 2010, 81(10): 1400–1433.

3. Deakin CD, Nolan JP, Sunde K, Koster RW. European Resuscitation Council Guidelines for Resuscitation 2010 Section 3: electrical therapies: automated external defibrillators, defibrillation, cardioversion and pacing. *Resuscitation* 2010, 81(10): 1293–1304.

4. Arntz H-R, Bossaert LL, Danchin N, Nikolaou NI. European Resuscitation Council Guidelines for Resuscitation 2010 Section 5: initial management of acute coronary syndromes. *Resuscitation* 2010, 81(10): 1353–1363.

5. de Caen AR, Kleinman ME, Chameides L, Atkins DL, Berg RA, Berg MD, et al. Part 10: paediatric basic and advanced life support: 2010 International Consensus on Cardiopulmonary Resuscitation and Emergency Cardiovascular Care Science with Treatment Recommendations. *Resuscitation* 2010, 81(1): e213–259.

6. Deakin CD, Morrison LJ, Morley PT, Callaway CW, Kerber RE, Kronick SL, et al. Part 8: advanced life support: 2010 International Consensus on Cardiopulmonary Resuscitation and Emergency Cardiovascular Care Science with Treatment Recommendations. *Resuscitation* 2010, 81(1): e93–174.

7. Wyllie J, Perlman JM, Kattwinkel J, Atkins DL, Chameides L, Goldsmith JP, et al. Part 11: neonatal resuscitation: 2010 International Consensus on Cardiopulmonary Resuscitation and Emergency Cardiovascular Care Science with Treatment Recommendations. *Resuscitation* 2010, 81(1): e260–287.

8. Sunde K, Jacobs I, Deakin CD, Hazinski MF, Kerber RE, Koster RW, et al. Part 6: defibrillation: 2010 International Consensus on Cardiopulmonary Resuscitation and Emergency Cardiovascular Care Science with Treatment Recommendations. *Resuscitation* 2010, 81(1): e71–85.

9. Bossaert L, O'Connor RE, Arntz H-R, Brooks SC, Diercks D, Feitosa-Filho G, et al. Part 9: acute coronary syndromes: 2010 International Consensus on Cardiopulmonary Resuscitation and Emergency Cardiovascular Care Science with Treatment Recommendations. *Resuscitation* 2010, 81(1): e175–212.

Chronic Obstructive Pulmonary Disease

1. Introduction

- Chronic obstructive pulmonary disease (COPD) is a chronic progressive disorder characterised by airflow obstruction.

- A diagnosis of COPD is usually made in the presence of airflow obstruction in people >35 years of age, who are or were previously smokers and may have one or more risk factors (refer to Table 3.33).

- Patients over 50 years of age who are long-term smokers with a history of exertional breathlessness and no other known cause of breathlessness should be treated as having COPD.

TABLE 3.33 – Signs/Symptoms of COPD

Signs/symptoms

- Exertional breathlessness.
- Chronic cough.
- Regular sputum production.
- Frequent winter 'bronchitis'.
- Wheeze.

- Patients with COPD usually present to the ambulance service with an acute exacerbation of the underlying illness. COPD is a concomitant/secondary illness in many incidents with other chief complaints.

- Some patients with COPD are at increased risk of hypercapnic respiratory failure (Type 2) and respiratory acidosis due to carbon dioxide retention. It is vital for any patient who has a history of this to know their baseline oxygen saturation levels (when well), to have an oximeter (where possible) and to be issued an 'alert card' by their specialist so that respiratory failure is not worsened by high levels of oxygen administration. Ambulance clinicians should be aware of the British Thoracic Society and **Oxygen** guidelines; however, these patients may require a tailored approach.

- Excessive oxygen administration in these patients can lead to:
  - Worsened ventilation-perfusion matching due to attenuation of hypoxic pulmonary vasoconstriction
  - Decreased binding affinity of haemoglobin for carbon dioxide
  - Decreased minute ventilation.

2. Incidence

- It is estimated that approximately 3 million people have COPD, affecting 2–4% of the population over 45 years of age. However, only 1.5% of the population are diagnosed with the condition.

- In the UK, COPD is the fifth leading cause of death and it is estimated that by 2020 it will be the third leading cause of death worldwide.

3. Severity and Outcome

- COPD results in disability and impaired quality of life, leading to 30,000 deaths per annum in the UK.

- COPD is the second leading cause of emergency admission in the UK, with 130,000 cases per annum and direct costs estimated at £800 million and indirect costs of £24 million.

4. Pathophysiology

- Airflow obstruction is the result of airway and parenchymal damage due to chronic inflammation.

- COPD increases the risk of co-morbidities such as lung cancer and cardiovascular disease.

- An acute exacerbation refers to a worsening of the patient's symptoms (refer to Table 3.34). There is no single feature that defines an exacerbation, although there are a number of known causes (refer to Table 3.36); however, in 30% of cases the cause is unknown.

- COPD patients generally have lower than normal SpO_2 levels, and British Thoracic Society oxygen guidelines should be followed to maintain a target saturation of 88–92% SpO_2.

- Some exacerbations are mild and self-limiting whilst others are more severe, potentially life-threatening and require intervention – not all features will be present (refer to Table 3.34).

- Some conditions may present with symptoms similar to an exacerbation of COPD – consider these when diagnosing an exacerbation of COPD (refer to Table 3.35).

TABLE 3.34 – Features of an Acute Exacerbation of COPD

Features

- Increased dyspnoea – particularly on exertion.
- Increased sputum volume/purulence.
- Increased cough.
- Upper airway symptoms (e.g. colds and sore throats).
- Increased wheeze.
- Chest tightness.
- Reduced exercise tolerance.
- Fluid retention.
- Increased fatigue.
- Acute confusion.
- Worsening of a previously stable condition.

(continued)

Chronic Obstructive Pulmonary Disease

TABLE 3.34 – Features of an Acute Exacerbation of COPD *(continued)*

Severe features

- Marked dyspnoea.
- Tachypnoea.
- Pursed-lips breathing.
- Use of accessory respiratory muscles (sternomastoid and abdominal) at rest.
- Acute confusion.
- New-onset cyanosis.
- New-onset peripheral oedema.
- Marked reduction in activities of daily living.

TABLE 3.35 – Conditions with Similar Features to an Acute Exacerbation of COPD

Features

- Asthma.
- Pneumonia.
- Pneumothorax.
- Left ventricular failure/pulmonary oedema.
- Pulmonary embolus.
- Lung cancer.
- Upper airway obstruction.
- Pleural effusion.
- Recurrent aspiration.

TABLE 3.36 – Causes of Exacerbation of COPD

Infections

- Rhinoviruses (common cold).
- Influenza.
- Parainfluenza.
- Coronavirus.
- Adenovirus.
- Respiratory syncytial virus.
- *C. pneumoniae.*
- *H. influenzae.*
- *S. pneumoniae.*
- *M. catarrhalis.*
- *S. aureus.*
- *P. aeruginosa.*

Pollutants

- Nitrogen dioxide.
- Particulates.
- Sulphur dioxide.
- Ozone.

5. Assessment and Management

For assessment and management of chronic obstructive pulmonary disease, refer to Table 3.37 and Figure 3.9.

TABLE 3.37 – ASSESSMENT and MANAGEMENT of: Chronic Obstructive Pulmonary Disease

Assess <C>ABCDE

- If any of the following **TIME-CRITICAL** features present:
  - major **<C>ABCDE** problems
  - extreme breathing difficulty (by reference to patient's usual condition)
  - cyanosis (although peripheral cyanosis may be 'normal' in some patients)
  - exhaustion
  - hypoxia (oxygen saturation <88%) unresponsive to oxygen (O_2) – some COPD patients normally have a lower than normal oxygen saturation (SpO_2) at baseline. It is important to ask if patients know what their baseline levels are, and if they have had problems with oxygen treatment previously.
- Start correcting any **<C>ABCDE** problems.
- Undertake a **TIME-CRITICAL** transfer to nearest appropriate receiving hospital.
- Continue patient management en-route.
- Provide an ATMIST information call.

Position

- Position the patient for comfort and ease of respiration, often sitting forwards, but be aware of potential hypotension.

Chronic Obstructive Pulmonary Disease

TABLE 3.37 – ASSESSMENT and MANAGEMENT of: Chronic Obstructive Pulmonary Disease *(continued)*

Ventilation

- Consider non-invasive ventilation if not responding to treatment.

Ask the Patient If They Have an Individualised Treatment Plan

- Follow the individualised treatment plan or alert card if available.
- The patient will often be able to guide their care.
- Alert cards outline emergency treatment, with specific target oxygen saturation as decided by the specialist, according to most recent investigations. As part of general history-taking and scene survey, ambulance clinicians should be mindful of the need to find out if such a card exists. Many patients may also have a special message passed from the GP surgery to the Ambulance Clinical Hub.
- A typical card will be similar to the one shown below, as recommended by the British Thoracic Society (BTS, 2017).

OXYGEN ALERT CARD

Name: _____

I have a chronic respiratory condition and I am at risk of having a raised carbon dioxide level in my blood during flare-ups of my condition (exacerbations)

Please use my _____% Venturi mask to achieve an oxygen saturation of

_____ % to _____ % during exacerbations of my condition

Use compressed air to drive nebulisers (with nasal oxygen a 2 l/min)
If compressed air is not available, limit oxygen-driven nebulisers to 6 minutes

---

Republished with kind permission of the British Thoracic Society. BTS Guideline for oxygen use in adults in healthcare and emergency settings 2017. Thorax Vol 72, Suppl 1.

- Patients with COPD can easily become anxious, making it feel harder to breathe. They may have received advice about using specific breathing control techniques to help reduce breathlessness; one example is pursed-lips breathing. Encourage the patient to use these techniques if appropriate and if the patient has found them helpful previously.

Specifically Assess:

Diagnosis

- Assess whether this is an acute exacerbation of COPD (refer to Table 3.34 for the features of COPD).
- Or another condition (refer to Table 3.35 and **Dyspnoea** for conditions with similar features to an acute exacerbation of COPD).

NB Chest pain and fever are uncommon symptoms of COPD – therefore consider other possible causes.

Airway

- Maintain airway patency.

NB Noises (e.g. 'bubbling' or wheeze) associated with breathing, indicating respiratory distress.

Bronchodilators

- Administer nebulised salbutamol (refer to **Salbutamol**).
- In severe cases, administer ipratropium bromide (refer to **Ipratropium Bromide**).
- If inadequate response after 5 minutes, a further dose of nebulised salbutamol may be administered.
- Ipratropium can only be administered ONCE; salbutamol may be repeated at regular intervals unless the side effects of the drug become significant.

NB Limit oxygen-driven nebulisation to 6 minutes. If journey time is significant, consider a further 6 minutes of nebulisation therapy ONLY if clinically indicated, but aim for a target saturation within the range of 88–92%.

(continued)

Chronic Obstructive Pulmonary Disease

TABLE 3.37 – ASSESSMENT and MANAGEMENT of: Chronic Obstructive Pulmonary Disease *(continued)*
Steroids
▪ Administer Prednisolone (refer to **Prednisolone**) or Hydrocortisone (refer to **Hydrocortisone**).
Respiratory Rate
▪ Measure and record respiratory rate.
Oxygen
If the primary illness in a patient with COPD requires high-concentration oxygen (refer to **Oxygen**), then this should **NOT BE WITHHELD**. The patient should be continually monitored closely for changes in respiratory rate and depth and the inspired concentration adjusted accordingly. In the short time that a patient is in ambulance care, hypoxia presents a much greater risk than hypercapnia in most cases.
▪ Measure oxygen saturation. Pulse oximetry, whilst important in COPD patients, will not indicate carbon dioxide (CO_2) levels which are assessed by capnography or, more commonly, blood gas analysis in hospital.
▪ Administer supplemental oxygen; aim for a target saturation within the range of 88–92% or the prespecified range – refer to the patient's individualised treatment plan or alert card if available.
NB The aim of oxygen therapy is to prevent life-threatening hypoxia – administer cautiously, as a proportion of COPD sufferers are chronically hypoxic and when given oxygen may develop increasing drowsiness and loss of respiratory drive. If this occurs, reduce oxygen concentration and support ventilation if required.
Pulse
▪ Measure and record pulse.
Blood Pressure and Fluids
▪ Measure and record blood pressure; if required, administer fluids (refer to **Intravascular Fluid Therapy in Adults** and **Intravascular Fluid Therapy in Children**).
Blood Glucose
▪ If appropriate, measure and record blood glucose for hypo/hyperglycaemia (refer to **Glycaemic Emergencies in Adults and Children**).
Temperature
▪ Measure and record temperature.
NEWS2
▪ These observations will enable you to calculate a NEWS2 Score (refer to **Sepsis**).
ECG
▪ If required, monitor and record 12-lead ECG. Assess for abnormality (refer to **Cardiac Rhythm Disturbance**).
Assess the Patient's Pain
▪ Where present, assess the **SOCRATES** of pain and record initial and subsequent pain scores.
▪ Consider analgesia if appropriate (refer to **Pain Management in Adults** and **Pain Management in Children**).
Documentation
▪ Complete documentation to include all clinical findings, advice from other clinicians, onward referral and worsening advice given.
Transfer
▪ Consider alternative care pathway where appropriate (refer to Table 3.38).
▪ Arrange a follow-up, such as visiting a nurse, a GP review or referral to other support before discharge.

Chronic Obstructive Pulmonary Disease

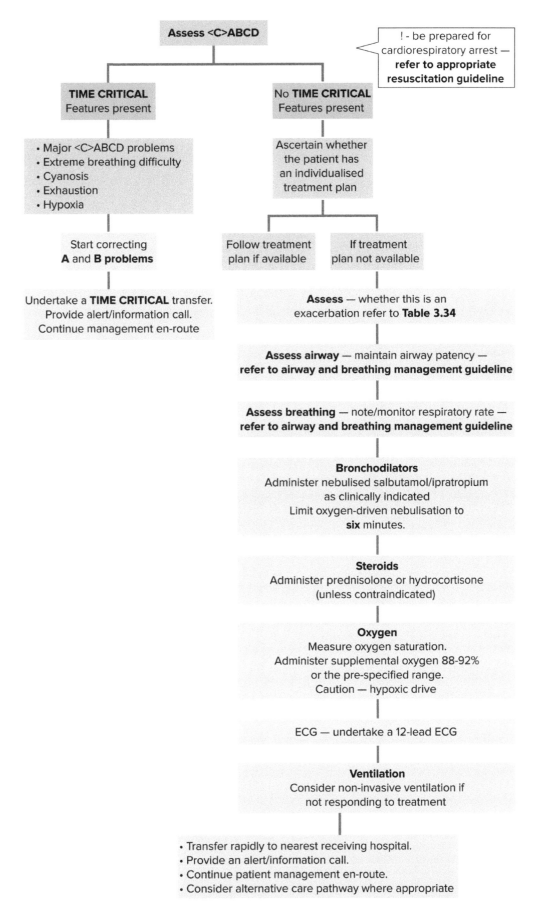

Figure 3.9 – Assessment and management of chronic obstructive pulmonary disease algorithm.

Chronic Obstructive Pulmonary Disease

TABLE 3.38 – Factors to Consider When Deciding Where to Treat A Person with COPD		
Factor	**Treat at home**	**Treat in hospital**
Able to cope at home	Yes	No
Breathlessness	Mild	Severe
General condition	Good	Poor/deteriorating
Level of activity	Good	Poor/confined to bed
Cyanosis	No	Yes
Worsening peripheral oedema	No	Yes
Level of consciousness	Normal	Impaired
Already receiving long-term oxygen therapy	No	Yes
Social circumstances	Good	Living alone/not coping
Acute confusion	No	Yes
Rapid rate of onset	No	Yes
Significant comorbidity (particularly cardiac disease and insulin-dependent diabetes)	No	Yes
SpO$_2$ <90%	No	Yes

KEY POINTS!

Chronic Obstructive Pulmonary Disease

- Early respiratory assessment (including oxygen saturation) is vital.
- If in doubt, provide oxygen therapy, titrating en-route, aiming for oxygen saturation of 88–92%.
- Provide nebulisation with salbutamol and assess response.

Bibliography

1. National Institute for Health and Clinical Excellence. *Chronic Obstructive Pulmonary Disease in over 16s: diagnosis and management.* London: NICE, 2018. Available from: https://www.nice.org.uk/guidance/ng115/chapter/Recommendations#managing-exacerbations-of-copd.

2. British Thoracic Society Emergency Oxygen Guideline Development Group. BTS Guideline for Oxygen Use in Adults in Healthcare and Emergency Settings. *Thorax: An International Journal of Respiratory Medicine.* 2017, 72: 1. Available from: https://www.brit-thoracic.org.uk/document-library/clinical-information/oxygen/2017-emergency-oxygen-guideline/bts-guideline-for-oxygen-use-in-adults-in-healthcare-and-emergency-settings/.

3. Rubin BK, Dhand R, Ruppel GL, Branson RD, Hess DR. Respiratory care year in review 2010. Part 1: Asthma, COPD, pulmonary function testing, ventilator-associated pneumonia. *Respiratory Care* 2011, 56(4): 488–502.

4. Austin MA, Wills KE, Blizzard L, Walters EH, Wood-Baker R. Effect of high flow oxygen on mortality in chronic obstructive pulmonary disease patients in pre-hospital setting: randomised controlled trial. *British Medical Journal* 2010, 341: c5462.

5. Austin MA, Wood-Baker R. Oxygen therapy in the pre-hospital setting for acute exacerbations of chronic obstructive pulmonary disease. *Cochrane Database of Systematic Reviews* 2006, 3. DOI: 10.1002/14651858.CD005534.pub2. Available from: http://www.mrw.interscience.wiley.com/cochrane/clsysrev/articles/CD005534/frame.html.

6. National Institute for Health and Clinical Excellence. *Chronic Obstructive Pulmonary Disease: Management of chronic obstructive pulmonary disease in adults in primary and secondary care (partial update)* (CG101). London: NICE, 2010. Available from: http://www.nice.org.uk/nicemedia/live/13029/49397/49397.pdf.

7. NHS Evidence. *COPD.* 2012. Available from: http://www.evidence.nhs.uk/topic/chronic-obstructive-pulmonarydisease?q=copd.

8. Ram FSF, Picot J, Lightowler J, Wedzicha JA. Non-invasive positive pressure ventilation for treatment of respiratory failure due to exacerbations of chronic obstructive pulmonary disease. *Cochrane Database of Systematic Reviews* 2004, 3. DOI: 10.1002/14651858.CD004104.pub3.

9. Schmidbauer W, Ahlers O, Spies C, Dreyer A, Mager G, Kerner T. Early pre-hospital use of non-invasive ventilation improves acute respiratory failure in acute exacerbation of chronic obstructive pulmonary disease. *Emergency Medicine Journal* 2011, 28(7): 626–627.

10. The Global Initiative for Chronic Obstructive Lung Disease. *Global Strategy for Diagnosis, Management, and Prevention of COPD.* 2011. Available from:

Chronic Obstructive Pulmonary Disease

http://goldcopd.org/gold-2017-global-strategy-diagnosis-management-prevention-copd/.

11. Uronis H, McCrory DC, Samsa G, Currow D, Abernethy A. Symptomatic oxygen for non-hypoxaemic chronic obstructive pulmonary disease. *Cochrane Database of Systematic Reviews* 2011, 6. DOI: 10.1002/14651858. CD006429.pub2. Available from: http://www.mrw. interscience.wiley.com/cochrane/clsysrev/articles/ CD006429/frame.html.

12. O'Driscoll BR, Howard LS, Davison AG, on behalf of the British Thoracic Society. BTS guideline for emergency oxygen use in adult patients. *Thorax* 2008, 63(suppl. 6): vi1–vi68.

13. Healthcare Commission. *Clearing the Air: A national study of chronic obstructive pulmonary disease.* London: Healthcare Commission, 2006.

SECTION **3** Medical Emergencies

Convulsions in Adults

1. Introduction

- A convulsion is an involuntary contraction and relaxation of the muscles producing rigidity and violent shaking of the body and limbs. Convulsions are often associated with altered/reduced consciousness (refer to **Altered Level of Consciousness**).

- The most common causes of convulsions are seizures in the context of epilepsy, provoked (acute symptomatic) seizures, psychogenic non-epileptic seizures (PNES), vasovagal syncope and cardiogenic events. The full list of causes is long and beyond the scope of this guideline. Other JRCALC guidelines are potentially relevant to the assessment of the convulsing patient and are cited here where appropriate.

- Eclampsia is a complication of pregnancy which may occur in women who are ≥20 weeks pregnant (including post-partum) and can give rise to epileptic seizures. Eclamptic seizures are beyond the scope of this guideline. Refer to **Pregnancy-induced Hypertension (including Eclampsia)** and **Magnesium Sulfate** for the assessment and management of convulsions in patients who are ≥20 weeks pregnant.

2. Epileptic Seizures

- Epileptic seizures are caused by abnormal electrical activity in the brain. There are many types of epileptic seizures. The manifestations of seizures depend on which part of the brain is affected. This guideline focuses on bilateral tonic-clonic seizures (BTCS), which are the most common type of seizure, and present as stiffening of the whole body (tonic phase), gradually merging into vigorous shaking (clonic phase). During a BTCS, patients typically have their eyes open and are unresponsive to commands or sensory stimuli. Most BTCS terminate within 90 seconds of their onset, and afterwards patients are often confused and/or drowsy.

- A BTCS that has not stopped after 5 minutes, or a series of such seizures without recovery in between which lasts for 5 minutes or more, is defined as convulsive status epilepticus (CSE). This is a medical emergency and requires rapid treatment. However, many patients with prolonged convulsions are having a psychogenic seizure, which can resemble a BTCS; see section 3. It may be difficult to distinguish between BTCS and PNES but some features are important in making this distinction (refer to Table 3.39).

- Seizures often start in only one part of the brain (a focal seizure) and then spread through the brain to cause a BTCS. Consciousness may be retained in focal seizures (also called an aura). The manifestations of all types of epileptic seizures are very diverse and their description is beyond the scope of this guideline which focuses on BTCS.[1,2]

- If a patient suffers focal motor seizures that last longer than 10 minutes and also has an impaired level of consciousness, then these should be treated in the same way as BTCS. However, the risk of long-term consequences is only likely to occur if the focal convulsion continues for over 60 minutes.

- Epilepsy is a chronic disorder in which patients are at increased risk of unprovoked seizures. Epileptic seizures also occur as 'provoked' (acute symptomatic) seizures caused by irritation of the brain, for instance by head injury, stroke, alcohol, hypoglycaemia, drug overdose or infection. The provoking factor may itself require emergency treatment.

- Many patients with epilepsy have an emergency care plan. They may also have a supply of emergency medication (usually midazolam), which can be administered by carers or healthcare professionals according to the care plan.

TABLE 3.39 – Features Which Help to Distinguish Between BTCS and PNES

Signs that favour Bilateral Tonic-Clonic (Epileptic) Seizures	Signs that favour Psychogenic Non-Epileptic Seizures
BTCS: during convulsion	**PNES: during convulsion**
Consistent, repeated, rhythmic myoclonic jerking	Fluctuating intensity/location
'Shock-like' movement	Brief pauses, tremor or slow flexion/extension movements
Arms & legs mostly synchronised/symmetrical	Arms & legs often not synchronised/symmetrical
Convulsion may spread from focal to generalised and tonic merging to clonic	Convulsion may move from one body area to another
Unresponsive (GCS 3 (4 if grunting))	May respond in some way (e.g. to speech, blink reflex or on NPA or IV insertion)
Lateral tongue-biting common	Tongue-biting rare/minor/involves tip

Convulsions in Adults

TABLE 3.39 – Features Which Help to Distinguish Between BTCS and PNES *(continued)*

Signs that favour Bilateral Tonic Clonic (Epileptic) Seizures	Signs that favour Psychogenic Non-Epileptic Seizures
Eyes often open	Eyes mostly shut (opening may be resisted)
Mouth often open	Mouth often shut
Pupils not reacting	Pupils reacting
No purposeful movements	May carry out purposeful movements
Low SpO$_2$ or cyanosis	Normal SpO$_2$, no cyanosis, ? hyperventilation
Typically short (<90 secs) or repeated without recovery between (constant prolonged rare)	May be prolonged (>3 mins)
Pelvic thrusting rare	Pelvic-thrusting common
Arching of the head, neck and spine rare	Arching of the head, neck and spine common
Clonic head movements to one side may occur	Side-to-side movements of the head/body
Initial scream, then grunting	Crying during/after convulsion
Plantar response may be abnormal (big toe up)	Plantar response normal (big toe flexed down)
BTCS: post-ictal	**PNES: post-ictal**
Gradual slowing down of convulsion	Rapid end to convulsion
Gradual post-ictal recovery	Rapid post-ictal recovery
Noisy laboured post-ictal breathing	Normal post-ictal breathing (or slow after hyperventilation)
BTCS: history	**PNES: history**
Onset under 10 years old	Onset over 15 years old
Alcohol misuse	Recurrent 'status epilepticus' (a misdiagnosis)
Provoked seizure (e.g. brain injury)	PTSD or psychological distress

3. Psychogenic Non-Epileptic Seizures (PNES)

- PNES are a common cause of prolonged convulsions. They are the most important differential diagnosis of epileptic convulsions in the emergency setting. PNES are usually an involuntary psychological response to distress and are commonly associated with a history of emotional trauma (abuse or neglect, potentially in childhood). Patients with PNES have commonly received an erroneous diagnosis of epilepsy and many are treated with antiepileptic drugs which are ineffective in this condition. Those who have received a diagnosis of PNES may know their condition by another name, e.g. non-epileptic attack disorder (NEAD), dissociative seizures, functional seizures, conversion disorder or pseudo-seizures.

- In contrast to convulsions caused by epilepsy, convulsive activity in PNES often continues for more than 5 minutes and PNES are commonly mistaken for status epilepticus. See Table 3.39 for a guide on distinguishing PNES from status epilepticus. Even prolonged PNES do not put the patient at risk of physiological derangement or brain damage. Emergency drug treatment is not effective and is potentially dangerous because it puts patients at risk of the side effects including respiratory depression, aspiration and death. Many patients with PNES have an emergency care plan which should be taken into account in decisions about treatment.

- Because of the similarity of PNES and CSE, it is important to note and record the characteristics of the convulsions as accurately as possible. This aids assessment and treatment during the convulsion but it also assists specialists in making the diagnosis in retrospect. For the same reason, families and carers may have been asked by specialists to video-record the events, and they should be encouraged to do so.

4. Syncope

- Vasovagal syncope (fainting) is the most common cause of transient loss of consciousness. It is caused by a temporary disruption to the supply of oxygen and glucose to the brain due to a fall in cerebral blood pressure. Vasovagal syncope usually happens when the person is upright, especially just after standing up, but it can occur whilst sitting especially when provoked by intercurrent illness, medical procedures, drugs, dehydration, alcohol and loss of bodily fluids, such as might occur with vomiting, bleeding

SECTION **3** Medical Emergencies

Convulsions in Adults

Convulsions in Adults

```
┌─────────────────────────────────┐
│   Is the convulsion ongoing      │
│      or has it stopped?          │
└─────────────────────────────────┘
```

| If the convulsion is **ongoing or recurrent**, refer to Table 3.40. | If the convulsion has **stopped**, refer to Table 3.41.

NB Even though convulsive movements have ceased, the patient may still be unresponsive. |

Figure 3.10 – Initial assessment and management of convulsions in adults.

or diarrhoea. In men, syncope is sometimes provoked by passing of urine while standing. People who faint usually feel dizzy and sweaty, get blurred vision and may experience distortion of hearing before they collapse. Brief but vigorous jerking may occur. This can mimic an epileptic seizure, although the jerking usually stops within less than 20 seconds, once normal cerebral circulation is restored. When the patient is supine, recovery is rapid and the patient may be able to hear what is going on around them before they can respond verbally. Patients may faint again if they sit up before their blood pressure and heart rate have stabilised.

- Syncope can also be caused by cardiac dysrhythmia (tachycardia or bradycardia), when it is known as cardiac syncope (refer to **Cardiac Rhythm Disturbance**), but this is much less common than vasovagal syncope. Cardiac syncope can occur whilst resting but it is more likely to occur during exercise. Pre-existing heart disease is a risk factor for cardiac syncope. Cardiac syncope can cause impairment of consciousness lasting for over 1 minute and decerebrate posturing (tonic extension of the limbs and neck), but is not likely to cause convulsive movements lasting longer than 20 seconds.

5. Alcohol

- Alcohol is an important cause of convulsions. Acute intoxication is a cause of reduced/lost consciousness. Alcohol withdrawal and delirium tremens is a cause of seizures and requires urgent medical treatment. Chronic alcohol overuse predisposes to seizures. Consider referring the patient to an alcohol misuse service as per locally agreed pathways.

6. Driving

- The DVLA has specific and legal regulations regarding convulsions and other causes of lost/altered consciousness. Epileptic seizures and the other conditions mentioned in this guideline are a common medical cause of collapse at the wheel. It is a legal requirement for drivers to inform the DVLA themselves if they have a medical condition that could affect driving.

- When it is appropriate, particularly when discharging a patient who is a driver and not conveying them to a healthcare facility, ambulance clinicians should:
  - advise the patient on the possible impact of their medical condition for safe driving ability.
  - advise the patient on their legal requirement to notify the DVLA about seizures.
  - document any of the above if it is discussed with the patient.

Note that the patient could be fined up to £1,000 if they do not tell the DVLA about a medical condition that affects their driving, and they could be prosecuted if they are involved in an accident as a result.

If an ambulance clinician is concerned that the patient cannot or will not notify the DVLA themselves, it would be appropriate to liaise with the patient's GP and to document these actions.

7. Assessment and Management

Assessment and management of convulsions varies according to whether the convulsion is ongoing/recurrent or has stopped; see Figure 3.10. If the convulsion is ongoing or recurrent, refer to Table 3.40. If the convulsion has stopped, refer to Table 3.41.

Convulsions in Adults

TABLE 3.40 – ASSESSMENT and MANAGEMENT of: ONGOING/RECURRENT Adult Convulsions

General

Assess <C>ABCDE

- Assess for, and simultaneously manage, immediately life-threatening conditions using the <C>ABCDE approach.

Correct Position

- Position the patient for safety and comfort. Protect from dangers, especially aspiration and head injuries, during the convulsion.

History

- Take a focused history while simultaneously managing **<C>ABCDE**. Establish key information from carers/witnesses (if there are any available). The history should be taken from the most appropriate person(s) and at the most appropriate time throughout the assessment/management of the patient. Consider all causes of convulsions, especially potential provoking factors for epileptic seizures. Try to establish:
  - an estimate of the duration of the convulsion.
  - whether the patient already has a diagnosis of epilepsy or PNES (and if there is a history of previous convulsions regardless of formal diagnoses made by doctors).
  - if this is an isolated seizure or if there has been a cluster of seizures.
  - whether any medication has already been administered to terminate the seizure.
  - if there were any symptoms preceding the seizure providing hints to its underlying cause and the need for additional emergency interventions (e.g. treatment of hypoglycaemia, thiamine deficiency, meningitis).
  - if the patient is pregnant and if the gestational age is ≥20 weeks, suspect eclampsia and refer to **Pregnancy-Induced Hypertension (including Eclampsia)** and **Magnesium Sulfate**.
  - relevant past medical history (including diabetes, hypertension, heart disease) and medication use.
  - alcohol intake.
  - potential provoking factors.

Observe/Inspect

- Observe and record types of movements (see Table 3.39).

Airway

Assess and Manage as Appropriate

- Consider an oropharyngeal airway but do not attempt to force an oropharyngeal airway into a convulsing patient if there is trismus or if it is not tolerated. Inability to tolerate an airway adjunct is suggestive of a GCS >3, which is not consistent with a BTCS. A nasopharyngeal airway can be a useful adjunct. Use caution in patients who may have a basal skull fracture or facial injury.

Breathing

Assess Breathing Rate and Quality

- BTCS cause cessation of effective respiration. PNES may involve breath-holding interspersed with periods of hyperventilation. Refer to **Hyperventilation Syndrome** guideline if relevant.

- For BTCSs administer high-concentration oxygen using a reservoir mask at 15 l/min, until a reliable oximetry measurement can be obtained; clinicians should then aim for an oxygen saturation of 94–98% (or 88–92% if the patient is at risk of hypercapnic respiratory failure, e.g. COPD). Refer to **Oxygen**.

- If assessment indicates this convulsion is PNES, then oxygen should **not** normally be administered; measure oxygen saturation and only administer oxygen if it is actually required (SpO_2 of 93% or less).

- In CSE, if pulse oximetry is low and/or end tidal CO_2 is high, and respirations are ineffective, then assist ventilations with a bag-valve-mask device (with suitable airway adjuncts, and supplemental oxygen); this may be difficult during a convulsion (but will be possible if there are pauses between convulsions, or in the post-ictal period).

(continued)

Convulsions in Adults

TABLE 3.40 – ASSESSMENT and MANAGEMENT of: ONGOING/RECURRENT Adult Convulsions *(continued)*

- Administration of medicines for the convulsion should not be delayed, as treating the convulsion can improve ventilation (indeed there is a higher rate of respiratory compromise in status epilepticus where patients are not treated with benzodiazepines than in those who are). Refer to Figure 3.13 and to **Midazolam** and **Diazepam**.

Circulation

Blood Pressure

- Measure BP as soon as possible. Consider eclampsia as a cause of hypertension if the patient is pregnant (gestational age ≥20 weeks). Refer to **Pregnancy-induced Hypertension (including Eclampsia)** and **Magnesium Sulfate**.

Heart Rate and Rhythm

- Monitor heart rate and rhythm. Cardiac dysrhythmia can cause transient loss of consciousness and convulsions (hypoxic seizures). However, sinus tachycardia is normal during epileptic seizures or PNES. Refer to **Cardiac Rhythm Disturbance** if relevant. Record a 12-lead ECG when possible where the diagnosis is unclear. Document your interpretation of the ECG.

- Rarely, epileptic seizures or status epilepticus can trigger abnormal heart rhythms requiring ECG monitoring or even defibrillation.

IV Access

- Assess the need for IV access, taking into account individual circumstances. Consider the possible need for IV administration of emergency drugs, taking into account the choice of drug and the alternative routes of administration.

Disability

Consciousness

- Assess consciousness using AVPU and GCS. Take special care to record how the patient responds to voice and provide an opportunity for the patient to respond by grunting or moving part of a limb (e.g. squeezing the hand of the examiner). Ongoing convulsions in patients who are responsive are likely to be PNES. Refer to Table 3.39.

Blood Glucose Level

- Measure capillary blood glucose and document the result. If glucose is <4 mmol/l, treat according to **Glycaemic Emergencies in Adults and Children**.

Exposure

Temperature

- Measure temperature. A raised temperature may indicate that the patient has an infection. Consider cerebral infections, especially meningococcal meningitis. Refer to **Meningococcal Meningitis and Septicaemia** if this is suspected. Epileptic seizures can cause a rise in body temperature in the absence of infection.

Injuries

- A head injury may be the cause of a convulsion, i.e. a provoked seizure. This may have occurred in the context of a major trauma or RTC. Treat the **Head Injury** and the convulsion in parallel.

- Convulsions may cause injuries. Treat injuries as appropriate. Common minor injuries are facial contusions, dental injuries, joint dislocation and trauma to the tongue and lips. These should be noted even if they do not require immediate treatment because they are important factors for specialists to consider when trying to make a diagnosis in retrospect.

Incontinence

- Urinary incontinence regularly occurs in epileptic seizures and PNESs. It is also reported by patients with vasovagal episodes (rarely). It is not a good discriminator between epileptic seizures and PNESs, but it is an important feature and it should be noted.

Convulsions in Adults

TABLE 3.40 – ASSESSMENT and MANAGEMENT of: ONGOING/RECURRENT Adult Convulsions *(continued)*

Rash

- Look for a non-blanching rash. A purpuric rash and fever is highly predictive of meningococcal infection/meningitis, which can cause seizures (refer to **Meningococcal Meningitis and Septicaemia**).

Pregnancy

- Examine the abdomen of female patients. Is there a palpable uterus that indicates a second/third-trimester pregnancy and the possibility of eclampsia? If so, refer to **Pregnancy-induced Hypertension (including Eclampsia)** and **Magnesium Sulfate**.

Description of the Seizure

- Because of the similarity of PNES to CSE it is important to note and record the characteristics of the convulsions as accurately as possible. This aids assessment and treatment during the convulsion, but it also assists specialists in making the diagnosis in retrospect. For the same reason, families and carers may have been asked by specialists to video-record the events, and they should be encouraged to do so.

Conveyance and Referral

- Most seizures will stop spontaneously. A small proportion will require emergency medical treatment for CSE; many will respond to this treatment and the seizure will terminate. A priority is therefore timely and effective delivery of a dose(s) of a benzodiazepine drug via the optimal route of administration and then appropriate supportive care. A small proportion of patients will not respond to benzodiazepine treatment and will require time-critical transport to hospital. Preparing and transferring the patient for conveyance is therefore a competing priority; decisions about how long to treat at the scene, when to transport and to what extent the treatment and conveyance can happen simultaneously need to be made on a case-by-case basis.
- The following factors should be taken into account:
  - Time since onset of seizure(s).
  - Diagnosis (status epilepticus, PNES, uncertainty).
  - Relative ease or difficulty of extricating the patient to the ambulance.
  - Distance from hospital and transport time.
  - Availability of an effective drug and route of administration.
  - Co-existing acute or chronic medical conditions.

TABLE 3.41 – ASSESSMENT and MANAGEMENT of: STOPPED Adult Convulsions

General

Assess <C>ABCDE

- Assess for, and simultaneously manage, immediately life-threatening conditions using the **<C>ABCDE** approach.
- Most patients will spontaneously make a full recovery after a convulsion. The aim for these patients is to support them as they recover. However, all patients should undergo a careful assessment once their convulsion has stopped to identify the small number with a serious underlying illness as well as those patients who have sustained serious injuries during the seizure.

Correct Position

- Position the patient for comfort and protect from dangers, especially aspiration if the patient remains obtunded. Consider placing in the recovery position.

(continued)

Convulsions in Adults

TABLE 3.41 – ASSESSMENT and MANAGEMENT of: STOPPED Adult Convulsions *(continued)*
■ History
■ Take a focused history, including previous episodes, while simultaneously managing **<C>ABCDE**. After an epileptic seizure, patients are often confused, drowsy and agitated. It can take minutes or hours for them to return to normal consciousness and they are unlikely to be able to give a reliable history immediately after a seizure. After a PNES and syncope, the recovery is usually more rapid. Establish key information from carers/witnesses (if there are any available). The history should be taken from the most appropriate person(s) and at the most appropriate time throughout the assessment/management of the patient. Consider all causes of convulsions, especially potential provoking factors for epileptic seizures. Try to establish: – an estimate of the duration of the seizure.   – whether the patient already has a diagnosis of epilepsy or PNES (and if there is a history of previous convulsions regardless of formal diagnosis).   – if this an isolated seizure or if there has been a cluster of seizures.   – whether any medication has already been administered to terminate the seizure.   – if there were any symptoms preceding the seizure providing hints to its underlying cause/need for additional emergency interventions (e.g. treatment of hypoglycaemia, thiamine deficiency, meningitis).   – if the patient is pregnant and if the gestational age is ≥20 weeks, suspect eclampsia and refer to **Pregnancy-induced Hypertension (including Eclampsia)** and **Magnesium Sulfate**.   – relevant past medical history (including diabetes, hypertension, heart disease) and medication use.   – alcohol intake.   – potential provoking factors.
Airway
Assess and Manage as Appropriate
■ Consider an oropharyngeal or nasopharyngeal airway.
Breathing
Assess Breathing Rate and Quality
■ Respiration usually rapidly returns to normal after cessation of a convulsion.
■ Measure oxygen saturations and only administer oxygen if it is actually required (SpO$_2$ of 93% or less). Refer to **Oxygen**.
■ If assessment indicates this convulsion is PNES, then oxygen should **not** normally be administered.
Circulation
Blood Pressure
■ Measure BP. Consider eclampsia as a cause of hypertension if the patient is pregnant (gestational age ≥20 weeks).
Heart Rate and Rhythm
■ Monitor heart rate and rhythm. Perform a 12-lead ECG if the diagnosis is unclear. Document your interpretation of the ECG. Cardiac arrhythmias are an important cause of transient loss of consciousness and suspected seizures, so an ECG is an important part of the assessment of a patient after a convulsion.
IV Access
■ Assess the risk of another convulsion and the potential need for IV access, taking into account individual circumstances. Consider the possible need for IV administration of emergency drugs, taking into account the choice of drug and the alternative routes of administration.
Disability

Convulsions in Adults

TABLE 3.41 – ASSESSMENT and MANAGEMENT of: STOPPED Adult Convulsions *(continued)*

Consciousness

- Assess consciousness using AVPU and GCS. If improving, wait 10 minutes and repeat. Take special care to record how the patient responds to voice, and provide an opportunity for the patient to respond by grunting or moving part of a limb (e.g. squeezing the hand of the examiner). Refer to Table 3.39.

- After an epileptic seizure, patients are often left confused, tired and aching (this is the post-ictal state). The confusion usually resolves relatively rapidly, leaving the patient alert with a GCS of 15/15. Tiredness, aching and amnesia may persist longer than this, but it is not a cause for concern.

Blood Glucose Level

- Measure capillary blood glucose and document the result. If glucose is <4 mmol/l, treat according to **Glycaemic Emergencies in Adults and Children**.

Exposure

Temperature

- Measure temperature. A raised temperature may indicate that the patient has an infection. Consider cerebral infections, especially meningococcal meningitis. Refer to **Meningococcal Meningitis and Septicaemia** if this is suspected. Epileptic seizures can also lead to a temporary rise in body temperature in the absence of infection.

Injuries

- Treat injuries as appropriate.

- A head injury may be the cause of a convulsion, i.e. a provoked seizure. This may have occurred in the context of a major trauma or RTC. Treat the head injury and the convulsion in parallel.

- Convulsions may cause injuries. Common minor injuries are facial contusions, dental injuries, joint dislocation and trauma to the tongue from biting. These should be noted even if they do not require immediate treatment because they are important factors for specialists to consider when trying to make a diagnosis in retrospect.

Incontinence

- Urinary incontinence regularly occurs in epileptic seizures and PNES. It is also reported by patients with vasovagal episodes (rarely). It is not a good discriminator between epileptic seizures and PNES, but it is an important feature and it should be noted.

Rash

- Look for a non-blanching rash. A purpuric rash and fever is highly predictive of meningococcal infection/meningitis, which can cause seizures. Refer to **Meningococcal Meningitis and Septicaemia**.

Pregnancy

- Examine the abdomen of female patients. Is there a palpable uterus that indicates a second/third-trimester pregnancy and the possibility of eclampsia? If so, refer to **Pregnancy-induced Hypertension (including Eclampsia)** and **Magnesium Sulfate**.

Description of the Seizure

- An accurate assessment, including a detailed description of events, is very important during and after a convulsion. Based on witness accounts and the events that you witnessed, write a detailed account of the events.

Conveyance and Referral

- All patients with a first seizure must be conveyed to hospital.

- The decision whether to convey a patient to hospital after a convulsion is difficult. The overall risk of adverse events is low, and most patients do not require the facilities of a hospital emergency department. But it is important to accurately identify those patients who do need transport to hospital. The following factors should be considered when making this decision:
  - Single or serial convulsions.
  - Known seizure disorder.
  - Extent of neurological recovery.
  - Level of support/supervision. Availability of suitable care pathways.

(continued)

Convulsions in Adults

- – Care plan.
- – Injuries.
- – Treatment with benzodiazepines (these patients should always be transported to hospital unless their care plan states otherwise).
- – Comorbidities including frailty.
- – The patient's wishes, assuming that they have mental capacity. Refer to **Mental Capacity Act 2005**.
- – Refer to **Pregnancy-induced Hypertension (including Eclampsia)**.
- ■ For patients who are not conveyed:
  - – Document the justification for the decision not to convey.
  - – Advise them to make an appointment with their epilepsy specialist or GP to discuss the events and provide them with a copy of the PRF if possible.
  - – Use an alternative care pathway if one is available, for example referral to an epilepsy specialist nurse team.
  - – Advise patients/carers to dial 999 if there are further convulsions.
  - – Provide written advice if possible or leave a relevant patient information leaflet.
  - – Advise the patient about driving and DVLA regulations.

8. Emergency Medical Treatment

First-dose benzodiazepines

Refer to **Midazolam** and **Diazepam**.

Other doses of benzodiazepines previously administered during this episode of care, for example by carers, should be considered and subtracted from the maximum cumulative dose unless there was clear evidence it was not absorbed.

Midazolam

- ■ If buccal midazolam is immediately available, use this (do not use PR diazepam or delay administration by attempting IV access).
- ■ Ambulance clinicians can administer the patient's own buccal midazolam provided they are competent to administer buccal medications and are familiar with midazolam's indications, actions and side effects, which are very similar to diazepam although midazolam is shorter acting.
- ■ Midazolam is probably more effective than diazepam.

Diazepam

- ■ If no midazolam is available, and IV access is unlikely to be obtained quickly, administer PR diazepam.
- ■ If IV access has previously been achieved, IV diazepam can be given instead.

After the 1st dose

- ■ Convulsive status epilepticus is an emergency, and can cause permanent brain damage or even death. If IV access is difficult then IO access (where available) should be used.
- ■ The aim should be to have IV access within 10 minutes of the first dose.

Second-dose benzodiazepines

- ■ If the convulsion is continuing **10 minutes** after the first benzodiazepine has been given, a dose of IV diazepam should be administered.
- ■ Only if IV or IO access has proved impossible should the second dose be given buccally (midazolam) or per rectum (PR) (diazepam).
- ■ Do not delay the second dose.
- ■ If the convulsion continues 10 minutes after the second dose, then seek senior clinical advice to consider:
  - – alternative diagnoses, including PNES.
  - – reasons for lack of effect, such as poor administration/absorption, patient size or inadequate dose.
  - – any access to alternative second-line anti-convulsant.
  - – the risks/benefits of a third dose of benzodiazepine. The risk of side effects increases with the number of doses and the effectiveness of the drug decreases over the duration of the convulsion.
- ■ Consider asking for senior clinical advice from a prescriber to consider a third dose of IV/IO benzodiazepine, if no alternative anticonvulsant available and the patient is still another 15 minutes or more from hospital, i.e. a total of 25 minutes from the end of last dose.
- ■ After prolonged convulsions or drug treatment, prepare for airway obstruction, respiratory depression, hypotension and cardiac arrhythmia, particularly if they have also received opiates, additional benzodiazepines or alternative central nervous system depressants.

Convulsions in Adults

CONVULSION(S) ONGOING OR RECURRENT

Refer to **Glycaemic Emergencies, Pregnancy Induced Hypertension, Cardiac Rhythm Disturbance, Hyperventilation Syndrome, Meningococcal Meningitis and Septicaemia, Altered Level of Consciousness, Overdose and Poisoning** and **Head Injury**

Continue to assess **<C>ABCDE**
Consider/treat cause:
hypoxia, hypoglycaemia (check blood glucose), epilepsy, PNES, eclampsia or convulsion provoked by: head injury, stroke, alcohol, drug overdose or infection
(refer to Table 3.39)

Impression:
Bilateral Tonic-Clonic Seizure (BTCS)

Impression:
Psychogenic Non-Epileptic Seizure (PNES)

Duration under 5 minutes

Duration 5 minutes or more **or** 3 or more convulsions in an hour, and **still convulsing**
STATUS EPILEPTICUS

Follow individualised treatment plan if available, otherwise follow algorithm

Follow individualised treatment plan if available, otherwise follow algorithm

Follow individualised treatment plan if available, otherwise follow algorithm

- Position for comfort
- Protect from harm
- Further treatment usually not required

Administer **1st benzodiazepine (consider drugs already administered)**

- Position for comfort
- Protect from harm
- Reassure patient & carers (assume the patient can hear)
- Attempt to communicate
- Oxygen **not** usually indicated (SpO₂)
- Do **not** give anti-convulsive drugs
- Consider family video recording
- Manage any hyperventilation

If no midazolam and IV access is unlikely to be obtained quickly, administer PR diazepam

1st DOSE BENZODIAZEPINE
(refer to midazolam/diazepam guideline)
No IV access:
Midazolam Buccal 10mg
or
Diazepam PR 20mg (10mg if 70 yrs and older)
or
IV access:
Diazepam IV 10mg (over 2 mins)

Use Buccal midazolam if available (do not use PR diazepam or delay administration of the first dose by attempting to obtain IV access if Buccal midazolam is available)

Attempt IV/IO access (if not already gained)

If still convulsing 10 minutes after 1st dose completed

2nd DOSE BENZODIAZEPINE
(refer to midazolam/diazepam guideline)
No IV/IO access:
Midazolam Buccal 10mg
or
Diazepam PR 10mg
IV/IO access:
Diazepam 10mg (over 2 mins)

Only give 2nd dose midazolam Buccal or diazepam PR if **NO IV/IO access possible**

After prolonged convulsions or drug treatment prepare for: respiratory depression, hypotension and/or cardiac arrhythmia

If still convulsing 10 minutes after 2nd dose benzodiazepine:
Seek senior clinical advice to consider diagnosis (is this a PNES?), and risk/benefit of 3rd dose IV/IO benzodiazepine (en-route) if **no** alternative anticonvulsant available **and** still another 15 minutes or more from hospital (i.e. total 25 minutes from end of last dose)

Figure 3.11 – Emergency medical treatment algorithm for adult convulsions: ongoing or recurrent.

Convulsions in Adults

KEY POINTS!

Convulsions in Adults

- Psychogenic non-epileptic seizures (PNES) are the most important differential diagnosis of epileptic convulsions.

- Most bilateral tonic-clonic seizures (BTCS) are self-limiting and do not require drug treatment.

- All patients with a first seizure should be conveyed to hospital.

- Diazepam is only indicated for patients with ongoing convulsions: patients who have prolonged convulsions (lasting 5 minutes or more), OR repeated convulsions (three or more in an hour), and who are CURRENTLY CONVULSING – not secondary to an uncorrected hypoxic or hypoglycaemic episode.

- Consider referral to an epilepsy specialist nurse team or an alternative care pathway for patients who are not conveyed.

- If the patient is pregnant and gestational age is ≥20 weeks, suspect eclampsia and refer to Pregnancy-induced Hypertension (including Eclampsia) and Magnesium Sulfate.

Bibliography

1. Falco-Walter JJ, Bleck T. Treatment of established status epilepticus. *Journal of Clinical Medicine* 2016, 5(5): 49.

2. Meierkord H, Boon P, Engelsen B, Göcke K, Shorvon S, Tinuper P, Holtkamp M, European Federation of Neurological Societies. EFNS guideline on the management of status epilepticus in adults. *European Journal of Neurology* 2010, 17(3): 348–355.

Convulsions in Children

1. Introduction

- Convulsions (also called 'tonic-clonic seizures' or 'fits') arise from abnormal electrical activity in the brain. They are usually **generalised** (affecting both sides of the body), but may also be **focal**, affecting just one side of the body. Fever is the commonest cause for convulsions (febrile convulsions) but they can also be caused by epilepsy, CNS infections (meningitis or encephalitis), hypoglycaemia, hypoxia, electrolyte imbalances, head injuries or (rarely) hypertension. Occasionally, cardiac arrest can be the presenting feature of an initial convulsion.

- Most convulsions stop within 4 minutes (>90%). After 5 minutes, a convulsion is unlikely to stop spontaneously. Prolonged fits become harder to stop with anticonvulsants. As a consequence, if a convulsion has not stopped within 5 minutes of its start, emergency (rescue) medication should be given.

- During febrile illnesses, small children (aged 6 months to 5 years) may develop febrile convulsions. These are not epilepsy. They can be seen in up to 1 in 20 children.

- A child having convulsions that are not triggered by fever requires further investigation.

2. Incidence

- 1 in 200 people have active epilepsy.

- It is twice as common in children as in adults.

- It can be related to another underlying condition such as cerebral palsy or a genetic disorder.

- Both meningitis and encephalitis cause fever and may cause convulsions (although these would not normally be classed as febrile convulsions).

3. Severity and Outcome

3.1 Febrile Convulsions

- 66% of children only ever have one febrile convulsion; the remainder may have further episodes during subsequent infections.

- 5% of children with febrile convulsions go on to develop epilepsy.

3.2 Convulsive Status Epilepticus (CSE)

- Convulsive status epilepticus (CSE) is the most common neurological emergency in children.

- 1 in 20 febrile convulsions present with CSE.

- 1 in 20 epileptic children have CSE (more common in children with Dravet syndrome and Lennox-Gastaut syndrome).

- A bilateral tonic clonic seizure (BTCS) that has not stopped after 5 minutes, or a series of such seizures without recovery in between which lasts for 5 minutes or more, is defined as CSE.

- Prolonged convulsions (45–60 minutes or more) can result in death (observed mortality rate: 4%). They can also cause serious and irreversible consequences such as stroke, learning difficulties, visual impairment, behavioural problems and epilepsy. Adverse outcomes are more common in young children (less than 5 years of age).

4. Assessment

(Refer to Table 3.42)

- Correct hypoxia and seek an underlying cause for the seizure. Ensure the child is not hypoglycaemic.

- Document if the child was unwell or feverish before the convulsion, any serious past medical history and any important events immediately preceding the convulsion (e.g. head injury).

- When managing a febrile convulsion, it is not sufficient to simply manage the convulsion. It is vitally important to seek and identify the underlying infection producing the child's fever, especially if managing in the community (although this should not delay immediate treatment priorities or hospital transport).

- Seizures are a feature of meningitis – if the seizure has stopped and the child's condition permits, look for clinical signs (e.g. the typical rash of meningococcal septicaemia (and treat when present)).

- Establishing that a convulsion has fully stopped can be difficult. Following a tonic-clonic convulsion, the repeated, regular, rhythmic jerks of the limbs (the clonic phase of the seizure) become less frequent and eventually stop. In the following minutes, the child may show some or all of the following post-ictal ('post-convulsion') features:
  - brief and irregular jerks of one or more limbs
  - eye deviation
  - nystagmus (jerky eye movements to one side and then back to the midline)
  - noisy breathing.

- Since these features do not **necessarily** mean the child is still convulsing, additional emergency (rescue) medication (benzodiazepines) should not be given.

- Even when the above features are found to be part of an ongoing seizure, they are not thought to be harmful.

- Conversely, further doses of benzodiazepines can cause significant respiratory depression and respiratory arrest. When uncertain, do not give further benzodiazepines but transfer the child rapidly to hospital, for further assessment and ongoing treatment.

Convulsions in Children

5. Management

(Refer to Table 3.42 and Figures 3.12 and 3.13)

- This follows <C>ABCDE priorities, treating the convulsion once ABC issues have been addressed.

- Manage airway, breathing and circulation as usual (also remember to measure the blood glucose, as hypoglycaemia can cause seizures). An oropharyngeal airway may be helpful to maintain airway patency (alternatively, if the jaw is clenched a nasopharyngeal airway may prove useful). Administer oxygen and treat shock in the usual way. Oxygen saturation monitoring and capnography (if available) should be applied.

- Children with epilepsy in the UK now carry individualised 'Epilepsy Passports', containing essential information about their epilepsy, their emergency care plan and key professional contacts. These should be located, where possible, without delaying treatment.

- Most convulsions stop spontaneously (within 4 minutes).

- Anticonvulsant treatment should be given if the convulsion **has lasted 5 minutes or more or if the child has had three or more focal or generalised convulsions in an hour**. Pre-hospital treatments include **buccal midazolam** and **diazepam** (both rectal and intravenous preparations). Buccal midazolam is more effective than rectal diazepam but often diazepam is the only drug available. Both drugs may cause respiratory depression although this is uncommon.

- Do not delay the first dose of anticonvulsant medication whilst attempting venous access, for example use buccal or rectal routes.

- Before administration, ensure that the appropriate anticonvulsant dose for the child's weight and age is chosen, giving the **full** dose at the appropriate times. It is **not** appropriate to either i) gradually 'titrate the dose upwards' or ii) only give a partial dose if the convulsion stops (even if the seizure has stopped, that full dose must be given). If this approach is followed, seizure recurrence is much less likely.

- A focal convulsion lasting longer than 5 minutes should be managed and treated in the same way as a generalised convulsion.

- If the convulsion is continuing 10 minutes after the first dose of medication has been given, a second dose of anticonvulsant can be given. Ideally, this should be given intravenously or intra-osseously e.g. **diazepam** IV/IO (refer to **Diazepam**) but if this is not possible a second dose can be given buccally or rectally. (This also applies if a carer has given the first dose of medication before the clinician arrives on scene.)

- In very rare cases, a child may continue in CSE 10 minutes after a second full dose of benzodiazepine. If at that point in time the hospital is still over 15 minutes away (total 25 minutes after the second dose), then seek clinical advice to consider a third dose of benzodiazepine. This must only be intravenous or intra-osseous.*

* Be ready to support ventilation, as respiratory depression may occur.

- Children may sometimes experience brief (i.e. <5-minute) repeated or 'serial' convulsions. Such children should be given an anticonvulsant if they have experienced three convulsions in an hour.

5.1 Hospital transfer

- Often it is safest to treat the convulsion before moving the child, although if the seizure has not stopped after one dose of anticonvulsant the child will have to be transferred while still convulsing.

- Pre-alert the hospital if the child continues to fit during the journey or appears to be otherwise very unwell.

- All children having their first convulsion should be transported to hospital for investigation.

- If the child has fully recovered and is a known epileptic, it may not be necessary to take them to hospital.

TABLE 3.42 – ASSESSMENT and MANAGEMENT of: Convulsions in Children

Assess <C>ABCD

Treat problems as they are found.

- The airway must be cleared – oropharyngeal or nasopharyngeal airways may be helpful.
- Administer high levels of supplemental oxygen (refer to **Oxygen**).
- Assist ventilations with a BVM if necessary.
- Check blood glucose level, and manage if low (refer to **Glycaemic Emergencies in Adults and Children**).
- Monitor vital signs.
- Manage the convulsion (see below).

Convulsions in Children

Medication

- Administer an anticonvulsant. The first choice anticonvulsant is usually given buccally (midazolam) or rectally (diazepam):

i. if the first convulsion lasts ≥5 minutes or

ii. if the child has another convulsion that lasts ≥5 minutes within 10 minutes of the end of the first convulsion or

iii. if the child continues to have brief (<5-minute) convulsions and has had three of these in a hour or has not regained consciousness between each convulsion.

Ask whether the child has their own supply of medication.

- If the child **has** their own supply of medication:
  - if the child has their own buccal midazolam this should be used.
  - ask whether they have already received a dose; if not, administer the patient's own buccal midazolam.*

- If the child does **not** have their own buccal midazolam medication:
  - (and they have not yet received an anticonvulsant) give **buccal midazolam** (if carried) or (if midazolam is not available) **rectal diazepam** (refer to **Midazolam/Diazepam**).*

- If the child **has already received an anticonvulsant** (e.g. rectal **diazepam** or buccal **midazolam**):
  - If the convulsion is continuing **10 minutes** after this first anticonvulsant, one dose of an intravenous or intra-osseous anticonvulsant should be given, e.g. **diazepam** IV/IO (refer to **Diazepam**).

- If it is not possible to gain intravenous or intra-osseous access for the second dose of medication, the child **should** be given another full dose of buccal or rectal medication, as continuing convulsive activity is more dangerous than the risk of side effects e.g. respiratory depression.

- In very rare cases, a child may continue in convulsive status epilepticus 10 minutes after a second full dose of benzodiazepine. If at that point in time the hospital is still over 15 minutes away (total 25 minutes after the second dose), then seek clinical advice to consider a third dose of benzodiazepine. This must only be intravenous or intra-osseous.*

* Be ready to support ventilation, as respiratory depression may occur.

Other Care

- Record the child's temperature.

- If transporting to hospital, ongoing assessments of ABCDEs and continuous ECG and oxygen saturation monitoring (and $EtCO_2$ if available) should be undertaken, continuing **oxygen** therapy as needed.

- If meningococcal septicaemia is diagnosed, treat with **benzylpenicillin** en-route to hospital (refer to **Benzylpenicillin Sodium**).

- A child who has suffered a seizure and has a fever is likely to be distressed, therefore Paracetamol should be considered (refer to **Paracetamol**).

- A febrile child should wear light clothing only. If the child begins to shiver (e.g. after stripping off all layers down to a nappy), this will potentially raise core temperature and will be counterproductive.

Transfer to Further Care

The following should all be transported to hospital:

- Any child who is still convulsing or in status epilepticus must be transferred to further care as soon as possible, preferably after the first dose of anticonvulsant – undertake a **TIME-CRITICAL** transfer, provide an alert/information call.

- Any child with suspected meningococcal septicaemia or meningitis – undertake a **TIME-CRITICAL** transfer, provide an alert/information call.

- All first febrile convulsions, even if the child has recovered.

- All children with seizures who have required more than one dose of anticonvulsant.

- Any child two years old or less who has had a seizure (even if totally recovered).

(continued)

SECTION 3 Medical Emergencies

Convulsions in Children

TABLE 3.42 – ASSESSMENT and MANAGEMENT of: Convulsions in Children *(continued)*

- Any child who has not fully recovered from their seizure. The following children may not require transport to hospital:
- Children following a febrile convulsion:
  - that is **not their first** and
  - **who have completely recovered** and
  - **where the carer is happy for the child not to be transported**

  may be left at home, providing that urgent review by the general practitioner (GP) or out-of-hours (OOH) GP is arranged to establish the cause of the fever. If this cannot be arranged by the attending crew, the child must be transported to hospital.

- Children who have recovered from a convulsion, are known to have epilepsy, have followed their normal pattern and have not required more than one dose of medication do not need to be transported if they are otherwise well and this is consistent with their care plan. A responsible adult must be with the child.

Convulsions in Children

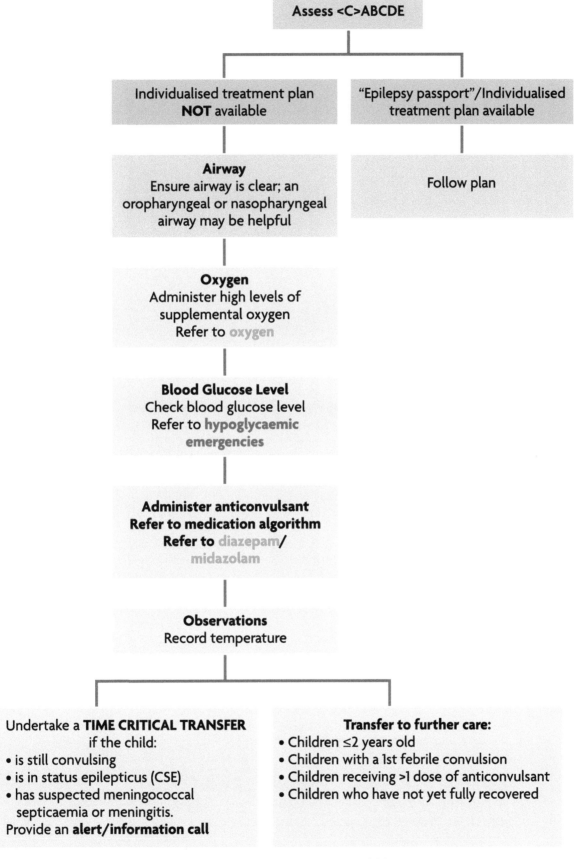

Assess <C>ABCDE

Individualised treatment plan NOT available

"Epilepsy passport"/Individualised treatment plan available

Airway
Ensure airway is clear; an oropharyngeal or nasopharyngeal airway may be helpful

Follow plan

Oxygen
Administer high levels of supplemental oxygen
Refer to oxygen

Blood Glucose Level
Check blood glucose level
Refer to **hypoglycaemic emergencies**

Administer anticonvulsant
Refer to medication algorithm
Refer to diazepam/ midazolam

Observations
Record temperature

Undertake a **TIME CRITICAL TRANSFER** if the child:
• is still convulsing
• is in status epilepticus (CSE)
• has suspected meningococcal septicaemia or meningitis.
Provide an **alert/information call**

Transfer to further care:
• Children ≤2 years old
• Children with a 1st febrile convulsion
• Children receiving >1 dose of anticonvulsant
• Children who have not yet fully recovered

Figure 3.12 – Assessment and management algorithm of convulsions in children.

Convulsions in Children

Figure 3.13 – Medication algorithm for convulsions in children.

Convulsions in Children

KEY POINTS!

Convulsions in Children

- Prolonged convulsions, called convulsive status epilepticus (CSE), are a medical emergency and may result in death or serious neurological impairments.

- Febrile convulsions are a very common cause for a childhood convulsion and occur between the ages of 6 months and 5 years.

- Most convulsions stop spontaneously within 4 minutes.

- A convulsion lasting 5 minutes (or more) should be treated with anticonvulsants.

- Buccal midazolam is the most widely available rescue medication used in childhood epilepsy.

- First-choice anticonvulsants are usually given buccally or rectally, with buccal midazolam being the preferred treatment option.

- Wherever possible, the second dose of anticonvulsant should always be given intravenously (e.g. diazepam).

- The full dose for the child's age must be given when treating a convulsion.

- A child should not usually receive more than two doses of pre-hospital anticonvulsant.

- Always consider (and actively seek) the underlying cause for the convulsion.

- All first convulsions must be transported to hospital.

Bibliography

1. National Institute for Health and Clinical Excellence. *The Epilepsies: The diagnosis and management of the epilepsies in adults and children in primary and secondary care* (CG137). London: NICE, 2012. Available from: https://nice.org.uk/guidance/CG137.

2. Woollard M, Pitt K. Antipyretic pre-hospital therapy for febrile convulsions: does the treatment fit? A literature review. *Health Education* 2003, 62(1): 23–28.

3. Yoong M, Chin RFM, Scott RC. Management of convulsive status epilepticus in children. *Archives of Disease in Childhood Education and Practice Edition* 2009, 94(1): 1–9.

4. The Status Epilepticus Working Party, Appleton R, Choonara I, Martland T, Phillips B, Scott R, et al. The treatment of convulsive status epilepticus in children. *Archives of Disease in Childhood* 2000, 83(5): 415–419.

5. Sadleir LG, Scheffer IE. Febrile seizures. *British Medical Journal* 2007, 334(7588): 307–311.

6. Baysun S, Aydin ÖF, Atmaca E, Gürer YKY. A comparison of buccal midazolam and rectal diazepam for the acute treatment of seizures. *Clinical Pediatrics* 2005, 44(9): 771–776.

7. Sadleir LG, Scheffer IE. Febrile seizures. *British Medical Journal* 2007, 334(7588): 307–311.

SECTION **3** Medical Emergencies

Dyspnoea

1. Introduction

- Dyspnoea is defined as 'a subjective experience of breathing discomfort that consists of qualitatively distinct sensations that vary in intensity'.

- Dyspnoea is an important clinical symptom that may indicate underlying pathology for a large range of conditions (refer to Table 3.43), particularly those affecting the respiratory and cardiac systems.

- Acute episodes of dyspnoea often have a pulmonary or cardiac cause. Asthma, cardiogenic pulmonary oedema, chronic obstructive pulmonary disease (COPD), pneumonia, cardiac ischaemia, and interstitial lung disease are common causes and account for approximately 85% of all ED cases of dyspnoea. In 15% of cases dyspnoea is unexplained.

TABLE 3.43 – Causes of Dyspnoea

Pulmonary causes	Cardiac causes	Other causes
Acute exacerbation of asthma.	Acute heart failure.	Anaphylaxis.
Bronchiectasis.	Cardiac arrhythmia.	Chemicals/poisons.
Acute exacerbation of COPD.	Cardiac tamponade.	Diabetic ketoacidosis.
Flail chest.	Ischaemic heart disease.	Diaphragmatic splinting.
Interstitial lung disease.	Myocardial infarction.	Hyperventilation.
Lung/lobar collapse.	Valvular dysfunction.	Panic attack/anxiety.
Massive haemothorax.	Pericarditis.	Severe hypovolaemia.
Pleural effusion.		Metabolic causes.
Pneumonia.		Obesity.
Pneumothorax.		Pain.
Pulmonary embolism.		Severe anaemia.
Upper airway obstruction.		End of life.
		Carbon monoxide exposure.

2. Severity and Outcome

- Dyspnoea is an important clinical symptom which in some circumstances can be severe or life-threatening. Dyspnoea varies in intensity and can be a distressing symptom, especially for patients at the end of life. **For details of the severity and outcome for specific conditions refer to individual guidelines.**

3. Pathophysiology

- Dyspnoea is a multi-dimensional process involving physiological and psychological systems. Table 3.44 details symptoms, signs and history associated with the potential causes of dyspnoea.

- The respiratory system is designed to match alveolar ventilation with metabolic demand. Disruption of this process may lead to the conscious awareness of breathing and dyspnoea. Dyspnoea is an uncomfortable sensation and may include chest tightness, air hunger, effortful breathing, the urge to cough and a sense of suffocation.

4. Assessment and Management

- Diagnosis of the underlying cause of the patient's presenting illness can be difficult, and may require in-hospital investigations. Assessment must include a detailed history and a thorough physical examination. For the assessment and management of patients with dyspnoea refer to Table 3.45.

TABLE 3.44 – Differential Diagnosis for Common Conditions

Condition	Symptoms	Signs	Auscultation or audible sounds	History
Acute exacerbation of asthma Refer to **Asthma in Adults and Children**	Dyspnoea Cough Unable to complete sentences	Wheeze Tachypnoea Tachycardia Pulsus paradoxus Hyperresonant chest Accessory muscle use	Decreased or absent breath sounds if severe Wheeze	Previous asthma Recent increase in inhaler use Allergen exposure

Dyspnoea

	TABLE 3.44 – Differential Diagnosis for Common Conditions *(continued)*			
Condition	**Symptoms**	**Signs**	**Auscultation or audible sounds**	**History**
Acute Coronary Syndrome, for example, STEMI or NSTEMI Refer to **Acute Coronary Syndrome**	Central chest pain for >15 minutes, constricting or crushing that radiates to arm/neck	Tachycardia Arrhythmia	Wheeze Crackles	Symptoms suggestive of ischaemic heart disease (IHD) or previous investigations for chest pain
Acute Heart Failure Refer to **Heart Failure**	Dyspnoea especially on exertion Orthopnoea/paroxysmal nocturnal dyspnoea Cough producing frothy, white or pink phlegm	Peripheral oedema Tachycardia	Rales Heart murmur Crepitations	Angina Hypertension History of heart failure, for example, left ventricular failure, right ventricular failure or cor pulmonale Valvular dysfunction or congenital heart problems
Anaphylaxis Refer to **Allergic Reactions including Anaphylaxis**	Dyspnoea Dysphagia Chest tightness	Tachycardia Tachypnoea Erythema Urticaria Angioedema Pharyngeal or laryngeal oedema	Decreased breath sounds Wheeze Stridor	Allergen exposure
Chronic Obstructive Pulmonary Disease (COPD) Refer to **Chronic Obstructive Pulmonary Disease**	Progressive dyspnoea Chest tightness Cough – purulent sputum	New-onset cyanosis Peripheral oedema Accessory muscle use Pursed lip breathing	Rales Wheeze	Smoking >35 years of age
End of life dyspnoea Refer to **End of Life Care**	Dyspnoea	Tachypnoea	Decreased breath sounds	Long term respiratory conditions such as COPD
Foreign Body Airway Obstruction (FBAO) Refer to **Foreign Body Airway Obstruction**	Dyspnoea Inability to speak Cough	Clutching at neck New-onset cyanosis	Stridor Wheeze	Eating – especially fish, meat, or poultry Illicit drug ingestion or substance misuse

(continued)

Dyspnoea

TABLE 3.44 – Differential Diagnosis for Common Conditions (continued)

Condition	Symptoms	Signs	Auscultation or audible sounds	History
Hyperventilation Refer to **Hyperventilation Syndrome**	Dyspnoea Acute agitation and anxiety Chest pain which may resemble angina pectoris Palpitations	Sudden dyspnoea Hyperpnoea Tachypnoea Numbness and tingling in the limbs and around the mouth		**NB** ensure other more serious conditions are excluded before considering this diagnosis
Pneumonia Refer to **Medical Emergencies in Adults – Overview** and **Medical Emergencies in Children – Overview**	Dyspnoea Fever Cough	Tachycardia	Rhonchi	Smoking IHD
Pneumothorax Rrefer to **Thoracic Trauma**	Dyspnoea Sudden onset pleuritic chest pain	Dyspnoea	Decreased breath sounds	Trauma Previous pneumothorax COPD Asthma Smoking Tall, thin stature
Pulmonary Embolism Refer to **Pulmonary Embolism**	Dyspnoea Pleuritic chest pain Cough or haemoptysis Possible DVT Leg oedema Syncope Fever	Tachycardia Tachypnoea Fever ECG: Non-specific ST wave changes Hypotension	Focal rales Crepitations	Prolonged immobilisation Recent surgery Thrombotic disease Active cancer

TABLE 3.45 – ASSESSMENT and MANAGEMENT of: Dyspnoea

NB Take a defibrillator at the earliest opportunity and keep this with the patient until handover.

Assess <C>ABCD

- If any of the following **TIME-CRITICAL** features present:
  - major **<C>ABCD** problems, refer to **Medical Emergencies in Adults – Overview** and **Medical Emergencies in Children – Overview**
  - extreme airway/breathing difficulty or cyanosis, refer to **Airway and Breathing Management**
  - features of life-threatening asthma, refer to **Asthma in Adults and Children**
  - features of tension pneumothorax or major chest trauma, refer to **Thoracic Trauma**
  - acute myocardial infarction, refer to **Acute Coronary Syndrome**
  - anaphylaxis, refer to **Allergic Reactions including Anaphylaxis**
  - foreign body airway obstruction, refer to **Foreign Body Airway Obstruction**
  - loss of consciousness, refer to **Altered Level of Consciousness**, then:

Dyspnoea

TABLE 3.45 – ASSESSMENT and MANAGEMENT of: Dyspnoea *(continued)*
▪ Start correcting **<C>ABCD** problems
▪ Undertake a **TIME-CRITICAL** transfer to the nearest receiving hospital.
▪ Continue patient management en-route.
▪ Provide an ATMIST information call.
Position
▪ Position the patient for comfort, usually sitting upright.
Ask the Patient If They Have an Individualised Treatment Plan
▪ Be aware that the patient may have a treatment plan or care plan.
▪ Patients with long term conditions will often be able to guide their care and have a care plan, ReSPECT form or DNACPR form in place.
If the patient is not TIME-CRITICAL
▪ Obtain a thorough history to help identify the cause of dyspnoea.
Specifically assess:
▪ Effort and effectiveness of ventilation – rate and depth.
▪ Medical Research Council (MRC) Dyspnoea Scale.
▪ Duration of difficulty breathing – sudden or gradual onset?
▪ Pain associated with breathing – any pattern of breathing/depth of respiration?
▪ Do certain positions exacerbate breathing (e.g. unable to lie down, must sit upright)?
▪ Does the patient have a cough?
▪ If yes, is the cough productive: – **sputum or bubbling**: consider infection or heart failure   – **frothy white/pink sputum**: consider acute heart failure   – **yellow/green sputum**: consider chest infection   – **haemoptysis**: consider PE, chest infection or carcinoma of the lung.
▪ Has the patient increased their medication recently?
▪ Signs of anaphylaxis: – Urticarial rash   – facial swelling   – circulatory collapse.
Percuss the Chest
To determine if there are collections of fluid in the lungs.
Auscultate the Chest
To determine adequacy of air entry on both sides of the chest.
To determine chest sounds: – audible wheeze on expiration – consider asthma, ACS, anaphylaxis, COPD or heart failure (especially in older patients with no history of asthma)   – audible stridor (upper airway narrowing) – consider anaphylaxis, or FBAO   – crepitations (fine crackling in lung bases) – ACS, heart failure   – rhonchi (harsher, rattling sound) indicating collections of fluid in larger airways – pneumonia.   – rales (clicking, rattling or crackling noises) – heart failure, COPD, pulmonary embolism
Consider Possible Causes Table 3.43 Table 3.44
▪ Refer to Table 3.43 and Table 3.44.
Known cause
▪ If the cause of dyspnoea is known follow relevant guideline, as per Table 3.44.

(continued)

SECTION **3** Medical Emergencies

Dyspnoea

TABLE 3.45 – ASSESSMENT and MANAGEMENT of: Dyspnoea *(continued)*

Unknown cause

- If cause of dyspnoea unknown refer to **Medical Emergencies in Adults – Overview** and **Medical Emergencies in Children – Overview** and follow management below.

Ventilation

Consider assisted ventilation at a rate of 12–20 breaths per minute if:

- SpO_2 is <90% on high concentration O_2.
- Respiratory rate is 30.
- Expansion is inadequate, refer to **Airway and Breathing Management**.

Fluid

- Administer fluid as required, refer to **Intravascular Fluid Therapy in Adults** and **Intravascular Fluid Therapy in Children**.

Pain Management

- Administer pain relief if indicated, refer to **Pain Management in Adults** and **Pain Management in Children**.

Transfer to Further Care

- All patients with an unexplained cause of dyspnoea.
- Where the cause is known refer to the releant guideline for care pathway.

TABLE 3.46 – MRC Dyspnoea Scale

Grade 1	Breathless only with strenuous exercise
Grade 2	Short of breath when hurrying on the level or up a slight hill
Grade 3	Slower than most people of the same age on a level surface OR Have to stop when walking at my own pace on the level
Grade 4	Stop for breath walking 100 meters OR After a walking few minutes at my own pace on the level
Grade 5	Too breathless to leave the house

Used with the permission of the Medical Research Council

KEY POINTS!

Dyspnoea

- **Is dyspnoea a result of respiratory, cardiac, both or other causes?**
- **Consider time-critical causes.**
- **Assess degree of dyspnoea and response to treatment.**
- **Consider possible causes and refer to relevant guidelines for assessment and management.**

Bibliography

1. Lansing RW, Gracely RH, Banzett RB. The multiple dimensions of dyspnea: review and hypotheses. *Respiratory Physiology and Neurobiology* 2009, 167(1): 53–60.

2. Nardi AE, Freire RC, Zin WA. Panic disorder and control of breathing. *Respiratory Physiology and Neurobiology* 2009, 167(1): 133–143.

3. Peiffer C. Dyspnea relief: more than just the perception of a decrease in dyspnea. *Respiratory Physiology and Neurobiology* 2009, 167(1): 61–71.

4. Parshall MB, Schwartzstein RM, Adams L, Banzett RB, Manning HL, Bourbeau J, et al. An official American Thoracic Society statement: update on the mechanisms, assessment, and management of dyspnea. *American*

Dyspnoea

Journal of Respiratory and Critical Care Medicine 2012, 185(4): 435–452.

5.   Michelson E, Hollrah S. Evaluation of the patient with shortness of breath: an evidence based approach. *Emergency Medicine Clinics of North America* 1999, 17(1): 221–237.

6.   Karras DJ, Sammon ME, Terregino CA, Lopez BL, Griswold SK, Arnold GK. Clinically meaningful changes in quantitative measures of asthma severity. *Academic Emergency Medicine* 2000, 7(4): 327–334.

7.   National Institute for Health and Clinical Excellence. *Chest Pain of Recent Onset: Assessment and diagnosis of recent onset chest pain or discomfort of suspected cardiac origin* (CG95). London: NICE, 2010. Available from: https://www.nice.org.uk/guidance/cg95.

8.   NHS Evidence. *Dyspnoea.* 2010.

9.   National Institute for Health and Care Excellence. *Angio-oedema and Anaphylaxis.* Clinical Knowledge Summaries. 2018. Available from: https://cks.nice.org.uk/angio-oedema-and-anaphylaxis#!diagnosissub:2.

10.   National Institute for Health and Care Excellence. *Chronic Obstructive Pulmonary Disease.* Clinical Knowledge Summaries. 2018. Available from: https://cks.nice.org.uk/chronic-obstructive-pulmonary-disease.

11.   National Institute for Health and Care Excellence. *Pulmonary Embolism.* Clinical Knowledge Summaries. 2015. Available from: https://cks.nice.org.uk/pulmonary-embolism#!diagnosissub.

SECTION **3** Medical Emergencies

Febrile Illness in Children

1. Introduction

- There are many important differences between children and adults in their anatomy, their physiology and their immunity, as well as differences in the types of illnesses they encounter and the ways these conditions present, develop and progress.

- The assessment and management of children poses many potential pitfalls for the unwary and inexperienced, and presents healthcare providers with significant challenges, whatever the setting.

- Children may struggle to verbalise and communicate their condition to you, adding to the challenges faced when assessing and caring for them.

1.1 'Major' and 'Minor' Childhood Illnesses

- Sick children are notoriously difficult to assess, except when they are obviously very ill or injured, with grossly deranged vital signs. The younger the child, the more difficult the assessment.

- Before considering 'minor' illnesses in children, it is crucial to both appreciate and understand that 'major' childhood illnesses (including life-threatening conditions such as meningococcal disease and sepsis) do not commonly present in extremis, but typically present with relatively innocent features that can easily be mistaken for minor illnesses.

- Children's vital signs may well be deranged when their illness (or injury) is advanced (significant), and these abnormalities should be readily detected. However, earlier in the same illness, these same children may appear relatively well and exhibit 'normal' physiology. There is a risk that the significance of these children's illnesses may not be appreciated if assessed early in the course of their illness.

- In critically ill children, temperature is not routinely recorded as part of the 'ABC' assessment as it delays treatment without altering management.

- Temperature should however be measured in the less-ill child, where it forms part of the picture of their illness and is an essential sign that informs clinical decision making.

- Staff should be familiar with NICE's *Feverish Illness in Children* guidance (on which this guideline is based).

1.2 Fever

- Normal body temperature is 37°C. A temperature of 38°C and above is likely to be significant.

- Fever is part of the immune system's response to infection and is not thought to be harmful (although lay people often assume that it is).

- It can herald a significant underlying infection, hence the importance of identifying its cause.

- Throughout most of childhood, the height of the fever bears little relationship to the gravity of the illness, although in babies aged under 6 months a high temperature is much more likely to be significant.

- When facing serious infections, small babies often have unstable body temperatures and may paradoxically present with a low body temperature.

- Febrile illnesses in children aged between 6 months and 5 years can produce a seizure – a febrile convulsion – following a rapid rise in body temperature (refer to **Convulsions in Children**).

- A child with a fever is a very common presentation. Such children may have a self-limiting viral condition or else another obvious cause, such as an ear infection or upper respiratory tract infection. However, for some febrile children no obvious cause will be found and a small number of these will have a serious illness.

- Ambulance clinicians have an important role to play in the reduction of the mortality rate for children with feverish illness, which remains higher in the UK than in many other European countries. The main priorities are to:
  - Identify any immediately life-threatening features.
  - Assess whether the child has (i) a serious illness requiring intervention or (ii) a self-limiting illness, without necessarily diagnosing a specific condition.
  - Determine a likely source of the illness to direct specific treatment.
  - Make appropriate management decisions based upon the results of the assessment.

- NICE defines a fever as 'an elevation of body temperature above the normal daily variation'. It recognises that this is often hard to define, as normal temperature varies depending on the individual, the body site where temperature is measured and the time of day.

2. Incidence

- Febrile illness is the most common medical problem in childhood. Younger children are the most vulnerable due to the immaturity of their immune systems. By the age of 18 months, an otherwise healthy child would be expected to have had around eight acute febrile illnesses.

3. Severity and Outcome

- Infectious diseases are a major cause of childhood mortality and morbidity.

- Most febrile illnesses are due to self-limiting viral infections requiring little or no intervention. However, fever is a common presenting feature of serious bacterial infections (SBI) such as meningitis, septicaemia, urinary tract infections and pneumonia, and distinguishing between a simple

Febrile Illness in Children

viral infection and a more serious bacterial infection is a real diagnostic challenge. 1% of the UK's under-5 population will have an SBI each year.

4. Assessment

4.1 Febrile Child Assessment

Carry out a primary survey immediately on any ill child to exclude any evidence of life-threatening illness. For the assessment and management of a febrile child, refer to Table 3.47.

- Use the traffic light system shown in Table 3.48 to support the assessment and management of the child.
- When assessing children with learning disabilities, take the individual child's learning disability into account when interpreting the traffic light table.

TABLE 3.47 – ASSESSMENT and MANAGEMENT of: a Febrile Child

Assess <C>ABCD

- If any of the following **TIME-CRITICAL** features are present:
  - Major **<C>ABCD** problems (refer to **Medical Emergencies in Children – Overview**).
  - Active seizure (refer to **Convulsions**).
- Start correcting any **<C>ABCD** problems.
- Undertake a **TIME-CRITICAL** transfer to nearest appropriate receiving hospital.
- Continue patient management en-route.
- Provide an ATMIST information call.

Respiratory Rate

- Measure and record respiratory rate. For specific ranges, refer to Table 3.50.

Pulse

- Measure and record pulse. For specific ranges, refer to Table 3.50.

Oxygen Saturation

- Monitor the patient's SpO$_2$; administer oxygen to achieve saturations of >92% if the patient presents as hypoxemic on air (refer to **Oxygen**).

Blood Pressure and Fluids

- Measure and record blood pressure; if required, administer fluids (refer to **Intravascular Fluid Therapy in Children**).

Blood Glucose

- If appropriate, measure and record blood glucose for hypo/hyperglycaemia (refer to **Glycaemic Emergencies in Adults and Children**).

Overall Assessment

- AVPU.
- Consider the overall impression of the child (e.g. playful, lively, disinterested, miserable, floppy etc.).
- Capillary refill.

Temperature

- Measure and record temperature.

Take and Record a Full History

- Length of illness.
- Other symptoms besides fever, specifically asking about:
  - urinary symptoms
  - abdominal pain
  - abnormal skin colour, cold hands and feet, muscle pains
  - headache, photophobia, neck stiffness
  - other complaints, such as a painful joints, sore throat, ear pain etc.

(continued)

Febrile Illness in Children

TABLE 3.47 – ASSESSMENT and MANAGEMENT of: a Febrile Child *(continued)*

- Is fluid intake adequate? A febrile child needs extra fluids to prevent dehydration.
- If they are vomiting, they may become dehydrated and be unable to absorb medication.
- Diarrhoea also increases fluid losses, increasing the risk of dehydration.
- Underlying (chronic) medical problems, including advice that the parent may have been given by specialists regarding actions to be taken if their child develops a fever. (This should include whether the child is under current investigation or management by a doctor.)
- Medications, antibiotics or steroids (or other drugs reducing immunity). To assess a child properly, you will need to be aware of the action of any drug they are taking as this may be relevant. If in doubt, this must be checked.
- Any other illness in the family, the nursery or school etc?
- Recent foreign travel – consider malaria or other tropical illness.

ECG

- If required, monitor and record 12-lead ECG. Assess for abnormality (refer to **Cardiac Rhythm Disturbance**).

Assess the Patient's Pain

- Where present, assess the SOCRATES of pain and record initial and subsequent pain scores.
- Consider analgesia if appropriate (refer to **Pain Management in Children**).

Documentation

- Complete documentation to include all clinical findings, advice from other clinicians, onward referral and worsening advice given.

TABLE 3.48 – Traffic Light System for Assessing Paediatric Fever

	Green – Low Risk	Amber – Intermediate Risk	Red – High Risk
Colour (of skin, lips or tongue)	- Normal colour	- Pallor reported by parent/carer	- Pale/mottled/ashen/blue
Activity	- Responds normally to social cues - Content/smiles - Stays awake or awakens quickly - Strong normal cry/not crying	- Not responding normally to social cues - No smile - Wakes only with prolonged stimulation - Decreased activity	- No response to social cues - Appears ill to a healthcare professional - Does not wake or if roused does not stay awake - Weak, high-pitched or continuous cry

Respiratory		- Nasal flaring
		- Tachypnoea: respiratory rate
		  – >50 breaths/minute, age 6–12 months
		  – >40 breaths/minute, age >12 months
		- Oxygen saturation ≤95% in air
		- Crackles in the chest
			- Grunting
			- Tachypnoea: respiratory rate >60 breaths/minute
			- Moderate or severe chest indrawing

Febrile Illness in Children

TABLE 3.48 – Traffic Light System for Assessing Paediatric Fever *(continued)*

Circulation and hydration	▪ Normal skin and eyes
	▪ Moist mucous membranes
		▪ Tachycardia:
		  – >160 beats/minute, age <12 months
		  – >150 beats/minute, age 12–24 months
		  – >140 beats/minute, age 2–5 years
		▪ Capillary refill time ≥3 seconds
		▪ Dry mucous membranes
		▪ Poor feeding in infants
		▪ Reduced urine output
			▪ Reduced skin turgor

Other	▪ None of the amber or red symptoms or signs	▪ Age 3–6 months, temperature ≥39°C ▪ Fever for ≥5 days ▪ Rigors ▪ Swelling of a limb or joint ▪ Non-weight-bearing limb/not using an extremity	▪ Age <3 months, temperature ≥38°C* ▪ Non-blanching rash ▪ Bulging fontanelle ▪ Neck stiffness ▪ Status epilepticus ▪ Focal neurological signs ▪ Focal seizures

*Some vaccinations have been found to induce fever in children aged under 3 months.

Note: The traffic light system does not seek to make a specific diagnosis but simply identifies which symptoms and signs should receive the highest priority, guiding subsequent management.

4.2 Temperature Measurement

▪ Any reported parental perception of a fever should be considered valid and taken seriously.

▪ Do not take temperatures orally in the under 5s. Even in older children, it may be easier to avoid using the oral method.

▪ In order to obtain an accurate temperature, an appropriate thermometer must be used:
- In children **under** 4 weeks of age, use an electronic thermometer placed in the child's axilla. **NB** The thermometer must be left in place for at least the minimum recommended time, otherwise it may under-record.
- In children **over** 4 weeks of age, use either an electronic thermometer or a tympanic thermometer.

▪ Earlier treatment with antipyretics (e.g. paracetamol, ibuprofen) must be considered, as it may mask the child's fever.

▪ Chemically sensitive strips placed on the forehead are inaccurate and should not be used.

▪ Mercury-containing, glass thermometers are no longer used, for safety reasons.

4.2.1 Important clinical points

Tachycardia frequently accompanies a fever and is suggestive of an underlying infection, while **tachypnoea** suggests an underlying respiratory illness.

A child's resting heart rate increases 10 bpm for every 1°C rise in body temperature.

A **disproportionate tachycardia** – i.e. above the accepted normal range (refer to Table 3.50) having taken account of the fever – is seen in early sepsis and meningococcal disease. Such children must receive further medical assessment.

Other features suggesting sepsis include cold hands and feet, abnormal skin colour and muscle pains in the legs.

Infants and small children with meningococcal disease rarely exhibit 'classical' textbook signs (**neck stiffness, photophobia** and **non-blanching rash**), but more commonly present with features

Febrile Illness in Children

that might suggest a non-specific viral illness such as an upper respiratory tract infection (URTI) or gastroenteritis.

In such circumstances, seek (and document) evidence to rule out the possibility of meningococcal disease.

- Conduct an assessment of dehydration (refer to **Paediatric Gastroenteritis**).

- Examine all other systems (including skin) to determine the source of the fever and estimate the disease severity.

- A positive sign must be 'seen' rather than assumed (e.g. otitis media cannot be diagnosed on a history of 'earache' alone). Direct visualisation of the tympanic membrane using an auroscope is required to diagnose otitis media.

- **NB It is possible for a child to have a common infection as well as a more serious underlying one; a child with coryza and runny nose could still have meningitis.**

4.3 Specific Febrile Illnesses

The following potential diagnoses must each be specifically considered; some typical signs and symptoms are shown in Table 3.49:

- **Meningococcal septicaemia** – often the child does not present as acutely as tradition would have it.

- **Meningitis** (pre-school children rarely have neck stiffness).

- **Urinary tract infection (UTI)** – UTIs are particularly common in babies and young children and can cause permanent kidney damage. UTIs can also progress to

life-threatening septicaemia. Symptoms can again be very non-specific and include: poor feeding, lethargy and abdominal pains. In hospital practice, clean catch urine samples are collected on every febrile child to exclude UTIs.

- **Pneumonia** – typical chest signs may be absent.

- **Herpes simplex encephalitis** – classical pointers include focal neurological signs and focal seizures.

- **Septic arthritis/osteomyelitis** – fever plus very tender swollen joint(s)/bone(s), with a refusal to weight-bear.

- **Kawasaki's disease** – a collection of signs including: fever for >5 days; cervical lymphadenopathy; mucosal changes in the upper respiratory tract (e.g. redness and cracked lips); peripheral limb changes (e.g. oedema, peeling skin); a non-specific, blanching 'measles-like' rash; and bilateral conjunctival redness.

5. Management

(Using the **Traffic Light System for Assessing Paediatric Fever** as shown in Table 3.48).

5.1 Red Traffic Light Features

Children with any of the NICE Red Traffic Light features or Red Flags must be conveyed to an ED with appropriate paediatric services for further specialist assessment.

Provide an ATMIST pre-alert and convey under emergency driving conditions where required. Consider sepsis or meningitis as possible causes and provide care en-route according to Trust/JRCALC guidelines.

TABLE 3.49 – Symptoms and Signs Suggestive of Specific Diseases	
Diagnosis to be considered	**Symptoms and signs in conjunction with fever**
Meningococcal disease	Non-blanching rash, particularly with one or more of the following: - an ill-looking child - lesions larger than 2 mm in diameter (purpura) - capillary refill time ≥3 seconds - neck stiffness
Bacterial meningitis	Neck stiffness Bulging fontanelle Decreased level of consciousness Convulsive status epilepticus
Herpes simplex encephalitis	Focal neurological signs Focal seizures Decreased level of consciousness

Febrile Illness in Children

TABLE 3.49 – Symptoms and Signs Suggestive of Specific Diseases *(continued)*

Diagnosis to be considered	Symptoms and signs in conjunction with fever
Pneumonia	Tachypnoea (respiratory rate >60 breaths/min, age 0–5 months; >50 breaths/min, age 6–12 months; >40 breaths/minute, age >12 months)
	Crackles in the chest
	Nasal flaring
	Chest indrawing
	Cyanosis
	Oxygen saturation ≤95%
Urinary tract infection	Vomiting
	Poor feeding
	Lethargy
	Irritability
	Abdominal pain and tenderness
	Urinary frequency or dysuria
Septic arthritis	Swelling of a limb or joint
	Not using an extremity
	Non-weight-bearing
Kawasaki disease	Fever for more than 5 days and at least four of the following:
	▪ bilateral conjunctival infection
	▪ change in mucous membranes
	▪ chnage in extremities
	▪ polymorphous rash
	▪ cervical lymphadenopathy

5.2 Amber Traffic Light Features

Children with amber traffic light features may be considered for an alternative treatment pathway. Children presenting with multiple amber features must be considered for hospital assessment.

Note: If a child has amber traffic light features and a decision is made **not** to transport the child OR a child has green traffic light features but a cause for the fever has not been found, the following 'safety nets' **MUST** be put in place:

▪ The patient MUST be discussed with a GP or paediatric healthcare professional, following local protocols, for urgent follow-up arrangements giving a specified time and place (e.g. for the child to be seen within the next 2–6 hours, exact timing to be decided by the attending staff).

▪ Direct verbal handover to the doctor is important but may not always be possible.

▪ The arrangements must be made by the attending ambulance staff.

▪ **It is not adequate to tell the parents to make their own arrangements to see the GP.**

5.3 Green Traffic Light Features

Children who have only green traffic light features may be managed at home. Record that the child has been assessed as having only green features on the patient clinical record and ensure that negative findings are noted to demonstrate the absence of amber or red features, e.g. no nasal flaring.

Ensure that parents/carers are provided with a patient information leaflet if one is available. They should receive specific, written worsening advice, including expectations on length of illness. Ensure that they are aware of the following:

▪ Suitable antipyretic interventions available.

Febrile Illness in Children

- The importance of offering the child regular fluids (if breastfeeding, then continue as normal).

- How to identify a non-blanching rash.

- Checking the child during the night.

- Keeping the child away from nursery/school while the fever persists and to notify the nursery/school of the illness.

- The common signs of dehydration:
  - sunken fontanelle
  - dry mouth
  - sunken eyes
  - absence of tears
  - poor overall appearance.

Advise parents/carers to seek further advice if:

- The child has a fit.

- The child develops a non-blanching rash.

- They are worried that the child is becoming dehydrated.

- Nappies are becoming drier or changed much less frequently.

- They feel that the child's health is getting worse.

- They are more worried than when they last received advice.

- The fever lasts longer than 5 days.

- They are distressed or concerned that they are unable to look after their child.

TABLE 3.50 – 'Normal' Paediatric Physiological Values

Age	Respiratory rate (bpm)	Heart rate (bpm)
<1 year	40–60	110–160
1–2 yrs	25–35	110–150
2–5 yrs	25–30	95–140
5–12 yrs	20–25	80–120
Over 12 yrs	15–20	60–100

Use local referral pathways to inform the child's GP as required. Arrange for infants and children presenting with unexplained fever of 38°C or higher to have a urine sample tested after 24 hours at the latest.

Important clinical points – antipyretics and antibiotics

- Tepid sponging is not recommended. Do not over- or under-dress a child with fever.

- Giving an **antipyretic** such as paracetamol or ibuprofen purely to treat the fever is not necessary, but parental sensitivities should be observed.

⚑ TABLE 3.51 – Red Flags

Febrile children fulfilling the following red flag criteria **must** be transported to hospital:

- Any febrile baby <1 month old (irrespective of the absolute temperature).

- Any febrile child <3 months old without an obvious cause (as a minimum, an urgent urine sample will be required).

- Any febrile child <3 years without an obvious cause, if a urine sample cannot be arranged at the time through the GP.

- Those with any signs of serious illness (refer to **Medical Emergencies in Children – Overview**).

- Any child with a significant fever but no localising symptoms or signs, who has received antibiotics within the last 48 hours (signs of meningitis can be masked by antibiotic use; so-called 'partially treated' meningitis).

- Any child on steroids or other medication known to suppress the immune system.

- Any child, regardless of age, where there is any doubt that they could be seriously ill.

- Any child where the social or psychological environment suggests that they may not receive adequate supervision or care if left at home.

- Those with a medical protocol saying that transport is necessary.

- An analgesic/antipyretic may help relieve misery and other unpleasant symptoms that often accompany febrile illnesses (e.g. aches, pains and other symptoms which the child is often unable to fully describe).

- Antipyretics do not protect against febrile convulsions. Giving antipyretics to a child who either has just had a seizure or is thought to be at risk of having a seizure has not been shown to be beneficial.

- Note: Antipyretics are effective, even in children with SBI. It would therefore be wrong to assume that a clinical improvement seen following an antipyretic excludes a serious underlying infection.

- Combinations of paracetamol and ibuprofen should not be given. Only consider alternating these agents if the distress persists or recurs before the next dose is due.

- Paracetamol is normally given every 6 hours and ibuprofen every 8 hours; care needs to be taken not to exceed the maximum dose of each drug in a 24-hour period. A treatment diary may be useful if the parents or carers find it difficult to remember which was the last drug given and at what time.

Febrile Illness in Children

■ **Antibiotics** should not be given to a febrile child where the diagnosis is not known. This can delay the subsequent diagnosis of a serious infection such as meningitis.

5.4 Febrile convulsions

Febrile convulsions commonly occur in children who are aged between 6 months and 3 years and who have a temperature greater than 38°C. Most febrile convulsions occur in those aged approximately 18 months, although children up to 5 years of age can be affected.

Ambulance clinicians must not apply the diagnosis of febrile convulsion to patients aged over 5 years; older children require a paediatrician to rule out other causes of the convulsion first.

For the management of active febrile convulsions, refer to **Convulsions in Children**.

KEY POINTS!

Febrile Illness in Children

■ **Febrile illness is the most common paediatric presentation and suggests underlying infection.**

■ **Always seek the underlying cause of the fever.**

■ **All febrile children must be assessed with a full history and examination.**

■ **Physiological parameters must be measured, documented and compared against age-specific, 'normal' values.**

■ **Significant tachycardia suggests sepsis.**

■ **Use the NICE 'traffic light' system.**

■ **The early features of serious infections are often non-specific (e.g. meningococcal disease often mimics URTIs and gastroenteritis).**

■ **Small children rarely exhibit the 'classical' meningococcal signs – neck stiffness, photophobia or non-blanching rash; these features are more likely in older children and teenagers. In all age groups, important early features include fever, cold hands and feet, abnormal skin colour and muscle pains or confusion.**

■ **Improvement following antipyretics does not rule out a serious underlying infection.**

■ **Antibiotics should not be blindly given to a febrile child where the diagnosis is not known.**

■ **Where a justifiable clinical reason not to transport a child to hospital has been found and a decision made to stay at home, these decisions must be carefully documented.**

■ **Provide a 'safety net', with written information, to any febrile child not transferred to hospital.**

■ **If uncertain, seek advice from either their GP or out-of-hours doctor.**

■ **The GP should be routinely informed of any consultation.**

Bibliography

1. National Collaborating Centre for Women's and Children's Health. *Urinary Tract Infection in Children: Diagnosis, treatment and long-term management* (CG54). London: Royal College of Obstetricians and Gynaecologists, 2007. Available from: http://www.nice.org.uk/nicemedia/pdf/CG54fullguideline.pdf.

2. Hanna CM, Greenes DS. How much tachycardia in infants can be attributed to fever? *Annals of Emergency Medicine* 2004, 43(6): 699–705.

3. Hay AD, Costelloe C, Redmond NM, Montgomery AA, Fletcher M, Hollinghurst S, et al. Paracetamol plus ibuprofen for the treatment of fever in children (PITCH): randomised controlled trial. *British Medical Journal* 2008, 337: a1302.

4. National Collaborating Centre for Women's and Children's Health. *Feverish Illness in Children: Assessment and initial management in children younger than 5 years* (CG47). London: National Institute for Health and Clinical Excellence, 2007.

5. National Collaborating Centre for Women's and Children's Health. *Patient's Information Sheet.* London: National Institute for Health and Clinical Excellence, 2007.

6. National Collaborating Centre for Women's and Children's Health. *Bacterial Meningitis and Meningococcal Septicaemia: Management of bacterial meningitis and meningococcal septicaemia in children and young people younger than 16 years in primary and secondary care* (CG102). London: National Institute for Health and Clinical Excellence, 2010. Available from: https://www.nice.org.uk/guidance/cg102.

7. Woollard M, Pitt K. Antipyretic pre-hospital therapy for febrile convulsions: does the treatment fit? A literature review. *Health Education* 2003, 62(1): 23–28.

8. Sharp A. Management of febrile convulsions within the pre-hospital environment. *Journal of Paramedic Practice* 2016, 8(9): 447–451.

Febrile Illness in Children

9.   National Institute for Health and Clinical Excellence. *Febrile Convulsions.* NICE Clinical Knowledge Summaries. NICE, 2013. Available from: https://cks.nice.org.uk.

10. National Institute for Health and Clinical Excellence. *Feverish Illness in Children: Assessment and Initial Management in children younger than five years.* NICE, 2013. Available from: https://www.nice.org.uk/guidance/cg160/resources/fever-in-children-younger-than-5-years-pdf-246224941765.

11. National Institute for Health and Care Excellence. *Fever in Under 5s: Assessment and initial management* [CG160]. London: NICE, 2017. Available from: https://www.nice.org.uk/guidance/cg160.

Gastrointestinal Bleeding

1. Introduction

Gastrointestinal (GI) bleeding is a common medical emergency accounting for 7,000 admissions per year in Scotland alone.

Gastrointestinal haemorrhage is commonly divided into:

▪ Upper gastrointestinal haemorrhage.

▪ Lower gastrointestinal haemorrhage.

2. Incidence

▪ Upper GI bleeding is more common than lower GI bleeding and is more prevalent in socioeconomically deprived areas.

▪ Upper GI bleeding accounts for up to 85% of gastrointestinal bleeding events.

3. Severity and Outcome

▪ The severity of gastrointestinal bleeding can range from clinically insignificant blood loss to significant life-threatening haemorrhage.

▪ Death is uncommon in patients less than 40 years of age; it is estimated that the overall mortality rate in the UK for patients admitted with acute GI bleeding is approximately 7%. The majority of deaths occur in older people, particularly those with comorbidities. There are many factors that are associated with a poor outcome, including liver disease, acute haemodynamic disturbance, clotting abnormalities, continued bleeding, haematemesis, haematochezia and elevated blood urea.

▪ Upper GI bleeding tends to be more severe and in extreme circumstances can rapidly lead to hypovolaemic shock.

4. Pathophysiology

▪ The upper gastrointestinal tract comprises the oesophagus, stomach and duodenum. For common causes of bleeding, refer to Table 3.52.

▪ The lower gastrointestinal tract comprises the lower part of the small intestine, the colon, rectum and anus. Common causes of bleeding include diverticular disease, inflammatory bowel disease, haemorrhoids and tumour.

4.1 ACUTE UPPER GI BLEEDING

▪ More than 50% of cases are due to peptic ulcers which, together with oesophagitis and gastritis, account for up to 90% of all upper GI bleeding in older people. Eighty-five percent of deaths associated with upper GI bleeding occur in persons older than 65 years.

▪ Patients presenting with upper GI bleeding may have a history of aspirin or non-steroidal anti-inflammatory drug (NSAID) use.

– Only 50% of patients present with haematemesis alone, 30% with melaena and 20% with haematemesis and melaena

– Patients with haematemesis tend to have greater blood loss than those with melaena alone. Patients older than 60 years account for up to 45% of all cases (60% of these are women).

TABLE 3.52 – Common Causes of Upper Gastrointestinal Bleeding

Common causes

▪ Peptic ulcers:
  – Duodenal ulcers
  – Gastric ulcers
▪ Oesophageal varices
▪ Gastritis
▪ Oesophagitis
▪ Mallory–Weiss tears
▪ Caustic poison
▪ Tumour

Peptic Ulcers

▪ Peptic ulcers are commonly associated with the use of aspirin, non-steroidal anti-inflammatory drugs, corticosteroids, anticoagulants, alcohol and cigarettes.

Oesophageal Varices

▪ It is estimated that variceal bleeding is the cause of 10% of cases. These patients can bleed severely, with up to 8% dying within 48 hours from uncontrolled haemorrhage. It is commonly associated with alcoholic cirrhosis and increased portal pressure (causing progressive dilation of the veins and protrusion of the formed varices into the lumen of the oesophagus). Spontaneous rupture of the varices will cause the patient to become haemodynamically unstable within a very short period of time due to large volumes of blood loss.

Mallory–Weiss Tears

▪ Approximately 10% are caused by oesophageal tears, which are more common in the young. Predisposing factors include hiatal hernia and alcoholism. Initiating factors are persistent coughing or severe retching and vomiting, often after an alcoholic binge; haematemesis presents after several episodes of non-bloody emesis. Bleeding can be mild to moderate.

Gastritis

▪ Drugs, infections, illnesses and injuries can cause inflammation of the lining of the stomach and lead to bleeding.

3 Medical Emergencies

SECTION

Gastrointestinal Bleeding

Oesophagitis

- Gastroesophageal reflux disease or alcohol can lead to inflammation and ulcers in the lining of the oesophagus which may lead to bleeding.

Tumour

- A tumour in the oesophagus, stomach or duodenum can cause bleeding.

4.2 ACUTE LOWER GI BLEEDING

Patients with a lower GI bleed commonly present with bright-red/dark blood with clots per rectum (PR); bright-red blood PR in isolation excludes upper GI bleeding in over 98% of cases (unless the patient appears hypovolaemic). Lower GI bleeding is less likely to present with signs of haemodynamic compromise, is more prevalent in men and also has a common history of aspirin or NSAID use. The mean age for lower GI bleeding is 63–77 years, with mortality around 4% (even serious cases have rarely resulted in death). Common causes include:

Diverticular disease

- Diverticular bleeding accounts for up to 55% of cases. Patients commonly present with an abrupt but painless PR bleed. The incidence of diverticular bleeding increases with age.

Inflammatory Bowel Disease

- Major bleeding from ulcerative colitis and Crohn's disease is rare. Inflammatory bowel disease accounts for less than 10% of cases.

Haemorrhoids

- Haemorrhoids account for less than 10% of cases. Bleeding is bright red and usually noticed on wiping or in the toilet bowl. The incidence is high in pregnancy, a result of straining associated with constipation and hormonal changes. Further evaluation may be needed if the patient complains of an alteration of bowel habit and blood mixed with the stool.

Tumour

- Tumour in the large bowel can cause bleeding.

Differential diagnosis

- Post-rectal bleeding can cause significant embarrassment for the patient and care must be taken when assessing female patients that per vaginum (PV) bleeding is excluded.

5. Assessment and Management

For the assessment and management of gastrointestinal bleeding, refer to Table 3.53.

TABLE 3.53 – ASSESSMENT and MANAGEMENT of: Gastrointestinal Bleeding

Assess <C>ABCD

- If any of the following **TIME-CRITICAL** features present:
  - major **<C>ABCD** problems (refer to **Medical Emergencies in Adults – Overview** and **Medical Emergencies in Children – Overview**).
  - haematemesis – large volume of bright-red blood
  - haemodynamic compromise
  - decreased level of consciousness.
- Start correcting any **<C>ABCD** problems.
- Undertake a **TIME-CRITICAL** transfer to nearest appropriate receiving hospital.
- Continue patient management en-route.
- Provide an ATMIST information call.

Assess Blood Loss

Where does the bleeding originate – upper or lower GI tract?

- **Haematemesis** – vomited fresh/dark red/brown/black or 'coffee ground' blood (depending on how long it has been in the stomach). Did this occur after an increase in intra-abdominal pressure (e.g. retching or coughing).
- Ascertain how many episodes of non-bloody emesis.
- **Melaena** – malodorous, liquid, black stool or bright-red/dark blood with clots PR. It can be difficult to estimate blood loss when mixed with faeces.
- Estimate blood loss – if not visible, ask the patient or relatives/carers to estimate colour/volume – PR blood loss is difficult to estimate. (**NB** The blood acts as a laxative, but repeated blood-liquid stool, or just blood, is associated with more severe blood loss than maroon/black solid stool.)
- If the patient has suffered unexplained syncope, this may indicate concealed GI bleeding. Ensure PV bleeding is excluded in females.

Gastrointestinal Bleeding

TABLE 3.53 – ASSESSMENT and MANAGEMENT of: Gastrointestinal Bleeding *(continued)*

History

- **When did the bleeding begin?**
- Is/has the patient:
  - currently taking or recently taken aspirin or NSAID?
  - currently taking iron tablets?
  - consumed food or drink containing red dye(s)?
  - currently taking beta-blockers or calcium-channel blockers – may mask tachycardia in the shocked patient?
  - currently taking or recently taken anticoagulatory or antiplatelet therapy?
- **Is there a history of:**
  - bleeding disorders?
  - liver disease?
  - abdominal surgery, in particular, abdominal aortic surgery?
  - alcohol abuse?
  - syncope?

Oxygen Saturation

- Monitor the patient's SpO$_2$; administer oxygen to achieve saturations of >94% if the patient presents as hypoxaemic on air; refer to **Oxygen**.

Respiratory Rate

- Measure and record respiratory rate.

Pulse

- Measure and record pulse.

ECG

- If required, monitor and record 12-lead ECG. Assess for abnormality (refer to **Cardiac Rhythm Disturbance**).

Assess the Patient's Pain

- GI bleeding is not generally associated with pain.
- Where present, assess the SOCRATES of pain and record initial and subsequent pain scores.
- Consider analgesia if appropriate (refer to **Pain Management in Adults** and **Pain Management in Children**).

Fluid

- Measure and record blood pressure; if required, administer fluids (refer to **Intravascular Fluid Therapy in Adults** and **Intravascular Fluid Therapy in Children**).
- Tranexamic acid is not indicated in GI haemorrhage due to a lack of current evidence for benefit.

Blood Glucose

- If appropriate, measure and record blood glucose for hypo/hyperglycaemia (refer to **Glycaemic Emergencies in Adults and Children**).

Temperature

- Measure and record temperature.

NEWS2

- These observations will enable you to calculate a NEWS2 score (refer to **Sepsis**).

Transfer to Further Care

- Continue patient management en-route.
- Provide an alert/information call.

Documentation

- Complete documentation to include all clinical findings, advice from other clinicians, onward referral and worsening advice given.

Gastrointestinal Bleeding

KEY POINTS!

Gastrointestinal Bleeding

- Haematemesis or melaena indicates an upper GI source.
- Bright-red or dark blood with clots per rectum indicates a lower GI source.
- Almost all deaths from GI bleeds occur in older people.
- Approximately 80% of all GI bleeds stop spontaneously or respond to conservative management.
- Tranexamic acid is not indicated in GI haemorrhage due to a lack of current evidence for benefit.

Bibliography

1. Bennett C, Klingenberg SL, Langholz E, Gluud LL. *Tranexamic acid for upper gastrointestinal bleeding (Review).* London: Cochrane Library and Wiley, 2014. Available from: https://www.cochranelibrary.com/cdsr/doi/10.1002/14651858.CD006640.pub3/epdf/standard.

2. Scottish Intercollegiate Guidelines Network. *Management of Acute Upper and Lower Gastrointestinal Bleeding* (Guideline 105). Edinburgh: SIGN, 2008.

3. Cappell MS, Friedel D. Initial management of acute upper gastrointestinal bleeding: from initial evaluation up to gastrointestinal endoscopy. *Medical Clinics of North America* 2008, 92: 491–509.

4. Edwards AJ, Maskell GF. Acute lower gastrointestinal haemorrhage. *British Medical Journal* 2009, 339: b4156.

5. Michels SL, Collins J, Reynolds MW, Abramsky S, Paredes-Diaz A, McCarberg B. Over-the-counter ibuprofen and risk of gastrointestinal bleeding complications: a systematic literature review. *Current Medical Research and Opinion* 2012, 28(1): 89–99.

6. Palmer K. Acute upper gastrointestinal haemorrhage. *British Medical Bulletin* 2007, 83(1): 307–324.

7. Szajerka T, Jablecki J. Upper gastrointestinal bleeding in a young female with AIDS: a case report. *International Journal of STD & AIDS* 2012, 23(3): e33–34.

8. van Leerdam ME. Epidemiology of acute upper gastro-intestinal bleeding. *Best Practice & Research in Clinical Gastroenterology* 2008, 22(2): 209–224.

9. Alkhatib AA, Elkhatib FA, Maldonado A, Abubakr SM, Adler DG. Acute upper gastrointestinal bleeding in elderly people: presentations, endoscopic findings, and outcomes. *Journal of the American Geriatrics Society* 2010, 58(1): 182–185.

10. Kent AJ, O'Beirne J, Negus R. The patient with haematemesis and melaena. *Acute Medicine* 2011, 10(1): 45–49.

Glycaemic Emergencies in Adults and Children

1. Introduction

- A person without diabetes maintains their blood glucose level within a narrow range.

- This is achieved by a balance between glucose entering the blood stream (from the gastrointestinal tract or from the breakdown of stored energy sources) and glucose leaving the circulation through the action of insulin.

- Increasingly, prevalence of both Type 1 and Type 2 diabetes is on the rise, in both adults and children. Type 1 diabetes, previously known as juvenile diabetes, is increasingly diagnosed in the adult population and there are known incidences of diagnosis of Type 2 diabetes in children. It is important to note that Type 2 diabetes is not always associated with severe obesity.

2. Considerations for Patients with Diabetes

2.1 Blood Glucose Monitors

- Prior to testing blood glucose, the patient's fingers must be cleaned using sterile water and a gauze swab. This prevents contamination of blood glucose results from residual deposits on the skin. Alco-wipes are not a suitable alternative as research suggests their use may adversely affect blood glucose readings. Rinsing hands thoroughly in tap water is an acceptable alternative.[1,2]

- Blood glucose monitors should be routinely checked for accuracy using control solutions as provided by manufacturers. Patients with Type 1 diabetes should have their own blood glucose monitors, and ambulance clinicians may encounter a wide variety of different devices, which may not be regularly checked. Therefore, it is recommended that clinicians use service-issue blood glucose monitors only.

- Patients with Type 2 diabetes may not have their own blood glucose monitor, and blood glucose levels may only be tested sporadically at their GP's surgery.

2.2 Blood Ketone Meters

Most Type 1 diabetes patients will have a blood ketone meter issued to them. These are operated in the same way as a blood glucose meter. If available, blood ketone meters may assist the ambulance clinician in determining diabetic ketoacidosis (DKA) in the hyperglycaemic patient.

- A blood ketone level of <0.6 mmol/l is normal.

- A blood ketone level of >0.6 mmol/l usually requires the patient to administer additional rapid-acting insulin as per 'sick-day rules' (see below).

- Ketone levels of >0.6 and <3.0 mmol/l may require hospital assessment in the presence of illness and/or vomiting. However, if the patient is able to reliably eat and drink and administer additional doses of rapid-acting insulin (as per 'sick-day rules'), it may be possible to avoid hospital attendance. In children, specialist diabetes teams should always be contacted for advice.

- A blood ketone level of >=3.0mmol/l is predictive of diabetic ketoacidosis and will require hospital assessment.

- Pregnant women with Type 1 diabetes are more prone to ketosis and thus ketoacidosis, even when glucose levels may be relatively normal.

- Ketoacidosis occasionally occurs in those with Type 2 diabetes during acute illness.[3,4] DKA has also been observed in those Type 2 patients who take a 'flozin tablet to control their diabetes (dapagliflozin, canagliflozin, empagliflozin). It is not uncommon for blood glucose levels to be relatively normal in this situation ('euglycaemic ketoacidosis'). While this is a rare complication of 'flozin treatment, consider ketoacidosis if the patient appears unwell or has symptoms suggestive of DKA.

2.3 Sick-day Rules

- Illness generally raises blood glucose levels and increases the risk of ketone body production. This can result in DKA if adequate insulin and hydration are not maintained.[5]

- Increased levels of stress hormones during illness may also contribute to high blood glucose levels. Diarrhoea and vomiting may reduce blood glucose levels, with a possibility of hypoglycaemia rather than hyperglycaemia. However, ketones (known as starvation ketones) may still be produced in significant quantities.

- NICE guidelines recommend that people with Type 1 diabetes mellitus (T1DM) should be provided with clear guidance for the management of diabetes during periods of illness. Thus many patients with T1DM will be able to competently manage transient episodes of hyperglycaemia at home. Timely and appropriate sick-day management may prevent progression to DKA and consequent admission to hospital.

General Sick-day Rule Principles

- Never stop the insulin.

- Insulin dosages may need to be increased or decreased depending on blood glucose or ketone levels. Most patients (or parents of paediatric patients) will be aware of the relevant correction dosages. Paediatric patients will be able to contact their specialist team for further advice and support if needed.

- Encourage fluids to prevent dehydration.

- Increase the frequency of monitoring of blood glucose levels. A minimum of one test every 2 hours is generally suggested.

Glycaemic Emergencies in Adults and Children

If available, blood ketone levels should also be closely monitored. Urinalysis for ketones is less reliable, taking longer to be detected and normalised, but in the absence of a blood ketone meter, urine ketones may still be used to guide patients on additional insulin doses.

2.4 Insulin Pumps

- Increasing numbers of Type 1 diabetes patients, especially children, now wear insulin pumps. These deliver a continuous flow of rapid-acting insulin via a subcutaneous cannula, combined with a bolus delivery at mealtimes to cover the carbohydrate content of the meal.

- At no time should these devices be removed or altered by ambulance clinicians.

- Due to the use of rapid-acting insulin, patients using insulin pump therapy will generally not need to consume a slow release carbohydrate, such as a biscuit or toast, once blood glucose levels have returned to normal. If in doubt, consult the patient or the child's caregivers.

- Patients using insulin pumps are at a high risk of DKA in cases of cannula blockage or pump failure. If needing to transfer a patient with Type 1 diabetes on insulin pump therapy, encourage the patient to bring a supply of pump consumables with them. Hospitals do not routinely stock insulin pump consumables, potentially risking an interruption in insulin delivery for the patient, which may lead to ketosis and DKA.

2.5 Continuous Glucose Monitors (CGMs) and Flash Glucose Monitoring

- These devices are also becoming more common. These are subcutaneous devices that read interstitial fluid glucose levels at approximately 5-minute intervals.

- These monitors cannot be relied on by ambulance clinicians in lieu of blood glucose testing, as interstitial glucose lags behind that of blood glucose and does not always give accurate readings.

2.6 Driving

- It is a legal requirement for drivers to inform the DVLA of their insulin-treated diabetes. Patients with Type 2 diabetes on tablet or non-insulin injectable therapy are not required to inform the DVLA of their condition. However, patients with Type 2 diabetes taking medication that may predispose them to hypoglycaemia (e.g. gliclazide, glipizide, glimepiride, glibenclamide, tolbutamide and metiglinide or repaglinide) are required to inform the DVLA if they have recurrent episodes of hypoglycaemia.[6]

- When it is appropriate – particularly when discharging a patient who is a driver after a hypoglycaemic episode and not conveying them

to a healthcare facility – ambulance clinicians should:

- – advise the patient on the impact of their medical condition for safe driving ability
- – advise the patient on their legal requirement to notify the DVLA if they have insulin-treated diabetes
- – document any of the above if it is discussed with the patient.

Note that the patient could be fined up to £1,000 if they do not tell the DVLA about a medical condition that affects their driving, and they could be prosecuted if they are involved in an accident as a result.

There are differences in requirements to report to the DVLA between Group 1 (cars and motorbikes) and Group 2 (bus or lorry) drivers and differences between Type 1 and Type 2 patients. Current legislation (January 2018)[7] states that:

- Nocturnal hypoglycaemic events do not require reporting to the DVLA.

- Those on insulin or who take tablets for diabetes that may predispose them to hypoglycaemia (as above) should, when assistance has been required to treat **DAYTIME** hypoglycaemia, report it to the DVLA **IF** episodes have occurred **within the past 12 months, and the last event has occurred within the last 3 months**, when this has been the:
  - – second episode (Group 1, car and motorbike) or
  - – first episode (Group 2, bus and lorry).

If an ambulance clinician is concerned that the patient cannot or will not notify the DVLA themselves after recurrent episodes of hypoglycaemia requiring assistance, it would be appropriate to liaise with the patient's GP and again, document these actions.

3. Hypoglycaemia

- Hypoglycaemia is the term used to describe low blood glucose levels.[8]

- In the patient with diabetes, the definition of hypoglycaemia is a blood glucose of <4.0 mmol/L.[9] This should not be confused with the lower level of <3.0 mmol/l used for patients without diabetes. There are three types of hypoglycaemia: mild, moderate and severe. In mild cases, the person can treat themselves, whereas in severe cases, third-party assistance will be required.

- Correction of hypoglycaemia is a medical emergency. If left untreated, hypoglycaemia may lead to the patient suffering permanent brain damage and may even prove fatal.

- Hypoglycaemia occurs when glucose metabolism is disturbed (refer to Table 3.54).

- Any person whose level of consciousness is decreased, who is having a convulsion, is seriously ill or is traumatised should have hypoglycaemia excluded.

Glycaemic Emergencies in Adults and Children

- Some patients can detect the early symptoms for themselves, but others may be too young or deteriorate rapidly and without apparent warning.

- Abnormal neurological features may occur, for example one-sided weakness, identical to a stroke.

- Signs and symptoms can vary from person to person. Symptoms may be masked due to medication or other injuries, for example with beta-blocking agents (refer to Table 3.55).

- The classical symptoms of hypoglycaemia may **NOT** be present, and children may have a variety of unusual symptoms with low blood glucose (refer to Table 3.55).

- In diabetes mellitus, hypoglycaemia is due to a relative excess of exogenously administered insulin over available glucose.

TABLE 3.54 – Risk Factors for Hypoglycaemia

Medical risk factors[10]	Lifestyle risk factors
- Insulin or other hypoglycaemic drug treatments. - Tight glycaemic control. - Previous history of severe hypoglycaemia. - Undetected nocturnal hypoglycaemia. - Long duration of Type 1 diabetes. - Duration of insulin therapy in Type 2 diabetes. - Lipohypertrophy at injection sites. - Impaired awareness of hypoglycaemia. - Preceding hypoglycaemia (<3.5 mmol/l). - Severe hepatic dysfunction. - Renal dialysis therapy. - Impaired renal function. - Inadequate treatment of previous hypoglycaemia. - Terminal illness. - Sepsis. - Endocrine illness (including Addisonian crisis). - Sudden cessation of peritoneal dialysis. - Hypothermia (especially in very young babies). - Sudden cessation of tube or IV feeding. - Very sick or traumatised children. - Very young babies (especially preterm). - Ketotic hypoglycaemia of infancy.	- Drug ingestion, e.g. oral hypoglycaemic drugs, beta-blockers, alcohol. - Inadequate carbohydrate intake. - Increased exercise (relative to usual)/excessive physical activity. - Irregular lifestyle (or supervision if the patient is a child). - Increasing age. - Excessive or chronic alcohol intake. - Early pregnancy. - Breastfeeding. - No or inadequate blood glucose monitoring.

TABLE 3.55 – Signs and Symptoms of Hypoglycaemia			**TABLE 3.55** – Signs and Symptoms of Hypoglycaemia *(continued)*	
- **Autonomic**[11,12]	- Sweating - Trembling/shaking - Palpitations/ pounding heart - Hunger		- **Neuroglycopenic**[13]	- Incoordination - Confusion - Speech difficulty - Drowsiness - Odd behaviour - Aggression/ combative behaviour - Fitting - Unconsciousness
- **General malaise**	- Headache - Nausea			

Glycaemic Emergencies in Adults and Children

3.1 Hypoglycaemia in the Absence of Diabetes

This is a rare occurrence with many different causes. It can generally be divided into two types:[14,15]

- **Reactive hypoglycaemia** – may be the result of gastrointestinal surgery or enzyme deficiency and may occasionally be found in patients with pre-diabetes as the body struggles to regulate insulin production.

- **Fasting hypoglycaemia** – may occur as a result of medication such as salicylates, certain antibiotics, pentamidine and quinine; with excessive alcohol intake, especially binge drinking; serious illnesses, especially those affecting the liver, heart or kidneys; hormonal abnormalities; or the presence of certain types of tumours, particularly those in the pancreas.

Note that hypoglycaemia in the absence of diabetes is diagnosed by the lower blood glucose of <3.0 mmol/l.

3.2 Impaired Awareness of Hypoglycaemia

- Impaired awareness (IA) arises in those whose perception of hypoglycaemia is reduced or absent and as such the possibility of severe hypoglycaemic events is increased. IA is more commonly associated with insulin therapy[16] and may be induced by recurrent hypoglycaemic episodes and/or strict glycaemic control, which cause a dampening of the sympathetic response.[17] It is the dampening or absence of any sympathetic response that leads to an under-recognition of the onset of hypoglycaemia, progression to neuroglycopenia and subsequently an inability to self-treat. The condition can be objectively identified using a number of validated tools[18] and is reversible for many through strict avoidance of hypoglycaemia for a period of weeks or months.[19,20,21]

- In the general population of those diagnosed with diabetes treated with insulin, the prevalence of IA varies between 8% and 25%[22] and increases with the duration of insulin therapy.[23] However, more recent evidence suggests the prevalence may be significantly higher (53% to 57%) in the ambulance service hypoglycaemia population.[24]

3.3 Assessment and Management of Hypoglycaemia

For the assessment and management of hypoglycaemia, refer to Tables 3.56 and 3.57 and Figure 3.14. The principles of assessment and management are essentially the same in adults and children both with and without diabetes. **NB** Note that the lower blood glucose level for hypoglycaemia in the patient without diabetes is 3.0 mmol/l.

TABLE 3.56 – ASSESSMENT and MANAGEMENT of: Hypoglycaemia
Assess <C>ABCD
▪ Start correcting <C>ABCD problems (refer to **Medical Emergencies in Adults – Overview** and **Medical Emergencies in Children – Overview**).
▪ Consider and look for medical alert/information signs (alert bracelets, chains and cards).
Assess Blood Glucose Level
▪ Measure and record blood glucose level (pre-treatment measure).
▪ Clean the patient's fingers prior to testing blood glucose levels as they may have been in contact with sugary substances (e.g. sweets). It is vital that fingers are cleaned with sterile water prior to obtaining a blood glucose reading and NOT alcohol wipes as these may give a false high reading.
▪ Glucagon may take 10 minutes to take effect and requires the patient to have adequate glycogen stores – thus, it may be ineffective if glycogen stores have been exhausted through, for example, frequent episodes of hypoglycaemia, alcohol use or poor carbohydrate content of diet. This is likely in any patients who have any NON-diabetic causes of hypoglycaemia, although it is worth trying.

Glycaemic Emergencies in Adults and Children

TABLE 3.56 – ASSESSMENT and MANAGEMENT of: Hypoglycaemia *(continued)*

Severe

Patient unconscious (GCS ≤8)/convulsing or very aggressive.

■ Check <C>ABCD and correct as necessary.

■ Administer IV glucose 10% over 15 minutes (refer to Glucose 10% for dosages).

■ Only administer glucagon IM if IV access is not possible (onset of action is 10 minutes but can take up to 15 minutes). Glucagon is less effective in those who take a sulphonylurea (e.g. gliclazide, glipizide, tolbutamide, glimepiride), are chronically malnourished or take excess alcohol, so IV glucose is preferred in these groups. **NB** IM glucagon to be given ONCE ONLY.

■ Keep nil by mouth as there is an increased risk of aspiration/choking.

■ Titrate to effect – an improvement in clinical state and glucose level should be observed rapidly.

■ Reassess blood glucose level after 10 minutes.

■ If <4.0 mmol/l, administer a further dose of IV 10% glucose.

■ Reassess blood glucose level after a further 15 minutes.

■ Consider rapid transfer to the nearest suitable receiving hospital if no improvement.

■ Monitor vital signs and conscious level en-route. Check glucose again if patient deteriorates, or half-hourly.

■ Provide a pre-alert/information call if necessary.

Mild to Moderate

Patient conscious, orientated, able to swallow.

■ If capable, cooperative and deemed to have a safe swallow, administer 15–20 grams of quick-acting carbohydrate, such as one of the following:
  - 5–7 Dextrosol® tablets (or 4–5 Glucotabs®) or
  - 1 bottle (60 ml) Glucojuice® or
  - 150–200 ml pure fruit juice, e.g. orange (avoid pure fruit juice if a renal dialysis patient because of potassium content) or
  - 1–2 tubes of 40% glucose gel or
  - 3–4 heaped teaspoons of sugar dissolved in water (**NB** this is not an effective treatment for patients taking acarbose as it prevents the breakdown of sucrose to glucose).

■ Do not give chocolate, as it is slower acting.

■ If **NOT** capable and cooperative, but able to swallow, administer 1–2 tubes of 40% glucose gel to the buccal mucosa or give IV glucose 10% or IM glucagon (refer to Glucagon) if IV access is not possible.

■ Re-assess blood glucose level after 10–15 minutes and ensure blood glucose level has improved to at least 4.0 mmol/l in addition to an improvement in level of consciousness.

■ If no improvement, repeat oral treatment up to three times in total. **NB** IM glucagon to be given **ONCE ONLY**.

■ If no improvement after three treatments or 30–45 minutes, give IV glucose 10% (refer to Glucose 10%).

■ Refer to Table 3.57.

■ Once blood glucose is >4 mmol/l, give a starchy snack, e.g. two biscuits, one slice of bread/toast, 200–300 ml glass of milk (not soya) or a normal meal if due (must contain carbohydrate).

■ **NB** Patients given glucagon require a larger portion of long-acting carbohydrate to replenish glycogen stores (double the suggested amount above).

■ **NB** Patients who self-manage their insulin pumps (CSII) may not need a long-acting carbohydrate.

■ Transfer to the nearest suitable receiving hospital if the patient requires further treatment, otherwise the patient can usually be safely left at home. If the patient is a child, ensure they are left with a responsible adult.

SECTION **3** Medical Emergencies

Glycaemic Emergencies in Adults and Children

TABLE 3.57 – Care Pathway

Patients who do not need conveyance to hospital

- The following patients may not need conveyance to hospital:
  - patients whose episode was mild or moderate and who are now fully recovered after treatment
  - patients with a sustained blood glucose level of >4.0 mmol/l
  - patients who have been able to eat/drink a glucose- and carbohydrate-containing food where relevant.
- If the patient is a child, they must be in the care of a responsible adult.
- Advise patients/carers to call for help if any symptoms of hypoglycaemia recur.
- Ambulance services must arrange for a message to be forwarded to a primary healthcare team or diabetes nurse as per local pathways. All patients with hypoglycaemia who require third-party assistance should be referred to a specialist diabetes team. Where these pathways do not exist, the patient's GP must be informed.
- Patient consent is not required in order to make a referral, although the patient should be informed that a referral is being made.
- Consider giving the patient and carers a patient information leaflet.
- Consider advising the patient about their responsibilities in relation to driving.

Patients who require further care

Consider conveying to hospital patients that are older, frail, have a low BMI, live alone or are on multiple medications.

- The following patients should be transferred to further care, with continuing patient management en-route:
  - patients who have had recurrent treatment within the previous 48 hours
  - patients whose episode was severe and who had a very slow response and recovery after treatment
  - patients taking **sulphonylureas (glibenclamide, glipizide, gliclazide, tolbutamide, glimepiride). These can be longer acting and result in a prolonged or recurrent hypoglycaemic event. Be aware that you may need to monitor these patients for a longer time period and use clinical judgement**
  - patients with no previous history of diabetes who have suffered their first hypoglycaemic episode
  - patients with a blood glucose level of ≤4.0 mmol/l after treatment
  - patients who have not returned to normal mental status within 10 minutes of treatment
  - patients with any additional disorders or other complicating factors (e.g. renal dialysis, chest pain, cardiac arrhythmias, Addison's disease, alcohol consumption, dyspnoea, seizures or focal neurological signs/symptoms)
  - patients with signs of infection (urinary tract infection, upper respiratory tract infection) and/or who are unwell ('flu-like symptoms).

4. Hyperglycaemia

- Hyperglycaemia is the term used to describe high blood glucose levels. Symptoms include unusual thirst (polydipsia), urinary frequency (polyuria) and tiredness. They are usually of slower onset in comparison to those of hypoglycaemia but can develop relatively quickly (days to weeks) in those with newly presenting Type 1 diabetes.
- Patients with diabetes mellitus are very likely to develop a raised blood glucose in response to infection and will have instructions as to how to deal with this – so called 'sick-day rules' (see above).
- Hyperglycaemia may also occur transiently in patients who are severely physically stressed (e.g. during a convulsion).

- It is important to distinguish a simple raised blood glucose from the condition of DKA, which is much more serious. A raised blood glucose is not a pre-hospital emergency unless DKA is present. However, the underlying reason for the raised blood glucose may well be an emergency in its own right.
- In adults, if capillary blood glucose is more than 7.8 mmol/l but less than 11.1 mmol/l, this may indicate that the patient is at risk of Type 2 diabetes; that they have non-diabetic hyperglycaemia (raised blood glucose levels but not in the diabetic range, also known as 'impaired glucose regulation') or 'stress hyperglycaemia' (transient rise in blood glucose levels due to acute illness in a patient without diabetes, which settles to normal after the acute illness has settled); or that they are taking medication that

Glycaemic Emergencies in Adults and Children

MILD	MODERATE	SEVERE
The patient is conscious, orientated and able to swallow.	The patient is conscious and able to swallow, but may be confused, disoriented and/or combative.	The patient is unconscious/fitting or combative or where there is increased risk of aspiration/choking.

MILD

- Give 15–20 g quick acting carbohydrate, such as:
  - 4–5 Glucotabs or
  - 1 bottle (60 ml) Glucojuice® or
  - 1–2 tubes 40% glucose gel or
  - 3–4 heaped teaspoons of sugar dissolved in water or
  - 150–200 ml pure fruit juice.

- Re-test blood glucose after 15 mins.

- If blood glucose remains <4 mmol/l, repeat above treatment up to twice more at 15-minute intervals until a blood glucose of >4 mmol/l is obtained.

- If blood glucose fails to rise >4 mmol/l AFTER 3 cycles of oral treatment (i.e. 45 mins), consider IV 10% glucose or IM glucagon.

MODERATE

If capable and cooperative:

- Give 15–20 g quick acting carbohydrate, such as:
  - 4–5 Glucotabs or
  - 1 bottle (60 ml) Glucojuice® or
  - 1–2 tubes 40% glucose gel or
  - 3–4 heaped teaspoons of sugar dissolved in water or
  - 150–200 ml pure fruit juice.

If **NOT** capable and cooperative, but able to swallow:

- Administer 1–2 tubes of glucose gel 40% to the buccal mucosa or give 1 mg glucagon IM (refer to **Glucagon**).

- Re-test blood glucose after 15 mins. If <4 mmol/l, repeat administration of 40% glucose gel. **NB** IM glucagon cannot be repeated.

- If 40% glucose gel cannot be administered due to patient disposition, consider IV 10% glucose (refer to **Glucose 10%**).

- If blood glucose remains <4 mmol/l, repeat above treatment up to twice more at 15-minute intervals until a blood glucose of >4 mmol/l is obtained.

SEVERE

- Check ABC and correct as necessary.

- Administer IV glucose 10% over 15 minutes (refer to **Glucose 10%** for dosages).

- If IV not possible administer IM glucagon (may take up to 15 minutes to work and IM glucagon ONCE ONLY).

- Re-assess blood glucose level after 10 minutes.

- If blood glucose remains <4.0 mmol/l, administer a further dose of IV 10% glucose.

- Repeat treatment until a blood glucose of >4 mmol/l is obtained.

- If no improvement, convey to nearest suitable receiving hospital.

- Check glucose again if patient deteriorates.

- Provide a pre-alert/information call if necessary.

Blood glucose level should now be 4 mmol/l or above.

- Once a blood glucose of >4 mmol/l is achieved, give a starchy snack, e.g. two biscuits; one slice of bread/toast; 200–300 ml glass of milk (not soya); a normal meal if due (must contain carbohydrate).
- **NB** Patients given glucagon require a larger portion of long-acting carbohydrate to replenish glycogen stores (double the suggested amount above).
- **NB** Patients who self-manage their insulin pumps (CSII) may not need a long-acting carbohydrate.
- In most cases patients who have fully recovered and maintain glucose levels >4 mmol/l will not require admission to ED.

If blood glucose is now >4 mmol/l, follow up treatment as described on the left.

Glucagon may take up to 15 minutes to work and can be ineffective in the very young, older people, undernourished patients or those with hepatic disease.
In patients with renal/cardiac disease, use IV fluids with caution.
Avoid fruit juice in renal failure. **Note:** the carbohydrate content of some commercially available glucose-containing drinks varies – individual product labels should be checked. Diet drinks may not contain sugar.

Figure 3.14 – Hypoglycaemic emergencies algorithm.

Source: http://www.diabetologists-abcd.org.uk/JBDS/JBDS_HypoGuideline_FINAL_280218.pdf.

causes a rise in blood glucose, e.g. steroids, anti-retrovirals.[25] Patients should be advised to see their GP for an HbA1c test to determine their risk of Type 2 diabetes.

- If patients have no symptoms of diabetes yet a capillary glucose of >=11.1 mmol/l, they should be directed to their GP for confirmatory tests for diabetes.

- If patients have typical osmotic symptoms such as excessive thirst, polyuria, tiredness, weight loss, thrush or recurrent infections, with capillary glucose >=11.1 mmol/l, that is diagnostic of diabetes, in which case follow the guidance on hyperglycaemia below.

- The majority of children who develop diabetes have Type 1 diabetes, the diagnosis and treatment of which is a medical emergency. In order to prevent these children developing DKA, prompt diagnosis is necessary as DKA is the principal cause of death in children with diabetes. Clinicians should maintain a high index of suspicion when presented with any generally ill child with a blood glucose >11 mmol/l and convey immediately to ED/Paediatric Assessment Unit (PAU). If blood glucose is 7–10.9 mmol/l, diabetes or hyperglycaemia due to illness should be considered and referred to/discussed with the patient's GP.[26]

- Type 1 diabetes can occur even in infants. These children may have blood glucose levels that are particularly difficult to control and may be very difficult to manage.

5. Diabetic Ketoacidosis (DKA)

- A relative lack of circulating insulin means that cells cannot take up glucose from the blood and use it to provide energy. This forces the cells to provide energy for metabolism from other sources, such as fatty acids.

- Omissions or inadequate dosage of insulin or other hypoglycaemic therapy may also contribute or be responsible. Some medications, particularly steroids, may greatly exacerbate the situation.

- Ketones are produced as a by-product of fatty acid metabolism in the liver. Ketones are acidic chemicals whose accumulation leads to the development of a metabolic acidosis. Ketone production ceases with insulin therapy, which allows the body to convert from fat to its preferred fuel substrate, glucose. Insulin with IV fluids allows the body to stop ketone production and excrete ketones via the urine, which explains why urine ketostix tests remain positive even after DKA has resolved.

- New onset Type 1 diabetes may present with DKA. More frequently it complicates intercurrent illness in a person with diabetes. Infections, myocardial infarction (which may be silent) or a stroke may precipitate the condition.

- Patients may present with one or more signs and symptoms and this should alert the pre-hospital provider to the possibility of hyperglycaemia and DKA (refer to Table 3.58).

- DKA may occur relatively rapidly in children, sometimes without a long history of the classical symptoms. The absolute blood glucose level is not a good indicator of the presence of DKA – some children with blood glucose levels in the >20 range may appear quite well and not have DKA.

- Where available, ketone measurement (blood or urine) is useful in the diagnosis of DKA.

- Patients with diabetes may present with significant dehydration, resulting in reduced fluid in both the vascular and tissue compartments. Often this has taken time to develop and will take time to correct.

- In adults, dehydration is very common in association with DKA and usually requires IV fluid resuscitation in line with intravascular fluid therapy guidelines (**Intravascular Fluid Therapy in Adults** and **Intravascular Fluid Therapy in Children**). Note that rapid fluid replacement into the vascular compartment can compromise the cardiovascular system, particularly where there is pre-existing cardiovascular disease and in the elderly. Gradual rehydration over hours rather than minutes is indicated.

- Children and young adults with DKA may also present with significant dehydration (refer to **Intravascular Fluid Therapy in Children**). Establish IV/IO access at scene, and commence fluids if shocked, giving an initial fluid bolus of 20ml/kg (over 15 minutes) whilst undertaking an urgent transfer and pre-alerting the ED. Further fluid may be required, using smaller volumes (a 10ml/kg bolus), but only after discussion with a senior clinician. When intravenous fluids are felt to be indicated in **NON-SHOCKED** patients with DKA, an initial 10 ml/kg bolus should be given (over 30 minutes).[27,28]

- Do not try to give oral fluids to children with DKA – they have a very high risk of aspiration.

Glycaemic Emergencies in Adults and Children

TABLE 3.58 – Signs and Symptoms of Hyperglycaemia and DKA	
Hyperglycaemia	**Diabetic ketoacidosis**
The symptoms of hyperglycaemia include: ▪ polyuria ▪ polydipsia ▪ weight loss ▪ lethargy ▪ recurrent infections especially thrush ▪ blurred vision ▪ fruity odour of ketones on the breath (resembling nail varnish remover) **NB** Not everyone can detect this odour. ▪ presence of ketones (measured) in the urine and/or blood ▪ hyperventilation	In addition to symptoms of hyperglycaemia, the patient presenting with DKA may also have: ▪ vomiting ▪ abdominal pain ▪ rapid breathing ▪ appear confused ▪ other autoimmune conditions that are more common in Type 1 diabetes, e.g. Addison's disease which can predispose to DKA ▪ dehydration, dry mouth and possible circulatory failure due to hypovolaemia ▪ Kussmaul breathing

The signs of ketoacidosis may include:

▪ A – reduced conscious level/coma – check airway.

▪ B – rapid deep-breathing (Kussmaul respiration).

▪ C – clinically dehydrated with possible circulatory failure due to hypovolaemia.

▪ D – reduced conscious level; check airway is protected. Aspiration may be a risk.

▪ E – appearing thin or exhibiting signs of dramatic weight loss; there may be evidence of diabetes complications, e.g. previous toe/foot amputation or foot ulceration. Consider pregnancy in women of child-bearing age. The fetus is very sensitive to ketosis in the mother.

TABLE 3.59 – ASSESSMENT and MANAGEMENT of: DKA in Adults and Children

Assess ABCD

▪ Start correcting ABC problems (refer to **Medical Emergencies in Adults – Overview** and **Medical Emergencies in Children – Overview**).

▪ Consider giving IV fluids if there is clear evidence of circulatory failure or dehydration (refer to **Intravascular Fluid Therapy in Adults** and **Intravascular Fluid Therapy in Children** and/or **Sodium Chloride 0.9%**).

▪ **DO NOT** delay at scene for fluid replacement.

If the patient is **TIME-CRITICAL:**

▪ Correct life-threatening conditions, airway and breathing on scene.

▪ Then commence transfer to nearest suitable receiving hospital.

▪ **NB** These patients have a potentially life-threatening condition – they require urgent hospital treatment including insulin and fluid/electrolyte therapy.

▪ Consider and look for medical alert/information signs (alert bracelets, chains, tattoos and cards).

Assess Blood Glucose Level

▪ Measure and record blood glucose level.

(continued)

3 Medical Emergencies | SECTION

Glycaemic Emergencies in Adults and Children

TABLE 3.59 – ASSESSMENT and MANAGEMENT of: DKA in Adults and Children *(continued)*

Assess for Signs of Dehydration

- Signs may include:
  - The skin of the forearm remains tented following a gentle pinch, only returning to its normal position slowly.
  - Dry mouth.
- In severe cases this may lead to hypovolaemic shock. If the patient is shocked, with poor capillary refill, tachycardia, reduced Glasgow Coma Score (GCS) and hypotension, then refer to **Intravascular Fluid Therapy in Adults** and **Intravascular Fluid Therapy in Children**.
- **DO NOT** delay at scene for fluid replacement.

Assess Heart Rhythm

- Undertake ECG.

Measure Oxygen Saturation (SpO$_2$)

- Administer supplemental oxygen if the patient is hypoxaemic, SpO$_2$ <94%.
- Refer to **Oxygen**.
- Provide a pre-alert/information call.
- If the patient has records of their blood glucose levels, ensure these accompany the patient.

6. Hyperosmolar Hyperglycaemic State (HHS) – previously Hyperglycaemic Hyperosmotic Non-Ketotic Coma (HONK)

- Hyperosmolar Hyperglycaemic State (HHS) is a complication of Type 2 diabetes and is defined by the presence of high blood glucose (>30 mmol/l), usually without the presence of ketones, with a resultant state of hyperosmolality. HHS patients are often elderly and present with several co-morbidities, but are always seriously ill. As such, HHS is a medical emergency and requires prompt recognition, treatment and urgent transfer to definitive care.

- The change of name from HONK to HHS acknowledges that the majority of patients presenting with this condition are not comatose but may still be seriously ill. It is important to note that these patients may be mildly ketotic.

TABLE 3.60 – Characteristics of and Risk Factors for HHS

Characteristics:	Risk factors:
Type 2 diabetes	Undiagnosed Type 2 diabetes
Hypovolaemia	Infection
Marked hyperglycaemia (>30 mmol/L) without significant hyperketonia or acidosis	Certain medication, in particular recent use of steroids, such as Prednisolone
Severely dehydrated and unwell	Co-existing disease
	Poor management of Type 2 diabetes
	Substance misuse

- While HHS has been commonly diagnosed in older patients, recent prevalence of diagnosis of Type 2 diabetes in both younger adults and children indicates the potential for increased numbers of HHS diagnoses across a broader age range.

6.1 Management

- Patients should undergo urgent transfer to definitive care.

- Patients should be encouraged to drink fluids, if able to tolerate without nausea.

- Consider administering IV 0.9% sodium chloride in line with intravascular fluid therapy guidelines to restore circulating volume and attempt to reverse dehydration (refer to **Intravascular Fluid Therapy in Adults** and **Intravascular Fluid Therapy in Children**). Care should be taken to prevent fluid overload, and risk of cerebral oedema must be considered.

Glycaemic Emergencies in Adults and Children

KEY POINTS!

Glycaemic Emergencies in Adults and Children

- Clean the patient's fingers prior to obtaining a blood glucose reading (using sterile water and gauze swab – rinsing hands thoroughly in tap water is an acceptable alternative).

- Follow the care pathway for managing patients.

- Glucagon may be used intramuscularly to treat hypoglycaemia if treatment with glucose is not possible.

- Patients whose hypoglycaemia is not due to diabetes may not respond well to glucagon.

- If GCS ≤13, consider IM glucagon or 10% IV glucose, refer to Glucose 10% and review patient's condition, titrate to effect.

Further Reading

Further important information and evidence in support of this guideline can be found in the Bibliography.[29,30,31,32,33,34,35,36,37,38,39,40]

Bibliography

1. Hirose T, Mita T, Fujitani Y, Kawamari R, Watada H. Glucose monitoring after fruit peeling: pseudohyperglycemia when neglecting hand washing before fingertip blood sampling. *Journal of Diabetes Care* 2011, 34: 596–597.

2. Ferretti DO, Martin KD. Isopropyl alcohol left on the skin falsely lowers capillary glucose values. *Journal of Clinical Outcomes Management* 2008, 15: 179–181.

3. Rosenstock J, Ferrannini E. Euglycemic diabetic ketoacidosis: a predictable, detectable, and preventable safety concern with SGLT2 inhibitors. *Diabetes Care* 2015, 38(9): 1638–1642.

4. Umpierrez GE, Smiley D, Kitabchi AE. Narrative review: ketosis-prone type 2 diabetes mellitus. *Annals of Internal Medicine* 2006, 144: 350–357.

5. Ng SM, Soni A, Agwu JC, Edge JA, Drew JH et al. *Sick Day Rules*. ACDC Clinical Guideline, version 3, 2015.

6. Driver and Vehicle Licensing Agency. *Diabetes Mellitus: Assessing fitness to drive*. 2016. Available from: https://www.gov.uk/guidance/diabetes-mellitus-assessing-fitness-to-drive.

7. Department for Transport. *Road Traffic*. Statutory Instruments 2017, No. 1208. Available from: http://www.legislation.gov.uk/uksi/2017/1208/pdfs/uksi_20171208_en.pdf.

8. Walden E, Stanisstreet D, Graveling A. *The Hospital Management of Hypoglycaemia in Adults with Diabetes Mellitus* [JBDS Guideline 1b, revised April 2018]. Available from: http://www.diabetologists-abcd.org.uk/JBDS/JBDS_HypoGuideline_Revised_v2_08052018.pdf.

9. Ng SM, Williams E, Ackland F, Burren C, Edge J et al. *Management of Hypoglycaemia in Children and Young People with Type 1 Diabetes*. ACDC Clinical Guideline, version 3, 2016.

10. Joint British Diabetes Societies. *The Hospital Management of Hypoglycaemia in Adults with Diabetes Mellitus*. 3rd edn. 2018. Available from: http://www.diabetologists-abcd.org.uk/JBDS/JBDS_HypoGuideline_Revised_v2_08052018.pdf.

11. Hepburn DA, Deary IJ, Frier BM. Classification of symptoms of hypoglycaemia in insulin-treated diabetic patients using factor analysis: relationship to hypoglycaemia unawareness. *Diabet Med* 1992, 9(1): 70–75.

12. Cox DJ, Gonder-Frederick L, Antoun B, Cryer PE, Clarke WL. Perceived symptoms in the recognition of hypoglycemia. *Diabetes Care* 1993, 16(2): 519–527.

13. Deary IJ, Crawford JR, Hepburn DA, Langan SJ, Blackmore LM, Frier BM. Severe hypoglycemia and intelligence in adult patients with insulin-treated diabetes. *Diabetes* 1993, 42: 341–344.

14. Laffel LMB, Wentzell K, Loughlin C, Tovar A, Moltz K, Brink S. Sick day management using blood 3-hydroxybutyrate (3-OHB) compared with urine ketone monitoring reduces hospital visits in young people with T1DM: a randomized clinical trial. *Diabetic Medicine* 2006, 23(3): 278–284.

15. Eckert-Norton M, Kirk S. Non-diabetic hypoglycaemia. JCEM 2013, 98(10): 39–40.

16. Graveling AJ et al. Impaired awareness of hypoglycaemia: a review. *Diabetes and Metabolism* 36: S64–S74.

17. Frier BM. Impaired awareness of hypoglycaemia. In BM Frier and M Fisher (eds) *Hypoglycaemia in Clinical Diabetes*. Oxford: John Wiley and Sons, 2007: 141–170.

18. Gold AE, Macleod KM, Frier BM. Frequency of severe hypoglycemia in patients with Type I diabetes with impaired awareness of hypoglycaemia. *Diabetes Care* 1994, 17(7): 697–703.

19. Cranston I, Lomas J, Amiel SA, Maran A, Macdonald I. Restoration of hypoglycaemia awareness in patients with long-duration insulin-dependent diabetes. *The Lancet* 1994, 344(8918): 283–287.

20. Dagogo-Jack S, Rattarasarn C, Cryer PE. Reversal of hypoglycaemia unawareness, but not defective glucose counter-regulation, in IDDM. *Diabetes* 1994, 43: 1426–1434.

21. Fanelli C, Pampanelli S, Epifano L, Rambotti AM, Vincenzo A et al. Long-term recovery from unawareness, deficient counterregulation and lack of cognitive dysfunction during hypoglycaemia, following institution of rational, intensive insulin therapy in IDDM. *Diabetologia* 1994, 37: 1265–1267.

Glycaemic Emergencies in Adults and Children

22. Geddes J, Schopman JE, Zammitt NN et al. Prevalence of impaired awareness of hypoglycaemia in adults with Type 1 diabetes. *Diabet Med* 2008, 25: 501–504.

23. Hepburn DA, Patrick AW, Eadington DW et al. Unawareness of hypoglycaemia in insulin-treated diabetic patients: prevalence and relationship to autonomic neuropathy. *Diabet Med* 1990, 7: 711–717.

24. Duncan EAS, Fitzpatrick D, Ikegwuonu T et al. Role and prevalence of impaired awareness of hypoglycaemia in ambulance service attendances to people who have had a severe hypoglycaemic emergency: a mixed-methods study. *BMJ Open* 2018, 8: e019522.

25. Sampson M, Haq M, Hanley S. New diagnosis of diabetes in inpatients [JBDS Guideline 14 – forthcoming]. Available from: https://abcd.care/joint-british-diabetes-societies-jbds-inpatient-care-group.

26. South West Paediatric Diabetes Network. *Referral and Ongoing Care for Children with Suspected Diabetes.* 2014. Available from: http://rms.kernowccg.nhs.uk/content/Referral%20and%20Ongoing%20Care%20for%20Children%20with%20suspected%20Diabetes.pdf.

27. Glaser N, Kuppermann N. Fluid treatment for children with diabetic ketoacidosis. *Paediatric Diabetes* 2019, 20: 10–14.

28. British Society for Paediatric Endocrinology and Diabetes. BSPED Interim Guideline for the Management of Children under the age of 18 years with Diabetic Ketoacidosis. 2020. Available from: https://www.bsped.org.uk/media/1745/bsped-dka-guidelines-no-dka-link.pdf.

29. National Institute for Health and Care Excellence. *Diagnosis and Management of Type 1 Diabetes in Children, Young People and Adults* [CG15]. London: NICE, 2004. Available from: https://www.nice.org.uk/guidance/cg15.

30. National Institute for Health and Care Excellence. *Diabetes in Pregnancy: Management from pre-conception to the postnatal period* [NG3]. London: NICE, 2015. Available from: https://www.nice.org.uk/guidance/ng3.

31. National Institute for Health and Care Excellence. *Diabetes (Type 1 and Type 2) in Children and Young People: Diagnosis and management* [NG18]. London: NICE, 2015. Available from: https://www.nice.org.uk/guidance/ng18.

32. National Institute for Health and Care Excellence. *Type 2 Diabetes in Adults: Management* [NG28]. London: NICE, 2015. Available from: https://www.nice.org.uk/guidance/ng28.

33. BCT Field, R Nayar, A Kilvert, M Baxter, J Hickey et al. A retrospective observational study of people with Type 1 diabetes with self-reported severe hypoglycaemia reveals high level of ambulance attendance but low levels of therapy change and specialist intervention. *Diabet Med* 2018. Available from: https://onlinelibrary.wiley.com/doi/pdf/10.1111/dme.13670.

34. Welsh Government. *Diabetes Delivery Plan for Wales 2016–2020.* Available from: https://gov.wales/topics/health/nhswales/plans/diabetes/?lang=en.

35. National Institute for Health and Care Excellence. *Sepsis: Recognition, diagnosis and early management* [NG51]. London: NICE, 2016. Available from: https://www.nice.org.uk/guidance/ng51.

36. National Institute for Health and Care Excellence. *Fever in Under 5s: Assessment and initial management* [CG160]. London: NICE, 2017. Available from: https://www.nice.org.uk/guidance/cg160.

37. Royal College of Paediatrics and Child Health. *National Paediatric Diabetes Audit Report 2015–16.* Available from: https://www.rcpch.ac.uk/work-we-do/quality-improvement-patient-safety/national-paediatrics-diabetes-audit.

38. Diabetes UK. *Do You Know the 4 Ts of Type 1 Diabetes?* Available from: https://www.diabetes.org.uk/Get_involved/Campaigning/4-Ts-campaign.

39. Joint British Diabetes Societies Inpatient Care Group. *The Management of the Hyperosmolar Hyperglycaemic State (HHS) in Adults with Diabetes.* 2012. Available from: http://www.diabetologists-abcd.org.uk/JBDS/JBDS_IP_HHS_Adults.pdf.

40. Stoner GD. Hyperosmolar hyperglycemic state. *Am Fam Physician* 171(9): 1723–1730.

Headache

1. Introduction

- Headache disorders are among the most common disorders of the nervous system and are a feature of both minor and major illness, which can prove challenging for a clinician.

- Most headaches are simple and not serious, but care must be taken to ensure that **TIME-CRITICAL** conditions are not missed.

- A detailed history is vital when dealing with headache, as the aetiology may go back hours, days, months or even years in relation to family history or childhood illness, e.g. tumours.

2. Incidence

- More than 10 million people in the UK suffer from headaches. Most headaches are not serious and can be treated with over-the-counter medicines and lifestyle changes such as getting more rest and drinking enough fluids. However, there are red flags in both history and examination that may indicate more concerning causes.

- The severity of headaches varies from patient to patient in terms of the pain the patient experiences. Although the pain may be the primary concern of the patient, it may not be associated with the severity of the underlying cause.

- The outcome for a patient presenting to ambulance services for headache will be as varied as the cause of the headache: the clinical significance of the headache and the progression are all dependent on the presenting factors.

3. Types of Headache

- Headaches can be broadly defined as primary or secondary:
  - **Primary headaches** are those which occur spontaneously (simple headaches); occur in response to a lifelong condition (e.g. migraines); are 'tension-type' headaches (various aetiologies); or are severe, short-lasting headaches (cluster headaches). These should not be considered as being pathophysiological as that is normal for the patient.
  - **Secondary headaches** are secondary to illness or injury and are pathological in origin, for instance head trauma (skull fracture); infective origin (i.e. meningitis); intracranial haemorrhage (i.e. spontaneous subarachnoid bleed or subdural bleed following trauma); or vascular (i.e. temporal arteritis).

- It is difficult to accurately differentiate between a simple headache, which requires no treatment, and a potentially more serious condition. Table 3.61 lists **'red flag'** symptoms that require the patient to undergo hospital assessment. **NB** This does not mean that any patient presenting without these symptoms is safe to be left at home.

- Consideration should be given to transferring all first presentations of severe headache to the emergency department for further investigation.

TABLE 3.61 – Red Flag Signs and Symptoms

⚑ Headache localised to the vertex, i.e. top of the head.

⚑ Escalating headache of an unusual nature.

⚑ Changed visual acuity.

⚑ Meningeal irritation, i.e. neck stiffness and photophobia.

⚑ Cranial nerve palsy.

⚑ Worsening headache with fever.

⚑ Sudden-onset or thunderclap headache reaching maximum intensity within 5 minutes.

⚑ New-onset neurological deficit, i.e. loss of function or altered sensation.

⚑ New-onset cognitive dysfunction.

⚑ Change in personality.

⚑ Impaired level of consciousness.

⚑ Recent head trauma, typically within the past three months.

⚑ Headache triggered by cough, Valsalva (trying to breathe out with nose and mouth blocked) or sneeze.

⚑ Headache triggered by exercise.

⚑ Orthostatic headache, i.e. a headache that changes with posture.

⚑ Symptoms suggestive of giant cell arteritis, which could include pain and tenderness over the temples, jaw pain while eating or talking and vision problems.

⚑ Symptoms and signs of acute narrow-angle glaucoma, i.e. red eye.

⚑ A substantial change in the characteristics of the headache.

⚑ Vomiting without other obvious cause.

⚑ Newly presenting ataxia, i.e. a neurological sign consisting of a lack of voluntary coordination of muscle movements.

⚑ Any evidence of a rash.

3.1 Migraine

- A migraine is a severe headache felt as a throbbing pain that is usually unilateral and frontal, often accompanied by nausea and vomiting. Some people also have other symptoms, such as sensitivity to light. Migraine is a common health condition, affecting about 15% of adults in the UK.

Headache

- There are several types of migraine, including:
  - **Migraine with aura**: this has the presence of a warning sign, known as an aura, before the migraine begins. About a third of people with a migraine have this. Warning signs may include visual problems such as flashing lights; stiffness in the neck, shoulders or limbs; or occasionally limb weakness or altered limb sensations. The migraine with aura may appear like a transient ischaemic attack (TIA) or stroke — great care is needed to differentiate between the two diagnoses; if there is any doubt, treat this as a TIA/stroke.
  - **Migraine without aura**: this is a headache without the signs and symptoms of an aura listed above.
  - **Migraine without headache**: also known as a silent migraine, this is when an aura or other migraine symptoms are experienced in the absence of a headache. Particular attention should be paid to this condition, as the symptoms can clearly mimic those of other conditions such as a TIA. If in any doubt, treat as a TIA/stroke.

- Migraines affect 1 in 4 women and 1 in 12 men in the UK. Some women find that migraine attacks are more frequent around the time of their menstruation, although this association has not been proven. Migraines usually begin in young adults. About 9 in 10 have their first migraine before they are 40 years old, although it is possible for migraines to begin later in life.

- Everyone will experience migraines differently. Some people have attacks frequently, up to several times a week. Other people only have a migraine occasionally and it is possible for years to pass between migraine attacks. Sometimes migraine attacks are associated with certain triggers, such as stress and certain foods.

3.2 Tension-type Headaches

- Tension-type headaches are the most common type of headache and the ones we think of as normal, everyday headaches. Most people are likely to have experienced them at some point. Up to 70% of the whole population will experience a tension headache during their lifetime; however, they are most prevalent up to the age of 30.

- Tension-type headaches may feel like a constant ache that affects both sides of the head and is often frontal. Patients may also complain of their neck muscles tightening and a feeling of pressure behind the eyes. The headaches usually last for 1 to 6 hours, but some people may have more persistent headaches that last for several days.

- Tension-type or chronic daily headaches can be caused by medication overuse or withdrawal. These should be considered to be secondary headaches.

- A tension-type headache is the most common symptom of mild carbon monoxide poisoning. Refer to **Overdose and Poisoning in Adults and Children**.

3.2.1 Medication-overuse Headaches

- Be alert to the possibility of medication-overuse headache in people whose headache developed or worsened while they were taking the following drugs for 3 months or more:
  - Triptans, opioids, ergots or combination analgesic medications on 10 days per month or more.
  - Paracetamol, aspirin or an NSAID, either alone or in any combination, on 15 days per month or more.

- The body gets used to the painkillers that are being taken. A rebound headache develops, particularly if patients have not taken a painkiller within a day or so of the last dose. Patients assume that they are suffering from a further tension headache or migraine and take a further dose of painkiller. When the effect of the painkiller wears off, another rebound headache develops and the cycle continues. Patients may start to take painkillers every day as a prophylactic measure to prevent headaches, which can further compound the problem.

3.3 Cluster Headaches

- Cluster headaches are excruciating attacks of pain in one side of the head, often felt behind the eye. Sufferers often call them 'suicidal headaches' because they are so severe. Cluster headaches begin unexpectedly and they are much more painful than migraines or any other type of headache.

- They are called cluster headaches because sufferers usually get one to three of the attacks every day, for several weeks or months, before they subside. A pain-free period will follow, which sometimes lasts months or years, before the headache attacks start again.

- Each cluster headache lasts between 15 minutes and 3 hours, but often less than 1 hour. They may start in the early hours of the morning and wake the person from sleep. Because of the intensity of the pain, some people will pace the room, rock or may even bang their head against the wall out of frustration, restlessness and despair.

- There are two types of cluster headaches:
  - **Episodic headache clusters** are separated by headache-free periods of 1 month or more.
  - **Chronic headache clusters** are separated by headache-free periods of less than 1 month, or are not separated at all. About 10% of cluster headache cases are chronic.

- Cluster headaches are rare and affect around 1 in 1,000 people. Anyone can be affected, but

Headache

approximately 80% of sufferers are male and most are smokers. It is not known what causes cluster headaches, but they are more common in autumn and spring. In some people, an attack can be triggered by drinking alcohol or an extreme increase in temperature, such as from exercising in hot weather.

3.4 Subarachnoid Haemorrhage

- Subarachnoid haemorrhage (SAH) is usually the result of bleeding from an aneurysm. It was previously thought to be mostly congenital but the cause is now considered to vary from genetic malformations of the elastic lamina to stressors such as hypertension and atherosclerosis.

- SAH affects 6–12 people per 100,000 of the population per year and constitutes about 6% of first strokes. Although SAH represents a small proportion of strokes, it tends to affect younger people, of whom about half die due to the episode.

- Risk factors include hypertension, smoking and excessive alcohol; however, the bigger the aneurysm, the more likely it is to bleed.

- The most characteristic feature is a sudden headache. This may last a few seconds or even a fraction of a second. Patients may even look round and accuse someone of hitting them on the back of the head.

- SAH should be considered in any patients presenting with sudden-onset, severe and unusual headache with or without any associated alteration in consciousness:
  - The headache is often diffuse.
  - The dominant feature is the severity, rather than the suddenness, of the headache, often being described as the most severe ever experienced.
  - It may last a week or 2.
  - Vomiting may occur; however, this does not distinguish it from other causes of headache.
  - Seizures occur in only about 7% of patients but, when they do, they are highly suggestive of a haemorrhage.

4. Assessment and Management

- For the assessment and management of headaches, refer to Table 3.62.

TABLE 3.62 – ASSESSMENT and MANAGEMENT of: Headache

Assess <C>ABCD

- Start correcting any <C>ABCD problems (refer to **Medical Emergencies in Adults – Overview** and **Medical Emergencies in Children – Overview**).

- Exclude the following or refer to the specific guidelines for:
  - **Stroke/Transient Ischaemic Attack**
  - **Head Injury**
  - **Glycaemic Emergencies in Adults and Children.**

- Consider carbon monoxide poisoning (refer to **Overdose and Poisoning in Adults and Children**).

Levels of Consciousness

- Assess AVPU:
  - **A** — Alert
  - **V** — Responds to voice
  - **P** — Responds to painful stimulus
  - **U** — Unresponsive.

- **NB** The only normal GCS is 15.

Respiratory Rate

- Measure and record respiratory rate.

Pulse

- Measure and record pulse.

Oxygen Saturation

- Monitor the patient's SpO_2; administer oxygen to achieve saturations of >94% if the patient presents as hypoxemic on air; refer to **Oxygen**.

Blood Pressure and Fluids

- Measure and record blood pressure; if required, administer fluids (refer to **Intravascular Fluid Therapy in Adults** and **Intravascular Fluid Therapy in Children**).

(continued)

Headache

TABLE 3.62 – ASSESSMENT and MANAGEMENT of: Headache *(continued)*
Blood Glucose
▪ If appropriate, measure and record blood glucose for hypo/hyperglycaemia (refer to **Glycaemic Emergencies in Adults and Children**).
Temperature
▪ Measure and record temperature.
NEWS2
▪ These observations will enable you to calculate a NEWS2 score (refer to **Sepsis**).
Record Pain Score
▪ Assess the **SOCRATES** of the pain: – **S**ite — where exactly is the pain?   – **O**nset — what was the patient doing when the pain came on?   – **C**haracter — what does the pain feel like?   – **R**adiates — where does the pain spread to?   – **A**ssociated symptoms — e.g. nausea, dizziness.   – **T**iming — how long has the patient had pain?   – **E**xacerbating/relieving factors — what makes it better or worse?   – **S**everity — obtain an initial pain score.
▪ Offer symptomatic pain relief for clinically benign headaches, using appropriate pain management drug therapy and taking into account the patient's preference, comorbidities and risk of adverse events.
▪ Consideration should therefore be given to initial management with NSAID and/or paracetamol, combined with onward referral for consideration of additional therapies, such as anti-emetics and triptans, EXCEPT in cluster headaches where paracetamol, NSAIDs, opioids, ergots or oral triptans should NOT be offered for the acute treatment. In this instance, the patient should be referred to their GP for onward management. Beware of making the diagnosis of cluster headaches, as it is very rare and other serious conditions may present in this way.
▪ Where medication overuse is the cause, advise the patient to stop taking all overused acute headache medication and to see their GP. It is best to stop abruptly rather than gradually. It is important to note that headache symptoms are likely to get worse in the short term before they improve and that there may be associated withdrawal symptoms.
▪ Avoid morphine due to potential side effects, which could worsen the patient's condition and/or hinder further assessment.
Key Questions for a Patient with Headache
▪ Is this the worst headache ever?
▪ Is it different from your usual headache?
▪ Is this a new headache?
Assess for Red Flag Symptoms (refer to Table 3.61)
▪ Multiple red flags significantly increase the risk of serious pathology.
▪ Undertake a TIME-CRITICAL transfer to the nearest suitable receiving hospital.
▪ Provide an alert or information call.
Documentation
▪ Complete documentation to include all clinical findings, advice from other clinicians, onward referral and worsening advice given.

▪ Patients may deteriorate rapidly if they have a space-occupying condition, e.g. a haemorrhage resulting in a mass effect.

▪ Clinicians must ensure that patients receive the safest pathway of care. It is always better to be cautious, especially in children and those patients who are on their own.

▪ **NB** Where patients are not conveyed, follow-up care **MUST** be arranged. Always liaise with the patient's GP (or out-of-hours doctor) to discuss onward care. Ensure that, where practicable, patients are not left alone while awaiting follow-up.

SECTION **3** Medical Emergencies

Headache

Headache

- It is preferable to be cautious when dealing with patients with headaches, as diagnosis can be challenging.

- Headaches with different or unusual characteristics are significant.

- Sufferers of migraines are at risk of serious intracranial events.

- With headache, blood pressure must be checked.

- Any headache is significant if it is persistent or if it is associated with altered conscious levels or unusual behaviour.

- Sinister headaches may or may not be accompanied by neurology. Do not exclude simply based on physical examination — HISTORY IS KEY.

- A tension-type headache is the most common symptom of mild carbon monoxide poisoning.

Bibliography

1. NHS Evidence. *Headache Assessment/Management: How Should I Assess Someone Presenting with a Headache?* Clinical Knowledge Summaries. London: NHS Evidence, 2010.

2. Scottish Intercollegiate Guidelines Network. *Diagnosis and Management of Headache in Adults* (Guideline 107). Edinburgh: SIGN, 2008. Available from: http://www.sign.ac.uk/assets/sign107.pdf.

3. The Headache Classification Subcommittee of the International Headache Society. *The International Classification of Headache Disorders.* 2nd edn. (ICHD-II). 1st revision. The International Headache Society, 2005.

4. World Health Organization. *Headache Disorders* (Fact sheet 277). Available from: http://www.who.int/mediacentre/factsheets/fs277/en, 2004.

Heart Failure

1. Introduction

- Heart failure is not a specific disease entity; rather, it is a clinical syndrome characterised by several clinical signs, symptoms and diagnostic findings. Heart failure is caused by a structural or functional cardiac abnormality, resulting in a reduced cardiac output and/or increased intra-cardiac pressures. The most common cause of heart failure in the UK is coronary artery disease, and many patients have had a myocardial infarction in their past medical history. Heart failure can also be caused by abnormalities of the valves, pericardium, endocardium, heart rhythm and conduction system.[1]

- It is important to recognise that heart failure is a long-term condition and many people live in the community with **chronic heart failure**, which is a generic term that means they have already been diagnosed with heart failure and are receiving treatment. People may develop **acute on chronic heart failure** (decompensated) if they already have a diagnosis of heart failure but develop worsening symptoms quite quickly, despite treatment.

- **Acute heart failure** may therefore represent a decompensation of stable chronic heart failure or may be the patient's first presentation of symptoms. As part of clinical history-taking, you may find the patient has had some preceding dyspnoea; they may also have chest pain and acute coronary syndrome or/and arrhythmias such as atrial fibrillation (refer to **Acute Coronary Syndrome**).

- Acute heart failure can present in three major forms:
  - **Acute pulmonary oedema**. This is the sudden development of interstitial oedema in the lungs with severe dyspnoea, with or without peripheral oedema. It may come on very suddenly or patients may have had some dyspnoea for weeks or days that suddenly worsens.
  - **Predominant peripheral oedema with or without pulmonary oedema**. The patient may have significant fluid-loading, with swollen legs, abdomen and scrotum, as well as elevated jugular venous pressure (JVP) and pleural effusions.
  - **Cardiogenic shock**. This is rare and occurs in 5–8% of cases of acute heart failure. The commonest cause in a new presentation of heart failure is STEMI, but this may be a decompensation of advanced chronic heart failure. These cases require rapid treatment.

- Patients with an existing diagnosis of heart failure may be known to or be currently under the care of a specialist multidisciplinary heart failure team. The team may include services such as rehabilitation, tertiary care, palliative care and community nursing care. Patients may have a personal, anticipatory care plan that details what should happen if their condition deteriorates.

- Heart failure patients in the palliative phase of their illness may develop decompensated heart failure, and it is important to refer to any palliative plans or pathways in place, including any DNACPR or ReSPECT forms. This is to ensure the patient's and/or their family's and carers' wishes are adhered to in an emergency.

- Acute heart failure is a life-threatening medical condition, so for all new cases and all chronic cases, unless there is an advanced care plan/palliative management in place, a TIME-CRITICAL transfer to hospital is required for urgent assessment and treatment, ideally at a hospital that has a coronary care unit.

1.1 Terminology

- There are many different terms and acronyms related to heart failure and some of them mean the same thing. Some terms are older and tend not to be referred to as often, but you may still see or hear them used.

- Some important terms are:
  - **Ejection fraction (EF):** The percentage of blood ejected by the ventricles relative to its filled volume.
  - **HFrEF:** Heart failure with reduced ejection fraction which is also referred to as LVSD – left ventricular systolic dysfunction. This is heart failure with an ejection fraction of <40%. There is reduced contractility of the left ventricle, so the heart is not able to pump blood around the body efficiently. Diagnosis is via an echocardiogram.
  - **LVSD:** Left ventricular systolic dysfunction, see also HFrEF above. This can be mild, moderate or severely impaired and is diagnosed usually on echocardiogram or MRI.
  - **HFpEF:** Heart failure with preserved ejection fraction, previously known as diastolic dysfunction. This is where on echocardiography the left ventricle is pumping well but it may have a problem relaxing and filling up with blood. The ejection fraction is ≥50%.
  - **HFmrEF:** Heart failure with a mid-ranged ejection fraction of 40–49%. This group of patients is in a 'grey area' and has elements of systolic and diastolic dysfunction.
  - **CCF:** Congestive cardiac failure. This is now an old-fashioned term and relates to people with both pulmonary and peripheral oedema. It involves the left and right ventricle.
  - **LVF:** Left ventricular failure. These patients tend to be breathless on exertion and may have signs of pulmonary oedema, including bi-basal crepitations on chest auscultation.

Heart Failure

They may also have signs of right-sided heart failure.

- **RVF:** Right ventricular failure. These cases have symptoms such as significant peripheral oedema, ascites, elevated JVP and pleural effusions. The lungs are often clear to auscultation.
- **De novo heart failure:** A term for the first presentation of heart failure. There has been no previous history or diagnosis of heart failure.
- **Cor pulmonale:** These cases have symptoms and signs of predominantly right heart failure but are primarily caused by chronic lung disease.

2. Incidence

Around 900,000 people in the UK have heart failure. It is estimated that there is also a similar number of patients with impaired heart function that have not yet been diagnosed with heart failure. Both the incidence and prevalence of heart failure increase steeply with age, with the average age at first diagnosis being 76 years. The prevalence of heart failure is expected to rise in the future as a result of an ageing population, improved survival of people with ischaemic heart disease and more effective treatments for heart failure.[2,3]

3. Severity and Outcome

- Acute heart failure carries an inpatient mortality of around 10%. In the long term, 27% of community heart failure patients are alive after 10 years.

4. Pathophysiology

- In HFrEF, reduced ejection fraction increases preload and results in left ventricular dilation to maintain stroke volume. This mechanism cannot be sustained, and ventricular remodelling occurs, reducing cardiac output.

- The signs and symptoms generated can be grouped together depending on whether the left or right side of the heart is involved. Left ventricular failure is the most common and most frequently caused by a previous myocardial infarction. Poor ventricular contraction occurs, and blood backs up into the lungs. This increases pulmonary vein hydrostatic pressure and subsequently causes fluid to enter the alveoli, seen as pulmonary oedema. The presence of this fluid causes a reduction in gas exchange (refer to Figure 3.15).

- Right heart failure is primarily caused by left heart failure but can also be caused in isolation by lung disease, such as COPD or pulmonary embolism as well as valvular disease. An increase in pressure in the pulmonary vasculature causes an increase in right ventricular afterload, resulting in ventricular hypertrophy, and subsequently leads to progressive dilation and eventual failure.

- This mechanism gives rise to the common signs and symptoms seen in a right-sided pathology – raised JVP, hepatomegaly, ascites and significant peripheral oedema.

4.1 Factors Triggering Acute Heart Failure

- An identifiable trigger/s causing the acute decompensation of heart failure can be found in two-thirds of cases. This is relevant as you may need to address two or more acute conditions at once. Some triggers, such as ischaemia and pneumonia, are associated with increased mortality risk. The commonest triggers are:
  - myocardial infarction
  - acute coronary syndrome
  - tachyarrhythmia, e.g. atrial fibrillation or ventricular tachycardia
  - infection, e.g. pneumonia, infective endocarditis or sepsis
  - excessive rise in blood pressure
  - non-adherence to medications
  - bradyarrhythmia
  - toxic substances, e.g. alcohol or recreational drugs
  - drugs, e.g. NSAIDs, corticosteroids, negative inotropic substances or cardiotoxic chemotherapeutics
  - exacerbation of chronic obstructive pulmonary disease
  - pulmonary embolism.

- Chest trauma, cardiac intervention, acute native or prosthetic valve incompetence secondary to endocarditis, aortic dissection or thrombosis are also causes.

5. Assessment and Management

- It can be difficult to differentiate heart failure from other causes of breathlessness, such as exacerbation of COPD, pulmonary embolism or pneumonia. Acute heart failure is frequently mistaken for sepsis as both can present with collapse and hypotension. If the patient has a history of heart failure or valve disease, STOP and THINK before administering intravenous fluids, as these can be harmful, especially if given quickly and in large amounts. A thorough history and physical examination of the patient is required. Assessment should focus on signs and symptoms associated with heart failure.

- Red flag indicators for heart failure are:
  - **Orthopnoea:** increased breathlessness on lying down. The patient may have slept in the chair on preceding nights.
  - **Paroxysmal nocturnal dyspnoea (PND):** waking up at night short of breath and relieved by sitting up.

Heart Failure

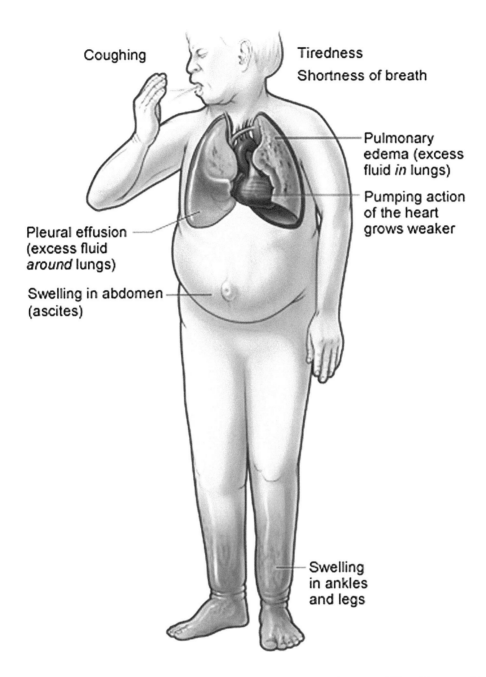

Coughing

Tiredness
Shortness of breath

Pulmonary edema (excess fluid *in* lungs)

Pumping action of the heart grows weaker

Pleural effusion (excess fluid *around* lungs)

Swelling in abdomen (ascites)

Swelling in ankles and legs

Figure 3.15 – Signs and symptoms of heart failure. Source: National Heart, Lung, and Blood Institute; National Institutes of Health; U.S. Department of Health and Human Services. Available from: https://www.nhlbi.nih.gov/health-topics/heart-failure.

- **New dyspnoea** with a past history of myocardial infarction/hypertension/angina.
- **New peripheral oedema**, accompanied by dyspnoea.
- **Coughing up pink frothy sputum**.

Patients with an existing diagnosis of chronic heart failure may be known to or be currently under the care of a specialist multidisciplinary heart failure team. These teams often know the patients well and can offer advice on treatment. If the patient is sufficiently stable and there is time to do so, contact the team for advice. Not

all chronic heart failure patients are palliative, and the majority should still be managed actively and conveyed to hospital. Good care plans, if available, should help decisions around need for conveyance to hospital.

Patients with advanced disease may have a personal or anticipatory care plan/end of life plan in place. This may be available by contacting a locally agreed directory of service or may be accessible electronically. For these patients, try to follow the care plan or contact the team for advice before admission. Following the care plan may involve assisting or instructing

Heart Failure

patients to take prescribed anticipatory medications such as extra oral diuretics, i.e. furosemide, bumetanide, bendroflumethiazide or metolazone, or taking the next dose early, in conjunction with a care plan/contact with the community team.

■ Currently, many more heart failure patients who are palliative or at the end of their life are cared for at home in their final days with the express wish to remain at home. Consider end of life plans and refer to **End of Life Care**.

■ Some patients with advanced heart failure may have a left ventricular assist device (LVAD), a mechanical pump that is implanted inside a person's chest to augment the weakened heart (refer to **Management and Resuscitation of Patients with Left Ventricular Assist Devices (LVADs)**).

■ Assessment and management of acute heart failure should focus on identifying the underlying cause, stabilisation and transport to the most appropriate facility (refer to Table 3.63 and Figure 3.16).

■ If conveyance to hospital is necessary, the patient should be conveyed rapidly to the most appropriate receiving hospital as per local pathways, preferably to a site with a cardiology department and/or CCU/ICU. Recent data suggest that acute heart failure might have a 'time-to-therapy' concept. Accordingly, pre-hospital management is considered a critical component of care. Many patients with acute heart failure have normal or high blood pressure at presentation and are admitted with symptoms and/or signs of congestion. This is quite unlike cardiogenic shock where low cardiac output leads to symptomatic hypotension and signs/symptoms of hypoperfusion, a circumstance that is relatively rare and associated with a particularly poor outcome. Therefore, it is important to note that appropriate therapy requires appropriate identification of the specific acute heart failure presentation. Caution must be noted regarding giving IV fluids for heart failure.

■ It is accepted that the diagnosis of acute heart failure is difficult, especially in the pre-hospital setting, and it is recognised that where doubt exists as to whether the condition is exacerbation of COPD rather than acute heart failure, administration of salbutamol may be considered (refer to **Dyspnoea** and **Medical Emergencies in Adults – Overview**).

TABLE 3.63 – ASSESSMENT and MANAGEMENT of: Acute Heart Failure
Assess <C>ABCD
■ Start correcting <C>ABC problems (refer to **Medical Emergencies in Adults – Overview**).
■ If the patient is **TIME-CRITICAL**:
– Correct life-threatening conditions, airway and breathing on scene.
– Then commence transfer to the nearest suitable receiving hospital.
– If the patient is in the palliative care stage, refer to their end of life pathway or anticipatory care plans and medicines. Be aware that a number of heart failure patients will have community DNACPR forms. Ask if the patient has an active DNACPR form.
– If the patient is stable and known to community heart failure services, consider contacting them for advice.
History
■ Document history and review any existing care plans for:
– HF diagnosis
– SOB/SOBOE
– chest pain
– COPD/asthma
– orthopnoea
– paroxysmal nocturnal dyspnoea.
Examination
■ Examine:
– heart rate
– blood pressure
– respiratory rate
– SpO_2

(continued)

Heart Failure

TABLE 3.63 – ASSESSMENT and MANAGEMENT of: Acute Heart Failure *(continued)*

- – oedema
- – auscultation.
- Non-invasive monitoring, including pulse oximetry, blood pressure, respiratory rate and a continuous ECG, should be instituted within minutes of patient contact and continued during transport to hospital.

Clinical Indicators of Potential Heart Failure

- Symptoms include dyspnoea, worsening cough, waking at night gasping for breath, breathlessness on lying down and anxiousness/restlessness.
- Fine crackling sounds (rales) are suggestive of pulmonary oedema, commonly heard in the lung bases, but may be heard over other lung fields as well. These crackles are often accompanied by expiratory wheeze.
- Coughing up of frothy sputum, white or pink (blood stained) in colour in decompensated heart failure.
- Although peripheral oedema is a common sign of heart failure, it is not specific to heart failure and may be a consequence of numerous pathologies. Peripheral oedema starts at the feet and extends up the body as the condition progresses. The patient may also have abdominal ascites and pleural effusion. People with venous insufficiency, obesity or lymphoedema may have chronic oedema.
- JVP provides an estimation of right atrial filling pressure as there are no valves between the right atrium and the internal jugular vein. It is accepted that assessment of JVP can be challenging, particularly in the pre-hospital environment. Assessment of JVP may be undertaken but should not delay treatment.

Oxygen

- Oxygen therapy is recommended for patients with acute heart failure.
- Target saturations 94–98%.
- Administer the initial oxygen dose until a reliable SpO_2 measurement is available, then adjust oxygen flow to aim for a target saturation within the range of 94–98% (refer to **Oxygen**).
- For all patients, sit the patient fully upright immediately. Doing so lowers left atrial pressure, the driving pressure for pulmonary oedema. Sitting the patient fully upright also reduces the abdominal pressure on the bases of the lungs by lowering the diaphragm and enables the patient to use accessory muscles fully. The importance of positioning cannot be overstated. The patient may be nearing exhaustion and will slump quickly so may need repositioning repeatedly during transfer to hospital.

ECG

- Record a 12-lead ECG.
- It is rare for patients with heart failure to have a normal ECG. Where no ECG abnormalities are identified, clinicians should consider the possibility of an alternative diagnosis.
- Where the ECG indicates that heart failure may be due to acute coronary syndrome, refer to **Acute Coronary Syndrome**.

SECTION 3 Medical Emergencies

Heart Failure

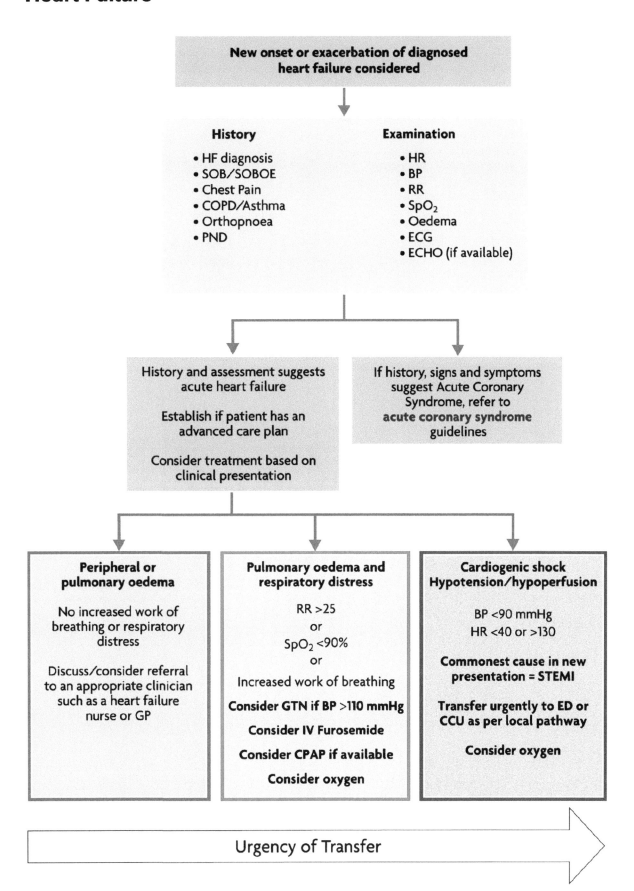

New onset or exacerbation of diagnosed heart failure considered

History
- HF diagnosis
- SOB/SOBOE
- Chest Pain
- COPD/Asthma
- Orthopnoea
- PND

Examination
- HR
- BP
- RR
- SpO$_2$
- Oedema
- ECG
- ECHO (if available)

History and assessment suggests acute heart failure

Establish if patient has an advanced care plan

Consider treatment based on clinical presentation

If history, signs and symptoms suggest Acute Coronary Syndrome, refer to **acute coronary syndrome guidelines**

Peripheral or pulmonary oedema

No increased work of breathing or respiratory distress

Discuss/consider referral to an appropriate clinician such as a heart failure nurse or GP

Pulmonary oedema and respiratory distress

RR >25
or
SpO$_2$ <90%
or
Increased work of breathing

Consider GTN if BP >110 mmHg

Consider IV Furosemide

Consider CPAP if available

Consider oxygen

Cardiogenic shock Hypotension/hypoperfusion

BP <90 mmHg
HR <40 or >130

Commonest cause in new presentation = STEMI

Transfer urgently to ED or CCU as per local pathway

Consider oxygen

Urgency of Transfer

Figure 3.16 – Heart failure algorithm.

Heart Failure

6. Therapies in Heart Failure

6.1 GTN

- Vasodilators are frequently used in heart failure for symptomatic relief; however, there is no robust evidence confirming their beneficial effects. They have dual theoretical benefit by decreasing venous tone (to optimise preload) and arterial tone (to decrease afterload). Consequently, they may also increase stroke volume. Vasodilators are especially useful in patients with hypertensive acute heart failure, whereas in patients with systolic BP <110 mmHg (or with symptomatic hypotension) they should be avoided. Vasodilators should be used with caution in patients with significant aortic stenosis.

6.2 Furosemide

- Furosemide has been the cornerstone of treatment of patients with both acute heart failure and chronic heart failure and signs of fluid overload and congestion for many years. Although there is little high-level evidence for or against its use to improve long-term mortality, it is required for symptomatic benefit. Diuretics increase renal salt and water excretion and have some vasodilatory effect. Initially, 40 milligrams of intravenous furosemide can be considered in acute heart failure patients, excluding cardiogenic shock. If the patient has chronic heart failure, consider reviewing the patient's care plan or contacting the local team/pathway. If the patient requires active management, do not delay conveyance to hospital. Depending on the severity of symptoms, the care plan may advise giving a short-term increase in oral diuretic therapy, particularly if not conveying to hospital.

6.3 Morphine

- Analysis of large heart failure registries suggests that the use of opiates in heart failure increases mortality. Therefore, opiates should not routinely be used but should be considered if the patient is complaining of chest pain. Patients with advanced heart failure under the care of a palliative care team may also have morphine listed as part of their routine care plan (refer to **End of Life Care**).

6.4 Continuous Positive Pressure Ventilation

- Continuous positive pressure ventilation (CPAP), if available, should be considered in patients with respiratory distress (respiratory rate >25 breaths/min, SpO_2 <90%) and started as soon as possible to decrease respiratory distress and reduce the rate of mechanical endotracheal intubation. With CPAP therapy, pressure remains constant through the inspiratory and expiratory phases.

- Prospective randomised controlled trials have demonstrated that CPAP improves survival to hospital discharge and decreases intubation rates.

- A systematic review of eight pre-hospital randomised trials of CPAP and BiPAP suggested that CPAP is the most effective treatment in terms of mortality and intubation rate compared to standard care. The effect of BiPAP on mortality and intubation rate was uncertain.

- The objective of non-invasive positive pressure ventilation (CPAP) is two-fold. The first is to 'splint' open collapsing alveoli and increase intra-alveolar pressure. The increase in pressure helps shift fluid present in the alveoli back into the pulmonary capillaries, thereby reducing pulmonary oedema. The second is to raise intrathoracic pressure throughout the respiratory cycle. This increase in intrathoracic pressure increases pressure in the vena cavae, and consequently serves to reduce filling pressures. Combined, these two actions reduce congestion.

Heart Failure

Heart Failure

- Acute heart failure is a life-threatening medical condition. For all new cases and all chronic cases, unless there is an advanced care plan or palliative management in place, a TIME-CRITICAL transfer to hospital is required for urgent assessment and treatment, ideally at a hospital that has a coronary care unit.

- If the patient has a history of heart failure or valve disease, STOP and THINK before administering intravenous fluids, as these can be harmful, especially if given quickly and in large amounts.

- Consider administering furosemide and/or GTN.

- In patients with systolic BP <110 mmHg, or with symptomatic hypotension, GTN/nitrates should be avoided.

- CPAP should be utilised where equipment and suitably trained clinicians are available.

- Pulmonary oedema can be difficult to differentiate from other causes of breathlessness, such as exacerbation of COPD, pulmonary embolism or pneumonia; therefore, a thorough history and physical examination are needed.

- Establish if the patient has a personal care plan or end of life plan and if they are being managed by a specialist heart failure team. Follow plans or liaise with other healthcare professionals to manage the patient appropriately.

- Initial management depends on the clinical presentation: acute pulmonary oedema, peripheral oedema, respiratory distress or cardiogenic shock.

Further Reading

Further important information and evidence in support of this guideline can be found in the Bibliography.[4,5,6,7,8,9]

Bibliography

1. Ponikowski P, Voors AA, Anker SD et al. 2016 ESC Guidelines for the diagnosis and treatment of acute and chronic heart failure: the Task Force for the diagnosis and treatment of acute and chronic heart failure of the European Society of Cardiology (ESC). *European Heart Journal* 2016, 37(27): 2129–2200.

2. National Institute for Health and Care Excellence. *Acute Heart Failure: Diagnosis and management* [CG187]. Manchester: NICE, 2014. Available from: https://www.nice.org.uk/guidance/cg187.

3. National Institute for Health and Care Excellence. *Chronic Heart Failure in Adults: Management* [CG108]. Manchester: NICE, 2010. Available from: https://www.nice.org.uk/guidance/cg108.

4. British Medical Association and the Royal Pharmaceutical Society. *British National Formulary 75 (BNF) March – September 2018.* London: The Pharmaceutical Press.

5. Goodacre S, Stevens JW, Pandor A et al. Prehospital noninvasive ventilation for acute respiratory failure: systematic review, network meta-analysis, and individual patient data meta-analysis. *Academic Emergency Medicine* 2014, 21: 960–970.

6. Vital FMR, Saconato H, Ladeira MT, Sen A, Hawkes CA et al. Non-invasive positive pressure ventilation (CPAP or bilevel NPPV) for cardiogenic pulmonary edema (Review). *Cochrane Database Systematic Review* 2013, CD005351.

7. Wakai A, McCabe A, Kidney R et al. Nitrates for acute heart failure syndromes. *Cochrane Database Systematic Review* 2013, CD005151.

8. Peacock WF, Emerman C, Costanzo MR et al. Early vasoactive drugs improve heart failure outcomes. *Congest Heart Fail.* 2009, 15: 256–264.

9. Vaswani A, Khaw HJ, Dougherty S et al. *Cardiology in a Heartbeat.* Banbury: Scion Publishing, 2016.

Heat Related Illness

1. Introduction

- Heat related illness is a relatively uncommon presenting condition to ambulance services but it can be life-threatening.
- Heat related illness can be **exogenous,** caused by environmental factors (e.g. the sun) or **endogenous** (e.g. drugs and exercise).
- Heat related illness is a continuum of heat related conditions (refer to Figure 3.17).

The management of heat related illness is supportive: refer to Table 3.67.

Figure 3.17 – Continuum of heat related illness.

Heat stress

- Heat stress is a mild form of heat illness, characterised by the features below (refer to Table 3.64). This level of heat disorder is often self-managed, but if left untreated can progress to more serious conditions.

TABLE 3.64 – Features of Heat Stress (European Resuscitation Council Guidelines)
Heat stress
■ **Temperature:** normal or mildly elevated.
■ **Heat oedema:** swelling of feet and ankles.
■ **Heat syncope:** vasodilation and dehydration causing hypotension.
■ **Heat cramps:** sodium depletion causing cramps.

Heat exhaustion

- A less severe heat illness than heat stroke, lacking the defining neurological symptoms of this condition. Symptoms are mainly due to excess fluid loss and electrolyte imbalance.

TABLE 3.65 – Features of Heat Exhaustion (ERC)
Heat exhaustion
■ Systemic reaction to prolonged heat exposure (hours to days).
■ Temperature >37°C and <40°C.

TABLE 3.65 – Features of Heat Exhaustion (ERC) *(continued)*
■ Headache, dizziness, nausea, vomiting, tachycardia.
■ Hypotension, sweating, muscle pain, weakness and cramps.
■ Haemoconcentration.
■ Hyponatraemia or hypernatraemia.
■ May progress rapidly to heat stroke.

Heat stroke

- A 'systemic inflammatory response' to a core body temperature >40°C in addition to a change in mental status and organ dysfunction (European Resuscitation Council Guidelines).

There are two types of heat stroke:

a. **Non-exertional heat stroke** due to very high external temperatures and/or high humidity; it tends to be more common in very hot climates. It tends to occur in the:

- older person
- very young
- chronically ill.

b. **Exertional heat stroke** is due to excess heat production. This tends to occur in:

- athletes including marathon and fun-runners
- manual workers
- firefighters
- military recruits.

TABLE 3.66 – Features of Heat Stroke (ERC)
Heat stroke
■ Core temperature ≥40°C.
■ Hot, dry skin (sweating is present in about 50% of cases of exertional heat stroke).
■ Early signs and symptoms are extreme fatigue, headache, fainting, facial flushing, vomiting and diarrhoea.
■ Cardiovascular dysfunction including arrhythmias and hypotension.
■ Respiratory dysfunction including acute respiratory distress syndrome (ARDS).
■ Central nervous system dysfunction including seizures and coma.
■ Liver and renal failure.
■ Coagulopathy.
■ Rhabdomyolysis.

Heat Related Illness

2. Incidence

The exact incidence of heat stroke is unknown, with many sufferers self-managing their condition. Mortality, in the absence of a heat wave is relatively low; in the United Kingdom it is estimated to be 40 deaths per million annually.

A variety of medications may predispose to the development of heat illness. In addition, individuals who take drugs of abuse (e.g. cocaine, ecstasy, amphetamines) and then engage in vigorous dancing in crowded 'rave' settings may also develop heat illness.

3. Severity and Outcome

- Heat stroke is a life-threatening emergency that requires prompt appropriate treatment, with estimates of mortality of 10–50%. Recovery from heat stroke even after appropriate treatment and rehabilitation may be incomplete and leave patients with persistent functional impairment.

- **Systemic effects** – heat stroke can lead to a variety of life-threatening systemic conditions including: disseminated intravascular coagulation, rhabdomyolysis, renal failure, hepatic necrosis, metabolic acidosis and decreased tissue perfusion, in addition to cerebral and cerebellar damage.

4. Pathophysiology

- In heat illnesses there is an imbalance in the metabolic production and subsequent loss of heat by the body. This increase in core body temperature has multiple undesirable effects on many body systems. Systemically this increased temperature leads to swelling and degeneration at both cellular and tissue levels.

- **Cellular changes** – at increased temperatures cellular organelles swell and stop functioning properly. Cell membranes become distorted, leading to unwanted increased permeability and inappropriate movement of ions into and out of cells. Red blood cells also change shape at elevated temperatures and their capacity to carry oxygen is decreased. At higher temperatures cells will also undergo inappropriate apoptosis and die.

5. Assessment and Management

- For the assessment and management of heat related illness refer to Table 3.67.

TABLE 3.67 – ASSESSMENT and MANAGEMENT of: Heat Related Illness

Assess <C>ABCD

- If any of the following **TIME-CRITICAL** features are present:
  - major **<C>ABCD** problems; refer to **Medical Emergencies in Adults – Overview** and **Medical Emergencies in Children – Overview**.
  - haemodynamic compromise
  - decreased level of consciousness, then:
- Start correcting any **<C>ABCD** problems.
- Undertake a **TIME-CRITICAL** transfer to nearest appropriate receiving hospital.
- Continue patient management en-route.
- Provide an ATMIST information call.

Assess

- Undertake physical examination and assess for the presence of features of heat related illness (refer to Tables 3.64–3.65).
- Remove the patient from the hot environment or remove cause if possible.
- Remove to an air-conditioned vehicle where available.
- Remove all clothing.
- Commence cooling with fanning, tepid sponging, water misting or with a wet sheet loosely over the patient's body.
- **NB** Consider other potential causes (e.g. diabetes or cardiac problems).

Temperature

- Measure and record:
  - The patient's core temperature.
  - If possible and time allows, measure the environmental temperature.

NB The core temperature may or may not be elevated, but patients may be tachycardic, hypotensive and/or sweating excessively.

(continued)

Heat Related Illness

TABLE 3.67 – ASSESSMENT and MANAGEMENT of: Heat Related Illness *(continued)*
Heat Stroke
Heat stroke is potentially fatal, and the patient needs to be cooled as an emergency.
▪ If cold or iced water is used, massaging of the skin may be needed to overcome cold-induced vasoconstriction and ensure effective heat loss.
▪ Apply ice packs, if available, wrapped in a thin cloth or towel to the patient's neck, axilla and groin.
NB Ice packs applied directly to the skin can cause frostbite.
▪ Transfer the patient with air conditioning turned on or with windows open.
NB Immersion in ice water is effective but usually not possible in the pre-hospital environment.
Respiratory Rate
▪ Measure and record respiratory rate.
Pulse
▪ Measure and record pulse.
Oxygen Saturation
▪ Monitor the patient's SpO$_2$; administer oxygen to achieve saturations of >94% if the patient presents as hypoxaemic on air; refer to Oxygen.
Blood Pressure and Fluids
▪ Measure and record blood pressure. If required, administer fluids. Refer to Intravascular Fluid Therapy in Adults and Intravascular Fluid Therapy in Children.
Blood Glucose
▪ Measure and record blood glucose for hypo/hyperglycaemia; refer to **Glycaemic Emergencies in Adults and Children**.
NEWS2
▪ These observations will enable you to calculate a NEWS2 Score; refer to **Sepsis**.
ECG
▪ If required, monitor and record 12-lead ECG. Assess for abnormality; refer to **Cardiac Rhythm Disturbance**.
Assess the Patient's Pain
▪ Where present, assess the **SOCRATES** of pain and record initial and subsequent pain scores.
▪ Consider analgesia if appropriate; refer to **Pain Management in Adults** and **Pain Management in Children**.
Transfer
▪ Transfer the patient to the nearest appropriate receiving hospital.
Documentation
▪ Complete documentation to include all clinical findings, advice from other clinicians, onward referral and worsening advice given.

Heat Related Illness

Heat Related Illness

- Heat exhaustion/heat stroke occurs in high external temperatures, as a result of excess heat production and with certain drugs. The higher the level of activity the lower the environmental temperature required to produce heat stroke.

- Do not assume that collapse in an athlete is due to heat – check for other causes.

- In heat exhaustion the patient may present with flu-like symptoms, such as headache, nausea, dizziness, vomiting, and cramps; the temperature may not be elevated.

- In heat stroke the patient will have neurological symptoms such as decreased level of consciousness, ataxia and convulsions, and the temperature will usually be elevated, typically >40°C.

- Remove the patient from the hot environment or remove cause, if possible, remove clothing and cool.

Bibliography

1. Soar J, Perkins GD, Abbas G, Alfonzo A, Barelli A, Bierens JJLM, et al. European Resuscitation Council Guidelines for Resuscitation 2010 Section 8: cardiac arrest in special circumstances: electrolyte abnormalities, poisoning, drowning, accidental hypothermia, hyperthermia, asthma, anaphylaxis, cardiac surgery, trauma, pregnancy, electrocution. *Resuscitation* 2010, 81(10): 1400–1433.

2. Bouchama A, Dehbi M, Mohamed G, Matthies F, Shoukri M, Menne B. Prognostic factors in heat wave related deaths: a meta-analysis. *Archives of Internal Medicine* 2007, 167(20): 2170–2176.

3. Pease S, Bouadma L, Kermarrec N, Schortgen F, Regnier B, Wolff M. Early organ dysfunction course, cooling time and outcome in classic heatstroke. *Intensive Care Medicine* 2009, 35(8): 1454–1458.

4. Allen A, Segal-Gidan F. Heat-related illness in the elderly. *Clinical Geriatrics* 2007, 15(7): 37–45.

5. Belmin J, Auffray J-C, Berbezier C, Boirin P, Mercier S, de Reviers B, et al. Level of dependency: a simple marker associated with mortality during the 2003 heatwave among French dependent elderly people living in the community or in institutions. *Age and Ageing* 2007, 36(3): 298–303.

6. Brody GM. Hyperthermia and hypothermia in the elderly. *Clinics in Geriatric Medicine* 1994, 10(1): 213–229.

7. Daniel V, Paladugu N, Fuentes G. Heat stroke and cocaine in an inner-city New York hospital. *Internet Journal of Emergency and Intensive Care Medicine* 2008, 11(1). DOI: 10.5580/157e.

8. de Galan BE, Hoekstra JBL. Extremely elevated body temperature: case report and review of classical heat stroke. *Netherlands Journal of Medicine* 1995, 47(6): 281–287.

9. Hausfater P, Megarbane B, Dautheville S, Patzak A, Andronikof M, Santin A, et al. Prognostic factors in non-exertional heatstroke. *Intensive Care Medicine* 2010, 36(2): 272–280.

10. Stafoggia M, Forastiere F, Agostini D, Biggeri A, Bisanti L, Cadum E, et al. Vulnerability to heat-related mortality: a multicity, population-based, case-crossover analysis. *Epidemiology* 2006, 17(3): 315–323.

11. Vicario SJ, Okabajue R, Haltom T. Rapid cooling in classic heatstroke: effect on mortality rates. *American Journal of Emergency Medicine* 1986, 4(5): 394–398.

12. Bernardo LM, Crane PA, Veenema TG. Treatment and prevention of pediatric heat-related illnesses at mass gatherings and special events. *Dimensions of Critical Care Nursing* 2006, 25(4): 165–171.

13. Guard A, Gallagher SS. Heat related deaths to young children in parked cars: an analysis of 171 fatalities in the United States, 1995–2002. *Injury Prevention* 2005, 11(1): 33–37.

14. Gutierrez G. Solar injury and heat illness: treatment and prevention in children. *Physician and Sportsmedicine* 1995, 23(7): 43–48.

15. Krous HF, Nadeau JM, Fukumoto RI, Blackbourne BD, Byard RW. Environmental hyperthermic infant and early childhood death: circumstances, pathologic changes, and manner of death. *American Journal of Forensic Medicine and Pathology* 2001, 22(4): 374–382.

16. Ohshima T, Maeda H, Takayasu T, Fujioka Y, Nakaya T. An autopsy case of infant death due to heat stroke. *American Journal of Forensic Medicine and Pathology* 1992, 13(3): 217–221.

17. Rossi R. Emergency treatment of an infant with heatstroke. *Notfallmedizin* 1993, 19(3): 109–111.

18. Wagner C, Boyd K. Pediatric heatstroke. *Air Medical Journal* 2008, 27(3): 118–122.

19. Martinez M, Devenport L, Saussy J, Martinez J. Drug-associated heat stroke. *Southern Medical Journal* 2002, 95(8): 799–802.

20. Aarseth HP, Eide I, Skeie B, Thaulow E. Heat stroke in endurance exercise. *Acta Medica Scandinavica* 1986, 220(3): 279–283.

21. Armstrong LE, Crago AE, Adams R, Roberts WO, Maresh CM. Whole-body cooling of hyperthermic runners: comparison of two field therapies. *American Journal of Emergency Medicine* 1996, 14(4): 355–358.

22. Binkley HM, Beckett J, Casa DJ, Kleiner DM, Plummer PE. National Athletic Trainers' Association position statement: exertional heat illnesses. *Journal of Athletic Training* 2002, 37(3): 329–343.

23. Clapp AJ, Bishop PA, Muir I, Walker IL. Rapid cooling techniques in joggers experiencing heat strain. *Journal of Science and Medicine in Sport* 2001, 4(2): 160–167.

24. Hansen RD, Olds TS, Richards DA, Richards CR, Leelarthaepin B. Infrared thermometry in the diagnosis and treatment of heat exhaustion. *International Journal of Sports Medicine* 1996, 17(1): 66–70.

Heat Related Illness

Heat Related Illness

25. Hee-Nee P, Rupeng M, Lee VJ, Chua W-C, Seet B. Treatment of exertional heat injuries with portable body cooling unit in a mass endurance event. *American Journal of Emergency Medicine* 2010, 28(2): 246–248.

26. McDermott BP, Casa DJ, O'Connor FG, Adams WB, Armstrong LE, Brennan AH, et al. Cold-water dousing with ice massage to treat exertional heat stroke: a case series. *Aviation Space and Environmental Medicine* 2009, 80(8): 720–722.

27. Centers for Disease Control and Prevention. Heat-related deaths among crop workers: United States, 1992–2006. *Morbidity and Mortality Weekly Report* 2008, 57(24): 649–653.

28. Maeda T, Kaneko S-Y, Ohta M, Tanaka K, Sasaki A, Fukushima T. Risk factors for heatstroke among Japanese forestry workers. *Journal of Occupational Health* 2006, 48(4): 223–229.

29. Tranter M. An assessment of heat stress among laundry workers in a Far North Queensland hotel. *Journal of Occupational Health and Safety Australia and New Zealand* 1998, 14(1): 61–63.

30. Yoshino K, Takano K, Nagasaka A, Shigeta S. An experimental study on the prediction of heat stress of workers in a hot environment. With special reference to the relation between wearing suits, work load and environmental temperature. *Japanese Journal of Industrial Health* 1987, 29(6): 466–479.

31. Angerer P, Kadlez-Gebhardt S, Delius M, Raluca P, Nowak D. Comparison of cardiocirculatory and thermal strain of male firefighters during fire suppression to exercise stress test and aerobic exercise testing. *American Journal of Cardiology* 2008, 102(11): 1551–1556.

32. Barr D, Gregson W, Reilly T. The thermal ergonomics of firefighting reviewed. *Applied Ergonomics* 2010, 41(1): 161–172.

33. Barr D, Gregson W, Sutton L, Reilly T. A practical cooling strategy for reducing the physiological strain associated with firefighting activity in the heat. *Ergonomics* 2009, 52(4): 413–420.

34. Giesbrecht GG, Jamieson C, Cahill F. Cooling hyperthermic firefighters by immersing forearms and hands in 10 degrees C and 20 degrees C water. *Aviation Space and Environmental Medicine* 2007, 78(6): 561–567.

35. Patel HC, Rao NM, Saha A. Heat exposure effects among firefighters. *Indian Journal of Occupational and Environmental Medicine* 2006, 10(3): 121–123.

36. Bedno SA, Li Y, Han W, Cowan DN, Scott CT, Cavicchia MA, et al. Exertional heat illness among overweight U.S. Army recruits in basic training. *Aviation Space and Environmental Medicine* 2010, 81(2): 107–111.

37. Bruce ASW, Tunstall C, Boulter MJ, Coneybeare A. A treatment algorithm for mass heat casualties. *Journal of the Royal Army Medical Corps* 2008, 154(1): 19–20.

38. Carter R III, Cheuvront SN, Sawka MN. A case report of idiosyncratic hyperthermia and review of U.S. Army heat stroke hospitalizations. *Journal of Sport Rehabilitation* 2007, 16(3): 238–243.

39. Gardner JW, Kark JA. Fatal rhabdomyolysis presenting as mild heat illness in military training. *Military Medicine* 1994, 159(2): 160–163.

40. Keatinge WR, Donaldson GC, Cordioli E, Martinelli M, Kunst AE, Mackenbach W, et al. Heat related mortality in warm and cold regions of Europe: observational study. *British Medical Journal* 2000, 321(7262): 670–673.

41. Epstein Y, Albukrek D, Kalmovitc B, Moran DS, Shapiro Y. Heat intolerance induced by antidepressants. *Annals of the New York Academy of Sciences* 1997, 813: 553–558.

42. Fijnheer R, Van De Ven PJG, Erkelens DW. Psychiatric medication as a risk factor for fatal heat stroke. *Nederlands Tijdschrift voor Geneeskunde* 1995, 139(27): 1391–1393.

43. Kao RL, Kelly LM. Fatal exertional heat stroke in a patient receiving zuclopenthixol, quetiapine and benztropine. *Canadian Journal of Clinical Pharmacology* 2007, 14(3): e322–325.

44. Kwok JSS, Chan TYK. Recurrent heat-related illnesses during antipsychotic treatment. *Annals of Pharmacotherapy* 2005, 39(11): 1940–1942.

45. Feldman KW, Mazor S. Ecstasy ingestion causing heatstroke-like, multiorgan injury in a toddler. *Pediatric Emergency Care* 2007, 23(10): 725–726.

46. Jenkins RD, Woodhouse KW. Drug-induced fever. *Adverse Drug Reaction Bulletin* 1999, 197: 751–754.

47. Kilbourne EM. Cocaine use and death during heat waves. *Journal of the American Medical* Association 1828, 279(22): 1828–1829.

48. Lan K-C, Lin Y-F, Yu F-C, Lin C-S, Chu P. Clinical manifestations and prognostic features of acute methamphetamine intoxication. *Journal of the Formosan Medical Association* 1998, 97(8): 528–533.

49. Dahmash NS, Al Harthi SS, Akhtar J. Invasive evaluation of patients with heat stroke. *Chest* 1993, 103(4): 1210–1214.

50. Graham BS, Lichtenstein MJ, Hinson JM, Theis GB. Nonexertional heatstroke. Physiologic management and cooling in 14 patients. *Archives of Internal Medicine* 1986, 146(1): 87–90.

51. LoVecchio F, Pizon AF, Berrett C, Balls A. Outcomes after environmental hyperthermia. *American Journal of Emergency Medicine* 2007, 25(4): 442–444.

52. Misset B, De Jonghe B, Bastuji-Garin S, Gattolliat O, Boughrara E, Annane D, et al. Mortality of patients with heatstroke admitted to intensive care units during the 2003 heat wave in France: a national multiple-center risk-factor study. *Critical Care Medicine* 2006, 34(4): 1087–1092.

53. Ramsey CB, Watson WA, Robinson WA. Effect of cooling time on survival in classical heatstroke. *Journal of Wilderness Medicine* 1993, 4(1): 27–31.

54. Varghese GM, John G, Thomas K, Abraham OC, Mathai D. Predictors of multi-organ dysfunction in heatstroke. *Emergency Medicine Journal* 2005, 22(3): 185–187.

55. Albukrek D, Bakon M, Moran DS, Faibel M, Epstein Y. Heat-stroke-induced cerebellar atrophy: clinical course, CT and MRI findings. *Neuroradiology* 1997, 39(3): 195–197.

56. Biary N, Madkour MM, Sharif H. Post-heatstroke parkinsonism and cerebellar dysfunction. *Clinical Neurology and Neurosurgery* 1995, 97(1): 55–57.

57. Deleu D, El Siddig A, Kamran S, Kamha AA, Al Omary IYM, Zalabany HA. Downbeat nystagmus following classical heat stroke. *Clinical Neurology and Neurosurgery* 2005, 108(1): 102–104.

58. Fink E, Brandom BW, Torp KD. Heatstroke in the super-sized athlete. *Pediatric Emergency Care* 2006, 22(7): 510–513.

59. Rav-Acha M, Shuvy M, Hagag S, Gomori M, Biran I. Unique persistent neurological sequelae of heat stroke. *Military Medicine* 2007, 172(6): 603–606.

SECTION 3 Medical Emergencies

Heat Related Illness

60. Sudhir U, Anil Kumar T, Srinivasan G, Punith K. Post-heat stroke cerebellar atrophy. *Journal, Indian Academy of Clinical Medicine* 2009, 10(1–2): 60–62.

61. Bazille C, Megarbane B, Bensimhon D, Lavergne-Slove A, Baglin AC, Loirat P, et al. Brain damage after heat stroke. *Journal of Neuropathology and Experimental Neurology* 2005, 64(11): 70–75.

62. Cleary M, Ruiz D, Eberman L, Mitchell I, Binkley H. Dehydration, cramping, and exertional rhabdomyolysis: a case report with suggestions for recovery. *Journal of Sport Rehabilitation* 2007, 16(3): 244–259.

63. Shafie H, Abd Wahab M, Masilamany M, Abu Hassan AA. Exertional heat stroke: a lucky bunch of overly motivated policemen! *Hong Kong Journal of Emergency Medicine* 2007, 14(1): 37–44.

64. Sharma HS, Hoopes PJ. Hyperthermia induced pathophysiology of the central nervous system. *International Journal of Hyperthermia* 2003, 19(3): 325–354.

65. Wang AYM, Li PKT, Lui SF, Lai KN. Renal failure and heatstroke. *Renal Failure* 1995, 17(2): 171–179.

66. Wexler RK. Evaluation and treatment of heat-related illnesses. *American Family Physician* 2002, 65(11): 2307–2315.

67. Yan Y-E, Zhao Y-Q, Wang H, Fan M. Pathophysiological factors underlying heatstroke. *Medical Hypotheses* 2006, 67(3): 609–617.

68. Bourdon L, Canini F, Saissy J-M, D'Aleo P, Koulmann N, Aubert M, et al. Exertional heatstroke: II – Pathophysiology. *Science and Sports* 2003, 18(5): 241–252.

69. Bouchama A, Hammami MM, Haq A, Jackson J, Al-Sedairy S. Evidence for endothelial cell activation/ injury in heatstroke. *Critical Care Medicine* 1996, 24(7): 1173–1178.

70. Lee SJ, Yang ES, Kim SY, Kim SY, Shin SW, Park J-W. Regulation of heat shock induced apoptosis by sensitive to apoptosis gene protein. *Free Radical Biology and Medicine* 2008, 45(2): 167–176.

71. Wang Z, Shi Q, Li S, Du J, Liu J, Dai K. Hyperthermia induces platelet apoptosis and glycoprotein 1b ectodomain shedding. *Platelets* 2010, 21(3): 229–237.

72. Al-Aska AK, Abu-Aisha H, Yaqub B. Simplified cooling bed for heatstroke. *The Lancet* 1987, 329(8529): 381.

73. Mundel T, Bunn SJ, Hooper PL, Jones DA. The effects of face cooling during hyperthermic exercise in man: evidence for an integrated thermal, neuroendocrine and behavioural response. *Experimental Physiology 2007*, 92(1): 187–195.

74. Sinclair WH, Rudzki SJ, Leicht AS, Fogarty AL, Winter SK, Patterson MJ. Efficacy of field treatments to reduce body core temperature in hyperthermic subjects. *Medicine and Science in Sports and Exercise* 2009, 41(11): 1984–1990.

75. Buono MJ, Jechort A, Marques R, Smith C, Welch J. Comparison of infrared versus contact thermometry for measuring skin temperature during exercise in the heat. *Physiological Measurement* 2007, 28(8): 855–859.

76. Gagnon D, Lemire BB, Jay O, Kenny GP. Aural canal, esophageal, and rectal temperatures during exertional heat stress and the subsequent recovery period. *Journal of Athletic Training* 2010, 45(2): 157–163.

77. Budd GM. Wet-bulb globe temperature (WBGT): its history and its limitations. *Journal of Science and Medicine in Sport* 2008, 11(1): 20–32.

78. Moran DS, Pandolf KB. Wet bulb globe temperature (WBGT): to what extent is GT essential? *Aviation Space and Environmental Medicine* 1999, 70(5): 480–484.

79. Smith JE. Cooling methods used in the treatment of exertional heat illness. *British Journal of Sports Medicine* 2005, 39(8): 503–507.

80. McDermott BP, Casa DJ, Ganlo MS, Lopez RM, Yeargin SW, Armstrong LE, et al. Acute whole-body cooling for exercise-induced hyperthermia: a systematic review. *Journal of Athletic Training* 2009, 44(1): 84–93.

81. Casa DJ, McDermott BP, Lee EC, Yeargin SW, Armstrong LE, Maresh CM. Cold water immersion: the gold standard for exertional heatstroke treatment. *Exercise and Sport Sciences Reviews* 2007, 35(3): 141–149.

82. Empana J-P, Sauval P, Ducimetiere P, Tafflet M, Carli P, Jouven X. Increase in out-of-hospital cardiac arrest attended by the medical mobile intensive care units, but not myocardial infarction, during the 2003 heat wave in Paris, France. [Erratum appears in *Critical Care Medicine* 2010, 38(2): 741.] *Critical Care Medicine* 2009, 37(12): 3079–3084.

83. Lacunza J, San Roman I, Moreno S, Garcia-Molina E, Gimeno J, Valdes M. Heat stroke, an unusual trigger of Brugada electrocardiogram. *American Journal of Emergency Medicine* 2009, 27(5): 634.e1–3.

84. Wakino S, Hori S, Mimura T, Miyatake S, Fujishima S, Aikawa N. A case of severe heat stroke with abnormal cardiac findings. *International Heart Journal.* 2005, 46(3): 543–550.

Hyperventilation Syndrome

1. Introduction

- Hyperventilation syndrome is defined as 'breathing in excess of metabolic requirements'.[1]

- It is characterised by an irregular and disorganised breathing pattern with an increased rate and depth of respirations, known as tachypnoea.[2]

- Hyperventilation has many causes, including a number of life-threatening conditions such as:
  - myocardial infarction
  - pulmonary embolism
  - diabetic ketoacidosis
  - asthma
  - sepsis.

- This guideline focuses on acute episodes of primary or idiopathic hyperventilation, which means there is no underlying cause.[3,4] This condition was initially termed Hyperventilation Syndrome (HVS), but more recently the term HVS has slowly disappeared in favour of:
  - Panic/anxiety attack
  - Panic/anxiety disorder
  - Dysfunctional breathing
  - Breathing pattern disorder.[5,6,7,8,9]

2. Incidence

- It is estimated that 6–10% of the general adult population may suffer from some form of HVS. The condition is more common in women.[6,7] Within UK ambulance services the prevalence of HVS is estimated to be 1%, which is comparable to estimates for emergency departments, which range from 0.3–6%.[10,11,3,12]

- HVS is rare in children, where the most likely cause is physical illness.

- Patients with HVS use a significant amount of hospital and emergency service resources because they frequently seek care in the emergency department or from paramedics due to fearing they are experiencing life-threatening emergencies.[11,13]

3. Severity and Outcome

- As per its definition, HVS has no organic cause and is self-limiting. No organic cause means that there is no underlying physical change to the patient's cells, tissues or organs which could account for the experienced symptoms. The signs and symptoms of HVS may be distressing for the patient but these will subside once a good respiratory pattern is established.

- Within the literature there are case study reports of apnoeic episodes following HVS, but these are rare.[14]

- **A diagnosis of HVS must be a diagnosis of exclusion of organic causes for hyperventilation.** This is due to the differential diagnoses of HVS including many life-threatening conditions with poor prognosis if the correct treatment is withheld. Potential differential diagnoses are listed in Table 3.68.

TABLE 3.68 – Differential Diagnoses of HVS by Body System[15,16,17,18]

BODY SYSTEM	DIFFERENTIAL DIAGNOSES	
Cardiovascular	Angina Aortic aneurysm Coronary artery disease Tachyarrhythmia	Myocardial infarction Pericarditis Heart failure
Neurological	Brain stem lesions Encephalitis Head trauma Mèniére's disease	Meningitis Stroke Vertigo
Respiratory	Asthma Chronic obstructive pulmonary disease Cystic fibrosis Interstitial lung disease	Lung tumour Pneumonia Pneumothorax Pulmonary embolism Pleural effusion
Gastrointestinal	Cholecystitis Liver failure Hiatus hernia	Liver cirrhosis Peptic ulcer

Hyperventilation Syndrome

TABLE 3.68 – Differential Diagnoses of HVS by Body System[15,16,17,18] *(continued)*

BODY SYSTEM	DIFFERENTIAL DIAGNOSES	
Endocrine	▪ Diabetic ketoacidosis ▪ Pheochromocytoma	▪ Thyrotoxicosis
Renal	▪ Kidney failure	
Environmental	▪ Heat or altitude acclimatisation	▪ Carbon monoxide poisoning
Other	▪ Anaemia ▪ Drug intoxication ▪ Drugs or caffeine (withdrawal) ▪ Pain	▪ Hypokalaemia ▪ Sepsis ▪ Serious aspirin overdoses ▪ Pregnancy

4. Pathophysiology

▪ The basic rhythm of respiration is controlled subconsciously by the medullary respiratory centre.[19] The automatic control of respiration can be overridden by anxiety, which causes central stimulation of the medullary respiratory centre's inspiratory area, leading to an increased rate and depth of respiration.[20]

▪ An increased rate and depth of respiration results in faster elimination of carbon dioxide through exhalation, causing a decrease in alveolar and arterial carbon dioxide known as hypocapnia.[18] Hypocapnia reduces the formation of hydrogen ions and bicarbonate ions in the blood, causing a rise in pH levels known as respiratory alkalosis.[21]

▪ Hypocapnia also causes constriction of cerebral arteries, thereby increasing vascular resistance and reducing blood flow to the brain.[18] This diminished cerebral perfusion may explain some of the neurological symptoms associated with HVS.[22]

▪ The physiological mechanisms by which many of the other HVS symptoms occur are not entirely clear, but they must nonetheless be seen as genuine consequences of physiological imbalances rather than figments of patients' imagination.[23]

▪ Signs and symptoms of HVS are wide-ranging and vague and can vary between patients. Experiencing the frightening symptoms of HVS may exacerbate patients' anxiety which promotes further hyperventilation, resulting in HVS symptoms entering a vicious cycle.

TABLE 3.69 – Signs and Symptoms of HVS by Body System[2,4,20,22]

BODY SYSTEM	SIGNS AND SYMPTOMS
Cardiovascular	Palpitations, tachycardia, arrhythmias, chest pain, blotchy flushing
Neurological	Paraesthesia (numbness and tingling of the mouth/lips/extremities), dizziness/unsteadiness/light-headedness, syncope, headache, blurred or tunnel vision, impaired concentration and memory
Respiratory	Tachypnoea, shortness of breath, tightness in chest/throat, frequent sighing, yawning, feeling of suffocation/choking
Gastrointestinal	Globus, dysphagia, epigastric discomfort, excessive air-swallowing, dry mouth, belching, flatulence, nausea
Musculoskeletal	Aching of the muscles of the chest, tremors, weakness, tetany of hands or feet (e.g. carpopedal spasm)
Psychological	Tension, anxiety, panic, feelings of unreality or disorientation, fear of dying, fear of losing control or going crazy, hallucinations, phobias
General	Fatigue, exhaustion, sleep disturbance, sweating, weakness, chills or heat sensations

Hyperventilation Syndrome

Hyperventilation Syndrome

5. Assessment and Management

For the assessment and management of hyperventilation syndrome, refer to Table 3.70 and Figure 3.18.

TABLE 3.70 – ASSESSMENT and MANAGEMENT of: Hyperventilation Syndrome
Assess <C>ABCD
<ul><li>If any of the following **TIME-CRITICAL** features present:</li><ul><li>major **<C>ABCD** problems</li><li>cyanosis</li><li>reduced level of consciousness (refer to **Altered Level of Consciousness**).</li><li>hypoxia (refer to **Oxygen**).</li></ul><li>Start correcting **<C>ABCD** problems.</li><li>Undertake a **TIME-CRITICAL** transfer to nearest receiving hospital.</li><li>Continue patient management en-route.</li><li>Provide an alert/information call.</li></ul>**NB** If any of the **TIME-CRITICAL** features listed above are present, it is unlikely to be due to hyperventilation syndrome and is more likely to be physiological hyperventilation, secondary to an underlying pathological process.
Individualised Treatment Plan
<ul><li>Ask the patient if they have an individualised treatment plan, and follow the plan if available.</li><li>The patient will often be able to guide their care.</li></ul>
History
⚠ **Always presume hyperventilation is secondary to hypoxia or another underlying respiratory or metabolic disorder until proven otherwise and such is a diagnosis of exclusion.**<ul><li>Cause of hyperventilation.</li><li>Previous episodes of hyperventilation.</li><li>Previous medical history.</li><li>Features of hyperventilation syndrome (refer to Table 3.68).</li><li>Did the patient's breathlessness occur at rest rather than exertion? This distinction points towards HVS.[24]</li></ul>
Differential Diagnosis
<ul><li>Refer to Table 3.68.</li></ul>
Basic Observations
<ul><li>Respiratory rate.</li><li>Peripheral oxygen saturations (SpO_2): apply pulse oximeter. **DO NOT** administer supplemental oxygen unless hypoxaemic (SpO_2 <94%) (refer to **Oxygen**). **NB** Low SpO_2 is not a presenting feature of HVS and will indicate an underlying clinical condition.</li><li>Heart rate.</li><li>Blood pressure.</li><li>Measure and record blood glucose for hypo/hyperglycaemia (refer to **Glycaemic Emergencies in Adults and Children**).</li><li>If required, monitor and record a 12-lead ECG and assess for abnormality (refer to **Cardiac Rhythm Disturbance**).</li><li>Temperature.</li><li>Respiratory rate and heart rate will likely be elevated in acute HVS patients alongside an abnormally high SpO_2 of 99%–100%.[25]</li></ul>

Hyperventilation Syndrome

TABLE 3.70 – ASSESSMENT and MANAGEMENT of: Hyperventilation Syndrome *(continued)*
Physical examination
▪ Auscultation of breath sounds to exclude physical causes of breathlessness as may be indicated by a wheeze or crackles.[24]
▪ Observation and palpation of the patient's chest may demonstrate paradoxical breathing associated with forced respiration, i.e. the abdomen retracts and upper chest expands on inhalation as supposed to normal abdominal protrusion and lower thorax expansion.[18]
▪ Refer to **Dyspnoea**.
Disease-specific Measurements
▪ Peak expiratory flow: readings should be compared with predicted values to exclude significant respiratory restriction.[18]
▪ ECG: temporary ECG changes can occur during acute episodes of HVS, and underlying cardiac conditions need to be excluded.[26]
Treatment
▪ Aim to restore a normal level of pCO_2 over a period of time by reassuring the patient and coaching them regarding their respirations.
▪ Practical ways to coach a patient's breathing include:
– asking the patient to count to two between each breath
– using distraction techniques
– asking the patient to slowly breathe in through their nose and out through their mouth.
▪ Try to remove the source of the patient's anxiety – this is particularly important in the management of children.
▪ Promote a good patient–clinician relationship: communicate to patients that you believe they are suffering with HVS, as this may offer sufficient reassurance and relief of anxiety which in turn will reduce the severity and frequency of symptoms.[27]
▪ Paper bag rebreathing has not been recommended since 1990 due to the risk of hypoxia.[28]
▪ Refer to **Mental Health Presentation: Crisis, Distress and Disordered Behaviour**.
Diagnosis
▪ There is a lack of agreement regarding specific HVS diagnostic criteria and no symptoms are absolutely diagnostic of HVS.[18]
Oxygen Saturation
▪ Apply pulse oximeter.
▪ **DO NOT** administer supplemental oxygen unless hypoxaemic (SpO_2 <94%) (refer to **Oxygen**).
▪ **NB** Low SpO_2 is not a presenting feature of HVS and will indicate an underlying clinical condition.
Breathing
▪ Consider auscultation of breath sounds during assessment of breathing.
▪ Aim to restore a normal level of pCO_2 over a period of time by reassuring the patient and coaching them regarding their respirations.
▪ Try to remove the source of the patient's anxiety – this is particularly important in the management of children.
▪ Refer to **Dyspnoea**.
Transfer
▪ Transfer to further care:
– Patients experiencing their first episode.
– Children aged <16 years.
– Known HVS sufferers whose symptoms have not settled or which re-occur within 10 minutes.
– Patients who have an individualised care plan and a responsible adult present may be considered for non-conveyance and managing at home according to local protocols.
– Provide details of local care pathways if symptoms re-occur.

3 Medical Emergencies

SECTION

Hyperventilation Syndrome

Assess ABCD

TIME CRITICAL features present

Major **ABCD** problems
Cyanosis.
Reduced level of consciousness.
Hypoxia.
NB If any **TIME CRITICAL** features are present it is unlikely to be due to hyperventilation syndrome and more likely to be a physiological hyperventilation, secondary to an underlying pathological process

Start correcting
A and **B problems**

Undertake a **TIME CRITICAL** transfer.
Provide alert/information call.
Continue management en-route

No **TIME CRITICAL** features present

Ascertain whether the patient has an individualised treatment plan

Follow treatment plan if available

If treatment plan not available

⚠ **Always presume hyperventilation is secondary to hypoxia or other underlying respiratory or metabolic disorder until proven otherwise**

Consider differential diagnosis such as:
• Heart failure – refer to heart failure.
• Acute asthma – refer to asthma.
• Chest infection – refer to medical emergencies.
• Pulmonary embolism – refer to pulmonary embolism.
• Diabetic ketoacidosis or other causes of metabolic acidosis – refer to glycaemic emergencies.
• Pneumothorax – refer to thoracic trauma.
• Drug overdose – refer to overdose and poisoning guidelines.
• Acute myocardial infarction – refer to acute coronary syndrome.

DO NOT administer supplemental O_2 unless hypoxaemic (SpO_2 <94%) – refer to oxygen.
NB Low SpO_2 – not a presenting feature – will indicate an underlying condition.

Reassure the patient.
Coach patients regarding their respirations.
Try to remove the source of the patient's anxiety, particularly in children

Transfer to further care
Patients experiencing their first episode.
Known HVS sufferers whose symptoms have not settled, or re-occur within 10 minutes. Children aged under 16 years Patients who have an individualised care plan and a responsible adult present may be considered for non conveyance and managing at home according to local protocols.
Provide details of local care pathways if symptoms re-occur

Figure 3.18 – Assessment and management of hyperventilation syndrome algorithm.

Hyperventilation Syndrome

KEY POINTS!

Hyperventilation Syndrome

- HVS is a diagnosis of exclusion.
- Differential diagnosis: many life-threatening medical conditions can cause hyperventilation.
- In children a medical cause is more likely than anxiety.
- Administer supplemental oxygen if hypoxaemic (SpO$_2$ <94%).
- Reassure the patient and coach their breathing.

Further Reading

Further important information and evidence in support of this guideline can be found in the Bibliography.[29,30,31,32,33,34,35,36,37,38,39,40,41,42]

Bibliography

1. Gardner WN. Hyperventilation: a practical guide. *Medicine* 2003, 31(11): 7–8.

2. Caroline N. *Emergency Care in the Streets.* 7th edn. Burlington, MA: Jones and Bartlett, 2016.

3. Pfortmueller CA, Pauchard-Neuwerth SE, Leichtle AB, Fiedler GM, Exadaktylos AK, et al. Primary hyperventilation in the emergency department: a first overview. *PLOS ONE* 2015, 10(6).

4. Clarke V, Townsend P. Respiratory assessment. In Blaber AY, Harris G. *Assessment Skills for Paramedics.* 2nd edn. Maidenhead: Open University Press, 2016: 14–46.

5. Kerr WJ, Gliebe PA, Dalton JW. 1938. Physical phenomena associated with anxiety states: the hyperventilation syndrome. *Cal West Med* 1938, 48(1): 12–16.

6. Thomas M, McKinley RK, Freeman E, Foy C. Prevalence of dysfunctional breathing in patients treated for asthma in primary care. *BMJ* 2001, 322(7294): 1098–1100.

7. Thomas M, McKinley RK, Freeman E, Foy C, Price D. The prevalence of dysfunctional breathing in adults in the community with and without asthma. *Prim Care Respir J* 2005, 14(2): 78–82.

8. Warburton CJ, Jack S. Can you diagnose hyperventilation? *Chron Respir Dis* 2006, 3(3): 113–115.

9. Todd S, Walsted ES, Grillo L, Livingston R, Menzies-Gow A, Hull JH. Novel assessment tool to detect breathing pattern disorder in patients with refractory asthma. *Respirology* 2017, 23: 284–290.

10. Wilson C, Harley C, Steels S. PP09 Pre-hospital diagnostic accuracy for hyperventilation syndrome. *Emerg Med J* 2017: 34:e3.

11. Coley KC, Saul MI, Seybert AL. Economic burden of not recognizing panic disorder in the emergency department. *J Emerg Med* 2009, 36(1): 3–7.

12. Greenslade JH, Hawkins T, Parsonage W, Cullen L. Panic disorder in patients presenting to the emergency department with chest pain: prevalence and presenting symptoms. *Heart Lung Circ* 2017, 26(12): 1310–1316.

13. Katerndahl DA, Realini JP. Where do panic attack sufferers seek care? *J Fam Pract* 1995, 40(3): 237–243.

14. Munemoto T, Masuda A, Nagai N, Tanaka M, Yuji S. Prolonged post-hyperventilation apnea in two young adults with hyperventilation syndrome. *BioPsychoSocial Medicine* 2013, 7(1): 9.

15. Pfeffer JM. The aetiology of the hyperventilation syndrome. *Psychother Psychosom* 1978, 30(1): 47–55.

16. Ong JR, Hou SW, Shu HT, Chen HT, Chong CF. Diagnostic pitfall: carbon monoxide poisoning mimicking hyperventilation syndrome. *Am J Emerg Med* 2005, 23(7): 903–904.

17. Brashear RE. Hyperventilation syndrome. *Lung* 1983, 161(1): 257–273.

18. Pizzorno JE, Murray MT, Joiner-Bey H. *The Clinician's Handbook of Natural Medicine.* 3rd edn. St Louis: Elsevier, 2016.

19. Aehlert B. *Paramedic Practice Today: Above and beyond.* Burlington, MA: Jones and Bartlett, 2011.

20. Porth CM, Litwack K. Disorders of acid-base balance. In Porth CM, Matfin G. *Pathophysiology: Concepts of altered health states.* 8th edn. Philadelphia: Lippinkott Williams & Wilkins, 2009: 805–825.

21. Khurana I. *Medical Physiology for Undergraduate Students.* New Delhi: Elsevier, 2012.

22. Evans RW. Unilateral paresthesias due to hyperventilation syndrome. *Pract Neurol* 2005: 65–68.

23. Chapman S, Robinson G, Stradling J, West S. *Oxford Handbook of Respiratory Medicine.* Oxford: Oxford University Press, 2009.

24. National Institute for Health and Care Excellence. *Breathlessness.* Clinical Knowledge Summaries. 2017. Available from: https://cks.nice.org.uk/breathlessness.

25. O'Driscoll BR, Howard LS, Earis J on behalf of the British Thoracic Society Emergency Oxygen Guideline Group. BTS guideline for oxygen use in adults in healthcare and emergency settings. *Thorax* 2017, 72: ii1–ii90.

26. Michaelides AP, Liakos CI, Antoniades C, Tsiachris DL, Soulis D, Dilaveris PE, Tsioufis KP, Stefanadis CI. ST-segment depression in hyperventilation indicates a false positive exercise test in patients with mitral valve prolapse. *Cardiology Research and Practice.* 2015. Available from: https://www.hindawi.com/journals/crp/2010/541781.

27. Boulding R, Stacey R, Niven R, Fowler SJ. Dysfunctional breathing: a review of the literature and proposal for classification. *Eur Respir Rev* 2016 25(141): 287–294.

28. Kishikawa M. Re-evaluation of paper bag rebreathing for hyperventilation syndrome. *International Conference*

Hyperventilation Syndrome

and Exhibition on Lung Disorders & Therapeutics. 2015. Available from: http://lung.conferenceseries.com/abstract/2015/re-evaluation-of-paper-bag-rebreathing-for-hyperventilation-syndrome.

29. Wilson C. Hyperventilation syndrome: diagnosis and reassurance. *Journal of Paramedic Practice* 2018, 10(9): 370–375.

30. American Psychiatric Association. Diagnostic and Statistical Manual of Mental Disorders. 5th edn. 2013. Available from: https://dsm.psychiatryonline.org/doi/book/10.1176/appi.books.9780890425596.

31. Malmberg LP, Tamminen K, Sovijärvi ARA. Orthostatic increase of respiratory gas exchange in hyperventilation syndrome. *Thorax* 2000, 55(4): 295–301.

32. Maguire CA, Robson AG, Pentland J, McAllister D, Innes JA. Smoking status predicts benefit from breathing retraining for hyperventilation. *Thorax* 2010, 65(suppl. 4): A157.

33. Gardner W. Orthostatic increase of respiratory gas exchange in hyperventilation syndrome. *Thorax* 2000, 55(4): 257–259.

34. Bazin KA, Moosavi S, Murphy K, Perkins A, Hickson M, Howard LS. Carbon dioxide sensitivity in patients with hyperventilation syndrome. *Thorax* 2010, 65(suppl. 4): A134.

35. van den Hout MA, Boek C, van der Molen GM, Jansen A, Griez E. Rebreathing to cope with hyperventilation: experimental tests of the paper bag method. *Journal of Behavioral Medicine* 1988, 11(3): 303–310.

36. Tavel ME. Hyperventilation syndrome: hiding behind pseudonyms? *Chest* 1990, 97(6): 1285–1288.

37. Saisch SGN, Wessely S, Gardner WN. Patients with acute hyperventilation presenting to an inner-city emergency department. *Chest* 1996, 110(4): 952–957.

38. Hornsveld HK, Garssen B, Fiedeldij Dop MJC, van Spiegel PI, de Haes J. Double-blind placebo-controlled study of the hyperventilation provocation test and the validity of the hyperventilation syndrome. *The Lancet* 1996, 348(9021): 154–158.

39. Gardner WN. The pathophysiology of hyperventilation disorders. *Chest* 1996, 109(2): 516–534.

40. Folgering H. The pathophysiology of hyperventilation syndrome. *Monaldi Archives for Chest Disease* 1999, 54(4): 365–372.

41. Callaham M. Hypoxic hazards of traditional paper bag rebreathing in hyperventilating patients. *Annals of Emergency Medicine* 1989, 18(6): 622–628.

42. The British Thoracic Society, Scottish Intercollegiate Guidelines Network. *British Guideline on the Management of Asthma* (Guideline 101). London/Edinburgh: BTS and SIGN, 2008 (revised May 2012). Available from: https://www.brit-thoracic.org.uk/document-library/clinical-information/asthma/btssign-asthma-guideline-2014/.

Hypothermia

1. Introduction

- Hypothermia is defined as a core body temperature below 35°C (refer to Figure 3.19). It is a potentially life-threatening condition and a reversible cause of cardiac arrest.

- Primary hypothermia is due to environmental exposure, with no underlying medical condition causing disruption of temperature regulation.

- Secondary hypothermia results from a medical illness lowering the temperature set-point.

- The speed of onset of hypothermia can vary:

i. **Acute hypothermia (immersion hypothermia)**
   - This occurs when a person loses heat very rapidly (e.g. by falling into cold water). It is associated with drowning. Acute hypothermia may also occur in a snow avalanche when it may be associated with asphyxia.

ii. **Subacute hypothermia (exhaustion hypothermia)**
   - This typically occurs in a hill walker who is exercising in moderate cold who becomes exhausted and is unable to generate enough heat. Heat loss will occur more rapidly in windy conditions or if the patient is wet or inadequately clothed. It may be associated with injury, frostbite or non-freezing cold injury. Do not forget that if one person in a group of walkers is hypothermic, others in the party who are similarly dressed and who have been exposed to identical conditions may also be hypothermic.

iii. **Chronic hypothermia**
   - In chronic hypothermia heat loss occurs slowly, often over days or longer. It most commonly occurs in the older person living in an inadequately heated house or the person who is sleeping rough. It can be associated with injury or illness (e.g. the patient who falls or has a stroke and who is on the floor overnight).

- Mixed forms of hypothermia may occur (e.g. the exhausted walker who collapses and falls into a stream).

1.1 Diagnosis

- In order to measure core body temperature accurately and make a diagnosis, a low-reading thermometer is required. However, most ambulance services do not carry low-reading thermometers. In the pre-hospital environment, measuring the patient's temperature using an oesophageal, bladder or rectal approach may not be practical. However, tympanic thermometry may not be reliable in cold environments (partly because the probe is not well insulated) or if the patient is in cardiac arrest, with no blood flow in the carotid artery.

- Because of the difficulty of diagnosing hypothermia in the pre-hospital environment, patients should be treated as having hypothermia if there is clinical suspicion of the diagnosis based on the risk factors in Table 3.71, the clinical history, examination and the presence of concurrent injuries or illness which may increase the likelihood of hypothermia.

TABLE 3.71 – Risk Factors for Hypothermia

Factors

- Older patients > 80 years due to impaired thermoregulation.

- Children due to their proportionately larger body surface area.

- Some medical conditions (e.g. hypothyroidism, stroke etc. due to impaired thermoregulation).

- Intoxicated patients (e.g. alcohol, recreational drugs).

- In association with drowning and in patients exposed to cold, wet and windy environments especially if inadequately dressed.

- Patients suffering from exhaustion.

- Injury and immobility.

- Decreased level of consciousness.

2. Incidence

- The true incidence is unknown but the ONS report fewer than 400 deaths per annum in England and Wales. However, it is suggested that hypothermia may be under-diagnosed in temperate climates such as the UK.

- Death from hypothermia is more common in those over the age of 70 and in males.

3. Pathophysiology

As the core body temperature falls, there may be:

- Progressive decrease in the level of consciousness (refer to **Altered Level of Consciousness**).

- Other brain dysfunction (e.g. slurring of speech, muscular incoordination).

- Slowing heart rate.

- Slowing respiratory rate.

- Development of cardiac arrhythmias, such as sinus bradycardia, atrial fibrillation, ventricular fibrillation and asystole.

- Cooling the body decreases oxygen demand and is protective for the brain and vital organs; therefore refer to the Hypothermia section within **Advanced Life Support** as good outcomes have resulted from prolonged resuscitation of hypothermic patients.

Hypothermia

4. Severity and Outcome

The severity of hypothermia can be classified as mild, moderate or severe depending on the patient's core body temperature (refer to Figure 3.19).

- However, in the pre-hospital environment, where appropriate thermometers and the skills to use them are often unavailable, it may be better to define the severity clinically (refer to Table 3.72).

Mild 35–32°C	Moderate 32–28°C	Severe <28°C

Figure 3.19 – Severity of hypothermia.

TABLE 3.72 – Clinical Stages of Hypothermia

Stage	Clinical Signs
I	Conscious and shivering.
II	Reduced conscious level; may or may not be shivering.
III	Unconscious; vital signs present.
IV	Apparent death; vital signs absent.

5. Assessment and Management

For the assessment and management of hypothermia, refer to Table 3.73.

TABLE 3.73 – ASSESSMENT and MANAGEMENT of: Hypothermia

Assess <C>ABCD

- If any of the following **TIME-CRITICAL** features are present:
  - major **<C>ABCD** problems, refer to **Medical Emergencies in Adults – Overview** and **Medical Emergencies in Children – Overview**.
  - haemodynamic compromise.
  - decreased level of consciousness.
  - cardiac arrest, then:
- Start correcting any **<C>ABCD** problems.
- Undertake a **TIME-CRITICAL** transfer to nearest appropriate receiving hospital or consider transfer to a hospital that provides extracorporeal life support (ECLS), as per local pathways.
- Continue patient management en-route.
- Provide an ATMIST information call.

Assess

- Undertake physical examination and assess for the presence of features of hypothermia (refer to Table 3.72): symptoms are often non-specific and can include ataxia, slurred speech, apathy, irrational behaviour and decrease in the level of consciousness (refer to **Altered Level of Consciousness**), heart rate and rhythm and respiratory rate.

Temperature

- Measure and record the patient's core temperature. Temperature measurement in the field is difficult, therefore it is important to suspect and treat hypothermia from the history and circumstances of the situation. Shivering peaks around 34°C and is minimal or stopped by 31–32°C. Shivering is a very effective way of raising body temperature BUT there must be adequate energy stores to fuel it.

SECTION 3 Medical Emergencies

Hypothermia

TABLE 3.73 – ASSESSMENT and MANAGEMENT of: Hypothermia *(continued)*

Warming

PREVENT FURTHER HEAT LOSS, as in the mildly hypothermic patient, preventing further heat loss will enable the patient to warm up by their own metabolism.

- Place in vehicle.
- Consider using foil blankets. Foil blankets work by reflecting radiated heat so are only useful in mild hypothermia. In severe hypothermia, minimal heat is radiated.
- Some foil blankets may only have one reflective surface so must be placed the right way round.
- If the patient is conscious, provide a hot drink/food if available and appropriate.
- **DO NOT** rub the patient's skin as this causes vasodilatation and may increase heat loss.
- **DO NOT** give the patient alcohol as this causes vasodilatation and may increase heat loss.
- Manage co-existing trauma or medical conditions as they arise (refer to appropriate **trauma/medical** guidelines).

Resuscitation

BEWARE: Severely hypothermic patients may initially appear to be dead but frequently have a very slow and weak pulse, very slow and shallow respirations, fixed dilated pupils and increased muscle tone. Dilated pupils can be seen in hypothermia and therefore should not be used as a sign of death.

- Rough handling can invoke cardiac arrhythmias (including VF and pulseless VT), so handle patients carefully.
- Airway – clear the airway.
- Ventilation – if there are no signs of respiration, ventilate with high concentrations of oxygen, but do NOT hyperventilate. A respiratory rate and tidal volume appropriate in normothermia is inappropriate in hypothermia (refer to appropriate **Resuscitation** guidelines).
- Signs of life – look for signs of life (palpate central artery, ECG monitoring etc.) for up to 1 minute.
- Cardiac arrest – refer to appropriate **Resuscitation** guidelines and additional information below. Remember that the rules for normothermic arrest must not be extrapolated completely to hypothermic arrest.
- Cardiac arrythmias (except VF) will usually revert spontaneously with re-warming and do not need treatment unless they persist after re-warming.

Respiratory Rate

- Measure and record respiratory rate.

Pulse

- Measure and record pulse.

Oxygen

- It is unlikely that SpO_2 can be reliably measured using a finger probe in a hypothermic patient. Oxygen should be given in all cases, and particularly if the patient is shivering and has co-morbidities, as the metabolic demand of intense shivering puts an extra burden on the heart. Administer 15 litres per minute until a reliable SpO_2 measurement can be obtained and then adjust oxygen flow to aim for target saturation within the range of 94–98% (refer to **Oxygen**).

Blood Pressure and Fluids

- Measure and record blood pressure. If required, administer fluids (preferably warm fluids). (Refer to **Intravascular Fluid Therapy in Adults** and **Intravascular Fluid Therapy in Children**).

Blood Glucose

- Measure and record blood glucose for hypo/hyperglycaemia (refer to **Glycaemic Emergencies in Adults and Children**).

NEWS2

- These observations will enable you to calculate a NEWS2 Score (refer to **Sepsis**).

ECG

- Monitor and record 12-Lead ECG. Assess for abnormality (refer to **Cardiac Rhythm Disturbance**).

(continued)

Hypothermia

TABLE 3.73 – ASSESSMENT and MANAGEMENT of: Hypothermia *(continued)*
Assess the Patient's Pain ▪ Where present, assess the **SOCRATES** of pain and record initial and subsequent pain scores. ▪ Consider analgesia if appropriate (refer to **Pain Management in Adults** and **Pain Management in Children**).
Transfer ▪ Transfer patients to the nearest appropriate receiving hospital. For patients with cardiac arrest, cardiovascular system instability (BP <90; irregular rhythm; ventricular arrhythmia), consider conveying to a hospital that provides ECLS, as per local pathways. ▪ In severe hypothermia with the presence of cardiac instability or arrest, the fastest way to re-warm patients is by extracorporeal warming – this may not be available in every hospital, so follow any local care pathways. Other patients can be re-warmed successfully by less invasive or non-invasive methods. ▪ Continue management en-route. ▪ Complete documentation.
Additional Information for Cardiac Arrest in Hypothermia While breathing continues, cardiac arrest has not occurred so do not start CPR. **Do not stop cardiac resuscitation in the field.** Follow the usual procedure (refer to appropriate **Resuscitation** guidelines) with the following minor changes: ▪ Hypothermia may cause chest wall stiffness, and ventilations and compressions may be more difficult. ▪ Drugs are less likely to be effective at low body temperatures: do not give ALS drugs if the core temperature is below 30°C. ▪ Defibrillation is less likely to be effective at low body temperatures: if VF persists after 3 shocks, delay further defibrillation until the core temperature is above 30°C. ▪ Hypothermia is protective and good outcomes have resulted from prolonged resuscitation of hypothermic patients. **Trauma** (refer to appropriate **Trauma** guidelines) – hypothermia worsens the prognosis of trauma patients, so it is important that patients who are initially normothermic are not allowed to become hypothermic. This may occur for example during a prolonged extrication from a road traffic collision or from the cooling of burns.
Documentation ▪ Complete documentation to include all clinical findings, advice from other clinicians, onward referral and worsening advice given.

KEY POINTS!

Hypothermia

▪ **Do not stop cardiac resuscitation in the field.**

▪ **Hypothermia is defined as a core body temperature below 35°C.**

▪ **Prevent further heat loss; wrap the patient appropriately, do not rub the skin or give alcohol.**

▪ **If cardiac arrest occurs, ALS drugs may not be effective; prolonged (hours) CPR will be required.**

Hypothermia

Bibliography

1. Gordon L, Paal P. Normothermic and hypothermic cardiac arrest – beware of Jekyll and Hyde. *Resuscitation* 2018, 129: e10–11.

2. Haverkamp FJC, Giesbrecht GG, Tan ECTH. The prehospital management of hypothermia – an up-to-date overview. *Injury* 2018, 49: 149–164.

3. Paal P, Gordon L, Strapazzon G, Brodmann Maeder M, Putzer G, Walpoth B, et al. Accidental hypothermia-an update: the content of this review is endorsed by the International Commission for Mountain Emergency Medicine (ICAR MEDCOM). *Scand J Trauma Resusc Emerg Med* 2016, 24: 111.

4. Truhlar A, Deakin CD, Soar J, Khalifa GE, Alfonzo A, Bierens JJ. European Resuscitation Council Guidelines for Resuscitation 2015. Section 8: cardiac arrest in special circumstances. *Resuscitation* 2015, 95: 148–201.

5. Caroselli C, Gabrieli A, Pisani A, Bruno G. Hypothermia: an under-estimated risk. *Internal and Emergency Medicine* 2009, 4(3): 227–230.

6. Strapazzon G, Procter E, Paal P, Brugger H. Pre-hospital core temperature measurement in accidental and therapeutic hypothermia. *High Alt Med Biol* 2014, 15(2): 104–111.

7. Ireland S, Endacott R, Cameron P, Fitzgerald M, Paul E. The incidence and significance of accidental hypothermia in major trauma—a prospective observational study. *Resuscitation* 2011, 82: 300–306.

8. Stroop R, Schone CH Grau Th. Incidence and strategies for preventing sustained hypothermia of crash victims during prolonged vehicle extrication. *Injury* 2019, 50: 308–317.

9. Waibel BH, Schlitzkus LL, Newell MA, et al. Impact of hypothermia (below 36°C) in the rural trauma patient. *J Am Coll Surg* 2009, 209: 580–588.

10. Shari S, Elliott AC, Gentilello L. Is hypothermia simply a marker of shock and injury severity or an independent risk factor for mortality in trauma patients? Analysis of a large national trauma registry. *J Trauma* 2005. 59: 1081–1085.

11. Eidstuen SC, Uleberg O, Vangberg G, Skogvoll E. When do trauma patients lose temperature – a prospective study. *Acta Aanes Scand* 2018, 62: 384–393.

12. Winkelmann M, Soechtig W, Macke C, et al. Accidental hypothermia as an independent risk factor or poor neurological outcome in older multiply injured patients with severe traumatic brain injury: a matched pair analysis. *Eur J Trauma Emerg Surg* 2019, 45: 255–261.

13. Trentzsche H, Huber-Wagner S, Hildebrand F, et al. Hypothermia for prediction of death in severely injured blunt trauma patients. *Shock* 2012, 37: 131–139.

14. Lapostolle F, Courvreur J, Koch FX, Savary D, et al. Hypothermia in trauma victims at first arrival of ambulance personnel: an observational study with assessment of risk factors. *Scand J Trauma Resus Emerg Med* 2017, 25: 43.

15. Khorsandi M, Dougherty S, Yound N, Kerslake D, Giordano V, Lendrum R, et al. Extracorporeal life support for refractory cardiac arrest from accidental hypothermia: a 1–year experience in Edinburgh. *J Emerg Med* 2016, 52: 160–168.

16. McCormack J, Percival D. HEMS advanced trauma team retrieval of a patient with accidental hypothermic cardiac arrest for ECMO therapy. *Resuscitation* 2016, 105: e23.

17. Ruttmann E, Dietl M, Kastenberger T, et al. Characteristics and outcome of patients with hypothermic out-of-hospital cardiac arrest: experience from a European trauma center. *Resuscitation* 2017, 120: 57–62.

18. Forti A, Brugnaro P, Crucitti M, Brugger H, Cipollotti G, Strapazzon G. Hypothermic cardiac arrest with full neurologic recovery after approximately nine hours of cardiopulmonary resuscitation: management and possible complications. *Ann Emerg Med* 2019, 73: 52–57.

Implantable Cardioverter Defibrillator

1. Introduction

- The implantable cardioverter defibrillator (ICD) has revolutionised the management of patients at risk of developing a life-threatening ventricular arrhythmia. Several clinical trials have testified to their effectiveness in reducing deaths from sudden cardiac arrest in selected patients, and the devices are implanted with increasing frequency.

- ICDs are used in both children and adults.

- ICD systems consist of a generator connected to electrodes placed transvenously into cardiac chambers (the ventricle, and sometimes the right atrium and/or the coronary sinus) (refer to Figure 3.20). The electrodes serve a dual function allowing the monitoring of cardiac rhythm and the administration of electrical pacing, defibrillation and cardioversion therapy. Modern ICDs are slightly larger than a pacemaker and are usually implanted in the left subclavicular area (refer to Figure 3.20). The ICD generator contains the battery and sophisticated electronic circuitry that monitors the cardiac rhythm, determines the need for electrical therapy, delivers treatment, monitors the response and determines the need for further therapy.

- The available therapies include:
  - Conventional programmable pacing for the treatment of bradycardia
  - Anti-tachycardia pacing (ATP) for ventricular tachycardia (VT)
  - Delivery of biphasic shocks for the treatment of ventricular tachycardia and ventricular fibrillation (VF)
  - Cardiac resynchronisation therapy (CRT) (biventricular pacing) for the treatment of heart failure.

- These treatment modalities and specifications are programmable and capable of considerable sophistication to suit the requirements of individual patients. The implantation and programming of devices is carried out in specialised centres. The patient should carry a card or documentation which identifies their ICD centre and may also have been given emergency instructions.

- The personnel caring for such patients in emergency situations are not usually experts in arrhythmia management or familiar with the details of the sophisticated treatment regimes offered by modern ICDs. Moreover, the technology is complex and evolving rapidly. In an emergency, patients will often present to the ambulance service or emergency department (ED) and the purpose of this guidance is to help those responsible for the initial management of these patients.

2. General Principles

- Some important points should be made at the outset.

- On detecting VF/VT, the ICD will usually discharge a maximum of eight times before shutting down. However, a new episode of VF/VT will result in the recommencing of its discharge sequence. A patient with a fractured ICD lead may suffer repeated internal defibrillation as the electrical noise is misinterpreted as a shockable rhythm.

- These patients are likely to be conscious with a relatively normal ECG rate.

- When confronted with a patient in cardiac arrest, the usual management guidelines are still appropriate (refer to **cardiac arrest** and **arrhythmia** guidelines). If the ICD is not responding to VF or VT, or if shocks are ineffective, external defibrillation/cardioversion should be carried out. Avoid placing the defibrillator electrodes/pads/paddles close to or on top of the ICD; ensure a minimum distance of 8 cm between the edge of the defibrillator paddle pad/electrode and the ICD site. Most ICDs are implanted in the left sub-clavicular position (refer to Figure 3.20) and are usually readily apparent on examination; the conventional (apical/right subclavicular) electrode position will then be appropriate. The anterior/posterior position may also be used, particularly if the ICD is right sided.

- Whenever possible, record a 12-lead electrocardiogram (ECG) and record the patient's rhythm (with any shocks). Make sure this is printed out and stored electronically (where available) for future reference. Where an external defibrillator with an electronic memory is used (whether for monitoring or for therapy), ensure that the ECG report is printed and handed to appropriate staff. Again, whenever

Figure 3.20 – Usual location of an ICD.

Implantable Cardioverter Defibrillator

possible, ensure that the record is archived for future reference. Record the rhythm during any therapeutic measure (whether by drugs or electricity). All these records may provide vital information for the ICD centre that may greatly influence the patient's subsequent management.

■ The energy levels of the shocks administered by ICDs (up to 40 Joules) are much lower than those delivered with external defibrillators (120–360 J). **Personnel in contact with the patient when an ICD discharges are unlikely to be harmed, but it is prudent to minimise contact with the patient while the ICD is firing.** Chest compression and ventilation can be carried out as normal, and protective examination gloves should be worn as usual.

■ Placing a ring magnet over the ICD generator can temporarily disable the shock capability of an ICD. The magnet does not disable the pacing capability for treating bradycardia. The magnet may be kept in position with adhesive tape if required. Removing the magnet returns the ICD to the status present before application. The ECG rhythm should be monitored at all times when the device is disabled. An ICD should only be disabled when the rhythm for which shocks are being delivered has been recorded. If that rhythm is VT or VF, external cardioversion/defibrillation must be available. With some models, it is possible to programme the ICD so that a magnet does not disable the shock capabilities of the device. This is usually done only in exceptional circumstances, and consequently such patients are rare.

■ The manufacturers of the ICDs also supply the ring magnets. Many implantation centres provide each patient with a ring magnet and stress that it should be readily available in case of emergency. With the increasing prevalence of ICDs in the community, it becomes increasingly important that emergency workers have this magnet available to them when attending these patients.

■ Decisions to apply a Do Not Attempt Cardio Pulmonary Resuscitation (DNACPR) order will not be made in the emergency situation by the personnel to whom this guidance is directed. Where such an order does exist, it should not be necessary to disable an ICD to enable the implementation of such an order.

■ Many problems with ICDs can only be dealt with permanently by using the programmer available at the ICD centre.

■ The guidelines should be read from the perspective of your position and role in the management of such patients. For example, the recommendation to 'arrange further assessment' will mean that the ambulance clinician should transport the patient to hospital. For ED staff, however, this might mean referral to the medical admitting team or local ICD centre.

■ Coincident conditions that may contribute to the development of arrhythmia (e.g. acute ischaemia worsening heart failure) should be managed as appropriate according to usual practice.

■ Maintain oxygen saturations above 94%.

■ Receiving ICD therapy may be unpleasant 'like a firm kick in the chest', and psychological consequences may also arise. It is important to be aware of these, and help should be available from implantation centres. An emergency telephone helpline may be available.

3. Management

■ The following should be read in conjunction with the treatment table (refer to Table 3.74) and algorithm (refer to Figure 3.21). Approach and assess the patient and perform basic life support according to current BLS guidelines.

Monitor the ECG	
3.1.	If the patient is in cardiac arrest.
3.1.1	Perform basic life support in accordance with current BLS guidelines. Standard airway management techniques and methods for gaining IV/IO access (as appropriate) should be established.
3.1.2	If a shockable rhythm is present (VF or pulseless VT) but the ICD is not detecting it, perform external defibrillation and other resuscitation procedures according to current resuscitation guidelines.
3.1.3	If the ICD is delivering therapy (whether by anti-tachycardia pacing or shocks) but is failing to convert the arrhythmia, then external defibrillation should be provided, as per current guidelines.
3.1.4	If a non-shockable rhythm is present, manage the patient according to current guidelines. If the rhythm is converted to a shockable one, assess the response of the ICD, performing external defibrillation as required.
3.1.5	If a shockable rhythm is converted to one associated with effective cardiac output (whether by the ICD or by external defibrillation), manage the patient as usual and arrange further treatment and assessment.

(continued)

Implantable Cardioverter Defibrillator

	Monitor the ECG *(continued)*
3.2.	If the patient is not in cardiac arrest.
3.2.1	Determine whether an arrhythmia is present.
3.2.2	If no arrhythmia is present:
	If therapy from the ICD has been effective and the patient is in sinus rhythm or is paced, monitor the patient, give O_2 and arrange further assessment to investigate the possibility of new myocardial infarction (MI), heart failure, other acute illness or drug toxicity/electrolyte imbalance etc.
	An ICD may deliver inappropriate shocks (i.e. in the absence of arrhythmia) if there are problems with sensing the cardiac rhythm or with the leads. Record the rhythm (while shocks are delivered, if possible), disable the ICD with a magnet, monitor the patient and arrange further assessment with help from the ICD centre. Provide supportive treatment as required.
3.2.3	If an arrhythmia is present:
	If an arrhythmia is present and shocks are being delivered, record the arrhythmia (while ICD shocks are delivered if possible) on the ECG. Determine the nature of the arrhythmia. Transport rapidly to hospital in all cases.
TACHYCARDIA	
3.2.3.1	If the rhythm is a **supraventricular tachycardia** (i.e. sinus tachycardia, atrial flutter, atrial fibrillation, junctional tachycardia, etc.) and the patient is haemodynamically stable and is continuing to receive shocks, disable the ICD with a magnet. Consider possible causes, treat appropriately and arrange further assessment in hospital.
3.2.3.2	If the rhythm is **ventricular tachycardia**:
	▪ Pulseless VT should be treated as cardiac arrest (3.1.2 above).
	▪ If the patient is haemodynamically stable, monitor the patient and convey to the emergency department.
	▪ If the patient is haemodynamically unstable, and ICD shocks are ineffective, treat as per VT guideline.
	▪ An ICD will not deliver antitachycardia pacing (ATP) or shocks if the rate of the VT is below the programmed detection rate of the device (generally 150 beats/min). Conventional management may be undertaken according to the patient's haemodynamic status.
	▪ Recurring VT with appropriate shocks. Manage any underlying cause (acute ischaemia, heart failure etc.). Sedation may be of benefit.
INAPPROPRIATE/INEFFECTIVE ICD FIRING	
3.2.3.3	A ring magnet placed over the ICD box will stop the ICD from firing and may be considered in conscious patients where the ICD shocks are ineffective and the patient is distressed. In ICDs that have a dual pacing function, the magnet will also usually change the pacing function to deliver a paced output of 50 beats/min.

TABLE 3.74 – ASSESSMENT and MANAGEMENT of: Patients Fitted with an ICD
Patient in Cardiac Arrest:
▪ Assess the patient
– Perform basic life support in accordance with current BLS guidelines.
– Standard airway management techniques.
– IV access (if required) should be used.
▪ Monitor the ECG.
Assess Rhythm:
▪ Shockable rhythm is present (VF or pulseless VT)
– **BUT** the ICD is not detecting it, perform external defibrillation and other resuscitation procedures according to current resuscitation guidelines.
– If the ICD is delivering therapy (whether by ATP or shocks) but is failing to convert the arrhythmia, then external defibrillation should be provided, as per current guidelines.

Implantable Cardioverter Defibrillator

TABLE 3.74 – ASSESSMENT and MANAGEMENT of: Patients Fitted with an ICD *(continued)*

- Non-shockable rhythm
  - Manage the patient according to current guidelines. If the rhythm is converted to a shockable one, assess the response of the ICD, performing external defibrillation as required.

- If a shockable rhythm is converted to one associated with effective cardiac output (whether by the ICD or by external defibrillation)
  - Manage the patient as usual and arrange further treatment and assessment.

Patient NOT in Cardiac Arrest

- Determine whether an arrhythmia is present.

If no arrhythmia is present

- If therapy from the ICD has been effective, the patient is in sinus rhythm or is paced:
  - Monitor the patient.
  - Administer oxygen and aim for a saturation above 94% (refer to **Oxygen**).
  - Arrange further assessment to investigate possibility of new myocardial infarction (MI), heart failure, other acute illness or drug toxicity/electrolyte imbalance etc.
  - An ICD may deliver inappropriate shocks (i.e. in the absence of arrhythmia) if there are problems with sensing the cardiac rhythm or problems with the leads:
  - Record the rhythm (while ICD shocks are delivered, if possible).
  - Disable the ICD with a magnet.
  - Monitor the patient.
  - Arrange further assessment with help from the ICD centre. Provide supportive treatment as required.
  - A ring magnet placed over the ICD box will stop the ICD from firing and may be considered in conscious patients where the ICD shocks are ineffective and the patient is distressed. In ICDs that have a dual pacing function, the magnet will also usually change the pacing function to deliver a constant paced output, dependent on the manufacturer.

If an arrhythmia is present

- If an arrhythmia is present and shocks are being delivered:
  - Record the arrhythmia (while ICD shocks are delivered, if possible) on the ECG.
  - Determine the nature of the arrhythmia.
  - Transport rapidly to hospital in all cases.

If the rhythm is **supraventricular** (i.e. sinus tachycardia, atrial flutter, atrial fibrillation, junctional tachycardia, etc.)

- If the patient is haemodynamically stable, and is continuing to receive shocks, disable the ICD with a magnet:
  - Consider possible causes, treat appropriately.
  - Arrange further assessment in hospital.

If the rhythm is **ventricular tachycardia**

- Pulseless VT should be treated as cardiac arrest (3.1.2 above).

If the patient is haemodynamically stable:

- Monitor the patient.
- Convey to the emergency department.

If the patient is haemodynamically unstable, and ICD shocks are ineffective, treat as per VT guideline.

- An ICD will not deliver ATP or shocks if the rate of the VT is below the programmed detection rate of the device. Conventional management may be undertaken according to the patient's haemodynamic status.

- For recurring VT with appropriate shocks, manage any underlying cause (acute ischaemia, heart failure etc.). Sedation may be of benefit.

3 SECTION **Medical Emergencies**

Implantable Cardioverter Defibrillator

Figure 3.21 – Implantable cardioverter defibrillator algorithm.

Implantable Cardioverter Defibrillator

Bibliography

1. Deakin CD, Nolan JP, Soar J, Sunde K, Koster RW, Smith GB, et al. European Resuscitation Council Guidelines for Resuscitation 2010 Section 4: adult advanced life support. *Resuscitation* 2010, 81(10): 1305–1352.

2. Koster RW, Baubin MA, Bossaert LL, Caballero A, Cassan P, Castren M, et al. European Resuscitation Council Guidelines for Resuscitation 2010 Section 2: adult basic life support and use of automated external defibrillators. *Resuscitation* 2010, 81(10): 1277–1292.

3. Nolan JP, Soar J, Zideman DA, Biarent D, Bossaert LL, Deakin C, et al. European Resuscitation Council Guidelines for Resuscitation 2010 Section 1: executive summary. *Resuscitation* 2010, 81(10): 1219–1276.

4. Deakin CD, Nolan JP, Sunde K, Koster RW. European Resuscitation Council Guidelines for Resuscitation 2010 Section 3: electrical therapies: automated external defibrillators, defibrillation, cardioversion and pacing. *Resuscitation* 2010, 81(10): 1293–1304.

5. Deakin CD, Morrison LJ, Morley PT, Callaway CW, Kerber RE, Kronick SL, et al. Part 8: advanced life support: 2010 International Consensus on Cardiopulmonary Resuscitation and Emergency Cardiovascular Care Science with Treatment Recommendations. *Resuscitation* 2010, 81(1): e93–174.

6. Sunde K, Jacobs I, Deakin CD, Hazinski MF, Kerber RE, Koster RW, et al. Part 6: defibrillation: 2010 International Consensus on Cardiopulmonary Resuscitation and Emergency Cardiovascular Care Science with Treatment Recommendations. *Resuscitation* 2010, 81(1): e71–85.

SECTION **3** Medical Emergencies

Low Back Pain (Non-traumatic)

1. Introduction

- This guideline applies to adults over 18 years old. It does **not** apply to patients that have experienced recent trauma causing their low back pain (including axial-loading mechanisms to top of head through spine). In these instances, refer to **Trauma Emergencies in Adults – Overview** and **Spinal Injury and Spinal Chord Injury**.

- Many people experience back pain at some point in their adult life. Most often, symptoms resolve within 6 weeks with conservative management, including appropriate analgesia, exercise and lifestyle advice. Radiographs are not normally required for acute non-traumatic musculoskeletal back pain in healthy individuals with good bone health.

- Ambulance services are frequently called to patients experiencing severe and debilitating acute low back pain. Assistance is often required for these patients; however, the high severity of the symptoms may frequently exceed the severity of the underlying diagnosis, which will often be non-sinister musculoskeletal pain.

- The likelihood of serious pathology increases with age, and caution is advised in patients over 50 years of age. Alternative diagnoses should be considered in all patients, regardless of age, particularly where symptoms are new or have recently changed. Specific causes of lower back pain that should be considered include cancer, infection, fragility fractures, renal colic, inflammatory disease, abdominal aortic aneurysm, pancreatitis, aortic dissection and ectopic pregnancy. Lower back pain is commonly encountered in pregnancy and the same clinical assessment should be performed, making special consideration of pregnancy-associated emergencies (refer to **Maternity Care (including Obstetric Emergencies Overview)**).

2. Incidence

- Low back pain is a common cause of calls to ambulance services in the UK.[1]

- In the United Kingdom, over 2.5 million people consult their GP every year due to back pain. Up to 60% of the population will experience back pain at some point in their adult life, with over 28% of adults over 25 years experiencing low back pain each month.[2]

- Patients may present with new onset lower back pain, or with exacerbations of known chronic pain. Between 3% to 7% of adults are chronically disabled by lower back pain.[3]

- Low back pain is a leading cause of sickness absence from work in the European workforce.[4] However, data suggest that over 70% of people have returned to work at 1 month from onset, and over 93% at 1 year.[5]

- Chronic back pain is associated with mental health issues contributed to by ongoing pain and disability.

3. Severity and Outcome

- Low back pain is subdivided by time frame into:
  - Acute low back pain: less than 4 weeks' duration.
  - Subacute lower back pain: 4 to 12 weeks' duration.
  - Chronic low back pain: lasting more than 12 weeks.

- Most low back pain is musculoskeletal in origin and is defined as pain and/or stiffness in the lumbosacral area of the back, between the bottom of the ribs and the top of the legs.[6] The symptoms may arise from many anatomical structures of the lower back and surrounding area.

- Non-specific low back pain is a well-recognised clinical entity that is diagnosed when the pain cannot be attributed to a specific cause but may likely be related to muscular, ligamentous, intervertebral disc or joint-related origins.[3,7]

- While patients may complain of isolated pain in the lumbosacral region of the spine, they may also encounter radiation of pain unilaterally to the buttocks or thighs, and this may extend beyond the knee.

4. Differential Diagnosis

4.1 Key Differential Diagnoses

- While most low back pain is musculoskeletal in origin, other causes of back pain must always be considered. These include (but are not limited to):
  - renal colic
  - aortic aneurysm
  - aortic dissection
  - pancreatitis
  - ectopic pregnancy.

- Abdominal examination must form part of the examination of patients with low back pain, and must be performed prior to making a diagnosis of musculoskeletal back pain.

4.2 Red Flag Symptoms in Musculoskeletal Pain

- Serious pathology as a cause of musculoskeletal conditions is considered rare but must be managed as an emergency or as urgent depending on local pathways.

- The majority of serious pathology affecting the spine (such as vertebral fractures, cauda equina syndrome, malignant metastatic disease, infection) will most commonly present with back

Low Back Pain (Non-traumatic)

pain. Serious pathologies such as these can involve other body systems.

- Consider serious pathology as a differential diagnosis to exclude where any of the following features are present:
  - escalating back pain and progressively worsening symptoms that have not responded to conservative management or analgesia
  - systemic illness (e.g. weight loss, fever)
  - night pain that prevents sleep, and/or difficulty in lying flat
  - saddle anaesthesia, disturbance of bladder or bowel function or bilateral sciatica
  - severe or progressive neurological deficit, motor weakness or paralysis.

5. Serious Pathologies (for Conveyance to Hospital)

5.1 Cauda Equina Syndrome (CES)

- Cauda equina syndrome (CES) is a rare but serious condition caused by compression to the nerve roots at the end of the spinal cord ('cauda equina' = 'horse's tail') typically at the levels from L2 to L5. It is a neurosurgical emergency requiring an urgent MRI scan to confirm or exclude the diagnosis. Where the diagnosis is confirmed, a neurosurgical strategy will typically involve emergency spinal decompressive surgery.
- CES should be suspected in people presenting with back pain. Specific symptoms to ask about include:
  - any changes in bladder or bowel function
  - bilateral sciatica (pain radiating down buttocks and thighs)
  - numbness or reduced sensation around or under the genitals, or around the anus
  - loss of anal tone (ability to squeeze anal muscles)
  - loss of sexual function.
- Care must be taken to enquire about these symptoms that may be embarrassing to patients, such as episodes of unexpected faecal incontinence or urinary retention, numbness affecting the perineum when they wipe themselves after going to the toilet or sensory disturbance affecting sexual function (including erectile dysfunction).

5.2 Metastatic Spinal Cord Compression (MSCC)

- Metastatic spinal cord compression (MSCC) occurs as a consequence of metastatic disease infiltrating the bones of the spine. It can lead to irreversible neurological damage.
- Symptoms can include:
  - banding pain (circulating around the torso)

- rapidly escalating pain
- disturbance of gait or coordination
- pain that is worsened on lying flat
- unremitting pain at night
- systemic illness associated with advanced malignancy.

- Metastatic disease of the spine can originate from many different primary cancers, including lung, bowel, breast, prostate and blood cancers such as lymphoma. Bony infiltration of the metastatic cancer can lead to collapse of the vertebral bones due to loss of their structural integrity (leading to pain) and can also lead to neurological symptoms from invasion or compression at the spinal canal.

5.3 Infection

- Infections can occur within the spine, notably at the level of the intervertebral discs (discitis) or as collection of pus within the epidural space (abscess). These are uncommon infections in healthy individuals with an uncompromised immune system. However, it is important to consider infection as a cause of unexplained back pain, especially in immune-compromised patients such as those on medications or treatment that reduce their immunity. Intravenous drug users and patients with known active or suspected tuberculosis are also at particular risk of spinal infection.
- Infection should be suspected in patients with back pain, alongside systemic symptoms such as:
  - fever
  - weight loss
  - general malaise/lethargy
  - unexplained tachycardia (patients in severe pain may be tachycardic until this is controlled).

5.4 Vertebral Insufficiency Fracture(s)

- Patients may present with sudden onset of pain localised to the spine, usually in the thoraco-lumbar region. This may occur after low-impact trauma, and may be a sharp, severe pain that is exacerbated by movement.
- Risk factors that may be associated with vertebral insufficiency fractures include:
  - a history of other fragility fractures (such as neck of femur or distal radius fractures)
  - osteoporosis
  - long-term steriod use
  - renal disease.

5.5 Cervical Spondylotic Myelopathy (CSM)

- In rare cases, cervical spondylosis (age-related degeneration) can progress to this syndrome, which is characterised by worsening neck pain, incoordination (e.g. difficulty with simple motor

Low Back Pain (Non-traumatic)

tasks such as fastening buttons), heaviness or weakness in arms or legs, pins and needles in arms, difficulty walking and bowel or bladder disturbance.

6. Urgent Conditions (May Be Appropriate for Community Management and/or Referral to Primary Care)

- In most instances, non-traumatic low back pain can be managed in the community with over-the-counter analgesic medications and simple exercises. Other conditions may be appropriate for management in the community but may nonetheless require investigation and support from primary care services. Ambulance clinicians should endeavour to contact a patient's own GP where possible (in-hours), and ensure that a copy of their assessment notes is available to the primary care services to access (as per local guidance and pathways).

- Patients should be provided with advice and guidance tailored to their needs and functional capabilities to empower them to provide self-care for their low back pain. This should include:
  - information relating to the nature of their back pain
  - encouragement to continue with normal activities and routines (where able).[8]

6.1 Rheumatological Conditions

- Osteoarthritis and rheumatoid arthritis may present with an acute flare or progression of symptoms affecting joints including the spine and sacro-iliac joints.

6.2 Known Primary or Secondary Cancers

- Red flag symptoms of MSCC or CES should be excluded (as previously described in section above); however, other patients with low back pain related to cancer may be appropriate for management in the community.

6.3 Acute Sciatica

- Sciatica is a painful syndrome caused by irritation or compression of the sciatic nerve that runs from the lower back to the feet. Sciatica is usually self-limiting within 4–6 weeks but may last longer. Symptoms may be exacerbated by movements such as bending, coughing or sneezing.

- Patients may complain of unilateral pain described as stabbing, burning or shooting in character, and may also encounter weakness, or tingling or numbness, to sensory areas of the buttock, back of leg, knee or foot.

7. Assessment and Management

- Taking a clear and thorough history is an essential part of the assessment in order to explore possible serious pathologies. This will require asking a range of questions, some of which may be intrusive or embarrassing, and so it should be explained to patients that these questions are important and relate to the symptoms of back pain.

- It may be helpful to explain that nerves supply all limbs and organs, and that the nerves at the lower part of the spine supply the bowel and bladder, as well as the patient's sexual function. It may be necessary to ask directly:
  - Have there been any episodes of incontinence (faeces or urine), or have they suffered urinary retention?
  - Have they been able to go to the toilet when they try to?
  - Have they been wet or soiled without knowing?
  - Does it feel different when they wipe themselves after going to the toilet?

- Ask how the patient is coping with the pain. This may be helpful in eliciting what they might be concerned about, and may also establish if the symptoms are exacerbating any chronic or acute mental health problems.

- Explain that medication and other substances can affect pain. Take a thorough social history, including a drug history of prescribed and non-prescribed drugs, alcohol and recreational substances. If necessary, refer to **Alcohol-use Disorders**.

TABLE 3.75 – ASSESSMENT and MANAGEMENT of: Low Back Pain

Assess CABCD

- If any of the following **TIME-CRITICAL** features are present:
  - Major **CABCD** problems (refer to **Medical Emergencies in Adults – Overview**).
- Start correcting any **CABCD** problems.
- Undertake a **TIME-CRITICAL** transfer to nearest appropriate receiving hospital.
- Continue patient management en-route.
- Provide an ATMIST information call.

Low Back Pain (Non-traumatic)

TABLE 3.75 – ASSESSMENT and MANAGEMENT of: Low Back Pain *(continued)*
Respiratory Rate
▪ Measure and record respiratory rate.
Pulse
▪ Measure and record pulse and heart rate.
Oxygen Saturation
▪ Monitor the patient's SpO$_2$; administer oxygen to achieve saturations of >94% if the patient presents as hypoxaemic on air (refer to **Oxygen**).
Blood Pressure
▪ Measure and record blood pressure.
Blood Glucose
▪ If appropriate, measure and record blood glucose for hypo/hyperglycaemia (refer to **Glycaemic Emergencies**).
Temperature
▪ Measure and record temperature.
NEWS2
▪ These observations will enable you to calculate a NEWS2 score.
ECG
▪ If required, monitor and record 12-lead ECG. Assess for abnormality (refer to **Cardiac Rhythm Disturbance**).
Assess the Patient's Pain
▪ Assessment of pain using SOCRATES and score pain using 0–10 rating (refer to **Pain Management**).
Assess for Other Possible Emergency Medical Causes of the Back Pain
▪ Assess the abdomen.
▪ Consider dissecting thoracic or abdominal aortic aneurysm, pancreatitis, renal colic, aortic dissection and ectopic pregnancy.
Assess for Any Red Flags
▪ Chest pain radiating through to the back.
▪ Known or suspected underlying serious pathology.
▪ Bladder/bowels disturbance (new retention or incontinence).
▪ Bilateral leg pain/pins and needles/numbness.
▪ Saddle paraesthesia.
▪ Banding pain (circulating around the whole torso)/pins and needles/numbness.
▪ Sudden onset of thoracic pain.
▪ Upper limb incoordination/heaviness.
▪ Gait incoordination.
▪ Jaw pain.
▪ Signs or suspicion of fracture.
▪ Persistent headache.
▪ Dizziness.
▪ Drop attack/blackout/collapse.
▪ Visual disturbance.
▪ Any signs of infection.
▪ Systemically unwell.
▪ Unremitting night pain.
▪ Escalating and worsening pain.

(continued)

Section 3 Medical Emergencies

Low Back Pain (Non-traumatic)

TABLE 3.75 – ASSESSMENT and MANAGEMENT of: Low Back Pain *(continued)*

Inspect the Patient

- What position is the patient when found?
- Can the patient sit?
- Can the patient stand?
- Can the patient lie flat?
- Can the patient mobilise?
- Can the patient evenly bear weight?
- Does the patient's spine have normal curvature, or do they have a kyphosis (bent forwards) or scoliosis (curved sideways)?
- Is the patient experiencing any muscle spasm?
- Does the patient have any areas of skin discolouration, rashes or swelling?
- Does the patient have any fasciculation (muscle twitch/involuntary muscle contraction)?

Palpation

- Palpate the spine for any bony tenderness, crepitus or unnatural alignment of spinal processes.
- Palpate sacroiliac joint and paravertebral muscles for pain/tenderness/spasm/swelling.

Assess for Paraesthesia (Pins and Needles)

See Figure 3.22.

- Where does the patient feel paraesthesia?
- Does the patient feel this constantly or intermittently?

Functional Assessment

- Ask patient to perform a straight leg raise – if this is painful, it usually indicates sciatic nerve irritation due to intervertebral disc disease.
- Assess and document range of movement/strength. Can patient mobilise and manage to undertake basic personal care?

Other Social and Psychological Factors to Assess (Yellow Flags)

- Mental health problems (mood/stress/anxiety/depression).
- Misuse of alcohol or medication misuse (prescription and non-prescription).
- Is the pain affecting activities of daily living (ADLs)?

Functional levels of exercise and activity

- Weight loss or weight gain.
- A belief that pain and/or activity is harmful.
- Social withdrawal.
- Have they been unable to work due to the pain?
- Lack of support at home.

What are the patient's expectations for their care?

- It is not uncommon for patient's to seek diagnostic imaging in the hope that this will remedy their symptoms, and it may be appropriate to counsel patients that emergency MRI imaging is not generally indicated in the absence of red flag signs or symptoms.
- Medication history, including non-prescribed and over the counter medication – what's been tried, dosages etc.

Documentation

- Complete documentation to include all clinical findings, advice from other clinicians, onward referral and worsening safety-net advice provided.

Low Back Pain (Non-traumatic)

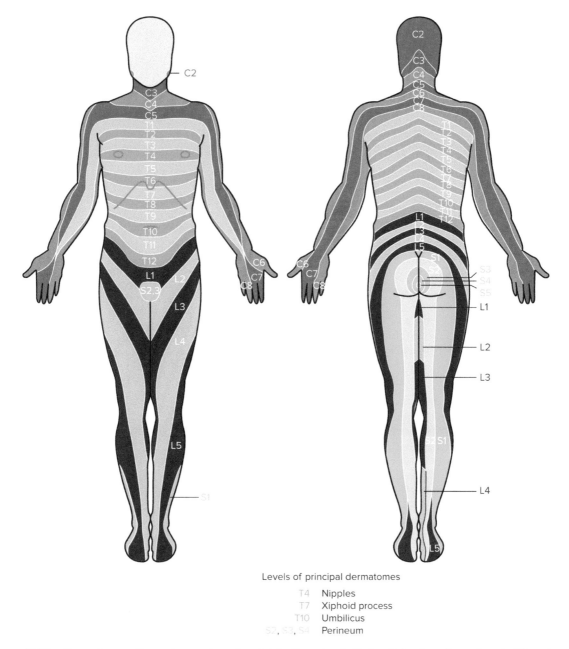

Levels of principal dermatomes

T4	Nipples
T7	Xiphoid process
T10	Umbilicus
S2, S3, S4	Perineum

Figure 3.22 – Dermatomes. Dermatomes show the distribution of pain that radiates from the spine at different levels.

8. Pain Management

Both pharmacological and non-pharmacological management options may be appropriate. As a general approach, the patient should be reminded that for simple low back pain their symptoms are likely to improve with a strategy of simple analgesia, gentle exercises and modification of lifestyle factors that may exacerbate the pain.

8.1 Pharmacological Management

▪ Refer to **Pain Management in Adults**. If a patient already has a pain management plan, they should be advised to follow this and to seek advice from a pharmacist as required.

▪ Current guidance suggests offering a non-steroidal anti-inflammatory (NSAID) such as ibuprofen as first-line pharmacological treatment in low back pain. Instruction to take gastro-protective medication is recommended, as these reduce stomach acid secretion and mitigate the small risk of GI bleeding that is increased with NSAIDs. Both ibuprofen and proton-pump inhibitors such as omeprazole can be bought over the counter in large stores or pharmacies, where additional advice will also be available.

▪ Ibuprofen is indicated for mild to moderate pain and inflammation. Refer to **Ibuprofen** for doses, indications and contraindications. Ibuprofen works as an anti-inflammatory at higher (400–600 mg) doses, and effects are usually noted within 30 minutes.

Low Back Pain (Non-traumatic)

Low Back Pain (Non-traumatic)

- Combined therapy with ibuprofen and paracetamol is a suitable initial strategy for the management of ongoing pain in most patients with low back pain. Patients should be counselled to take the medications regularly while experiencing the pain, rather than reactively if the pain is too severe. This will enable them to move and exercise more freely, a key component to recovery.

- If NSAIDs are contra-indicated or not tolerated, a weak opiate such as codeine is suggested, with or without paracetamol (co-codamol). Strong opiates such as morphine are not recommended for the treatment of acute non-traumatic low back pain.

- If pain is severe and uncontrolled, other analgesia may be necessary. However, in chronic or acute-on-chronic pain, additional analgesia may not be beneficial and can lead to increased dependency. Therefore, a cautious approach is advised for additional analgesics. When required, prescribing support may be required via a referral to the patient's GP, out-of-hours service, prescribing pharmacist or other local appropriate care pathway.

- Entonox or methoxyflurane may be useful to help a person from the floor to a standing position to facilitate assessment and examination. Patients may require reassurance to overcome the apprehension of movement when in severe pain, and may feel 'trapped' on the floor or on low furniture. Once patients have been mobilised to a more comfortable position, they should be advised to remain on high-backed chairs or standing up while the pain remains very severe.

8.2 Non-pharmacological Management

- There is limited evidence of benefit for the use of warm or cold compresses, but some patients will seek to apply hot-water bottles or ice packs to their lower back.

- Patients should be advised that muscular relaxation is a key part of easing low back pain. Bed rest is not advised and will delay recovery, as it prevents them from moving freely and regularly. Patients should be encouraged to maintain their normal activities as much as they are able to tolerate, and should be reassured that it is highly unlikely that gentle activities would aggravate their pain or cause injury.

- Personalised care should be provided for patients with chronic pain, recognising new symptoms, understanding patients' concerns and perceptions regarding their pain and managing expectations around being conveyed to an emergency department and diagnostic imaging.

- It may be necessary to counsel the patient that they may remain in pain but that further pain relief may not be helpful, and that the goal is not to resolve the pain but to control it such that they are able to undertake activity.

- Patients may be advised to refer themselves for local physiotherapy (if this is available locally).

- If pain is not settling after 4–6 weeks, patients should seek further support from primary care services.

9. Simple Exercises – Advice

- Patients can be encouraged to perform regular, simple exercises to aid pain management and relieve stiffness and pain. Various NHS websites have a suite of exercises that be accessed for guidance, e.g. https://www.nhs.uk/conditions/back-pain/treatment/.

- Consider the appropriateness of different exercises for each patient. For instance, older patients may be advised to undertake exercises on the bed rather than on the floor.

- Simple exercises should be advised for patients with confirmed musculoskeletal (non-traumatic) low back pain that are not being conveyed to hospital. The exercises below should be done three times per day, consisting of two sets of five repetitions.

9.1 Simple Exercises

- Patients should be advised to try walking little and often and should remain as active as possible.

Knees to chest:

1. Lie on your back, with your knees bent and feet flat on the floor or bed.

2. Bring one knee up and use your hands to pull it gently towards your chest.

Figure 3.23 – Simple 'knees to chest' exercise.

Figure 3.24 – Simple 'knee-rolling' exercise.

Low Back Pain (Non-traumatic)

3. Hold the leg in position for 5 seconds, and then relax.

4. Repeat this exercise with the other knee.

5. Do the exercise five times on each side.

Knee rolling:

1. Lie on your back, with your knees bent and your feet together.

2. Roll your knees to one side, keeping your shoulders flat on the bed or floor, and hold for 10 seconds.

3. Roll your knees back to the starting position, and then over to the other side and repeat.

4. Do this exercise three times on each side.

10. Safety-netting

- All safety-netting advice should be documented. The patient should be advised to contact their GP if pain is not settling within 4–6 weeks.

- Specific advice should be given to patients advising them to seek urgent help (i.e. attend an urgent treatment centre or emergency department) if they encounter any of the following symptoms:

  - New motor weakness affecting the lower limbs.
  - New onset of severe pain and/or new pins and needles/numbness affecting both legs.
  - Loss of sensation, numbness or pins and needles to inner thighs, genitals, anus or buttocks.
  - Altered sensation when wiping themselves after toileting.
  - New difficulty when trying to urinate, control urinary flow or new incontinence.
  - New loss of sensation when they pass urine.
  - New uncertainty regarding whether their bladder is full or empty.
  - Inability to control a bowel motion/faecal incontinence.
  - Loss of sensation when passing a bowel motion.
  - New change or inability to achieve an erection or ejaculate.
  - New altered sensation in genitals during sexual intercourse.

Further Reading

BMJ Best Practice. *Musculoskeletal Lower Back Pain*. 2020. Available from: https://bestpractice.bmj.com/topics/en-gb/778.

Booton P, Cooper C, Easton G, Harper M. *General Practice at a Glance*. Chichester: Wiley Blackwell, 2013.

Brotzman B, Manske R. *Clinical Orthopaedic Rehabilitation*. 3rd edn. Philadelphia: Mosby Elsevier, 2011.

Chartered Society of Physiotherapy. *Back Pain*. 2022. Available from: https://www.csp.org.uk/conditions/back-pain.

Dynamic Health. *Cauda Equina*. 2021. Available from: https://www.eoemskservice.nhs.uk/advice-and-leaflets/lower-back/cauda-equina.

Finucane LM, Downie A, Mercer C et al. International framework for red flags for potential serious spinal pathologies. *Journal of Orthopaedic & Sports Physical Therapy* 2020, 50(7): 350–371. Available from: https://www.jospt.org/doi/pdf/10.2519/jospt.2020.9971.

Henschke N, Maher CG, Refshauge KM et al. Prognosis in patients with recent onset low back pain in Australian primary care: inception cohort study. *BMJ* 2008, 337.

Hopcroft K, Forte V. *Symptom Sorter*, 6th Ed. Oxon: CRC Press, 2020.

NHS Mental Health. *Mental Health Services*, 2022. Available from: https://www.nhs.uk/mental-health/nhs-voluntary-charity-services/charity-and-voluntary-services/get-help-from-mental-health-helplines/.

RCGP. National Collaborating Centre for Primary Care (UK). *Low Back Pain: Early management of persistent non-specific low back pain*. London: Royal College of General Practitioners (UK), 2009. (NICE Clinical Guidelines, No. 88.) 2, Introduction. Available from: https://www.ncbi.nlm.nih.gov/books/NBK11709/.

Simon C, Everitt H, van Dorp F, Burkes M. *Oxford Handbook of General Practice*. 4th edn. Oxford: Oxford University Press, 2014. [p. 1288 of e-book]

The Christie NHS Foundation Trust. *MSCC Service Education Red Flag Card*. 2019. Available from: https://www.christie.nhs.uk/media/1125/legacymedia-1201-mscc-service_education_mscc-resources_red-flag-card.pdf.

Versus Arthritis. *Back Pain*. 2022. Available from: https://www.versusarthritis.org/about-arthritis/conditions/back-pain/.

Low Back Pain (Non-traumatic)

Bibliography

1. Capsey M, Cormac R, Alexanders J, Martin D. Ambulance service use by patients with lower back pain: an observational study. *British Paramedic Journal* 2022, 6(4): 11–17. https://doi.org/10.29045/14784726.2022.03.6.4.11.

2. Macfarlane GJ, Beasley M, Jones EA, Prescott GJ, Docking R, Keeley P, McBeth J, Jones GT; MUSICIAN study team. The prevalence and management of low back pain across adulthood: results from a population-based cross-sectional study (the MUSICIAN study). *Pain* 2012, 153(1): 27–32. doi: 10.1016/j.pain.2011.08.005. Epub 2011 Oct 5. PMID: 21978663.

3. National Institute for Health and Care Excellence (NICE). *Back Pain – Low (without radiculopathy).* 2022. Available from: https://cks.nice.org.uk/topics/back-pain-low-without-radiculopathy/.

4. Bevan S, Quadrello T, McGee R et al. *Fit for Work? Musculoskeletal Disorders in the European Workforce.* The Work Foundation Report, 2012.

5. Wynne-Jones G, Cowen J, Jordan JL et al. Absence from work and return to work in people with back pain: a systematic review and meta-analysis. *Occupational and Environmental Medicine* 2014, 71: 448–456.

6. Dionne CE, Dunn KM, Croft PR et al. A consensus approach toward the standardization of back pain definitions for use in prevalence studies. *Spine* 2008, 33(1): 95–103.

7. Deyo RA, Jarvik JG and Chou R. Low back pain in primary care. *BMJ* 2014, 349.

8. National Institute for Health and Care Excellence (NICE). *Low Back Pain and Sciatica in over 16s: Assessment and management* [NG59], 2016. Available from: https://www.nice.org.uk/guidance/ng59.

SECTION **3** Medical Emergencies

Management and Resuscitation of Patients with Left Ventricular Assist Devices (LVADs)

1. Introduction

- Left ventricular assist devices (LVADs) are implanted pumps used to replace or supplement cardiac function. The pump augments blood flow by draining blood from the left ventricle and ejecting it into the aorta. The pump is internally implanted but is powered by external batteries (or a mains transformer) and has an external controller, which is worn or carried by the patient (refer to Figure 3.25).

- Clinical trials have established the efficacy of LVAD therapy for advanced heart failure.[1,2,3,4] Ongoing technological improvements and a growing mismatch between the demand for donor hearts for transplantation and their supply have resulted in a progressive increase in the number of patients receiving LVAD support in the UK.[5,6]

HeartMate battery worn externally in holster

HeartMate battery worn externally in holster

Aorta

Heart

Power lead

Percutaneous lead exiting body

HeartMate II LVAD or "heart pump"

Power lead

HeartMate II LVAS System Controller

Figure 3.25 – Typical arrangement of the LVAD components.

Management and Resuscitation of Patients with Left Ventricular Assist Devices (LVADs)

In January 2016, 207 adult patients were receiving LVAD therapy in the UK, 184 (89%) as outpatients. These numbers are predicted to increase. There are a number of children with LVADs, mostly teenagers.

- There are four types of LVAD system suitable for adults which are implanted in the UK. These devices are implanted by, and currently managed by, the six UK adult cardiac transplant centres.

- LVAD recipients are normally ambulatory adult outpatients who, despite subnormal exercise capacity,[7] may travel extensively within the UK. However, LVAD failure is a life-threatening emergency.[8,9,10,11,12] This dependency arises for two reasons:
  - If the LVAD does not operate, the already dysfunctional left ventricle may not be able to generate an adequate cardiac output to sustain life.
  - As the device contains no valves, if it fails there is retrograde blood flow through it during ventricular diastole, further limiting systemic perfusion.[13] Moreover, LVAD outpatients are vulnerable to other complications,[14,15] particularly stroke,[16] bleeding,[17,18] systemic infection and LVAD thrombosis.[19,20,21,22]

- Patients discharged with an LVAD device undergo an extensive package of familiarisation and training, which includes training of relatives/friends. It is fundamentally important where a trained family member or friend is on scene that they are involved in attempts to rectify the condition. They will be familiar with the exact device the patient has implanted. However, LVAD recipients are often unaccompanied in the community and therefore will not always be accompanied by a trained companion.

- On discharge, patients are presented with a patient-specific protocol (PSP). These are often shared with local ambulance services and may be flagged on control room systems. It should be noted that the patient could be mobile and may not be at their home address or that the PSP may not be readily accessible.

- Patients discharged with an LVAD will normally have spare batteries with them, along with a spare control unit. All LVAD equipment must be conveyed with the patient to hospital. Wherever possible, a family member/friend who is trained and familiar with the device should also accompany the patient to hospital.

2. Assessment

- The algorithms given in Figures 3.26–28 are intended only for use with LVAD recipients who have experienced sudden clinical deterioration. For clinically compromised LVAD recipients, where the LVAD has been non-functional for more than a few minutes, restarting the LVAD carries a theoretical risk of release of thrombus from the LVAD and embolic stroke. However, this risk may be offset by bidirectional blood flow through the non-functional LVAD[13] and systemic anticoagulation. In a patient who is critically ill or in circulatory arrest, the balance of risk and benefit favours restarting a non-functioning LVAD. If LVAD non-function is suspected in a patient who is not severely compromised, immediate advice should be sought from the VAD centre (see Section 7 for contact details).

2.1 Assessment of Airway and Breathing

- The assessment starts with a rapid evaluation of the patient's responsiveness and breathing. In an unresponsive patient who is not breathing normally despite an open airway, that is, not breathing or giving only infrequent 'agonal' gasps (the features usually used to identify cardiac arrest),[23] ambulance clinicians should consider that a likely cause is that the LVAD has stopped and should proceed to the assessment of circulation. In the patient who is breathing normally, administration of oxygen and assessment to identify other respiratory conditions should follow standard guidelines.

2.2 Assessment of Circulation

- This part of the assessment starts by determining if the LVAD is running. Unresponsiveness and absence of normal breathing usually implies circulatory arrest.

- In an LVAD recipient, sudden failure of the LVAD is the cause most likely to be corrected by prompt, appropriate intervention.

- Sudden LVAD failure does not always cause circulatory arrest, so in an LVAD patient who is very ill but breathing, it is still important to check at this stage whether the LVAD is running.

- Clinicians should minimise delay by avoiding futile repeated attempts to palpate a pulse and record the arterial BP and oxygen saturation, as these may be difficult or impossible to detect in compromised LVAD recipients.

- A loud alarm coming from the controller is likely to indicate a stopped LVAD, unless its display shows another explanation.

- If no alarm is sounding, LVAD failure is still a possibility (due to alarm battery depletion or alarm failure), so a stethoscope should be placed over the apex of the heart to listen for a humming sound. Absence of a humming sound indicates that the LVAD is not working. If a loud alarm is sounding (with no other cause shown) or the pump is inaudible via stethoscope, the clinician is directed to Algorithm 2 (LVAD troubleshooting) (refer to Figure 3.27).

Management and Resuscitation of Patients with Left Ventricular Assist Devices (LVADs)

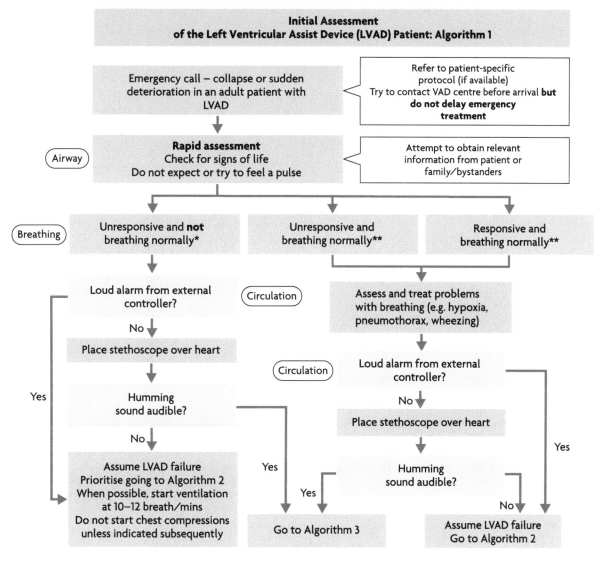

Initial Assessment of the Left Ventricular Assist Device (LVAD) Patient: Algorithm 1

Emergency call – collapse or sudden deterioration in an adult patient with LVAD

Refer to patient-specific protocol (if available)
Try to contact VAD centre before arrival **but do not delay emergency treatment**

(Airway)

Rapid assessment
Check for signs of life
Do not expect or try to feel a pulse

Attempt to obtain relevant information from patient or family/bystanders

(Breathing)

Unresponsive and **not** breathing normally*

Unresponsive and breathing normally**

Responsive and breathing normally**

Loud alarm from external controller?

(Circulation)

Assess and treat problems with breathing (e.g. hypoxia, pneumothorax, wheezing)

No → Place stethoscope over heart

(Circulation)

Loud alarm from external controller?

Humming sound audible?

No → Place stethoscope over heart

No ↓

Humming sound audible?

Yes →

Assume LVAD failure
Prioritise going to Algorithm 2
When possible, start ventilation at 10–12 breath/mins
Do not start chest compressions unless indicated subsequently

Yes → Go to Algorithm 3

Yes →

No →

Assume LVAD failure
Go to Algorithm 2

Yes →

* 'Not breathing normally' means not breathing or making only agonal gasps
** 'Breathing normally' includes breathlessness, rapid breathing and wheezing

Figure 3.26 – Algorithm 1 – Initial assessment of the LVAD patient.

2.3 LVAD Troubleshooting

- If the LVAD has stopped, the most effective resuscitation manoeuvre is to restart it without delay. Operation of the LVAD is dependent on:

1 secure connection of an external controller to the percutaneous cable (driveline) of the implanted blood pump
AND

2 the supply of power to the external controller, either via a rechargeable battery or via mains power.

- The percutaneous driveline usually exits the skin over the abdomen to the right of the umbilicus.

- All adult LVADs in use in the UK have two power connections to the controller, both of which are usually connected, although only a single working power source is needed for the LVAD to operate. This allows replacement of one power source without interrupting LVAD operation.

- The controller and batteries may be carried in a bag, contained within pockets of the patient's clothing or belt-mounted.

- If the LVAD is not running, first check the external components of the LVAD. The clinician should open the LVAD bag containing the controller and batteries to expose the contents, and check that all connections to the controller are fully engaged and secure.

- Next, check the battery charge by pressing a button on the battery that illuminates a display similar to a fuel gauge. If the battery charge level is low, the power source must be changed. Depleted batteries should be replaced with charged ones or with a mains power supply. If a mains power supply is in use and potentially defective, the device should be switched to a charged battery.

- If these measures fail to restart the LVAD, it is presumed that the controller is defective.

Management and Resuscitation of Patients with Left Ventricular Assist Devices (LVADs)

LVAD Troubleshooting: Algorithm 2
Use when directed from Algorithm 1
(see Figures 3.29–3.32 for information on the different LVAD types)

Circulation

Aorta

LVAD

Driveline

Battery

Battery

Controller

Schematics of the four current LVAD systems are provided with these algorithms and show how to disconnect and reconnect the external components
Refer to Figures 3.29–3.32

No humming sound heard in chest or loud alarm from LVAD

↓

Assume LVAD not working – try to restart

↓

Expose controller, power source and driveline

↓

Ensure driveline is firmly attached to controller

↓

Ensure that all connections between the controller and a working power source (charged battery or mains power) are secure

↓

Assess battery charge by pressing charge indicator button on battery
Replace discharged batteries with charged battery or mains power adaptor

↓

LVAD restarted?
Humming sound audible?

No →

Attach a charged battery (or mains power) to spare controller
Detach driveline from old controller and connect it to new controller

↓

LVAD restarted?
Humming sound audible?

Yes →

Yes ↓

No ↓

Consider cable fracture
Quickly but gently manipulate driveline to try to restore broken contact
If successful, stabilise driveline with tape

→ Go to Algorithm 3

Figure 3.27 – Algorithm 2 – LVAD troubleshooting.

The spare controller (carried by the patient at all times) should be connected to a charged battery (or mains power). Then, the driveline should be disconnected from the presumed-defective controller and connected to the replacement controller whereupon the LVAD should restart.

■ If these actions do not restart the LVAD, the possibility of cable fracture within the driveline causing loss of electrical continuity should be considered. If this is suspected, gentle manipulation of the driveline may restore LVAD operation, in which case the driveline should be stabilised (using tape).

Management and Resuscitation of Patients with Left Ventricular Assist Devices (LVADs)

- If the LVAD cannot be restarted, or in the unlikely event that an LVAD patient is found in an unconscious state with a non-functioning LVAD that cannot be restarted and no spare equipment, the clinician should proceed to Algorithm 3 (Figure 3.28) and the VAD centre should be contacted using a telephone number located:
  - on an identification card or bracelet
  - on an Immediate Action Notice, in an envelope in the bag with the controller in use
  - on the LVAD controller itself
  - in an emergency bag carried separately by the patient.

- Where the specific VAD centre cannot be contacted, the ambulance crew should contact the operations centre and attempts can be made to contact the local VAD centre for further advice and support. **If the clinician cannot rapidly establish which VAD centre the patient is from, they should call the nearest VAD centre for further advice and support.**

- Active LVAD audible alarms are often accompanied by warning messages, which may be displayed on the controller screen. Such messages either indicate an LVAD fault, which may cause rapid clinical deterioration, or may be indicative of a clinical problem causing LVAD parameters to fall outside the normal operating range. Alarm messages thus facilitate diagnosis of LVAD-related or medical issues and should be reported to the VAD centre co-ordinator who can provide appropriate advice.

3. Ensuring Adequate Circulation

- Whether the LVAD was found to be running, or an attempt has been made to restart a non-functioning LVAD, Algorithm 3 (Figure 3.28) should always be followed irrespective of clinical status and aims to ensure an adequate circulation. This includes checking the underlying cardiac rhythm, looking for signs of adequate perfusion and treating if necessary. Subsequently, the patient should be assessed for disabilities (e.g. stroke, glucose, drugs) and examined for evidence of bleeding and infection. Finally, transfer arrangements are made in consultation with the VAD centre.

3.1 Cardiac Rhythm Management

- Many LVAD recipients also have a cardiac resynchronisation therapy (CRT) pacemaker and, in some, their device incorporates an implantable cardiac defibrillator (ICD). Some have an ICD without CRT. An ICD would be expected to deliver a shock in the event of ventricular fibrillation (VF) or rapid ventricular tachycardia (VT).

- If a patient is unresponsive, and has VF or VT (with ICD not present or ineffective), immediate defibrillation (VF) or cardioversion (VT) is indicated.

- Some LVAD recipients without ICDs may be temporarily tolerant of what would normally be considered to be life-threatening ventricular arrhythmia (VF or VT) because LVAD operation is ECG independent and passive blood flow through the right heart and pulmonary circulation may sustain enough venous return to the LVAD to maintain systemic blood flow and consciousness.[24] A responsive patient with VT or VF should be transported to hospital for urgent treatment. If the patient becomes unresponsive during an episode of VT or VF prior to arrival at hospital, they should receive immediate defibrillation or cardioversion.

3.2 Circulatory Assessment and Observations

- Ambulance clinicians should look for clinical signs of an adequate circulation (e.g. capillary refill time less than 2 seconds, absence of pallor/cyanosis). Emergency treatment must not be delayed while repeated attempts are made to measure arterial BP or pulse oximetry in LVAD patients; contemporary pumps produce continuous (non-pulsatile) blood flow, resulting in an attenuated arterial pulse pressure, which typically renders ineffective usual sphygmomanometry[25] and pulse oximetry.[26,27] If arterial BP can be recorded, hypotension is a normal finding in LVAD recipients; a mean arterial BP between 60 and 90 mmHg would be considered acceptable.

3.3 Chest Compressions

- There is controversy as to whether chest compressions should be applied to LVAD recipients. The disagreement centres on safety, efficacy and when to start chest compressions.

- Evidence of compression efficacy in the presence of an LVAD is tenuous. Unsurprisingly, long periods of compressions were associated with poor outcomes. Short periods of compressions appeared to be associated with favourable outcomes, in keeping with a low risk of harm to an LVAD patient receiving CPR briefly, provided definitive treatment of the cause of circulatory arrest is not delayed.[28]

- It is reasonable to conclude that the balance of risks favours delivery of high-quality chest compressions by ambulance clinicians to LVAD recipients with out-of-hospital circulatory arrest either if attempts to restart an LVAD have failed or as a temporising measure until definitive intervention is possible, for example while searching for missing emergency LVAD equipment to restart an LVAD that is not running. Patients receiving CPR should have ECG monitoring in standard fashion; those with recurrent VF or VT should receive immediate defibrillation. Adrenaline can be given during CPR according to standard ALS guidelines.

Management and Resuscitation of Patients with Left Ventricular Assist Devices (LVADs)

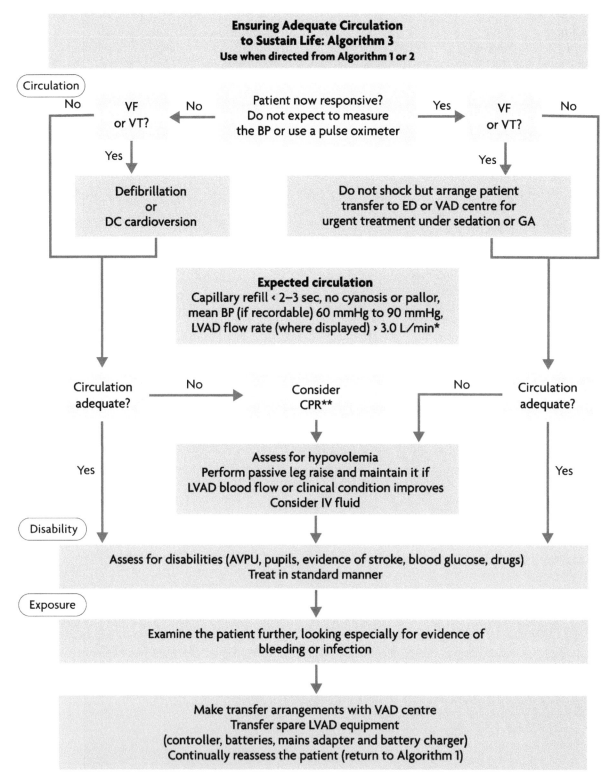

Figure 3.28 – Algorithm 3 – Ensuring adequate circulation.

3.4 Consider Hypovolaemia

- Hypovolaemia can reduce LVAD flow to critical levels. If this is the case, chest compressions should be commenced prior to the assessment of hypovolaemia. Otherwise, hypovolaemia can be assessed and treated without CPR.

- Hypovolaemia may be recognised by the display showing low LVAD flow (<3 L/min), with or without an audible alarm.

- Risk factors for hypovolaemia include a history of bleeding (notably gastrointestinal).

Management and Resuscitation of Patients with Left Ventricular Assist Devices (LVADs)

- When hypovolaemia is suspected, intravenous fluids should be given. Sustained passive elevation of the legs may provide a transient increase in venous return and help to maintain perfusion until the fluid has been administered.[26,29,30] If passive leg raising is followed by a transient increase in flow rate through the LVAD (sometimes for less than a minute), this supports the likely need for intravenous fluid.

- Positive responses to fluid administration include an increase in the displayed LVAD flow rate and clinical evidence of improved circulation. However, administration of excessive fluid can potentiate right heart failure; further advice can be provided by the VAD centre.

4. Transfer to Hospital

- Whether a patient should be transported to the local ED or to the VAD centre should be determined by dialogue with the VAD centre. This decision will depend on the patient's clinical condition and by logistical considerations.

- Appropriately trained caregivers should be encouraged to accompany the patient during ambulance transfer to hospital.

- It is of paramount importance that all emergency LVAD equipment (including the spare controller, rechargeable batteries, mains power adapter and battery charger) is transferred to hospital with the patient, as sustained LVAD function is dependent on the availability of these components.

- It is important to monitor the patient continuously during transfers, as clinical deterioration can be sudden.

5. Advance Decisions to Refuse Treatment and Do-Not-Attempt-CPR Decisions

- There is evidence of sporadic initiation of advance statements (living wills) or Advance Decisions to Refuse Treatment (England and Wales) (ADRTs) in UK LVAD outpatients. More frequently, do-not-attempt-CPR (DNACPR) decisions have been recorded by healthcare professionals for LVAD inpatients, typically with participation of the patient in the decision making process if they have the capacity, otherwise their family or authorised representative.[31] The increasing international use of LVADs for destination therapy in more elderly patients has focused debate on end-of life care planning, with more patients preferring to die in their home rather than in hospital.[32]

- It is recommended that the existence and location of advance statements, ADRTs and recommendations about CPR and/or other life-sustaining treatments should be recorded in the PSP. Unless there is a valid and applicable advance statement, ADRT or other recommendations warranting a different response in a community setting, the measures recommended in these guidelines may be assumed to be appropriate for any critically ill LVAD recipient.

6. Schematics of LVAD Types

Four different types of LVADs are implanted in the UK. Schematics of these different devices are included for reference purposes.

Management and Resuscitation of Patients with Left Ventricular Assist Devices (LVADs)

Press button to illuminate charge indicator

Battery

Controller

Black — Black

Driveline — Blue

Battery

If alarm message is displayed on controller, press arrow button to the right of screen to display flow rate

BATTERY DISCONNECTION

Rotate ring in direction of 'RELEASE' arrow and pull plug out

DRIVELINE DISCONNECTION

Pull back white rubber sleeve

Grip grooved section of silver plug and pull out without twisting

BATTERY RECONNECTION

Align arrow with white dot and push battery plug into controller power socket

DRIVELINE RECONNECTION

Align red dots and push driveline plug into controller

Figure 3.29 – Medtronic Inc. (formerly Heartware Inc.) HVAD.

Management and Resuscitation of Patients with Left Ventricular Assist Devices (LVADs)

1. Depress button to release battery from holder

2. Remove battery

3. Click replacement battery into holder

Battery

Battery

Press button to illuminate charge indicator

Controller

Driveline

DRIVELINE DISCONNECTION

1. Rotate ring to unlock

2. Press and hold button

3. Pull out driveline

DRIVELINE RECONNECTION

1. Align black markers and push plug into socket

2. Rotate ring to lock

CONTROLLER POWER LEAD DISCONNECTION

1. Rotate locking ring in direction shown until free

2. Pull power lead out without twisting

CONTROLLER POWER LEAD RECONNECTION

1. Align plug and socket
2. Carefully push together
3. Gently tighten locking ring

Figure 3.30 – LVAD type – Abbott Inc. (formerly Thoratec Inc.) HeartMate II, original version.

Management and Resuscitation of Patients with Left Ventricular Assist Devices (LVADs)

Battery

1. Depress button to release battery from holder

2. Remove battery

3. Click replacement battery into holder

Battery

Press button to illuminate charge indicator

Controller

Press button twice to display flow rate in l/min

Driveline

DRIVELINE DISCONNECTION

1. Rotate catch 90° anticlockwise

2. Press red button and pull driveline plug from controller

CONTROLLER POWER LEAD DISCONNECTION

1. Rotate locking ring in direction shown until free

2. Pull power lead out without twisting

DRIVELINE RECONNECTION

Align markings as shown. Insert driveline and rotate catch clockwise by 90° to lock

Figure 3.31 – LVAD type – Abbott Inc. (formerly Thoratec Inc.) HeartMate II, pocket controller version.

Management and Resuscitation of Patients with Left Ventricular Assist Devices (LVADs)

Battery

1. Depress button to release battery from holder

2. Remove battery

3. Click replacement battery into holder

Battery

Driveline

Press button to illuminate charge indicator

Controller

HeartMate3™

Press button twice to display flow rate in l/min

DRIVELINE DISCONNECTION

1. Rotate catch 90° anticlockwise

2. Press red button and pull driveline plug from controller

CONTROLLER POWER LEAD DISCONNECTION

1. Rotate locking ring in direction shown until free

OFF

2. Pull power lead out without twisting

OFF ⟷ ON

DRIVELINE RECONNECTION

Align markings as shown. Insert driveline and rotate catch clockwise by 90° to lock

Figure 3.32 – LVAD type – Abbott Inc. (formerly Thoratec Inc.) HeartMate 3.

Management and Resuscitation of Patients with Left Ventricular Assist Devices (LVADs)

7. Contact Details for Ventricular
Assist Device Implantation
Centres

Centre	Service	Emergency Number	Hospital Switchboard
Birmingham, QEII	Adult	07920530026	0121 371 2000
Cambridge, Royal Papworth	Adult	01223 639300 Direct line for transplant coordinator	01223 638000
Glasgow, Golden Jubilee	Adult	0141 951 5784	0141 951 5000
London, Great Ormond Street	Paediatric	**Mon** to **Fri** 0800–1600 0207 405 9200 Ext. 5807 **Out of hours** Cardiology 0207 405 9200 Ext. 1632 **OR** bleep 0548	0207 405 9200
London, Harefield	Adult	07805768819	01895 823737
Manchester, Wythenshawe	Adult	0161 998 7070 **Ask for the VAD coordinator on call**	0161 998 7070
Newcastle, Freeman	Adult	0191 244 8444	0191 233 6161
	Paediatric	**Working hours:** 0191 244 8961 **Out of hours:** Ward 23, PICU 0191 213 7023 0191 213 7028	0191 233 6161

Ambulance services should use the emergency number in the first instance and, if there is no response, should ring the hospital switchboard and ask for the VAD coordinator, or alternative speciality, as detailed.

KEY POINTS!

Management and Resuscitation of Patients with LVADs

- The number of patients fitted with an LVAD is increasing and will continue to increase.
- LVADs are implanted by and currently managed by the six UK adult cardiac transplant centres.
- LVAD failure is a life-threatening emergency.
- A responsive patient with VT or VF should be transported to hospital for urgent treatment following discussion with the VAD centre.
- Measurement of BP and arterial saturation is challenging but hypotension is a normal finding in LVAD recipients. A mean arterial BP between 60 and 90 mmHg would be considered acceptable.
- Whether a patient should be transported to the local ED or to the VAD centre should be determined by dialogue with the VAD centre.
- All emergency LVAD equipment, including the spare controller, rechargeable batteries, mains power adapter and battery charger, must be transferred to hospital with the patient.

Management and Resuscitation of Patients with Left Ventricular Assist Devices (LVADs)

Acknowledgements

These algorithms were first published in the *Emergency Medicine Journal* and are republished with permission.

Bowles CT, Hards R, Wrightson N, Lincoln P, Kore S, Marley L, Dalzell JR, Raj B, Baker TA, Goodwin D, Carroll P, Pateman J, Black JJM, Katternhorn P, Faulkner M, Parameshwar J, Butcher C, Mason M, Rosenberg A, McGovern I, Weymann A, Gwinnutt C, Banner NR, Schueler S, Simon AR and Pitcher DW. Algorithms to guide ambulance clinicians in the management of emergencies in patients with implanted rotary left ventricular assist devices. *Emergency Medicine Journal* 2017, 34: 842–850.

We would like to gratefully acknowledge the contribution of John JM Black, Christopher T Bowles and Mark Faulkner to this JRCALC guideline.

Bibliography

1. Slaughter MS, Rogers JG, Milano CA et al. Advanced heart failure treated with continuous-flow left ventricular assist device. *N Engl J Med* 2009, 361: 2241–2251.

2. Aaronson KD, Slaughter MS, Miller LW et al. Use of an intrapericardial, continuous flow, centrifugal pump in patients awaiting heart transplantation. *Circulation* 2012, 125: 3191–3200.

3. Miller LW, Pagani FD, Russell SD et al. Use of a continuous-flow device in patients awaiting heart transplantation. *N Engl J Med* 2007, 357: 885–896.

4. Birks EJ, Tansley PD, Hardy J et al. Left ventricular assist device and drug therapy for the reversal of heart failure. *N Engl J Med* 2006, 355: 1873–1884.

5. Emin A, Rogers CA, Parameshwar J et al. Trends in long-term mechanical circulatory support for advanced heart failure in the UK. *Eur J Heart Fail* 2013, 15: 1185–1193.

6. National Health Service. *Annual Report on Ventricular Assist Devices*. London: National Health Service Blood and Transplant, 2015.

7. Jakovljevic DG, McDiarmid A, Hallsworth K et al. Effect of left ventricular assist device implantation and heart transplantation on habitual physical activity and quality of life. *Am J Cardiol* 2014, 114: 88–93.

8. Bischof D, Graves K, Genoni M et al. Fatal disconnection of a ventricular assist device in an out-of-hospital setting. *Emerg Med J* 2012, 29: 247–248.

9. Cubillo EI, Weis RA, Ramakrishna H. Emergent reconnection of a transected left ventricular assist device driveline. *J Emerg Med* 2014, 47: 546–551.

10. Schima H, Stoiber M, Schlöglhofer T et al. Repair of left ventricular assist device driveline damage directly at the transcutaneous exit site. *Artif Organs* 2014, 38: 422–425.

11. Man survives after LVAD battery almost fails. *J Emerg Med Serv* 2010. Available from: http://www.jems.com/articles/2010/08/man-survives-after-lvad-batter-0.html.

12. Tigges-Limmer K, Schönbrodt M, Roefe D et al. Suicide after ventricular assist device implantation. *J Heart Lung Transpl* 2010, 29: 692–694.

13. Noor MR, Ho CH, Parker KH et al. Investigation of the characteristics of Heartware HVAD and Thoratec Heartmate II under steady and pulsatile flow conditions. *Artif Organs* 2016, 40: 549–560.

14. MacGowan GA, Schueler S. Right heart failure after left ventricular assist device implantation: early and late. *Curr Opin Cardiol* 2012, 27: 296–300.

15. Patil NP, Sabashnikov A, Mohite PN et al. De novo aortic regurgitation after continuous-flow left ventricular assist device implantation. *Ann Thorac Surg* 2014, 98: 850–857.

16. Harvey L, Holley C, Roy SS et al. Stroke after left ventricular assist device implantation: outcomes in the continuous-flow era. *Ann Thorac Surg* 2015, 100: 535–541.

17. Islam S, Cevik C, Madonna R et al. Left ventricular assist devices and gastrointestinal bleeding: a narrative review of case reports and case series. *Clin Cardiol* 2013, 36: 190–200.

18. Bhat P, Nassif ME, Vader JM et al. Epistaxis in patients with left ventricular assist devices – incidence, risk factors, and implications. *J Heart Lung Transpl* 2014, 33: S246.

19. Stulak JM, Davis ME, Haglund N et al. Adverse events in contemporary continuous flow left ventricular assist devices: a multi-institutional comparison shows significant differences. *J Thorac Cardiovasc Surg* 2016, 151: 177–189.

20. Koval CE, Thuita L, Moazami N et al. Evolution and impact of drive-line infection in large cohort of continuous-flow ventricular assist device recipients. *J Heart Lung Transpl* 2014, 33: 1164–1172.

21. Starling RC, Moazami N, Silvestry SC et al. Unexpected abrupt increase in left ventricular assist device thrombosis. *N Engl J Med* 2014, 370: 33–40.

22. Najjar SS, Slaughter MS, Pagani FD et al. An analysis of pump thrombus events in patients in the HeartWare ADVANCE bridge to transplant and continued access protocol trial. *J Heart Lung Transpl* 2014, 33: 23–34.

23. Resuscitation Council. Resuscitation Guidelines 2015. *Adult Basic Life Support and Automated External Defibrillation*. Available from: https://www.resus.org.uk/resuscitation-guidelines/adult-basic-life-support-and-automated-external-defibrillation/.

24. Busch MC, Haap M, Kristen A et al. Asymptomatic sustained ventricular fibrillation in a patient with left ventricular assist device. *Ann Emerg Med* 2011, 57: 25–28.

25. Bennett MK, Roberts CA, Dordunoo D et al. Ideal methodology to assess systemic blood pressure in patients with continuous-flow left ventricular assist devices. *J Heart Lung Transpl* 2010, 29: 593–594.

26. Bramstedt KA, Simeon DJ. The challenges of responding to 'high-tech' cardiac implant patients in crisis. *Prehosp Emerg Care* 2002, 6: 425–432.

27. Moazami N. Patients with a ventricular assist device need special considerations. *J Emerg Med Serv* 2012. Available from: https://www.jems.com/articles/print/volume-37/issue-2/patient-care/patients-ventricular-assist-device-need.html.

28. Shinar Z, Bellezzo J, Stahovich M et al. Chest compressions may be safe in arresting patients with left ventricular assist devices (LVADs). *Resuscitation* 2014, 85: 702–704.

Management and Resuscitation of Patients with Left Ventricular Assist Devices (LVADs)

29. Powell KR, Flattery MP, Cei LF et al. Pre-hospital care for VAD patients: where are the gaps? *J Heart Lung Transpl* 2015, 34: S23.

30. Shah KB, Cei LF, Pinney SP et al. Emergency care for patients with continuous flow left ventricular assist devices. *J Heart Lung Transpl* 2014, 33: S220–221.

31. MacIver J, Ross HJ. Withdrawal of ventricular assist device support. *J Palliat Care* 2005, 21: 151–156.

32. Brush S, Budge D, Alharethi R et al. End-of-life decision making and implementation in recipients of a destination left ventricular assist device. *J Heart Lung Transpl* 2010, 29: 1337–1341.

Meningococcal Meningitis and Septicaemia

1. Introduction

- Meningococcal disease is the leading cause of death by infection in children and young adults and can kill a healthy person of any age within hours of their first symptoms.

2. Incidence

- In England and Wales, the incidence of meningococcal disease is falling, with around 750 cases being reported each year (decreased incidence attributed to the efficacy of Men C and Men B vaccines).

3. Pathophysiology

- Two clinical categories are described, although they often overlap:

1 meningitis.
2 septicaemia.

- In meningitis, the meninges covering the brain and spinal cord are infected by bacteria causing inflammation.

- In septicaemia, bacteria invade the bloodstream, releasing toxins and producing a clinical picture of shock and circulatory collapse. Deterioration can be rapid and may be irreversible, with treatment becoming less effective by the minute. Early recognition and prompt treatment improves clinical outcomes.

- A minority of patients will have pure septicaemia and it is these patients who carry the worse prognosis.

4. Severity and Outcome

- The mortality from septicaemia can be up to 40% but if recognised early, resuscitated aggressively and managed on ITU, mortalities of less than 5% can be achieved.

5. Assessment and Management

- These presentations should be managed in the same way as any other form of severe sepsis, with a <C>ABCD approach and a **TIME-CRITICAL** transfer to hospital with an ATMIST pre-alert. Refer to **Sepsis**.

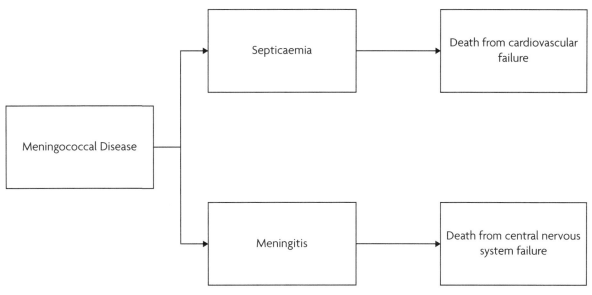

Figure 3.33 – Meningococcal meningitis and septicaemia.

TABLE 3.76 – ASSESSMENT AND MANAGEMENT of: Meningococcal Meningitis and Septicaemia

Assess <C>ABCD:

- If any of the following **TIME-CRITICAL** features are present:
  - Major **<C>ABCD** problems (refer to **Medical Emergencies in Adults – Overview** and **Medical Emergencies in Children – Overview**).
  - Seizures.
  - Rash – progressive petechial rash becoming purpuric – like a bruise or blood blister.
  - Start correcting any **<C>ABCD** problems.
- Undertake a **TIME-CRITICAL** transfer to nearest appropriate receiving hospital.
- Continue patient management en-route.
- Provide an ATMIST information call.

(continued)

Meningococcal Meningitis and Septicaemia

TABLE 3.76 – ASSESSMENT AND MANAGEMENT of Meningococcal Meningitis and Septicaemia *(continued)*

Clinical Findings

- The patient may have been previously unwell with non-specific symptoms, for example:
  - Irritability.
  - Pyrexia.
  - 'Flu-like' symptoms.

- The patient may be 'unwell' and deteriorate rapidly. In some individuals the meningococcal bacteria cross the blood – brain barrier, producing inflammation and swelling in the meninges and the brain tissue itself. This causes raised intracranial pressure, which can lead to neurological damage and death.

- The main symptoms of meningitis are due to central nervous system dysfunction. They may be very hard to assess and parents' anxieties about their child's condition must always be taken seriously.

- 'Classic' features (neck stiffness, photophobia and haemorrhagic rash) should be sought and can help you make the diagnosis when present. However, an absence of these signs should not be taken as evidence that meningococcal disease has been excluded. Do not be falsely reassured!

- Clinical features include:
  - Fever (may be masked by peripheral shutdown or antipyretics).
  - Cold, mottled skin (especially extremities). The skin may rarely be warm and flushed; features of 'warm shock'.
  - Raised respiratory rate and effort.
  - O_2 saturations – reduced or unrecordable (poor perfusion).
  - Raised heart rate.
  - Capillary refill time >2 seconds.
  - Pain in joints, muscles and limbs.
  - Rash – progressive petechial rash becoming purpuric – like a bruise or blood blister. **NB** These rashes are often not present at presentation.
  - Headache.
  - Vomiting, abdominal pain and diarrhoea.
  - Drowsiness/confusion.
  - Rigors.
  - Seizures.
  - Photophobia (less common in young children).
  - Neck stiffness (less common in young children).

The Rash

- The classic description of a haemorrhagic, non-blanching rash (may be petechial or purpuric) is only seen in approximately 40% of infected children.

- In pigmented skin it can be helpful to look at the conjunctiva under the lower eyelid.

- Early signs and symptoms are often subtle.

- Septicaemia: rashes do not necessarily develop at the same rate as the septicaemia.

- The rapidly evolving, haemorrhagic rash described in textbooks may be a very late sign – by the time this rash is present, resuscitation attempts may be too late.

- Up to 30% of cases start with a blanching pink rash, which fades with pressure, before becoming purpuric later.

- The rash may be absent.

The 'glass' or 'tumbler' test

- A petechial or purpuric rash does not blanch/fade when pressed with a glass tumbler.

- **NB** If the 'glass' test is negative, do not assume that meningococcal disease has been excluded.

SECTION **3** Medical Emergencies

Meningococcal Meningitis and Septicaemia

Specific Clinical Features

▪ Neck stiffness is rarely seen (but is more common in older children, teenagers and adults, being quite rare in pre-school children – the age group most at risk of infection). Small children often present with non-specific signs such as nausea, vomiting, loss of appetite, sore throat and coryzal symptoms – features that might otherwise suggest a diagnosis of viral illness.

Benzylpenicillin

▪ Where the patient meets the indication for administration of **Benzylpenicillin Sodium**, and where the clinician has a high index of suspicion of bacterial meningococcal septicaemia, even without the presence of a rash, benzylpenicillin should be administered.

▪ **NB** Meningococcal septicaemia can progress rapidly – early antibiotic administration is associated with better outcomes.

▪ Withhold benzylpenicillin only when there is a clear history of anaphylaxis after a previous dose; a history of a rash following penicillin is not a contraindication.

▪ In the unlikely event of an allergic reaction following administration of benzylpenicillin, manage according to **Allergic Reactions including Anaphylaxis**.

▪ Administer benzylpenicillin en-route to further care.

Respiratory Rate

▪ Measure and record respiratory rate.

Pulse

▪ Measure and record pulse.

Oxygen Saturation

▪ Monitor the patient's SpO_2; administer oxygen to achieve saturations of >94% if the patient presents as hypoxemic on air; refer to **Oxygen**.

Blood Pressure and Fluids

▪ Measure and record blood pressure; if required, administer fluids (refer to **Intravascular Fluid Therapy in Adults** and **Intravascular Fluid Therapy in Children**).

▪ Hypovolaemia complicating meningococcal septicaemia will require fluid resuscitation.

▪ **DO NOT** delay at scene for fluid replacement; cannulate and give fluid en-route to hospital wherever possible.

Blood Glucose

▪ If appropriate, measure and record blood glucose for hypo/hyperglycaemia (refer to **Glycaemic Emergencies in Adults and Children**).

Temperature

▪ Measure and record temperature.

NEWS2

▪ These observations will enable you to calculate a NEWS2 Score (refer to **Sepsis**). A National Paediatric Early Warning Score is still in development.

ECG

▪ If required, monitor and record 12-lead ECG. Assess for abnormality (refer to **Cardiac Rhythm Disturbance**).

Assess the Patient's Pain

▪ Assess the **SOCRATES** of pain and record initial and subsequent pain scores.

▪ Consider analgesia if appropriate (refer to **Pain Management in Adults** and **Pain Management in Children**).

Documentation

▪ Complete documentation to include all clinical findings, advice from other clinicians and onward referral.

Meningococcal Meningitis and Septicaemia

Figure 3.34 – Management algorithm for patients with suspected meningococcal disease.

* If bacterial meningitis is suspected and urgent
transfer is not possible, administer antibiotics even
in the absence of a non-blanching rash.

Meningococcal Meningitis and Septicaemia

6. Risk of Infection to Ambulance Personnel

- Meningococcal bacteria do not survive outside the nose and throat.

- Ambulance personnel directly exposed to large respiratory particles, droplets or secretions from patients with meningococcal disease should be offered preventative antibiotics. Such exposure is unlikely to occur unless working in very close proximity to the patient (e.g. inhaling droplets coughed or sneezed by the patient, or when undertaking airway management).

- Public Health will provide post-exposure antibiotics for meningococcal contacts who may otherwise be at increased risk of infection.

KEY POINTS!

Meningococcal Meningitis and Septicaemia

- **Meningococcal disease is the leading cause of death from infection in children and young adults. It can kill a healthy person of any age within hours of their first symptoms.**

- **Two clinical categories are described – meningitis and septicaemia – although they often overlap.**

- **Non-specific symptoms, such as pyrexia or a 'flu-like' illness, may be the only clinical features at first presentation.**

- **A non-blanching rash should be sought, suggestive of meningococcal septicaemia (not universally present).**

- **A TIME-CRITICAL transfer should be undertaken whenever meningococcal disease is suspected (irrespective of the presence or absence of a rash).**

- **Administer benzylpenicillin if septicaemia is suspected. The illness progresses rapidly and early antibiotics can improve outcomes.**

Bibliography

1. National Institute for Health and Clinical Excellence. Feverish Illness in Children: Assessment and Initial Management in children younger than five years. NICE, 2013. Available from: https://www.nice.org.uk/guidance/cg160.

2. National Institute for Health and Clinical Excellence. *Meningitis – Bacterial meningitis and meningococcal disease.* London: NICE, 2019. Available from: https://cks.nice.org.uk/meningitis-bacterial-meningitis-and-meningococcal-disease.

3. Meningitis Research Foundation. *Lessons from Research for Doctors in Training: Recognition and early management of meningococcal disease in children and young people.* Bristol: MRF, 2004. Available from: https://www.meningitis.org/healthcare-professionals/resources.

4. National Collaborating Centre for Women's and Children's Health. *Bacterial Meningitis and Meningococcal Septicaemia: Management of bacterial meningitis and meningococcal septicaemia in children and young people younger than 16 years in primary and secondary care* (CG102). London: National Institute for Health and Clinical Excellence, 2010. Available from: https://www.nice.org.uk/guidance/cg102.

5. Thompson MJ, Ninis N, Perera R, Mayon-White R, Phillips C, Bailey L, et al. Clinical recognition of meningococcal disease in children and adolescents. *The Lancet* 2006, 367(9508): 397–403.

6. Strang JR, Pugh EJ. Meningococcal infections: reducing the case fatality rate by giving penicillin before admission to hospital. *British Medical Journal* 1992, 305(6846): 141–143.

7. Riordan FA, Thomson AP, Sills JA, Hart CA. Who spots the spots? Diagnosis and treatment of early meningococcal disease in children. *British Medical Journal* 1996, 313(7067): 1255–1256.

8. Scottish Intercollegiate Guidelines Network. *Management of Invasive Meningococcal Disease in Children and Young People* (Guideline 102). Edinburgh: SIGN, 2008.

9. Chief Medical Officer. *Meningococcal infection* (letter, PL/CMO/99/1). London: Department of Health, 1999.

10. Hart CA, Thomson AP. Meningococcal disease and its management in children. *British Medical Journal* 2006, 333(7570): 685–690.

11. Hahne SJ, Charlett A, Purcell B, Samuelsson S, Camaroni I, Ehrhard I, et al. Effectiveness of antibiotics given before admission in reducing mortality from meningococcal disease: systematic review. *British Medical Journal* 2006, 332(7553): 1299–1303.

12. Meningitis Research Foundation. *Meningococcal Septicaemia: Identification & management for ambulance personnel*, 2nd edition. Bristol/Edinburgh/Belfast: Meningitis Research Foundation, 2008.

13. Cartwright K, Reilly S, White D, Stuart J. Early treatment with parenteral penicillin in meningococcal disease. *British Medical Journal* 1992, 305(6846): 143–147.

14. Booy R, Habibi P, Nadel S, de Munter C, Britto J, Morrison A, et al. Reduction in case fatality rate from meningococcal disease associated with improved healthcare delivery. *Archives of Disease in Childhood* 2001, 85(5): 386–390.

3 Medical Emergencies

SECTION

Meningococcal Meningitis and Septicaemia

15. Pollard AJ, Cloke A, Glennie L, Faust SN, Haines C, Heath PT, et al. *Management of Meningococcal Disease in Children and Young People*. 7th edition. Bristol/Edinburgh/Belfast: Meningitis Research Foundation, 2010. Incorporates NICE *Bacterial Meningitis and Meningococcal Septicaemia* (CG102). Distributed in partnership with NICE.

16. Health Protection Agency. *Meningococcal Reference Unit Isolates of Neisseria Meningitidis: England and Wales, by region, age group & epidemiological year, 2000–2001 to 2009–2010*. London: HPA, 2010.

17. Surtees SJ, Stockton MG, Gietzen TW. Allergy to penicillin: fable or fact? *British Medical Journal* 1991, 302(6784): 1051–2.

18. Carcillo JA, Davis AL, Zaritsky A. Role of early fluid resuscitation in pediatric septic shock. *Journal of the American Medical Association* 1991, 266(9): 1242–1245.

SECTION

3

Medical Emergencies

Mental Capacity Act 2005

1. Introduction

- The Mental Capacity Act 2005 (MCA) was implemented in England and Wales to provide protection and powers to individuals aged 16 years and over who may lack capacity to make some (or all) decisions for themselves. It is also for people working with or caring for them. It applies to public and private locations.

2. What Is the MCA?

- The MCA empowers individuals to make their own decisions where possible and protects the rights of those who lack capacity. Where an individual lacks capacity to make a specific decision at a particular time, the MCA provides a legal framework for others to act and make that decision on their behalf, in their best interests. This includes decisions about their care and/or treatment.

3. What Is Mental Capacity?

- 'Capacity' is 'the ability of an individual to make decisions regarding specific elements of their life' (MCA, 2005) and it is crucial within the pre-hospital emergency care environment since everything done to/for a conscious patient requires their consent. Patients must have mental capacity in order to give (or withhold) consent and, apart from situations where the Mental Health Act 1983 (MHA) applies, mental capacity is central to determining whether treatment and care can be given to someone who refuses.

- The MCA defines a lack of capacity as:

  '*For the purposes of this Act, a person lacks capacity in relation to a matter if at the material time he is unable to make a decision for himself in relation to the matter because of an impairment of, or a disturbance in the functioning of, the mind or brain*' (MCA, 2005).

- For the person's wishes to be overridden there must be evidence that some impairment or disturbance of mental functioning exists, rendering the person unable to make an informed decision at the time it needs to be made. In simple terms, 'capacity' is the ability to a make a decision at the time it needs to be made.

4. Responsibilities under the Act

- Ambulance staff have a formal duty of regard to the Act and the Code of Practice, and every ambulance trust should, as best practice, have a formal process (i.e. a policy/protocol) for establishing the capacity of patients to give, or withhold, consent for assessment, treatment and/or being transported for further care, when required.

- There must always be a presumption of capacity. In every situation, staff must assume that a person can make their own decision(s) unless it is found, on balance of probabilities, that they are unable to do so.

- Doubts about mental capacity may arise for many reasons, including the person's behaviour, their circumstances or concerns raised by someone else. Approximately 2 million people in England and Wales may lack capacity to make decisions for themselves because of:
  - dementia
  - learning disabilities
  - mental health problems
  - stroke and brain injuries
  - temporary impairment due to medication, intoxication, injury or illness.

- Staff must always act in the best interests of any person who lacks capacity; but if the impairment is temporary you should consider if it is safe to wait until the patient regains capacity before acting on their behalf.

5. Key Principles

- The MCA has five Key Principles which emphasise the fundamental concepts and core values of the Act. These must be considered and applied when you are working with, or providing care or treatment for, people who lack capacity.

- They are:

  1. Every person must be assumed to have capacity unless it is proved otherwise.

     This means that you cannot assume that someone is unable to decide for themselves just because they have a particular medical/neurological condition, disability or because of their age. The Human Rights Act protects individuals' autonomy and the threshold for over-riding this is high.

  2. People must be supported as much as possible to make a decision before anyone concludes that they cannot make their own decision.

     This means that you should make every effort to encourage and support the person to make the decision for themselves. If a lack of capacity is established, it is still important that you involve the person as much as possible in making decisions.

  3. A person should not be considered as unable to make a decision solely because they make an unwise decision.

     This means that capacity should not be confused with an assessment of the reasonableness of the person's decision. A person is entitled to make a decision that others might perceive to be unwise, eccentric or irrational, *as long as they have the capacity to do so.*

     However, it is important to note that when an apparently irrational decision is based on a misperception of reality (e.g. someone experiencing hallucinations/delusions/disordered thinking), rather than a different

Mental Capacity Act 2005

value system to that held by the assessor, then the patient may not truly be able to understand. This would lead to doubts about their ability to make a decision and an assessment should be completed.

4. Any act done, or decision made, on behalf of someone who lacks capacity must be done, or made, in their best interests.

   This means that anything done for, or on behalf of, a person who lacks mental capacity must be done in their best interests, which should be assessed by the decision maker, drawing upon all reasonably ascertainable and relevant information.

5. Before making a decision, or acting on behalf of someone who lacks capacity, a decision maker must consider if the outcome could be achieved effectively in a less restrictive manner.

   The Act does not mandate the use of the 'least-restrictive' option; instead, you must consider options that interfere less with the patient's rights and freedom of action while still achieving the objective of the decision/Act in hand. Make sure that whatever you do, you do not limit their freedom of movement any more than is necessary.

6. Helping People to Make Decisions for Themselves

- When a person in your care needs to make a decision, you must start from the assumption that the person has capacity to make the decision in question (Principle 1). You should make every effort to encourage and support the person to make the decision themselves (Principle 2) and you will have to consider a number of factors to assist in the decision making process.

- These could include:
  - Does the person have all the relevant information needed to make the decision? If there is a choice, has all the information been given on the alternatives? This should include information about the nature of the decision, the risks and benefits of choosing either way and the implications of not making a decision.
  - Could the information be explained or presented in a way that is easier for the person to understand? Help should be given to communicate information wherever necessary. For example, a person with a learning disability might find it easier to communicate using pictures, photographs or sign language.
  - Where it is safe to defer a decision, are there particular times of the day when a person's understanding is better, or is there a particular place where they feel more at ease and able to make a decision? For example, if a person becomes drowsy soon after they have taken

their medication, this would not be a good time for them to make a decision.
  - Can anyone else help or support the person to understand information or make a choice? For example, a relative, carer, friend or advocate.

- When there is reason to believe that a person lacks capacity to make a decision, you should consider the following:
  - Has everything been done to help and support the person to make the decision?
  - Does the decision need to be made without delay?
  - If not, is it possible to wait until the person does have the capacity to make the decision for him/herself?

7. Assessing Capacity

- There are several questions to consider when you are assessing a person's capacity:
  - What is the decision that needs to be made?
  - Is the person able to make that decision? (Functional Test)
  - Is there an impairment of, or disturbance in the functioning of, the person's mind or brain (this can be temporary or permanent)? (Diagnostic Test)
  - Is the impairment or disturbance sufficient to cause the person to be unable to make that particular decision at the relevant time? (Causative Nexus)

- A person may be mentally incapable of making the decision in question either because of a long-term mental disability or because of temporary factors such as unconsciousness, confusion or the effects of fatigue, shock, pain, anxiety, anger, alcohol or drugs (or drug withdrawal). When possible, attempts should be made to enhance capacity by, for example, pain management.

- Assessments of capacity are 'functional', and are related to the individual decision that needs to be made – at the time it needs to be made (i.e. can the person complete the functions required to make the decision, thus demonstrating they have capacity?). The more serious or complex the decision, the greater the level of capacity required. If an adult is mentally capable of making the decision, then his or her decision about whether to receive treatment or care must be respected, even if a refusal may risk permanent injury to that person's health or even lead to premature death (unless he or she is mentally disordered and can be treated under the MHA). Refusals of treatment can vary in importance. Some may involve a risk to life or of irreparable damage to health; others may not. What matters is whether, at the time in question, the patient has capacity to make that decision.

SECTION 3 Medical Emergencies

Mental Capacity Act 2005

- Causative nexus refers to a direct link between the inability to make a decision and the impairment/disturbance identified. For example, a patient may not be able to understand information because they are unconscious. Such determinations help to support and evidence a reasonable belief that at the time of the assessment, the patient lacked capacity. The absence of causative nexus can also help to identify where the patient is under undue external influence, or simply making an unwise decision.

- Remember that an unwise decision made by a person does not itself indicate a lack of capacity. Most people will be able to make most decisions, even when they have a diagnosis that may seem to imply that they cannot. This is a general principle that cannot be over-emphasised. The more complex the decision is, the greater the level of capacity required to make it.

- When consent is refused by a competent adult, the least you should do is:
  - Respect the patient's refusal as much as you would their consent.
  - Make sure that the patient is fully informed of the implications of refusal.
  - Involve other members of the healthcare team (as appropriate).
  - Ensure this is clearly and fully documented in the patient's records.

- Local policy may require additional elements. **If there is uncertainty as to the consequences of an act of self-harm, then it should be assumed that the consequences will be serious.**

- When an individual is reasonably believed to lack capacity to make the decision required, ambulance staff have a legal duty to act in that person's best interests – unless a valid and applicable Advance Decision to Refuse Treatment (ADRT) is in place.

- Figure 3.35 outlines the assessment process. Assessors must be able to show how their assessment was completed if required later on and details must be included in the patient's clinical record.

7.1 Alcohol and Substance Use

- When determining if there is an impairment of the mind or brain, the consumption of alcohol or use of illicit substances is often a complicating factor. This does not necessarily mean that the patient is not aware of their behaviour, or aware of the decisions they make, but it may mean that they are less aware/concerned about the consequences than they would otherwise be. Judging capacity in such circumstances is difficult and subjective, but the patient's safety is paramount, so consideration should be given to

balancing the risk of getting the determination of capacity wrong against the clinical risk of non-intervention.

8. Best Interests and Decision Making

- If a person has been assessed as lacking capacity, then any action taken or any decision made for – or on behalf of – that person must be made in their best interests (Principle 4).

- 'Best Interest Assessors' (BIA) are appointed to assist in making complex decisions for those who are unable to do so for themselves (e.g. when deciding on long-term treatment for a medical condition, or on where to live).

- There is a significant difference between making a 'best interest' decision involving a BIA and making a decision that is in the best interests of the patient in an emergency. BIAs are required to consider a wide range of elements when making such a decision on someone else's behalf. In emergencies, where there is limited or no information available, it will often be in a patient's best interests for urgent treatment to be provided without delay.

- Key factors which you must consider when working out what is in the best interests of a person who lacks capacity (whenever possible) include:

- *Identify all relevant circumstances.*

- Try to identify all the things that the person would consider if they were making the decision or acting for themselves.

- *Find out the person's views.*

- Try to find out the views of the person who lacks capacity, including:
  - Their past and present wishes and feelings – these may have been expressed verbally, in writing or through behaviour or habits (e.g. an ADRT).
  - Any beliefs and values (e.g. religious, cultural, moral or political) that would be likely to influence the decision in question.
  - Any other factors the person themselves would be likely to consider if they were making the decision or acting for themselves.

- Relatives/friends/carers may be able to assist with this.

- *Avoid discrimination.*
  - Do not make assumptions about someone's best interests simply based on the person's age, appearance, condition or behaviour.

- *Assess whether the person might regain capacity.*
  - Consider whether the person is likely to regain capacity. If so, can the decision wait until then? It may be that the person lacks capacity to make a decision to accept initial

Mental Capacity Act 2005

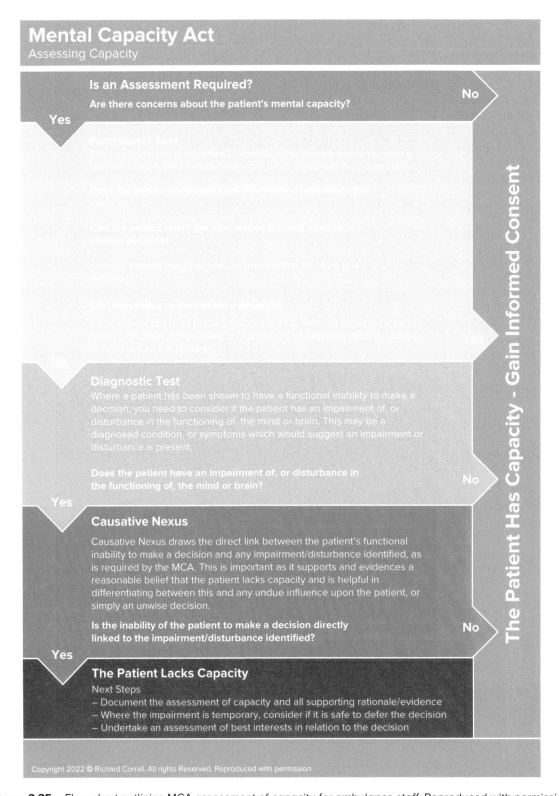

Mental Capacity Act
Assessing Capacity

Is an Assessment Required?
Are there concerns about the patient's mental capacity?

No

Yes

Functional Test

Diagnostic Test
Where a patient has been shown to have a functional inability to make a decision, you need to consider if the patient has an impairment of, or disturbance in the functioning of, the mind or brain. This may be a diagnosed condition, or symptoms which would suggest an impairment or disturbance is present.

Does the patient have an impairment of, or disturbance in the functioning of, the mind or brain?

No

Yes

Causative Nexus
Causative Nexus draws the direct link between the patient's functional inability to make a decision and any impairment/disturbance identified, as is required by the MCA. This is important as it supports and evidences a reasonable belief that the patient lacks capacity and is helpful in differentiating between this and any undue influence upon the patient, or simply an unwise decision.

Is the inability of the patient to make a decision directly linked to the impairment/disturbance identified?

No

Yes

The Patient Lacks Capacity
Next Steps
– Document the assessment of capacity and all supporting rationale/evidence
– Where the impairment is temporary, consider if it is safe to defer the decision
– Undertake an assessment of best interests in relation to the decision

The Patient Has Capacity - Gain Informed Consent

Figure 3.35 – Flow chart outlining MCA assessment of capacity for ambulance staff. Reproduced with permission of R Corrall.

treatment but, having received that treatment, regains capacity to refuse further treatment/intervention (including transport to hospital).

■ *If the decision concerns life-sustaining treatment.*
  – This should not be motivated in any way by a desire to bring about the person's death.

– Always check for an advance decision to refuse treatment – if the person has previously made arrangements for withholding life-sustaining treatment (when they had capacity to do so) this should be recorded in an ADRT. If a **valid and applicable** ADRT is found, it must be respected, and treatment withheld.

SECTION **3** Medical Emergencies

Mental Capacity Act 2005

- *Consult others.*
  - As far as possible, the decision maker must consult other people (e.g. family, friends, carers, Lasting Power of Attorney) if it is appropriate to do so, and take into account their views as to what would be in the best interests of the patient lacking capacity.
- *Avoid restricting the person's rights.*
  - Use the least-restrictive intervention.
- *Take all of this into account.*
  - Whenever possible, weigh up all of these factors in order to work out what is in the person's best interests.
- Section 5 of the MCA Code of Practice (CoP) outlines specific actions taken by ambulance staff (and others) that will be protected from liability and includes the following:
  - Carrying out diagnostic examinations and tests (to identify an illness, condition or other problem).
  - Providing professional medical, dental and similar treatment.
  - Giving medication.
  - Taking someone to hospital for assessment or treatment.
  - Providing nursing care (whether in hospital or the community).
  - Carrying out any other necessary medical procedures (e.g. taking a blood sample) or therapies (e.g. physiotherapy or chiropody).
  - Providing care in an emergency.

9. Restraint and Deprivation of Liberty

- In some cases, restraint, or restriction of the person's liberty, may be necessary to carry out acts of care or treatment under Section 5. Section 6 of the MCA, however, imposes some limitations on how Section 5 can be applied.
- Restraint is defined in Section 6 of the MCA as:
  - the use, or threat, of force where an incapacitated person resists, and any restriction of liberty or movement, whether or not the person resists.
- Restraint, or restrictions, on an incapacitate individual's liberty can be justified under the MCA, provided:
  - The person lacks capacity and restraint is in their best interests.
  - Restraint is used to prevent harm to the person.
  - It is proportionate to the seriousness of the harm.
- The least-restrictive method must be used for the shortest amount of time.
- Any power to restrain a person as a result of the MCA does not interfere with any other existing powers of arrest for criminal offences or powers under the Mental Health Act 1983.
- Deprivation of liberty is defined in case law (known as the acid test) as being any person who is subject to continuous control or supervision and is not free to leave. The nature and degree of any restriction, as well as the length of time it is applied, will impact on what may be considered a deprivation of liberty.
- However, the distinctions between restraining or restricting an individual, and depriving them of their liberty, are not always easy to identify. For example, it is possible to 'deprive' someone of their liberty not just by physical confinement, but also by virtue of the level of control exercised over an individual's movements.
- The concepts of restraint, restriction and deprivation of liberty are best understood as existing on the same continuum, with deprivation of liberty involving a higher degree or intensity of restrictions over that individual. Ultimately, the concept is one to be interpreted in view of the specific circumstances of that individual at the time.
- Deprivation of liberty without lawful justification is prohibited under Article 5 of the European Convention on Human Rights. There is a distinction between restraining or *restricting* an individual's movements and depriving that individual of their liberty.
- Most patients within the pre-hospital environment will not require any form of deprivation of liberty; however, in some cases the nature of their need for emergency life-sustaining treatment, or treatment to prevent a serious deterioration in the condition, may require it. In such situations, Section 4b of the MCA may provide a framework to deprive a person of their liberty in an emergency, subject to some pre-requisite conditions.
- Within hospital and care home settings, DoLS exist to protect the human rights of people who lack capacity to consent to arrangements for their care or treatment, and who might need to be deprived of their liberty (e.g. a person who has dementia may need to have doors locked to prevent them walking away from where they live and getting lost or coming to harm as a result).
- In simple terms, any person who is subject to regular and recurrent restrictions of their liberty should be considered for DoLS. Under this process, safeguards are put in place to keep the person safe; this includes regular review of the need for restriction. DoLS only apply to an individual at a stated location (address). If the person moves to another address (e.g. goes into hospital), then a new DoLS application will be required by the agency caring for them; DoLS authority will not be required during transit from one place to another.

Mental Capacity Act 2005

10. Use of Restraint by Ambulance Staff

- Ambulance staff are obliged under the MCA to act in the best interests of/for patients who lack capacity, even when the patient refuses treatment or is abusive, threatening or violent.

- The MCA also protects carers from liability when 'reasonable force' is required to ensure that patients lacking capacity receive care that is in their best interests, or to protect them from further harm. As stated previously, Section 6 of the Act defines restraint as the use or threat of force where an incapacitated person resists, and any restriction of liberty or movement, whether or not the person resists.

- Ambulance staff have limited training in this aspect. Minimal restraint (i.e. reasonable force) can be used in cases where patients lack capacity and there is no perceived risk of harm to the ambulance crew. If the behaviour of the patient exceeds what the crew can safely manage, then assistance must be requested in line with local policy (this does not necessarily have to be police).

- A dynamic risk assessment should always be completed prior to the use of any form of restraint, recording decisions and actions in the patient clinical record.

- Ambulance staff should always monitor the physical well-being of the patient and should be familiar with the information elsewhere in this guidance pertaining to **Acute Behavioural Disturbance**, which may result after prolonged forcible restraint.

11. Record-keeping

- Decision-makers should ensure that where a capacity assessment is undertaken, this is recorded in the individual's care and treatment record in line with local policy. This should include as a minimum:
  - The reasons an assessment of capacity was required.
  - What decision the assessment of capacity relates to.
  - The information provided to the person to support their understanding of the decision.
  - Any functional inability to make a decision identified and evidence to support this.
  - The nature and severity of any impairment/disturbance identified.
  - Evidence supporting the link between the inability to make a decision and the impairment/disturbance.
  - A clear statement as to whether you reasonably believe the patient to have capacity or not in light of the assessment.

- Where a patient lacks capacity:
  - Whether a valid and applicable ADRT exists.
  - The factors considered as part of the best interests decision.
  - The names and relationships of those you consult with as part of a best interests decision making process.
  - The identified decision or action.

- If the person was restrained or deprived of their liberty, the following should also be recorded:
  - Why restraint/deprivation of liberty was required.
  - An assessment of the restraint (including any force used), that this was in the person's best interests, that less-restrictive options were considered and how long any restraint/deprivation lasted.
  - Who was involved.

- It is recognised that it may not be possible to complete full details in an emergency situation, but do remember that it is not sufficient to say a patient does not have capacity without detailing how that decision was reached. A written record of the ambulance crew assessment and outcome must be made at the earliest opportunity.

- Ambulance trusts should monitor and audit capacity assessments, best interest assessments and any restraint or deprivation of liberty to ensure compliance with legislation, statutory codes of practice and national guidance.

12. Transfer and Continuing Care of the Patient

- Ambulance staff must complete a clinical record (in line with local policy) with the normal clinical information, including full details of the capacity assessment, risk factors and – where relevant – actions agreed with others, such as the transport method and a description of any restraint applied by either ambulance staff or others.

- Consider if a pre-alert to the receiving hospital/unit is required, and complete if necessary.

- Ambulance staff must provide a full clinical handover at hospital and a copy of the completed patient clinical record. Emergency department (ED) staff must be informed that the patient has been brought to ED using the provisions of the MCA. ED staff may need to re-assess the patient's capacity to make a decision regarding staying for further care, assessment and/or treatment.

13. Other Mental Capacity Act Safeguards

- The MCA includes other safeguards to protect vulnerable people who have reduced capacity and those using the Act to care for them.

Mental Capacity Act 2005

- Briefly, these include (amongst others):
  - **Lasting Power of Attorney (LPA)**
- An individual can give another person the authority to make a decision on their behalf if/when they become unable to do so. This is achieved by establishing an LPA. Once activated, the LPA can make decisions that are as valid as one made by the person. There are two types – Health and Wellbeing and Property and Financial Affairs. The LPA should always act in the best interests of the person.
  - **Advance Decisions to Refuse Treatment (ADRT)**
- Allow people to refuse treatment, providing that the decision to do so was made when the person had capacity.
- To make a valid ADRT the person must:
  - Be at least 18 years of age.
  - Have capacity to make the decision.
  - Make a decision that is specific and able to be complied with (i.e. outline in detail what they want to refuse and the circumstances in which it can be refused).
- The ADRT doesn't need to be in writing, unless it relates to life-sustaining treatment – in which case it must be in writing and witnessed.
- An ADRT is only valid and applicable when all of the conditions described are met and the person lacks capacity to make the decision themselves.
- If ambulance staff are not aware of an ADRT's existence when caring for someone who lacks capacity, then they should continue to act in the best interests of the patient.
  - **Court of Protection**
- Makes decisions on financial or welfare matters for people who can't make decisions at the time they need to be made and have no one appropriate to do this for them. Most cases are heard by district judges and a senior judge, but they are sometimes heard by High Court judges.
  - **Court Deputies**
- People who are appointed by the Court of Protection to act on behalf of a person with reduced capacity when there is no LPA. Court Deputies have similar powers to those of an LPA.
  - **Independent Mental Capacity Advocates (IMCAs)**
- IMCAs are a legal right for people over 16 who lack capacity and do not have an appropriate family member or friend to represent their views. An IMCA can be used to assist with decisions regarding serious medical treatment or a change of accommodation.
- The position taken in this guideline is that staff of the ambulance services should refer to their employers any questions or concerns they might have as regards gaining lawful consent from their patients or regarding the application of the relevant legislation (and associated codes of practice) that applies in the jurisdiction in which they work for assessing, caring for and treating apparently incapacitous persons.
- Readers should be aware that there are different laws relating to capacity and consent, and there is different mental health primary and secondary legislation in England and Wales, Northern Ireland and Scotland. This guideline cannot cover in detail any of that legislation, the associated codes of practice and governmental guidance. Therefore, it provides a very brief overview of some facets of the process in England and Wales.

Bibliography

1. Department of Constitutional Affairs. *The Mental Capacity Act 2005*. London: The Stationery Office, 2005.

2. Parliament of the United Kingdom. *The Mental Health Act 1983 (amended 2007)*. London: The Stationery Office, 2007.

3. Department of Constitutional Affairs. *Mental Capacity Act Code of Practice*. London: The Stationery Office, 2007.

4. Department of Health. *Reference Guide to Consent for Examination or Treatment. 2nd edition*. London: The Stationery Office, 2009.

5. S Willis, R Dalrymple. *Fundamentals of Paramedic Practice: A Systems Approach*. Oxford: Wiley-Blackwell, 2015.

6. National Collaborating Centre for Mental Health. *Self-Harm: The Short-Term Physical and Psychological Management and Secondary Prevention of Self-Harm in Primary and Secondary Care*. Leicester: British Psychological Society, 2004.

7. Department of Health. *Positive and Proactive Care: Reducing the Need for Restrictive Interventions*. London: The Stationery Office, 2014.

8. Ministry of Justice *The Human Rights Act 1998*. London: The Stationery Office, 1998.

9. Ministry of Justice. *Mental Capacity Act 2005: Deprivation of Liberty Safeguards – Code of Practice to Supplement the Main Mental Capacity Act 2005 Code of Practice*. London: The Stationery Office, 2008.

Mental Health Presentation: Crisis, Distress and Disordered Behaviour

1. Introduction

An ambulance clinician is often faced with behaviour that has made carers or bystanders concerned. Problematic behaviour is not in itself diagnostic of mental illness. There are three common problematic behaviours which may have multiple causes:

1 Violence and aggression, which has many underlying causes, including conflict, criminal intent, head injury, intoxication, metabolic disturbance, hypoxia and major mental illness.[1]

2 Treatment refusal and leaving against professional advice: this can seem counterintuitive and may be a decision made with or without capacity. Assessing a person's capacity to make decisions likely to lead to a clinical decline or even death in these circumstances can be difficult, as they may not be engaging in the decision making process.[2]

3 Self-harm and suicidality: these may seem the most obvious behaviours linked to mental illness but equally occur acutely in previously well people in high stress or distress situations, in people with autism and intellectual disability or as part of drug, alcohol or gambling use disorders.[3]

It is therefore important that ambulance clinicians do not leap to the conclusion that the problematic behaviour is due to mental illness and assume that the pathway of care should be by way of the 'health-based place of safety'. It is important to consider that intoxication by alcohol and/or drugs is a more common cause of both problematic behaviour and psychotic presentation.

Medical and trauma conditions need to be excluded and access to the right care, including appropriate investigations, arranged.

People with severe and enduring mental disorders will most often be known to their primary care and specialist mental health services, have a care plan that includes information on their '**relapse signature**' (the usual signs and symptoms each person has when relapsing) and statements about the care and treatment that works for them when presenting in crisis.

2. Management in the Pre-hospital Emergency Care Setting

- Ambulance clinicians may well be the first contact that a person with a mental health problem has with health services; we need to recognise the importance of our role. Patients will present in a variety of ways, but they will almost all be experiencing significant distress at the time. Successfully managing the distress (however this is displayed) will be key to ensuring a safe and satisfactory outcome for the patient.

- Whatever underlying mental health condition a patient may have, when in distress it is likely to manifest as an emotional response – it is this emotion that the ambulance clinician has to manage in order to establish a rapport and provide good-quality care for the patient.

- Understanding the basic components of an emotion will help to identify possible reasons for certain behaviours, and facilitate appropriate ways of managing them – for example, to reduce anxiety or anger. Being able to understand why a person is behaving in a certain way will make it easier to manage the situation safely and professionally.

- In 2011, Richards and Whyte outlined the ABC Model of Emotion,[4] which describes what an emotion is by breaking it down into three constituent parts – **autonomic, behavioural** and **cognitive** – that interact and influence each other.

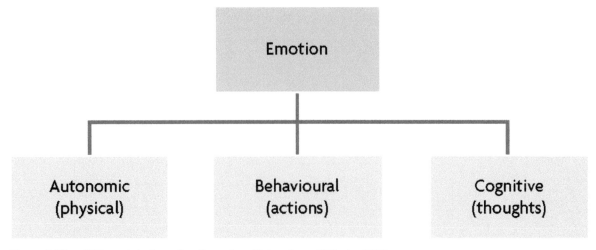

Figure 3.36 – ABC model of emotion (based on Richards and Whyte, 2011).

Mental Health Presentation: Crisis, Distress and Disordered Behaviour

3. Transporting Patients Detained Under the MHA

- Detained patients being transferred by ambulance (from a public or private place) should have an escort (this is **not** usually the approved mental health professional), along with authority to convey and completed 'Section' papers. The attending ambulance clinician will escort the patient in most cases.

- In the case of a Section 136, patients should normally be transported by ambulance and should **always** be accompanied by the police officer who has detained them; the police officer should remain with the patient during the journey.

- For transfers between mental health facilities, an escort from the ward should normally be present. Section papers (or copies) should also be present.

- Mental wellbeing does not just mean the absence of mental illness/distress/disorder. People who have been diagnosed with a mental disorder can be mentally well and lead a productive, fulfilling life. Equally, bereavement can produce responses similar to the symptoms of depression in a person who is not diagnosed with a mental disorder; bereavement is recognised as a normal response to a significant life event. Mental wellbeing is affected by an individual's mood and this is subject to fluctuation on a daily basis.

- The World Health Organization (WHO) has defined mental health as 'a state of well-being in which every individual realises his or her own potential, can cope with the normal stresses of life, can work productively and fruitfully, and is able to make a contribution to her or his community'.[5]

- When a person is unable to do this because of their emotional state, they are often said to be experiencing a mental disorder. The most common types of mental disorders are:
  - anxiety conditions
  - depression and severe mood change conditions
  - psychosis
  - personality disorders
  - high expressed emotional states.

4. Terminology

- **Mental disorder** – an umbrella term used to describe many different mental/psychological diagnoses and symptoms. The Mental Health Act 1983 (revised in 2007) defines mental disorder as 'any disorder or disability of the mind'. This includes mental illness and learning disability.[6]

Figure 3.37 – A mental health continuum.

- **Mental illness/mental ill health/mental health problems** – all used to describe common ailments across the full spectrum of diagnosed clinical conditions (e.g. depression, anxiety, bipolar disorder, phobias, obsessive compulsive disorder, personality disorders and schizophrenia).

- **Mental distress** – often used to describe the personal experience, or presentation, of an individual who may (or may not) have been diagnosed with a mental illness.

5. Context

- At any given time in the UK at least 1 in 4 people will be experiencing a diagnosed mental illness, and even more will be living with symptoms of an undiagnosed condition.[7]

- In England, 1 in 6 people report a common mental health problem (e.g. depression/anxiety) in any given week.[8]

- The most extreme outcome for some people experiencing mental distress is death by suicide. In the UK (according to the most recent figures), there were 6,188 suicides registered in 2015. This equates to more than one death per hour over the course of a year.[9]

- The majority of people diagnosed with a common mental illness are treated in the community within primary care.

- However, there are many generic and specialist secondary services available for people diagnosed with a mental illness that cannot be managed effectively in the community. These are provided by the NHS and private companies.

- For both groups of patients, additional help and support can be accessed via a number of national and/or local charities and self-help groups.

- Statutory NHS services are most often provided in three distinct age groups (within community and inpatient settings):
  - Child and Adolescent Mental Health Services (CAMHS)
  - services for adults of working age (18–65 years)
  - services for older people (aged over 65).

- Specialist services include (this is not an exhaustive list):
  - eating disorders
  - personality disorders
  - rehabilitation
  - forensic.

Mental Health Presentation: Crisis, Distress and Disordered Behaviour

6. Treatments

- Broadly, treatment will fall into one or more of the following categories:
  - **Talking therapy** – there are a wide range of talking therapies, but common ones include counselling and cognitive behavioural therapy (CBT).
  - **Medication** – based on symptoms and depending on need. Most commonly prescribed are anxiolytics, antidepressants and antipsychotics.
  - **Relaxation/mindfulness**.
  - **Electro-convulsive therapy** (ECT) may benefit a small number/percentage of patients.

7. Assessment and Management

TABLE 3.77 – Key Skills to Utilise During an Assessment of the Patient	
NB These lists are not exhaustive	
▪ Observation (in addition to the primary survey)	Consider the environment: ▪ Appearance– is the person appropriately dressed for the time of year/day/venue? Clean or unkempt? ▪ Non-verbal cues. ▪ Weapons? Other risks?
▪ Communication	▪ Questions should be easily understood, non-leading and asked one question at a time. ▪ Effective communication is fundamental to successfully working with someone who presents in crisis with a mental health problem.
▪ De-escalation of acute distress	▪ Remain calm and non-judgemental. ▪ Employ empathy, non-confrontation, threat minimisation, compromise and distraction.
▪ Screening	Assess: – behaviour – appearance – speech and rapport – mood/affect – cognition – thoughts – hallucinations/delusions – insight – risk to self/others.

7.1 Communication

- Gaining an understanding of the patient's situation (and their perception of the situation) is vital in assessing their immediate needs and achieving an appropriate/safe outcome.
- Consideration should be given to the following question types when communicating with the patient:
  - **Open questions** leave the respondent free to answer as they wish. They are broad in nature but are more time-consuming, and answers may contain irrelevant but valuable and unexpected information. They encourage the respondent to talk, leaving the questioner free to observe, listen and learn.
  - **Closed questions** place restrictions on the respondent. There is usually only one correct answer. They give the questioner control over the situation and they provide focus.
  - **Probing** questions are designed to encourage the respondent to enlarge or expand on their initial responses. They are often the follow-up question to find out more about a certain aspect, or to clarify understanding.

Mental Health Presentation: Crisis, Distress and Disordered Behaviour

TABLE 3.78 – Types of Question	
▪ General 'open' questions	▪ What's happened today to make you call for help? ▪ How are you feeling?
▪ Specific 'open' questions	▪ When did the increased anxiety/low mood/suicidal thoughts start? ▪ What coping strategies have you used/tried?
▪ 'Probing' questions	▪ Can you explain what you mean? ▪ And then what happened? ▪ What did you think would happen?
▪ 'Closed' questions	▪ Have you taken any medication? ▪ Have you called your CPN/support worker?

7.2 Key Aspects to Note During Assessment

▪ Does the patient have capacity to make specific decisions regarding their current situation (e.g. consent/withholding consent for proposed intervention or treatment)? If there are any doubts, an ambulance mental capacity assessment should be completed in line with local policy.

▪ A patient **HAS** capacity only if they can:

1 understand information about the decision to be made

2 retain that information in their mind

3 use or weigh up the information as part of the decision making process

4 communicate their decision (in whatever way they usually communicate).

▪ If a person lacks capacity in any of these areas, then (on the balance of probabilities) this represents a lack of capacity.[10]

▪ Are there any safeguarding issues (e.g. suicidal patient, patient is single parent, patient is frail elderly)? Remember that people in distress are vulnerable to abuse from others. Complete a safeguarding referral in line with local policy.

8. Common Causes of Mental Distress

8.1 Anxiety

▪ Anxiety is a normal feeling, usually experienced temporarily in a situation that is threatening or difficult. Recurrent/persistent episodes of anxiety for no apparent reason become a problem, interfere with life and can damage physical health.[11]

TABLE 3.79 – ABC of Anxiety		
A – Autonomic	**B – Behavioural**	**C – Cognitive**
▪ Increased respiration. ▪ Increased heart rate/palpitations. ▪ Sweating. ▪ Nausea/gastrointestinal disturbance. ▪ Frequency of micturition/urgency. ▪ Shaking/tremor. ▪ Dry mouth.	▪ Rubbing palms/hands. ▪ Pacing/restlessness. ▪ Shouting. ▪ Withdrawn. ▪ Avoidance. ▪ Increased consumption of alcohol and/or recreational drugs. ▪ **NB** Not all 'behaviours' are within the control of the patient while in a heightened emotional state.	▪ Fear (of the unknown) – 'What's happening?'. ▪ Panic – 'Something awful is going to happen'. ▪ Inability to concentrate. ▪ Not in control – 'I can't control this'. ▪ 'I'm dying'. ▪ Unable to focus on their current situation.
Things which happen automatically and are not within the person's control.	Actions/behaviours which the person may exhibit.	Thoughts experienced by the person.
This is not an exhaustive list. It has been used to briefly illustrate the ABC Model of Emotion.		

Mental Health Presentation: Crisis, Distress and Disordered Behaviour

- During an episode of heightened anxiety, simple strategies include:
  - staying with the person
  - encouraging them to sit
  - reassuring the person
  - demonstrating control of the situation; being firm but caring
  - encouraging the person to breathe in and out slowly
  - considering the environment; how much is noise and external stimulation influencing the anxiety? Can this be reduced?
  - ascertaining if this has happened previously, in which case does the patient have any appropriate coping skills? If so, encourage the patient to use them.
  - considering separation if there is an audience or relative/carer adding to the distress.

8.3 Depression

- Most people have periods of low mood from time to time, but these usually resolve spontaneously. Persistent low mood over a prolonged period of time is often indicative of an underlying depression.

- Depression is very common; one person in every five will experience an episode of depression during the course of their lifetime, ranging from mild (low mood, but not severe enough to impact normal activities of daily living) to severe and life-threatening (making the person feel suicidal and worthless). Some people with severe depression will experience psychotic episodes.[12]

TABLE 3.80 – ABC of Depression

A – Autonomic	B – Behavioural	C – Cognitive
Decreased appetite.	Anxious, upset.	Poor concentration.
Increased sensitivity to pain.	Withdrawn.	Low self-esteem and confidence.
Reduced/weakened immune system.	Poor eye contact.	Reduced motivation.
Insomnia; or sleeping more than usual.	Changes in normal sleep pattern.	Feeling worthless.
Tearful for no apparent reason.		Difficulty making decisions.
		Suicidal ideation (not in all cases).
		Pessimism.
		Impaired memory.

This is not an exhaustive list. It has been used to briefly illustrate the ABC Model of Emotion.

- During an episode of depression, simple strategies include:
  - being patient
  - adopting a non-judgemental approach
  - gaining an understanding of the person's situation
  - listening carefully to what the patient is saying
  - taking any threats or warnings of suicide seriously.

8.2 Self-harm

- Definition: self-poisoning or self-injury, irrespective of the apparent purpose of the act.[13]

- Self-harm is **NOT** classified as a specific mental disorder; however, a history of self-harm can be a strong predictor for repeated self-harm and completion of suicide. It is more commonly used as a way for a person to cope with life, rather than a failed attempt to end it; and there are many reasons why a person self-harms. Some examples are listed below:
  - release or catharsis
  - making an emotional pain a 'real' physical pain
  - having control when feeling out of control

  - as a self-punishment.

- A large part of the work for the ambulance clinician is likely to be centred on the physical nature of the self-harm. However, talking about the self-harm is vital as part of the assessment; it acknowledges what has happened and with this it communicates to the person that you are not rejecting them. This often helps reduce feelings of shame and stigma, which can help maintain self-harm.

- When working with someone who has self-harmed it is important that these factors are addressed:
  - What led up to it? (I.e. what was the trigger – interpersonal stressors and/or situational aspects?)
  - What was the intent of the act?
  - What was the motivation?
  - Was it planned or impulsive?
  - Are there practical protective factors in place to reduce the risk of harm occurring? (See IPAP Tool.)

- These questions may overlap somewhat with a suicide risk assessment; but ambulance clinicians should be aware to separate these two aspects and to treat each accordingly.

Mental Health Presentation: Crisis, Distress and Disordered Behaviour

TABLE 3.81 – Tips on Talking to Someone About Self-harm[14]	
Do . . .	**Don't . . .**
■ Actively listen. ■ Provide support and reassurance. ■ Encourage the use of any positive coping strategies. ■ Treat the patient with dignity and respect.	■ Minimise the person's feelings or problems. ■ Use statements that don't take the patient's pain seriously (such as 'but you've got a great life' or 'things aren't that bad'). ■ Try to solve the patient's problems for them. ■ Touch the patient (e.g. hug them or hold their hand/arm) without their permission. ■ Use terms such as 'self-mutilator', 'self-injurer' or 'cutter' to refer to the patient. ■ Accuse the patient of attention seeking. ■ Make the patient feel guilty about the effect their self-injuring is having on others. ■ Set goals or pacts.

8.4 Suicide

■ The act of suicide may be an act in isolation, or it may be after a lonely introspective mental journey, usually occurring gradually, progressing from suicidal thoughts, to planning then attempting (or rehearsing) suicide and finally dying. But, with the right help, many people who have been on a suicidal path do recover completely and go on to lead happy and fulfilling lives. However, some high lethality survivors do describe acting on impulse, often following acute loss or bereavement – of partner, parent, child, job, freedom – or when they have felt they had a problem they couldn't solve any other way.

■ The clinical and risk assessments should therefore each time be specific to the individual in front of us in crisis. Debt, bereavement, guilt, shame and hopelessness are the strongest predictors of suicidal risk, with ongoing clinical plans needed to reduce the risk for that individual.

■ Suicide warning signs include:[15]
  – expressions of hopelessness or helplessness
  – an overwhelming sense of shame or guilt
  – a dramatic change in personality or appearance
  – behaving 'out of character'
  – altered eating or sleeping habits
  – a serious drop in college or work performance
  – a lack of interest in the future
  – written or spoken notice of intention to end own life
  – giving away possessions or putting affairs in order
  – sudden unexplained 'recovery'.

■ A person is at a **higher risk** of completing suicide if they:
  – are male, aged 40–44 years
  – have made previous suicide attempts
  – have a family history of suicide
  – have been diagnosed with a mental disorder
  – have recently been discharged from a psychiatric hospital
  – are socially isolated
  – have been unemployed for more than 1 month
  – are homeless
  – have a debilitating or terminal illness
  – have a drug, alcohol or gambling addiction
  – have prison custody impending.

■ If the patient appears to be distressed and feeling hopeless, you must ask the question directly, in a compassionate way and at the right time – is the patient considering taking their life? Appropriate questioning can open a window – possibly for the first time – on that journey, and allow the individual to express their fears and accept support. It is therefore vital that ambulance clinicians are able to communicate effectively and identify key risks with a patient who is feeling suicidal.

■ The key to assessing risk within any situation is to ask questions. These should be clear, unambiguous and single. Do not use euphemisms. Adopting a sensitive but fairly direct approach is usually best. For example:
  – Are you thinking about killing yourself? **OR**
  – Are you thinking about suicide?
    (Asking these questions will not make somebody more likely to kill themselves.)

■ If the patient denies any suicidal ideation (and this is consistent with the patient's presentation), the clinical assessment can continue without further risk assessment; but always advise the patient to seek further medical attention should this change.

Mental Health Presentation: Crisis, Distress and Disordered Behaviour

- If the answer is 'yes', it is important to assess the level of risk at that time. The IPAP Suicide Risk Assessment Tool is a simple process to use (see Table 3.82).

TABLE 3.82 – IPAP Suicide Risk Assessment Tool	
Intent	Is the patient experiencing suicidal thoughts now? Explore: - Content. - Frequency. - Intrusiveness.
Plan	Has the patient made any plans? - What are they? - Are they practical? - Have they been rehearsed? - Is there access to the means, and are the means readily available?
Action	Has any action been taken, present or past? - **Present:** Has the patient carried out any acts in anticipation of death (e.g. putting their affairs in order, hoarding medication)? - **Past:** History of mental illness, previous suicide attempt, self-harm or substance misuse = higher risk of completing suicide.
Protective measures (**LACK** of these increases the risk)	What support does the patient have access to now? - Family. - Friends. - Health/social care service?
NOTE: Always consider the above in conjunction with other known risk factors such as age, gender, employment status and significant life events (e.g. relationship breakdown/divorce, bereavement, childbirth).	
IPAP – Suggested actions	
No thoughts of killing self.	Routine appointment with GP. Ring Samaritans on 116 123 if the patient would like to speak to someone. This is a free 24/7 number. If symptoms worsen, contact emergency care.
Some/vague thoughts. No plan.	Patient must be seen by a mental health practitioner. Consider:
Thoughts and/or vague plan.	- Mental Health Pathways, access to mental health services, crisis teams or crisis cafes etc. - Contact the GP for an urgent appointment. - GP triage or similar.

Mental Health Presentation: Crisis, Distress and Disordered Behaviour

TABLE 3.82 – IPAP Suicide Risk Assessment Tool *(continued)*	
Repeated thoughts and/or specific plan. Access to means.	Patient must be seen by a mental health specialist practitioner as soon as possible. If known to local mental health services, contact the care co-ordinator. If not known, contact local urgent access services or GP. If none available, take the patient to the emergency department (ED). If the patient has attempted suicide, take them to ED.
Persistent thoughts of killing self.	

Myth Busting – Common Untrue Assumptions About Suicide

- People who talk about suicide won't really do it.
- Anyone who tries to kill themselves must be mentally ill.
- If someone is determined to kill themselves, there is nothing you can do.
- People who kill themselves were unwilling to seek help.
- Talking about suicide may give someone the idea.

IPAP Suicide Risk Assessment

- IPAP is a basic suicide risk assessment process that can be used by non-mental health professionals to identify and assess the presence of suicidal risk. IPAP stands for intent, plan, action and protective measures; it is a structured method for completing a basic suicide risk assessment.
- Risk assessment – in mental health terms – is about identifying and considering a range of factors that may suggest an increased probability of an event or incident happening (e.g. suicide).
- Assessment should include examination of past incidents (both the context and detail) in the light of the current circumstances, which will inform and influence the subsequent management plan.
- IPAP uses key elements of various evidence-based suicide risk assessment tools used throughout the UK. It is a simple process, ideal for use in the pre-hospital emergency care environment, and will assist in identifying risk factors required to formulate a safe and effective care plan for patients who have expressed suicidal ideation. This will identify the key issues required at handover to other health/social care agencies and/or professionals.
- IPAP should be used to help inform immediate management on scene, not to act as part of a long-term measure of the patient's condition.

Mental Capacity

If the mental capacity of a person who is feeling suicidal has been impaired by the effects of alcohol or drugs, or by that person's emotional distress, clinicians must be satisfied that these temporary factors are operating to such a degree that the assumption of mental capacity is overridden.[10] Refer to Key Aspects to Note During Assessment.

Risk Management

Risk management is a statement of plans and allocation of responsibility (where appropriate) to support, contain or respond to the risk(s) identified.

Formulating and agreeing a plan of action provides challenges and opportunities for both the clinician and patient. Consent and collaboration need to be at the heart of the decision making process.

The components of the plan of action should include:

- The immediacy and severity of the risk.
- Service options – what the ambulance service can provide. What mental health specific services are available in the area?
- What the patient wants.
- Duty of care – particularly with issues of confidentiality. Professionals have a duty of care to balance confidentiality with the need to know, particularly regarding colleagues from other agencies. The issue of confidentiality is further clouded by the duty of care you hold to others, to pass on information to (or about) a third party you know to be at risk.

Some strategies to help care for a suicidal patient are:

- Ask directly about suicide, e.g. are you thinking about suicide – don't use euphemisms like 'harm yourself' or 'do something stupid'.
- Your primary role is to listen intently – not at this stage to direct or to make plans for the person.
- Ask the person to tell you their story. Listen carefully and without distraction – they will often talk about positives in their life as well as the crisis situation they are in today.
- When someone mentions positive things, e.g. relationships, pets, plans for tomorrow, reflect these things back, amplify these things and highlight that there are things or moments when they have been happy.

Mental Health Presentation: Crisis, Distress and Disordered Behaviour

- Ask the person if they would be prepared to think about how they could keep themselves safe for now – and what it would take to help them to keep safe.

- Try to focus on the here and now.

- Think about resources around the person – neighbours, friends, family, connections and support that can help to keep the person safe.

- Write the safety plan down with the person and ask them to keep adding ideas on how they might keep themselves safe.

- Make the environment safe – people will often tell you about the means of suicide they are contemplating, and may be willing for you to remove the means from their home, e.g. medications.

- Work with the person to identify what helps to soothe them, e.g. music, baths, walks, talking to others.

- Identify people who might be able to offer immediate support and who can help to implement the safety plan.

8.5 Mania

- Definition: unusually happy with exaggerated thoughts, feelings and behaviours affecting many aspects of life.[16]

- Common reasons for mania include substance abuse, bipolar disorder, schizoaffective disorder or an organic condition.

- During an episode of mania, simple strategies include:
  - remaining calm; avoid raising your voice or speaking fast
  - avoiding sudden/abrupt movements
  - trying not to restrict the patient's movements unless essential for safety
  - not responding in a challenging manner to the patient
  - considering the environment, how much noise and external stimulation may be influencing the situation – can this be reduced?

8.6 Acute Psychosis

- The term acute psychosis is used to describe symptoms or experiences that happen together. Each person will have different symptoms; the common feature is that they are not experiencing reality like most other people.[17]

- Common reasons include substance abuse, schizophrenia, bipolar disorder and psychotic depression.

TABLE 3.83 – ABC of Mania

A – Autonomic	B – Behavioural	C – Cognitive
Increased respiration.	Rubbing palms/hands.	Very happy and excited.
Increased heart rate/palpitations.	Pacing/restlessness.	Feeling more important than usual.
Sweating.	Shouting.	Feeling full of energy.
Nausea/gastrointestinal disturbance.	Short-tempered/irritable.	Auditory hallucinations.
Dilated pupils.	Aggressive.	Belief that they have special powers.
Flushed face.	Speaking very quickly and changing the subject frequently.	Racing thoughts.
	Laughing inappropriately.	
	Unwilling/unable to sleep.	
	Agitated.	
	Unable to relax.	
	Increase in consumption of alcohol or recreational drugs.	
	Over-familiarity.	
	Increased sexual activity.	
	Overspending.	

This is not an exhaustive list. It has been used to briefly illustrate the ABC Model of Emotion.

Mental Health Presentation: Crisis, Distress and Disordered Behaviour

TABLE 3.84 – ABC of Acute Psychosis		
A – Autonomic	**B – Behavioural**	**C – Cognitive**
▪ Increased respiration. ▪ Increased heart rate/palpitations. ▪ Sweating. ▪ Dilated pupils. ▪ Flushed face.	▪ Aggressive/suspicious/pre-occupied. ▪ Hyperactive. ▪ Very intense eye contact – or no eye contact at all. ▪ Intrusive conduct. ▪ May be extremely withdrawn. ▪ Shouting/swearing/laughing inappropriately. ▪ Placing hands over ears. ▪ Evidence (and/or self-reports) of hallucinations. ▪ Increase in consumption of alcohol or recreational drugs.	▪ Appears pre-occupied. ▪ Obsessive or disordered thinking. ▪ Sudden loss of train of thought, resulting in an abrupt pause in conversation or activity. ▪ Displaying unusual beliefs or delusional (unrealistic) ideas about themselves, others or the world in general (e.g. that there is a special/secret meaning in TV programmes/vehicles passing on a road/printed documents, or that someone is trying to poison/control them). ▪ Altered perception of reality – unable to distinguish their thoughts and ideas from reality. ▪ Believes that their thoughts can be read, changed or removed from their minds.
This is not an exhaustive list. It has been used to briefly illustrate the ABC Model of Emotion.		

▪ During an episode of acute psychosis, simple strategies include:
  - remaining calm; avoid raising your voice or speaking fast
  - reassuring the patient that you want to help them
  - avoiding sudden/abrupt movements
  - accepting that any hallucinations or delusions are very real to the patient
  - trying not to restrict the patient's movements unless essential for safety
  - not responding in a challenging manner to the patient
  - remembering it is the patient's symptoms that cause the fear/suspicion/paranoia, and doing all you can to reduce these and reassure the patient
  - taking any threats or warnings seriously, particularly if the patient believes they are being persecuted.[18]

8.7 Personality Disorders

▪ The Royal College of Psychiatrists (RCPsychs) describes 'personality' as a collection of characteristics – or traits – that individuals develop as they mature from children to adults.[19] These are unique and include ways that each individual thinks, feels and behaves in response to any given situation.

▪ An individual's personality is usually fully developed by the late teens or early 20s and will remain consistent throughout the rest of life. An important aspect of a developed personality is the ability to get on with other people (this requires empathy and self-awareness), but for some this does not happen, and certain personality traits make life difficult – both for the person and those around them.

▪ Several personality 'disorders' have been described and, according to the RCPsychs, research suggests that they tend to fall into three groups, according to their emotional 'flavour':
  - **Cluster A** – odd or eccentric.
  - **Cluster B** – dramatic, emotional or erratic.
  - **Cluster C** – anxious or fearful.[20]

▪ People with any type of personality disorder can be stigmatised because of their diagnosis. They can attract fear, anger and disapproval rather than compassion, support and understanding. This is both unfair and unhelpful.[21]

8.8 Emotionally Unstable Personality Disorder

▪ One of the most common types of personality disorder that ambulance clinicians encounter is from Cluster B – emotionally unstable personality disorder (often referred to as EUPD).

Mental Health Presentation: Crisis, Distress and Disordered Behaviour

- People diagnosed with this condition:
  - are impulsive
  - find it hard to control their emotions
  - feel bad about themselves
  - often self-harm and/or attempt suicide
  - describe feeling 'empty'
  - make relationships quickly, but easily lose them
  - can be very demanding
  - can feel paranoid or depressed
  - may hear noises or voices when stressed.
- Treatment for EUPD may involve individual or group psychotherapy, usually carried out by specially trained professionals within a community mental health setting. If required, appropriate medication may be prescribed for any specific symptoms associated with the condition (e.g. antipsychotics for auditory hallucinations).
- Treatment in an emergency situation will depend entirely on the presenting symptoms of the patient at the time.

Hints and tips when caring for someone with EUPD:

- Remain calm and non-judgemental.
- Use the ABC Model of Emotion to manage emotional aspects of the patient's presentation.
- Remember that EUPD is a diagnosed condition and your patient is unwell – not 'just' being manipulative and 'wasting' your time.
- The person with EUPD may not be able to verbalise how they are feeling, so won't be able to explain to you why they are feeling, or behaving, a certain way.
- Remember that the person with EUPD is responsible for his or her own actions and behaviours.
- Stick to professional boundaries and those outlined in a care plan if available. People with EUPD respond better to clear – and firm – boundaries.
- Do not engage in bargaining.
- Refer to a recent care plan if available.
- Consult with a specialist mental health professional if available.
- Use a locally agreed alternative care pathway if available (and necessary).
- Simple strategies include:
  - listening actively
  - focusing on the emotions, not the words
  - remaining calm
  - validating the patient's experience.

- As with any patient presenting with mental distress, clear communication is essential in achieving a safe and effective outcome for your patient.

8.9 Dementia

- Dementia is the name given to a group of diseases that affect the brain and share a common set of symptoms. Dementia is a progressive illness that can affect any area of the brain and have a significant impact upon the lives of a patient and their relatives and carers.
- There is currently no known cure for dementia; however, there are a number of medications that are used to alleviate symptoms and prolong the quality and length of the patient's life.
- Dementia is a growing issue in the UK, with numbers of sufferers expected to be in excess of 1 million by 2025. The rate of 'early onset dementia' in those under the age of 65 is also increasing.[22]
- The most commonly encountered forms of dementia include Alzheimer's disease and vascular dementia.
- Other types of dementia include Lewy body dementia, Fronto-temporal lobe dementia, Creutzfeldt–Jakob disease, HIV-related cognitive impairment, Parkinson's-related dementia and young onset dementia.[23]
- **Korsakoff's or alcohol-related brain damage** – Although sharing many common symptoms with dementia and often used in the same context, Korsakoff's is not a type of dementia. Brain damage can be caused by consistent alcohol misuse, resulting in many of the symptoms similar to dementia. If diagnosed early and managed well, progression can sometimes be halted, unlike dementia.[24]

TABLE 3.85 – Common Medications for Dementia

Treatment of cognitive symptoms	<ul><li>Acetylcholinesterase inhibitors (or cholinesterase inhibitors) act to slow or reduce the progression of symptoms.</li><li>Donepezil hydrochloride, rivastigmine and galantamine.</li></ul>

Mental Health Presentation: Crisis, Distress and Disordered Behaviour

TABLE 3.85 – Common Medications for Dementia *(continued)*	
Reduction of symptom progression and severity	NMDA receptor antagonists (N-methyl-D-aspartate receptor antagonist). Memantine hydrochloride.
Treatment of non-cognitive symptoms (e.g. aggression, hallucinations, depression)	Antipsychotic medications and benzodiazepines (used with caution due to side effects). Antidepressants, hypnotics.

Dementia and Mental Capacity

- Patients with dementia generally experience a decline in their abilities over time. Therefore, the need to take into consideration a patient's capacity should not be underestimated (refer to **Mental Capacity Act 2005**).

- A diagnosis of dementia does not mean that the patient lacks capacity, and all measures must be taken to ensure correct assessment and treatment. Check for the presence of an advance directive or living will, power of attorney, end of life plan or ReSPECT form, and if the patient is currently subject to a section of the Mental Health Act or a deprivation-of-liberty order.

- Any visit to hospital can be distressing and unpleasant, but in the case of a person with dementia it can be significantly more distressing. Consider whether the patient needs to be conveyed to hospital and, if so, what specific issues and concerns they may have. Refer to local pathways, GPs and community care services when possible to avoid hospital attendances.

- When thinking about admission to hospital for a person living with severe dementia, carry out an assessment that balances their current medical needs with the additional harms they may face in hospital, for example:
  - disorientation
  - a longer length of stay
  - increased mortality
  - increased morbidity on discharge
  - delirium
  - the effects of being in an impersonal or institutional environment.

- When thinking about admission to hospital for a person living with dementia, take into account:
  - any advance care and support plans
  - the value of keeping them in a familiar environment.

Communication

- Dementia causes damage to the areas of the brain that affect an individual's ability to communicate, retain information, make decisions or problem solve, eventually even on a very basic level. This can, and often does, lead to anxiety, frustration and fear. Communicating effectively with someone who has dementia is a skill that, if used properly, can make a considerable difference to experience and outcome for patients.

- Each patient with dementia must be treated as an individual with their own specific set of needs. Ensure patients are included and informed and that consent is gained whenever possible to reduce their anxiety and fears.

- Care home staff, family, carers and friends should be asked to help provide a detailed history and can determine the changes in a patient from their normal state. Those who know the patient best should be asked to help you with assessing, moving, handling and treating a patient and helping them to understand what is happening.

TABLE 3.86 – Tips for Communicating with Patients with Dementia
Consider the potential barriers to effective communication.
Consider carefully what language and questions can be used to minimise confusion and worry.
Ask simple questions one at a time and wait for an answer appropriately.
Reduce distractions such as noise and activity.
Use non-verbal communication such as tone of voice, posture and body position, making sure you appear approachable and non-threatening.
Using the person's name, make eye contact and appropriate touch.
Encourage the person to focus upon and communicate with you.
Take your time, try not to rush conversation.
Do not finish their sentence or presume you already know the answer.
Create a friendly and respectful rapport and environment.
Don't become frustrated.

Safeguarding

- Safeguarding issues should be considered for every encounter with a patient with dementia.

Mental Health Presentation: Crisis, Distress and Disordered Behaviour

Patients who live alone or who depend upon carers/relatives may be at a greater risk of abuse or neglect.

Carers and families may also be at risk themselves and require additional support.

Early Intervention and Diagnosis

Ambulance clinicians can often be the first to recognise the signs and symptoms of dementia before diagnosis or referral has taken place. Early diagnosis and intervention is shown to slow the progression of a number of symptoms.

Assessment tools could be considered such as the Mini-Mental State Examination for the clinician to consider the need for a full assessment. Therefore, all clinicians should consider making a referral or signposting patients with potential undiagnosed dementia using local pathways.[25]

9. Pregnancy and Mental Health

During pregnancy the mind changes as well as the body. It is important to consider that mothers during and after pregnancy may be particularly at risk of mental health illness. This includes mothers with pre-existing mental health problems, or those whose mental health illness is a result of pregnancy. Post-natal depression affects 10–15% of women who have recently given birth.

The 2015 report *MBRRACE-UK: Mothers and Babies: Reducing Risk through Audits and Confidential Enquiries across the UK* showed that almost a quarter of women who died between 6 weeks and 1 year after pregnancy died from mental health-related causes. One in seven women died from suicide.

Women who present with any of the 'Red Flag' presentations described in Table 3.87 **MUST** be referred urgently to a specialist perinatal mental health team.[10] Refer to **Safeguarding Adults at Risk**.

TABLE 3.87 – Post-natal Depression: Red Flag Signs

⚑ Recent significant change in mental state or emergence of new symptoms

⚑ New thoughts or acts of violent self-harm

⚑ New and persistent expressions of incompetency as a mother or estrangement from the infant.

Refer to local pathways and consider the need for conveyance to ED or an alternative care facility. Consider safeguarding issues and referral.

10. Pathways for Referral

It is recommended that providers of pre-hospital care have clear policies and procedures that set out the routes for onward referral to other agencies within their locality, such as:

Direct consultation with a mental health professional – via Ambulance Trust Clinical Contact Centre (or equivalent), or locally agreed referral routes with statutory mental health service providers. This may include:
– community mental health teams (usually during normal working hours)
– crisis or other out-of-hours teams (outside of normal working hours)
– hospital mental health liaison services.

Locally agreed alternative care pathways – to avoid use of emergency departments where other clinical pathways would be more appropriate.

If the patient is already known to local mental health services:

Ask to see a copy of their care plan and follow the recommendations/advice, as appropriate.

Contact their care co-ordinator (during normal office hours).

11. Physical Interventions/Safe Holding

It is beyond the scope of this guidance to prescribe fidelity to any particular training model for physical interventions/safe holding, or to mandate the depth and degree of training that each Trust must adopt to safely discharge its duties to protect patients, staff and the public. This must be determined locally based on current national guidance, a training needs analysis and assessment of risk.

Physical interventions broadly fall into three areas, these being:

1 Disengagement techniques often referred to as breakaway techniques which are skills designed to effect physical disengagement and escape from an assailant.

2 Physical restraint techniques often described as safe holding, which are manual holds and interventions to restrict the movement of an individual who may present a risk to self or others. These techniques will require a minimum of two staff to deploy safely.

3 Mechanical restraint, which describes techniques to restrict movement, using implements designed for the purpose, e.g. cuffs used by law enforcement agencies. The use of mechanical restraints is not appropriate for ambulance services.

Mental Health Presentation: Crisis, Distress and Disordered Behaviour

These techniques are all potential interventions that should only be deployed when verbal de-escalation techniques have proved ineffective, and where restraint techniques are deployed, following formal assessment under the guidance of the Mental Capacity Act (MCA) or Mental Health Act.

Where staff training in these areas is considered appropriate, the following guidelines should be regarded as mandatory:

1 All training programmes must be accredited and delivered by a certified physical interventions tutor, who has attended the requisite refresher training to continue practice.

2 Training programmes must include training in verbal de-escalation skills and interventions.

3 Training must form part of a rolling programme where appropriate refresher training intervals are mandated.

4 Training programmes and interventions must follow the guiding principles of NICE guideline NG10 and ideally BILD accreditation.

5 It is important to distinguish that physical intervention skills training in the ambulance service is primarily related to decision making under the MCA where the threshold is a risk of serious harm or a life-threatening condition. Physical restraint is only occasionally a consideration under the Mental Health Act and where safe to do so following a risk assessment.

6 Any planned intervention needs to be assessed considering risk and the consequence of doing nothing, and the risk of the least-restrictive physical intervention.

Ambulance staff are obliged under the MCA to act in the best interests of/for patients who lack capacity, even when the patient refuses treatment or is abusive, threatening or violent.

The MCA also protects carers from liability when 'reasonable force' is required to ensure that patients lacking capacity receive care that is in their best interests; or to protect them from further harm. As stated previously, Section 6 of the Act defines restraint as the use, or threat, of force where an incapacitated person resists, and any restriction of liberty or movement, whether or not the person resists.

Ambulance staff have limited training in this aspect. Minimal restraint (now known as 'safer holding') can be used in cases where patients lack capacity and there is no perceived risk of harm to the ambulance crew. If the behaviour of the patient exceeds what the crew can safely manage, then assistance must be requested in line with local policy (this does not necessarily have to be police).

A dynamic risk assessment should always be completed prior to the use of any form of safer holding and these decisions and actions must be recorded in the patient clinical record.

Ambulance staff should always monitor the physical well-being of the patient and should be familiar with ambulance service information related to acute behavioural disturbance and safer holding.

Conclusion

■ Fundamental to the management of any mental health incident is the approach taken by the health professional involved. Often what patients remember is not the advice tendered, but the warmth, empathy and concern of the healthcare professional who looked after them at a time of distress. These qualitative aspects of the intervention are particularly important when supporting patients with mental health concerns.

■ Staff who are able to establish rapport, manage distress and provide reassurance are more likely to elicit true expressions of feelings and worries from the patient, and this facilitates an effective assessment to formulate a safe outcome.

12. Traffic Light Tool for Assessing Mental Health

12.1 Low Mood

Persistent low mood may be an indicator of underlying depression (RCPsychs, 2017).

TABLE 3.88 – Traffic Light Assessment Tool for Low Mood

	Green	Amber	Red
	Low risk	Medium risk	High risk
Behaviour Verbal and non-verbal signs	Calm, relaxed. Appropriate eye contact, body language and conduct.	Anxious, upset. Tearful for no apparent reason. Withdrawn. Poor eye contact. Reduced motivation. Changes in normal sleep pattern.	Withdrawn. Little or no eye contact. No motivation. Extremely tired.

(continued)

Mental Health Presentation: Crisis, Distress and Disordered Behaviour

TABLE 3.88 – Traffic Light Assessment Tool for Low Mood *(continued)*

	Green Low risk	Amber Medium risk	Red High risk
Appearance	Attire is functional and appropriate to situation. No recent self-harm.	Evidence of reduced self-care. Signs of recent self-harm.	Attire may be appropriate or inappropriate to situation. Unkempt, evidence of poor hygiene. Recent self-harm.
Speech and rapport with others	Appropriate. Able to follow the flow of conversation. Positive attitude towards others. Normal rate and volume of speech. Spontaneous conversation.	Mild/minor difficulties following flow of conversation. Slower rate/volume of speech. Limited spontaneous conversation but able to answer questions using full sentences.	Poor. Unable to follow the flow of conversation. Negative attitude towards self and others. Unable to articulate thoughts clearly. Altered rate and/or volume of speech. Monosyllabic answers to questions.
Mood	Low/flat. Noticed some impact on daily life.	Continuous low mood/sadness. Blunted. Flat. Varies, inappropriate to the situation at times. Lost interest in things previously enjoyed. Anxious. Significant impact on daily life.	Feels numb. Flat. Hopeless. Helpless. Low self-esteem. Irritable and intolerant of others. Finds it impossible to cope with daily life.
Cognition	Orientated to time, place and person. Short-term memory intact (able to retain and recall information). Able to concentrate and follow simple instructions.	Orientated to time, place and person. Difficulty retaining and recalling information. Some difficulty following simple instructions or making decisions. Future appears bleak.	Orientated to time, place and person. Unable to concentrate or follow simple instructions. Difficulty making any decision. Can see no future.
Thoughts	No evidence (or self-reports) of suicidal thoughts.	Occasional/fleeting thoughts of suicide.	Appears pre-occupied. Frequent, recurring thoughts of suicide. Feeling guilt-ridden.
Insight	Understands and accepts their current situation and the need to receive further assessment/treatment.	Some understanding of their current situation. Unsure about need for further assessment/treatment.	Does not understand their current situation and the need to receive further assessment/treatment. Feels like nothing will help.
Risk to self/others People diagnosed with severe depression are much more likely to attempt suicide than the general population (NHS Choices, 2016).	None apparent. No previous history of mental disorder/self-harm/suicide attempt.	Moderate risk to self (suicide/self-harm). Previous history of mental disorder/self-harm/suicide attempt.	Evidence of risk to self and/or others, e.g. threats to harm self/others. Previous history of mental disorder, self-harm or suicide attempts. History of alcohol/drug misuse or dependence. Recent significant life event.

Mental Health Presentation: Crisis, Distress and Disordered Behaviour

TABLE 3.88 – Traffic Light Assessment Tool for Low Mood *(continued)*

	Green Low risk	Amber Medium risk	Red High risk
Recommended intervention:	**No further action required. Routine appointment with GP. Contact 111 or GP if symptoms deteriorate.**	**Complete IPAP Suicide Risk Assessment. Urgent psychiatric assessment. Contact care coordinator if known to local services, or GP if not known. OOH GP.**	**Complete IPAP Suicide Risk Assessment. Urgent psychiatric assessment. Contact care coordinator if known to local services, or GP if not known. Consider an OOH GP.**

12.2 Anxiety

'Anxiety is a normal feeling, usually experienced temporarily in a situation that is threatening or difficult. Recurrent/persistent episodes of anxiety for no apparent reason become a problem, interfere with life and can damage physical health' (RCPsychs, 2017).

Common triggers for anxiety: Saying something that could offend someone. Getting stuck on public transport/in a lift. Arriving somewhere late. Fearing something could go wrong. Forgetting to do something important. Not being able to control what's happening now or in the future. Wondering if loved ones are upset with you. Making a mistake at work that will result in being judged by others. Looking stupid in a social setting. Feeling anxious about being anxious.

TABLE 3.89 – Traffic Light Assessment Tool for Anxiety

	Green Low risk	Amber Medium risk	Red High risk
Behaviour Verbal and non-verbal signs	Calm, relaxed. Appropriate eye contact, body language and conduct.	Anxious, upset. Tearful for no apparent reason. Withdrawn. Poor eye contact. Reduced motivation. Changes in normal sleep pattern.	Withdrawn. Little or no eye contact. No motivation. Extremely tired.
Appearance	Attire is functional and appropriate to situation. No recent self-harm.	Evidence of reduced self-care. Signs of recent self-harm.	Attire may be appropriate or inappropriate to situation. Unkempt, evidence of poor hygiene. Recent self-harm.
Speech and rapport	Appropriate. Able to follow the flow of conversation. Positive attitude towards others. Normal rate and volume of speech. Spontaneous conversation.	Mild/minor difficulties following flow of conversation. Slower rate/lower volume of speech. Limited spontaneous conversation but able to answer questions using full sentences.	Poor. Unable to follow the flow of conversation. Negative attitude towards self and others. Unable to articulate thoughts clearly. Altered rate/volume of speech. Monosyllabic answer to questions.

(continued)

Mental Health Presentation: Crisis, Distress and Disordered Behaviour

TABLE 3.89 – Traffic Light Assessment Tool for Anxiety *(continued)*

	Green Low risk	Amber Medium risk	Red High risk
Mood/affect	Low/flat. Noticed some impact on daily life.	Continuous low mood/sadness. Blunted. Flat. Varies, inappropriate to the situation at times. Lost interest in things previously enjoyed. Anxious. Significant impact on daily life.	Feels numb. Flat. Hopeless. Helpless. Low self-esteem. Irritable and intolerant of others. Finds it impossible to cope with daily life.
Cognition	Orientated to time, place and person. Short-term memory intact (able to retain and recall information). Able to concentrate and follow simple instructions.	Orientated to time, place and person. Difficulty retaining and recalling information. Some difficulty following simple instructions or making decisions. Future appears bleak.	Orientated to time, place and person. Unable to concentrate or follow simple instructions. Difficulty making any decision. Can see no future.
Thoughts	No evidence (or self-reports) of suicidal thoughts.	Occasional/fleeting thoughts of suicide.	Appears pre-occupied. Frequent, recurring thoughts of suicide. Feeling guilt-ridden.
Insight	Understands and accepts their current situation and the need to receive further assessment/treatment.	Some understanding of their current situation. Unsure about need for further assessment/treatment.	Does not understand their current situation and the need to receive further assessment/treatment. Feels like nothing will help.
Risk to self/others People diagnosed with severe depression are much more likely to attempt suicide than the general population (NHS Choices, 2016).	None apparent. No previous history of mental disorder/self-harm/suicide attempt.	Moderate risk to self (suicide/self-harm). Previous history of mental disorder/self-harm/suicide attempt.	Evidence of risk to self and/or others (e.g. threats to harm self/others). Previous history of mental disorder/self-harm/suicide attempt. History of alcohol/drug misuse/dependence. Recent significant life event.
Recommended intervention:	**No further action required. Routine appointment with GP. Contact 111 or GP if symptoms deteriorate.**	**Complete IPAP Suicide Risk Assessment. Urgent psychiatric assessment. Care coordinator if known to local services. GP if not known. OOH GP.**	**Complete IPAP Suicide Risk Assessment. Emergency psychiatric assessment. Local Crisis Resolution/Home Treatment Team. ED as a last resort or when treatment for medical condition is required.**

Mental Health Presentation: Crisis, Distress and Disordered Behaviour

12.3 Mania

Unusually happy, with exaggerated thoughts, feelings and behaviours affecting many aspects of life (RCPsychs, 2017). Common reasons include: substance induced, bipolar disorder, schizoaffective disorder or an organic condition.

TABLE 3.90 – Traffic Light Assessment Tool for Mania

	Green Low risk	Amber Medium risk	Red High risk
Behaviour Verbal and non-verbal signs	Calm, relaxed. Appropriate eye contact, body language and conduct.	Unable to sit still for long. Pacing.	Agitated. Pacing. Unable to relax. Increase in consumption of alcohol or recreational drugs.
Appearance	Attire is functional and appropriate to situation. No recent self-harm.	Evidence of reduced self-care. Signs of recent self-harm.	Attire may be appropriate or inappropriate to situation. Unkempt, evidence of poor hygiene. Recent self-harm.
Speech and rapport	Appropriate. Able to follow the flow of conversation. Positive attitude towards others. Normal rate and volume of speech. Spontaneous conversation.	Mild/minor difficulties following flow of conversation. Faster rate of speech than normal. Very 'chatty'.	Unable to follow the flow of conversation. Intolerant/threatening attitude towards others. Unable to articulate thoughts clearly. Altered rate/volume of speech. Speaking very quickly, frequently switching from one topic of conversation to another without any clear link.
Mood/affect	Happy/euphoric. Noticed some impact on daily life.	Persistent happiness. Increased energy. Decreased need for sleep/food. Significant impact on daily life.	Feeling very happy, elated or overjoyed most of the time. Feeling full of energy/self-important/full of great new ideas and having important plans. Easily distracted. Easily irritated or agitated. Impatient with others. Impossible to cope with daily life.
Cognition	Orientated to time, place and person. Short-term memory intact (able to retain and recall information). Able to concentrate and follow simple instructions.	Orientated to time, place and person. Difficulty retaining and recalling information. Some difficulty following simple instructions or making decisions.	Not orientated to time, place and person. Unable to concentrate or follow simple instructions.

(continued)

3 Medical Emergencies

Mental Health Presentation: Crisis, Distress and Disordered Behaviour

TABLE 3.90 – Traffic Light Assessment Tool for **Mania** *(continued)*

	Green Low risk	**Amber** Medium risk	**Red** High risk
Thoughts	No evidence (or self-reports) of suicidal thoughts or disordered thinking/perception of reality.	Racing. Full of important plans.	Easily distracted. Obsessive, or disordered, thinking. Flight of ideas (racing thoughts, switching from one aspect to another very quickly with no clear links evident). Unusual beliefs or delusional (unrealistic) ideas about themselves, others or the world in general (e.g. that they have special powers, are a celebrity or a very important public figure). Altered perception of reality – unable to distinguish their own thoughts and ideas from reality.
Hallucinations/ delusions			Being delusional, having hallucinations and disturbed or illogical thinking
Insight	Understands and accepts their current situation and the need to receive further assessment/treatment.	Some understanding of their current situation. Unsure about need for further assessment/ treatment.	Does not understand their current situation and the need to receive further assessment/ treatment.
Risk to self/others People diagnosed with bipolar disorder are 20 times more likely to attempt suicide than the general population (NHS Choices, 2016).	None apparent. No previous history of mental disorder/self-harm/suicide attempt.	Moderate risk to self (suicide/self-harm). Previous history of mental disorder/self-harm/suicide attempt.	Doing things that often have disastrous consequences – such as spending large sums of money on expensive and sometimes unaffordable items. Making decisions or saying things that are out of character and that others see as being risky or harmful.
Recommended intervention:	**No further action required. Routine appointment with GP. Contact 111 or GP if symptoms deteriorate.**	**Complete IPAP Suicide Risk Assessment if suicidal ideation present. Urgent psychiatric assessment. Care coordinator if known to local services. GP if not known. OOH GP.**	**Complete IPAP Suicide Risk Assessment if suicidal ideation present. Emergency psychiatric assessment. Local Crisis Resolution/ Home Treatment Team. ED as a last resort or when treatment for medical condition is required.**

Mental Health Presentation: Crisis, Distress and Disordered Behaviour

12.4 Psychosis

Term used to describe symptoms or experiences that happen together. Each person will have different symptoms; the common feature is that they are not experiencing reality like most other people (RCPsychs, 2017).

Common reasons include: substance induced, schizophrenia, bipolar disorder and psychotic depression.

TABLE 3.91 – Traffic Light Assessment Tool for Psychosis

	Green Low risk	Amber Medium risk	Red High risk
Behaviour Verbal and non-verbal signs	Calm, relaxed. Appropriate eye contact, body language and conduct.	Anxious, upset, unable to settle. Inappropriate body language. May be withdrawn. Increase in consumption of alcohol or recreational drugs.	Aggressive/suspicious/pre-occupied. Hyperactive. Too intense eye contact – or no eye contact at all. Intrusive conduct. May be extremely withdrawn. Shouting/swearing/laughing inappropriately.
Appearance	Attire is functional and appropriate to situation. No recent self-harm.	Evidence of reduced self-care. Signs of recent self-harm.	Attire is inappropriate to situation. Unkempt, evidence of poor hygiene. Recent self-harm.
Speech and rapport	Appropriate. Able to follow the flow of conversation. Positive attitude towards others. Normal rate and volume of speech. Spontaneous conversation.	Mild/minor difficulties following flow of conversation. Ambivalent attitude towards others – may be fearful/suspicious of certain people. Altered rate/volume of speech (e.g. too fast or too slow).	Poor. Unable to follow the flow of conversation. Negative/suspicious/threatening attitude towards others. Unable to articulate thoughts clearly. Altered rate/volume of speech (e.g. too fast or too slow). Frequent changes to the topic of conversation, to unrelated topics or to whatever they observe in front of them. Using nonsense words or very mixed up sentences ('word salad').
Mood/affect	Altered. Noticed some impact on daily life.	Incongruous. Blunted. Varies, inappropriate to the situation at times. Significant impact on daily life.	Flat. Labile. Euphoric. Inappropriate to the situation most of the time. Impossible to cope with daily life.
Cognition	Orientated to time, place and person. Short-term memory intact (able to retain and recall information). Able to concentrate and follow simple instructions.	Orientated to time, place and person. Difficulty retaining and recalling information. Some difficulty following simple instructions.	Not orientated to time, place and person. Unable to concentrate or follow simple instructions.

(continued)

SECTION **3** Medical Emergencies

Mental Health Presentation: Crisis, Distress and Disordered Behaviour

TABLE 3.91 – Traffic Light Assessment Tool for Psychosis *(continued)*

	Green Low risk	Amber Medium risk	Red High risk
Thoughts	No evidence (or self-reports) of disordered thinking or unusual beliefs.	Evidence of some disordered thinking and/or unusual beliefs. Some suspicion about certain things, or people, may be evident.	Appears pre-occupied. Has obsessive, or disordered, thinking. Sudden loss in their train of thought, resulting in an abrupt pause in conversation or activity. Displays unusual beliefs or delusional (unrealistic) ideas about themselves, others or the world in general (e.g. that there is a special/secret meaning in TV programmes/vehicles passing on a road/printed documents, or that someone is trying to poison/control them). Altered perception of reality – unable to distinguish their own thoughts and ideas from reality.
Hallucinations/ delusions	No evidence (or self-reports) of hallucinations/delusions.	Previous history of hallucinations/delusions. Patient may feel that they themselves are not real or that the situation they are in is not real.	Evidence (and/or self-reports) of hallucinations. Visual/auditory hallucinations are the most common (individual to the patient). Patient believes that their thoughts can be read, changed or removed from their minds.
Insight	Understands and accepts their current situation and the need to receive further assessment/treatment. Understands how their behaviour impacts on others.	Some understanding of their current situation. Unsure/suspicious about need for further assessment/treatment.	Does not understand their current situation and the need to receive further assessment/treatment, nor how their behaviour impacts on others.
Risk to self/others As 1 in 10 people with psychosis die by suicide, it is important not to miss any symptoms of depression (RCPsychs, 2017).	None apparent.	Moderate risk to self (suicide/self-harm).	Evidence of risk to self and/or others (e.g. threats to harm self/others).

Mental Health Presentation: Crisis, Distress and Disordered Behaviour

	Green Low risk	Amber Medium risk	Red High risk
TABLE 3.91 – Traffic Light Assessment Tool for Psychosis *(continued)*			
Recommended intervention:	**No further action required. Contact 111 or GP if symptoms deteriorate.**	**Complete IPAP Suicide Risk Assessment if suicidal ideation present. Urgent psychiatric assessment. Care coordinator if known to local services. GP if not known. OOH GP.**	**Complete IPAP Suicide Risk Assessment if suicidal ideation present. Emergency psychiatric assessment. Local Crisis Resolution/Home Treatment Team. ED as a last resort or when treatment for medical condition is required.**

Bibliography

1. eLearning for Health. *Violence and Agression.* Leeds: Health Education England, 2016. Available from: http://portal.e-lfh.org.uk/Component/Details/432728.

2. eLearning for Health. *Suicide and Self-Harm.* Leeds: Health Education England, 2016. Available from: https://portal.e-lfh.org.uk/Component/Details/448052.

3. eLearning for Health. *Abscond and Treatment Refusal.* Leeds: Health Education England, 2016. Available from: http://portal.e-lfh.org.uk/Component/Details/439829.

4. Richards D, Whyte M. Reach Out. *National Programme Student Materials to Support the Delivery of Training for Psychological Wellbeing Practitioners Delivering Low Intensity Interventions.* London: Rethink Mental Illness, 2011.

5. World Health Organization. *Promoting Mental Health: Concepts, emerging evidence, practice (Summary Report).* Geneva: WHO, 2004.

6. Parliament of the United Kingdom. *The Mental Health Act 1983 (amended 2007).* London: The Stationery Office, 2007.

7. McManus S, Meltzer H, Brugha TS, Bebbington PE, Jenkins R. *Adult Psychiatric Morbidity in England, 2007: Results of a household survey.* London: The NHS Information Centre for Health and Social Care, 2009.

8. McManus S, Bebbington P, Jenkins R, Brugha T (eds). *Mental Health and Wellbeing in England: Adult psychiatric morbidity survey 2014.* Leeds: NHS Digital, 2016.

9. Scowcroft E. *Samaritans Suicide Statistics Report 2017.* Surrey: Samaritans, 2017, p. 6.

10. Ministry of Justice. *The Mental Capacity Act 2005 Code of Practice 2007.* London: The Stationery Office, 2005. Available from: https://www.gov.uk/government/publications/mental-capacity-act-code-of-practice.

11. Royal College of Psychiatrists. *Anxiety, Panic and Phobias – Information leaflet.* London: RCPsychs, 2018.

12. Royal College of Psychiatrists. *Depression: Key facts.* London: RCPsychs, 2015.

13. National Institute for Health and Care Excellence. *Clinical Practice Guideline No 23: Self-harm.* The British Psychological Society & the Royal College of Psychiatrists. London: NICE, 2004.

14. Mental Health First Aid. *Self-injury First Aid Guideline.* Melbourne: MHFA, 2014.

15. Mental Health First Aid. *Suicide First Aid Guideline.* Melbourne: MHFA, 2014.

16. Royal College of Psychiatrists. *Bi-Polar Disorder – Information leaflet.* London: RCPsychs, 2015.

17. Royal College of Psychiatrists. *Psychosis – Information leaflet.* London: RCPsychs, 2017.

18. Mental Health First Aid. *Psychosis First Aid Guideline.* Melbourne: MHFA, 2008.

19. Royal College of Psychiatrists. *Personality Disorder.* London: RCPsychs, 2018.

20. Royal College of Psychiatrists. *Personality Disorder: Key facts.* London: RCPsychs, 2016.

21. eLearning for Health. *Personality Disorder.* Leeds: Health Education England, 2016. Available from: http://portal.e-lfh.org.uk/Component/Details/421730.

22. Alzheimers Research UK. *Dementia Symptoms.* Cambridge: Alzheimers Research UK, 2018. Available from: https://www.alzheimersresearchuk.org/about-dementia/types-of-dementia/frontotemporal-dementia/symptoms/.

23. National Institute for Health and Care Excellence. *Dementia: Assessment, management and support for people living with dementia and their carers* [NG97]. London: NICE, 2018.

24. Alzheimers Research UK. *Frontotemporal Dementia.* Cambridge: Alzheimers Research UK, 2018. Available from: https://www.alzheimersresearchuk.org/about-dementia/types-of-dementia/frontotemporal-dementia/symptoms/.

25. PAR Inc. *Mini-Mental State Examination.* Florida: PAR Inc, 2009. Available from: https://www.parinc.com/products/pkey/237.

SECTION 3 Medical Emergencies

Non-Traumatic Chest Pain/Discomfort

1. Introduction

- Chest pain is one of the most common symptoms of acute coronary syndrome (ACS).

- It is also a common feature in many other conditions such as aortic dissection, chest infection with pleuritic pain, pulmonary embolus, reflux oesophagitis, indigestion and simple musculoskeletal chest pain.

- There must be a high index of suspicion that any chest pain is cardiac in origin.

- There are a number of specific factors that may help in reaching a reasoned working diagnosis, and applying appropriate management measures to the patient. ACS cannot be excluded on clinical examination alone (refer to **Acute Coronary Syndrome**).

- Do not assess symptoms differently in women and men or patients from different ethnic groups.

2. Assessment and Management

Assessing the type of pain is particularly important in the management of non-traumatic chest pain. For the types of pain typical for each cause, refer to Table 3.92.

TABLE 3.92 – Descriptions of Non-traumatic Chest Pain

Features which suggest a diagnosis of myocardial ischaemia include:

- Central chest pain.

- Crushing or constricting in nature.

- Persists for >15 minutes.

- Pain may also present in:
  - the shoulders
  - upper abdomen
  - referred to the neck, jaws and arms.

Features which suggest a diagnosis of stable angina include:

- Pain is typically related to exertion and tends to last minutes but should it persist for >15 minutes, or despite usual treatment, ACS is more likely.

Features of pleuritic-type pain:

- Stabbing.

- Generally one-sided.

- Worse on breathing in.

- Usually have cough with sputum.

- Raised temperature (>37.5°C) indicative of infection.

Features of indigestion-type pain:

- Central.

- Related to food.

- May be associated with belching and burning.

NB Some patients with ACS may also suffer indigestion-type pain and belching.

Features of muscular-type pain:

- Sharp/stabbing.

- Worse on movement.

- Often associated with tenderness on palpation.

Features of aneurysm-type pain:

- Sudden, severe pain.

- Pulsing sensation in the abdomen (like a heartbeat).

- Sudden, intense and persistent abdominal or back pain, which can be described as a tearing sensation.

- Pain that radiates to the back or legs.

Non-Traumatic Chest Pain/Discomfort

For the assessment and management of non-traumatic chest pain/discomfort, refer to Table 3.93.

TABLE 3.93 – ASSESSMENT and MANAGEMENT of: Non-Traumatic Chest Pain/Discomfort
NB A defibrillator must always be taken at the earliest opportunity to patients with symptoms suggestive of a myocardial infarction. Remain with the patient until handover to hospital staff.

Assess <C>ABCD
 	
▪ If any of the following **TIME-CRITICAL** features are present:
   – Major <C>ABC problems (refer to **Medical Emergencies in Adults – Overview** and **Medical Emergencies in Children – Overview**).
   – Suspected ACS, especially ST-segment-elevation myocardial infarction (STEMI) (refer to **Acute Coronary Syndrome**).
   – Aortic dissection.
▪ Start correcting any **<C>ABCD** problems.
▪ Undertake a **TIME-CRITICAL** transfer to the nearest appropriate receiving hospital.
▪ Continue management en-route.
▪ Provide an ATMIST information call.

ECG ▪ If required, monitor and record 12-lead ECG. Assess for abnormality (refer to **Cardiac Rhythm Disturbance**). **NB** For non-traumatic chest pain, an ECG should be taken as soon as practically possible to diagnose a STEMI requiring immediate conveyance to a centre able to provide Primary Percutaneous Coronary Intervention. **NB** DO NOT exclude an ACS when patients have a normal resting 12-lead ECG – a normal ECG cannot reliably exclude ACS.
Assess for Specific Accompanying Features ▪ Nausea/vomiting. ▪ Sweating. ▪ Pallor. ▪ Cough. ▪ Breathlessness – **NB** If breathlessness is a predominant symptom/sign with tightness in the chest, then causes of breathlessness must also be considered (refer to **Dyspnoea**).
Undertake a Clinical Assessment Specifically for: ▪ Heart failure. ▪ Cardiogenic shock. ▪ Ask the patient if they have a previous history of coronary heart disease.

Other Conditions
 	
▪ If clinical examination and a 12-lead ECG make a diagnosis of ACS less likely, assess for other acute conditions such as:
   – pulmonary embolism (refer to **Pulmonary Embolism**).
   – aortic dissection
   – pneumonia (refer to **Medical Emergencies in Adults – Overview** and **Medical Emergencies in Children – Overview**).

Respiratory Rate ▪ Measure and record respiratory rate.
Oxygen Saturation ▪ Monitor the patient's SpO_2; administer oxygen to achieve saturations of >94% if the patient presents as hypoxemic on air (refer to **Oxygen**).

(continued)

Non-Traumatic Chest Pain/Discomfort

TABLE 3.93 – ASSESSMENT and MANAGEMENT of: Non-Traumatic Chest Pain/Discomfort (continued)
Blood Pressure and Fluids
▪ Measure and record blood pressure; if required, administer fluids (refer to **Intravascular Fluid Therapy in Adults** and **Intravascular Fluid Therapy in Children**).
Blood Glucose
▪ If appropriate, measure and record blood glucose for hypo/hyperglycaemia (refer to **Glycaemic Emergencies in Adults and Children**).
Temperature
▪ Measure and record temperature.
NEWS2
▪ These observations will enable you to calculate a NEWS2 Score (refer to **Sepsis**).
Assess Patient's Pain
▪ For the features of specific types of pain, refer to Table 3.92.
▪ Where present, assess the **SOCRATES** of pain and record initial and subsequent pain scores.
▪ Consider analgesia if appropriate (refer to **Pain Management in Adults** and **Pain Management in Children**).
Documentation
▪ Complete documentation to include all clinical findings, advice from other clinicians, onward referral and worsening advice given.

KEY POINTS!

Non-traumatic Chest Pain/Discomfort

▪ **Most chest pain is not ACS – but this possibility needs to be excluded rapidly.**

▪ **Is there another life-threatening cause (e.g. aortic dissection)?**

▪ **Have a low threshold for recording a 12-lead ECG.**

▪ **A normal ECG cannot reliably exclude ACS.**

Bibliography

1. National Institute for Health and Clinical Excellence. *Chest Pain of Recent Onset: Assessment and diagnosis of recent onset chest pain or discomfort of suspected cardiac origin* (CG95). London: NICE, 2010. Available from: https://www.nice.org.uk/guidance/cg95.

2. Porter A, Snooks H, Youren A, Gaze S, Whitfield R, Rapport F et al. 'Covering our backs': ambulance crews' attitudes towards clinical documentation when emergency (999) patients are not conveyed to hospital. *Emergency Medicine Journal* 2008, 25(5): 292–295.

3. NHS. *Abdominal aortic aneurysm.* London: NHS, 2017. Available from: https://www.nhs.uk/conditions/abdominal-aortic-aneurysm.

Overdose and Poisoning in Adults and Children

1. Introduction

Overdose and poisoning is a common cause of calls to the ambulance service. When dealing with overdose and poisoning, advice is available online from TOXBASE®: https://www.toxbase.org. Consult your local procedures on how to use TOXBASE. An app containing searchable, offline access to the TOXBASE® database is available free to NHS users. A 24-hour, seven-day telephone advice line is also available from the National Poisons Information Service: 0344 892 0111.

1.1 Overdose and Poisoning

Exposure may occur by ingestion, inhalation, topical absorption, injection, inoculation or radiation of a quantity of a substance(s) and may result in mortality or morbidity.

Common agents include:

- Consumer products, for example washing powders, washing-up liquids, fabric cleaning liquid/tablets, bleaches, hand gels, screen-washes, anti-freeze, de-icers, silica gel, batteries, petroleum distillates, white spirit (e.g. paints and varnishes), descalers and glues. Exposure in children generally occurs as a result of ingestion but can arise from eye and skin contact; exposure can arise via multiple routes.
- Pharmaceutics, for example paracetamol, ibuprofen, co-codamol, aspirin, tricyclic antidepressants, selective serotonin uptake inhibitors (SSRIs), beta-blockers (atenolol, sotalol, propranolol), calcium channel blockers, benzodiazepines, opioids, iron tablets, cocaine and amphetamines.
- Naturally occurring poisons, toxins and venoms, for example snake envenomation and poisonous plants, including foxglove, laburnum, laurel, iris, castor oil plant and *Amanita phalloides*. For further details of poisonous plants, refer to TOXBASE®.
- Alcohol.
- Chemicals (refer to **CBRN**).
- Cosmetics.

Exposure may be:

- Accidental – This typically occurs in young children aged under 5 years, and ingestion of tablets and household products is most common, although almost anything, however unpalatable, may be ingested. Fortunately, the vast majority of ingestions and exposures in young children result in no or very mild symptoms. Many common ingestions involve low toxicity substances. Exploratory ingestion may raise the possibility of safeguarding concerns, as a result of either inadequate supervision or the nature of the ingested substance, even in the absence of a toxic effect on the child. If suspected, this must be reported (refer to **Safeguarding Children** and **Safeguarding Adults at Risk**).
- Intentional – Attempted poisoning as an act of deliberate self-harm. Over-the-counter medicine (e.g. paracetamol) or prescribed drugs are commonly used, although deliberate exposure to any substance, irrespective of actual toxicity, with the expectation or intent of self-harm is significant. Poisoning may also result from intentional exploratory risk-taking behaviour, for example with alcohol or recreational drugs, or as a result of solvent misuse. The expectation of effect is important. The patient does not need to be unwell for this to be a concern.
- Non-accidental (or deliberate) by a third party – This type of poisoning is extremely unlikely to be detected by the ambulance service, but if it is suspected it must be reported (refer to **Safeguarding Adults at Risk** and **Safeguarding Children**).

2. Incidence

- It is difficult to estimate the exact number of overdose and poisoning incidents that occur, as not all cases are reported. In 2016/2017, there were 43,611 poison-related telephone queries involving patients to the National Poisons Information Service. Approximately one-third of these concerned children under the age of five. Most of these incidents were accidental and occurred in the home.

3. Severity and Outcome

- There are a number of factors that affect severity and outcome following exposure; in particular, age and weight of the patient, toxicity of the agent, quantity, route of exposure and co-morbidities or physical injury.
- In patients that self-harm, death commonly results from airway obstruction and respiratory arrest, secondary to a decreased level of consciousness.
- Overdoses including slow-release medicines may have a delayed clinical effect.

4. Pathophysiology

- The toxic effect following exposure will depend primarily on the individual substance. For details of the effects of specific substances, refer to TOXBASE®.

5. Assessment and Management

For the assessment and management of overdose and poisoning, refer to Tables 3.94 and 3.95.

Overdose and Poisoning in Adults and Children

TABLE 3.94 – ASSESSMENT and MANAGEMENT of: Overdose and Poisoning in Adults and Children
Safety First – **DO NOT put yourself in danger** – carry out a dynamic risk assessment and undertake measures to preserve your own safety. **Avoid mouth-to-mouth ventilation.**

Assess <C>ABCD
 	
▪ The majority, perhaps up to 80%, of poisoned patients can be effectively managed by addressing the following **TIME-CRITICAL** features:
  – major **<C>ABCD** problems (refer to **Medical Emergencies in Adults – Overview** and **Medical Emergencies in Children – Overview**)
  – cardiac and respiratory arrest (refer to **Section 2 – Resuscitation**)
  – decreased level of consciousness – **NB** Most poisons that impair consciousness also depress respiration (refer to **Altered Level of Consciousness**)
  – respiratory depression (refer to **Airway and Breathing Management**)
  – arrhythmias (refer to **Cardiac Rhythm Disturbance**)
  – hypotension <70 mmHg systolic
  – convulsions (refer to **Convulsions in Adults** and **Convulsions in Children**)
  – hypothermia (refer to **Hypothermia**)
  – swallowed crack cocaine.
▪ Start correcting any **<C>ABCD** problems.
▪ Undertake a **TIME-CRITICAL** transfer to nearest appropriate receiving hospital.
▪ Continue patient management en-route.
▪ Provide an ATMIST information call.

Oxygen ▪ If indicated, administer high levels of supplemental oxygen, particularly in cases of carbon monoxide poisoning or inhalation of irritant gases (refer to **Oxygen**). ▪ Apply pulse oximeter. ▪ Patients with paraquat or bleomycin poisoning may be harmed by supplemental oxygen, so avoid oxygen unless the patient is hypoxaemic. Target saturation 85–88%.

Respirations
 	
▪ Monitor respirations.
▪ Consider assisted ventilation if:
  – SpO_2 is <90% after administering high levels of oxygen for 30–60 seconds
  – respiratory rate is 30 bpm
  – expansion is inadequate.

Naloxone ▪ Opiates such as morphine, heroin, etc. can cause respiratory depression; in cases of respiratory depression consider naloxone; monitor vital signs closely. **NB** Repeated doses of naloxone may be required (refer to **Naloxone Hydrochloride**).
Blood Pressure ▪ Hypotension is common in severe cases of poisoning. ▪ Monitor blood pressure. ▪ In cases of drug-induced symptomatic hypotension, consider intravascular fluid (refer to **Intravascular Fluid Therapy in Adults** and **Intravascular Fluid Therapy in Children**).
ECG ▪ Undertake continuous cardiac monitoring. A 12-lead ECG may be of diagnostic value and a rhythm strip is required for continuous monitoring in cases involving cardiotoxic drugs, such as beta-blockers, rate-limiting calcium channel blockers and digoxin. Several classes of antidepressants such as tricyclic antidepressants, antipsychotics, anticonvulsants, theophylline and stimulant drugs of misuse, such as cocaine, are also potentially cardiotoxic in overdose.

Overdose and Poisoning in Adults and Children

TABLE 3.94 – ASSESSMENT and MANAGEMENT of: Overdose and Poisoning in Adults and Children *(continued)*

Blood Glucose Level

- Measure blood glucose level – especially in cases of alcohol intoxication, which is a common cause of hypoglycaemia (<4.0 mmol/l).
- Correct blood glucose level (refer to **Glycaemic Emergencies in Adults and Children Glucagon** and **Glucose 10%**).

NB Glucagon is often not effective in overdoses, with the exception of beta-blocker overdose.

Substance

- Consider activated charcoal (refer to **Activated Charcoal**).
- Ascertain what has been ingested/inhaled/absorbed/injected – ask relatives, friends, work colleagues etc.
- Examine the patient for odours, needle marks, pupil abnormalities, signs of corrosion in the mouth.
- Estimate the quantity, for example by counting empty packets.
- Ascertain what, if any, treatment has been given.
- Document the time the incident occurred.
- **NEVER induce vomiting.**
- Refer to Table 1.02 for specific management of certain toxins.
- If possible, take and hand over to staff at the hospital:
  - a sample of the ingested substance
  - all substances found at the scene, whether thought to be involved or not
  - medicine containers
  - a sample of vomit, if present. Important information can be gained by contacting TOXBASE®, and local protocols should be followed to enable this.
- Consider deliberate poisoning or inadequate supervision (refer to **Safeguarding Children** and **Safeguarding Adults at Risk**).

Chemical Exposure

- If exposure to chemical substance is suspected, refer to **CBRN** for management.

Thermoregulation

- Hypo- or hyperthermia can occur. Consider the need for active cooling, particularly if the body temperature is >39° or if there are features of heat stroke (refer to **Heat Related Illness** and **Hypothermia**).

Assess the Patient's Pain

- Where present, assess the **SOCRATES** of pain and record initial and subsequent pain scores.
- Consider analgesia if appropriate (refer to **Pain Management in Adults** and **Pain Management in Children**).

Mental Health Assessment

- In cases of self-harm, assess the patient's emotional and mental state – undertake a rapid mental health assessment. Where appropriate, conversations should occur alone initially, to maintain confidentiality and help build trust (refer to **Mental Health Presentation: Crisis, Distress and Disordered Behaviour**).
- Do not delay treatment, but if possible, document the following information:
  - the patient's home environment
  - the patient's social and family support network
  - the patient's emotional state and level of distress
  - the events leading to the incident.

(continued)

Overdose and Poisoning in Adults and Children

Transfer to Further Care

- For certain patients, urgent transfer to further care may be appropriate, for example:
  - deliberate self-poisoning
  - patients who are symptomatic
  - patients who have ingested poisons with a delayed action such as aspirin, iron, paracetamol, tricyclic antidepressants, co-phenotrope and all modified-release preparations
  - where the type of poison is not known
  - all children and young people who have or may have been exposed to a potentially toxic substance
  - all patients suffering an opioid overdose whether or not they have responded to naloxone – the effects of respiratory depression opioid overdose can last 4–5 hours and may be further prolonged in cases involving a sustained release preparation or a long-acting opiate, such as methadone.

- Methadone has a longer half-life, which can be greater than 24 hours in regular users, and this should be considered when assessing patients and advising on whether to attend hospital.

- In cases of self-harm, even if the substance (or amount of substance) is considered harmless, if the patient does not require emergency treatment, but a mental health assessment may be required, consider alternative pathways (e.g. specialist mental health service) as per local protocol. **NB This decision should take into account the patient's preferences, and the views of the receiving service.**

- Following an exploratory ingestion, some **patients may be considered safe to be left at home if:**
  - the substance is verified by TOXBASE®/NPIS as harmless
  - the incident is/was accidental
  - there is a responsible adult present and there are no safeguarding concerns
  - advice is given to seek medical advice if the patient becomes unwell
  - arrangements have been made to inform the health visitor or GP.

NB Seek further advice should there be any doubt.

- In adults that refuse to go to hospital, the reason for refusal should be determined and information about the potential consequences of not receiving further care provided.

- If the person still refuses care that is felt to be in their best interests, an assessment of their mental capacity may be required (refer to **Mental Capacity Act 2005**) and consideration given as to whether an assessment for compulsory admission under the Mental Health Act is needed (refer to **Mental Health Presentation: Crisis, Distress and Disordered Behaviour**).

- If necessary, seek medical advice and inform the patient's GP – follow local protocol.

6. Specific Substance Management

The clinical features, signs and symptoms listed below are not exhaustive, especially if there have been multiple drug exposures. The lists of common or street names for drugs are similarly non-exhaustive. Visit www.talktofrank.com for an A-to-Z glossary of street names.

TABLE 3.95 – Specific Substance Management

Alcohol Ethanol	
Signs and symptoms	Nausea, vomiting, slurred speech, confusion, ataxia, convulsions, unconsciousness, hypotension.
Description	Alcohol intoxication is a common emergency, especially in young adults, and is usually a transient problem. Alcohol poisoning follows the consumption of excessive amounts of alcohol. It can be fatal, so should be taken seriously. It is not uncommon in teenagers.
Effects	Can cause severe hypoglycaemia, even in teenagers. Adulteration of ethanol with toxic alcohols, such as ethylene glycol or methanol, may occur.

Overdose and Poisoning in Adults and Children

TABLE 3.95 – Specific Substance Management *(continued)*

▪ Management	▪ Alcohol intoxication may cause alcohol-induced hypoglycaemia. Correct the blood glucose level (refer to **Glycaemic Emergencies in Adults and Children**). Other relevant guidelines are **Glucose 10%** and **Glucagon**, although glucagon is often not effective in overdoses. **ALWAYS** check the blood glucose levels in any child or young person with a decreased conscious level, especially in children and young adults who are 'drunk', as hypoglycaemia (blood glucose <4.0 mmol/l) is common and requires treatment with oral glucose or glucose 10% IV (refer to **Glycaemic Emergencies in Adults and Children**).
	▪ When alcohol is combined with drugs in overdose, it may pose a major problem. For example, when combined with opiate drugs or sedatives, it will further decrease the level of consciousness with increased risk of respiratory depression and aspiration of vomit. In combination with paracetamol, chronic alcohol excess increases the risk of liver damage.

Amphetamines

Methamphetamine. Street names: Bennies and Billy Whizz.

▪ Signs and symptoms	▪ Mood swings, extreme hunger, sleeplessness and hyperactivity.
▪ Description	▪ Amphetamines were developed in the 1930s and have been medically prescribed in the past for diet control and as a stimulant.
	▪ Administration: – They can be swallowed, sniffed or, rarely, injected. Onset approximately 30 minutes. Lasts for several hours. Used with other drugs or alcohol, the effects are magnified.
▪ Effects	Increases energy levels, confidence and sociability. **Cardiovascular** ▪ Tachycardia can lead to heart failure even in healthy individuals (refer to **Cardiac Rhythm Disturbance**). ▪ Hypertension can produce pinpoint haemorrhages in skin, especially on the face, and even lead to stroke. **Central nervous system** ▪ 'High' feelings, panic, paranoia which can lead to mental ill-health in the long term, poor sleep and hyperpyrexia. **Gastrointestinal** ▪ Liver failure.
▪ Management	▪ **Vital signs** – Monitor pulse, blood pressure, cardiac rhythm. ▪ **Agitation** – Agitation can be challenging and difficult to manage and there are a number of options, including safe holding techniques or the use of appropriate medications. Advanced/specialist paramedics may have received additional training in this area. Refer to local procedures. ▪ **Convulsions** (refer to **Convulsions in Adults** and **Convulsions in Children**) – In cases of seizures due to amphetamine toxicity, administer the full dose of diazepam (refer to **Diazepam**). ▪ **Cardiac rhythm disturbance** – Narrow-complex tachycardia with cardiac output is best left untreated. ▪ **Hypertension** – If systolic BP >220 and diastolic BP >140 mmHg in the absence of longstanding hypertension, seek medical advice. ▪ **Hypotension** – Correct hypotension by raising the foot of the trolley and/or by the administration of intravascular fluid (refer to **Intravascular Fluid Therapy in Adults** and **Intravascular Fluid Therapy in Children**). ▪ **Hyperthermia** – Rapid transfer to hospital; actively cool en-route if the body temperature is elevated (refer to **Heat Related Illness**).

(continued)

Overdose and Poisoning in Adults and Children

TABLE 3.95 – Specific Substance Management *(continued)*

Benzodiazepines

Diazepam, lorazepam, temazepam, flurazepam, alprazolam (xanax). Street names: Benzos, Jellies, Moggies, Mazzies.

Signs and symptoms	Decreased level of consciousness, respiratory depression, hypotension.
Management	Refer to Table 3.94 for management.
	Consider **Activated Charcoal**.

Beta-blockers

Medicines ending in '....olol' such as: propranolol, atenolol, bisoprolol, metoprolol.

Signs and symptoms include:	Cardiac: bradyarrhythmia, hypotension, VT, cardiac arrest.
	CNS effects: drowsiness, confusion, dilated pupils, CNS depression, respiratory depression, seizures, coma.
	Other: seizures, bronchospasm, pulmonary oedema, hyperkalaemia, hypoglycaemia.
Management	ABCDE.
	Continuous ECG monitoring – check for increased QRS duration, heart block.
	Bradycardia: conventional management (including atropine: refer to **Cardiac Rhythm Disturbance**).
	Hypotension: position head down, consider fluids.
	Bronchospasm: consider salbutamol (refer to **Salbutamol**).
	Seizures: conventional management (refer to **Convulsions in Adults**).
	Measure blood glucose (hypoglycaemia is more common in children with beta-blocker overdose).

Button batteries and magnets

	Button batteries and magnets are high-risk objects and require imaging. Anyone who has ingested a button battery or magnet should attend their nearest emergency department.
	Small powerful magnets (also known as neodymium or 'super strong', rare-earth magnets) are sold as toys, decorative items and fake piercings, and are becoming increasingly popular. Unlike traditional magnets, these extra-strength magnets are small in volume but powerful in magnetism and are easily swallowed. The magnets are often brightly coloured and can be of a variety of shapes such as balls, cylinders, discs, ellipses and bars, and are usually less than 6 mm in diameter.
	Ingestion of extra-strength magnets should be conveyed to Emergency Department as a medical emergency.
	Incidents have been identified where patients experienced a delay in assessment or treatment particularly where ingestion was unknown or unwitnessed and this has also led to missed diagnosis.
	Button battery or magnet ingestion affects all age groups, although most cases involve children under the age of six who mistake the object for a sweet, or older people with confusion or poor vision who mistake the object for a pill.
	Older children and adults may ingest batteries or magnets as a means of self-harming.
	Ingestion of button batteries and magnets can cause serious harm and death and larger batteries can become lodged in the oesophagus.

Overdose and Poisoning in Adults and Children

TABLE 3.95 – Specific Substance Management *(continued)*

	■ Severe tissue damage results from a build-up of sodium hydroxide (caustic soda) due to the electrical current discharged from the battery, causing burns, often in the oesophagus, which can then cause erosion into major blood vessels, resulting in catastrophic haemorrhage.
	■ Symptoms of tissue damage such as haematemesis, haemoptysis and respiratory difficulties can manifest up to 28 days after ingestion of the battery.
	■ Removal of the battery alone may be insufficient action to prevent further damage, with further symptoms manifesting later; patients need expert input, careful monitoring and follow-up.
	■ Consider ingestion in unwell patients with gastrointestinal symptoms.
	■ Consider the possibility of rare-earth magnet or button battery ingestion or aspiration in patients with: – airway obstruction, wheezing or noisy breathing, stridor, coughing – drooling – vomiting – chest discomfort – difficulty swallowing, decreased appetite, refusal to eat, choking or gagging when eating or drinking – abdominal pain.
	■ The ingestion of a single rare-earth magnet is unlikely to cause significant harm. However, if multiple magnets are ingested, or if a magnet is swallowed along with a metal object, significant injury can occur. Ingestion of a magnet with a button battery is a **TIME-CRITICAL** emergency. Magnets can attract each other across layers of bowel to cause ischemia and pressure necrosis of the gut and serious complications. The types of injuries have included ulceration, necrosis, perforation, rupture, stricture, fistula, haemorrhage, mediastinitis, gastric outlet or bowel obstruction, volvulus, sepsis and death. Urgent assessment and treatment is therefore vital.
	■ Abdominal symptoms may not manifest for weeks after ingestion of magnets, however intestinal injury can occur early, within 8–24 hours following ingestion, despite the patient often remaining well.

Calcium-channel blockers diltiazem, verapamil

■ Signs and symptoms	■ Bradycardia, hypotension, seizures.
■ Effects	■ Overdose may lead to cardiac arrest. ■ Overdose of sustained release preparations can lead to delayed onset of symptoms, including arrhythmias, hypotension, shock and sudden cardiac collapse.
■ Management	■ Refer to Table 3.94 for management. ■ Continuous ECG monitoring. **NB** Immediate-release preparations: problems are unlikely to develop in patients that are asymptomatic where the time interval is greater than 6 hours from time of ingestion. ■ Consider **Activated Charcoal**.

Carbon monoxide poisoning

■ Signs and symptoms	■ Disorientation, decreased consciousness, unconscious, unexplained headaches. **NB** The supposed cherry-red skin colouration in carbon monoxide poisoning is rarely seen in practice **and normally precedes mortality**. ■ Refer to Table 3.96.

(continued)

Overdose and Poisoning in Adults and Children

TABLE 3.95 – Specific Substance Management *(continued)*

	▪ Any patient found unconscious or disorientated in an enclosed space, for example a patient involved in a fire in a confined space (although smoke inhalation/CO poisoning is normally secondary to inhalation injury), where ventilation is impaired or a source of incomplete combustion is present, e.g. defective heating boiler, open flames, BBQ or exhaust fumes from a fuel-driven device (generator, chain saw, angle grinder, etc.).
▪ Effects	▪ Long-term low-level exposure is just as debilitating and as much a risk to health as short-term acute exposure and is often misdiagnosed.
▪ Management	▪ Any pregnant patient that is suspected of CO poisoning or any level of smoke inhalation should be transported to hospital, as the fotus has a higher affinity to CO and other toxins than the mother.
	▪ Refer to Table 3.97. Remove patient and responders from the scene where CO may be present.

Cocaine

Powder cocaine, crack cocaine. Street names: Charlie, crack, toot, freebase.

▪ Signs and symptoms	▪ Hyperexcitable, agitated, irritable and sometimes violent behaviour. Sweating. Dilated pupils.
▪ Description	▪ Cocaine is a powerfully reinforcing psychostimulant. Crack is made from cocaine in a process called freebasing.
	▪ Administration:
	– Cocaine comes in the form of a powder that is almost always 'cut' or mixed with other substances. It can be: snorted through the nose, rubbed into the gums, smoked or injected.
	– Crack comes in the form of solid rocks, chips or chunks that are smoked.
▪ Effects	▪ Induces a sense of exhilaration, euphoria, excitement and reduced hunger in the user primarily by blocking the re-uptake of the neurotransmitter dopamine in the midbrain, which blocks noradrenaline uptake causing vasoconstriction and hypertension.
	NB Crack cocaine is pure and therefore more potent than street cocaine; it enters the bloodstream more quickly and in higher concentrations. Because it is smoked, crack cocaine's effects are felt more quickly and they are more intense than those of powder cocaine. However, the effects of smoked crack are more short-lived than those of snorted powder cocaine. It is highly addictive even after only one use.
	▪ The symptoms of a cocaine overdose are intense and generally short-lived. Although uncommon, people do die from cocaine or crack overdose, particularly following ingestion (often associated with swallowing 'evidence').
	▪ All forms of cocaine/crack use can cause coronary artery spasm, myocardial infarction and accelerated ischaemic heart disease, even in young people.
	▪ Various doses of cocaine can also produce other neurological and behavioural effects such as:
	– dizziness
	– headache
	– movement problems
	– anxiety
	– insomnia
	– depression
	– hallucinations.
	▪ The unwanted effects of cocaine or crack overdose may include some or all of the following:
	– tremors
	– dangerous or fatal rise in body temperature
	– delirium

Overdose and Poisoning in Adults and Children

TABLE 3.95 – Specific Substance Management *(continued)*

	– hypertension – tachycardia and dysrhythmia – myocardial infarction – cardiac arrest – seizures including status epilepticus – stroke – kidney failure.
Management	Transfer patient rapidly to hospital. Administer supplemental oxygen (refer to **Oxygen**). Consider assisted ventilation at a rate of 12–20 breaths per minute if: – SpO$_2$ is <90% on high concentration O$_2$ – respiratory rate is >30 breaths per minute – expansion is inadequate. Undertake a 12-lead ECG – if the patient has a 12-lead ECG suggestive of myocardial infarction and a history of recent cocaine use, administer nitrates but do not administer thrombolysis. Administer aspirin and GTN if the patient complains of chest pain (refer to **Aspirin** and **Glyceryl Trinitrate**). **Chest pain** – Administer diazepam if the patient has severe chest pain (refer to **Diazepam**). In symptomatic cocaine toxicity, titrate diazepam slowly to response. **Convulsions** (refer to **Convulsions in Adults** and **Convulsions in Children**) – In cases of seizures due to cocaine toxicity, administer the full dose of diazepam (refer to **Diazepam**). **Hypertension** – If systolic BP >220 and diastolic BP >140 mmHg in the absence of longstanding hypertension, seek medical advice. **Hyperthermia** – Actively cool if the body temperature is elevated. **NB** Swallowed crack cocaine represents a severe medical emergency and needs **URGENT** transportation to hospital **EVEN IF ASYMPTOMATIC**.
Corrosive injuries[14]	
Mechanism of injury	Corrosives can injure any biological surface that they meet. The corrosive effects are a function of both the oxidizing capacity and the pH of the solution.
Signs and symptoms	Either strong acids or strong alkalis may cause pain, blistering, penetrating necrosis and coagulating burns. Cardiovascular collapse and metabolic acidosis may occur secondary to an extensive corrosive injury.
Management	**Ingestion** of a corrosive should be managed by an urgent assessment of the airway and the cardiovascular system. If there is evidence of oedema of the upper airway, early intubation or tracheotomy should be considered. **Inhalation** may occur directly in the presence of a volatile corrosive or indirectly through the aspiration of gastric contents. The upper airway should be assessed for potential injury. If there is evidence of oedema of the upper airway, early intubation or tracheotomy should be considered. Injury to the lower airway may result in a pneumonitis or acute respiratory distress syndrome. **Skin** contact with a corrosive should be treated by urgent irrigation with water for 20–60 minutes and be assessed and treated as a thermal burn. Any contaminated clothing should be removed. Personal protective equipment should be worn. **Eye** contact with a corrosive should be treated with urgent irrigation with water or normal saline for 10–15 minutes.

(continued)

3 Medical Emergencies

Overdose and Poisoning in Adults and Children

TABLE 3.95 – Specific Substance Management *(continued)*

Cyanide

Signs and symptoms	Confusion, drowsiness, decreased level of consciousness, dizziness, headache, convulsions.
Management	Cyanide poisoning requires specific treatment – seek medical advice. Provide full supportive therapy and transfer immediately to hospital. Provide an alert/information call.
	Cyanide poisoning can occur in patients exposed to smoke in a confined space (e.g. house fire). Remove the patient from the source and administer continuous supplemental oxygen in as high a concentration as possible. If there are signs of decreased levels of consciousness, transfer immediately to hospital. Provide an alert/information call.
	In cases of CBRNE, the HART/SORT team will provide guidance.
	Poisoning may occur in certain industrial settings. Cyanide 'kits' should be available, and the kit should be taken to hospital with the patient. The patient requires injection with dicobalt edetate or administration of the drug hydroxycobalamin or sodium thiosulphate.

Foreign bodies

Description	The majority of swallowed objects are low-risk objects and can be managed conservatively.
Effects	Large objects (>6 cm long or 2.5 cm wide) may obstruct the gut – these patients should be transferred to hospital.
Management	There is no need for transfer to hospital for patients who:
	– give a reliable history of ingestion of a small, low-risk object
	– look well and are pain free
	– have no respiratory distress
	– can eat and drink
	– have no significant past medical history.
	The patients/carers should be advised to seek medical advice if the patient develops:
	– breathing problems
	– abdominal pain
	– fever
	– vomiting
	– inability to tolerate food and drink.
	NOTE: any patient who has ingested a button battery (or small magnet) must be conveyed to hospital, even if they are symptom free.

Iron

Signs and symptoms	Nausea, vomiting blood, diarrhoea, black stools, metallic taste, convulsions, dizziness, flushed appearance, decreased level of consciousness, non-cardiac pulmonary oedema.
Effects	Iron pills are regularly used by large numbers of the population, including pregnant mothers. In overdose, especially in children, they are exceedingly dangerous.
	They may cause extensive damage to the liver and gut and these patients will require hospital assessment and treatment.
	NB Charcoal is contra-indicated as it does not absorb iron.

Ketamine and ketamine analogues

Street names: K, Cat, Kit-Kat, Special K, Vitamin K, Ket

Signs and symptoms	Sedation, loss of consciousness and respiratory depression.
Description	Administration: can be sniffed or injected.

Overdose and Poisoning in Adults and Children

TABLE 3.95 – Specific Substance Management *(continued)*

Effects	Dissociative anaesthetic.
	Cardiovascular
	▪ Tachycardia can lead to heart failure even in healthy individuals (refer to **Cardiac Rhythm Disturbance**).
	▪ Hypertension can produce pinpoint haemorrhages in skin, especially on the face, and even lead to stroke.
	Central nervous system
	▪ Hallucinations, coma, long-term memory problems and 'flashbacks'.
	Urogenital
	▪ Bladder irritation and incontinence.
Management	▪ **Vital signs** – Monitor pulse, blood pressure, cardiac rhythm.
	▪ **Agitation** – Agitation can be challenging and difficult to manage and there are a number of options, including safe holding techniques or the use of appropriate medications. Advanced/specialist paramedics may have received additional training in this area. Refer to local procedures.
	▪ **Cardiac rhythm disturbance** – Narrow complex tachycardia with cardiac output is best left untreated.
	▪ **Hypertension** – If systolic BP >220 and diastolic BP >140 mmHg in the absence of longstanding hypertension, seek medical advice.
	▪ **Hypotension** – Correct hypotension by raising the foot of the trolley and/or by the administration of intravascular fluid (refer to **Intravascular Fluid Therapy in Adults** and **Intravascular Fluid Therapy in Children**).

Lysergic acid

Street names: diethylamide (LSD), 'acid', blotter, dots and mushrooms.

Description	▪ A 'mind-altering drug' that alters the brain's perception of things.
	▪ Discovered in 1943, and was used in the 1960s as a 'recreational drug'.
	▪ Administration:
	– LSD is produced on patches of blotting paper, called tabs or trips, often with printed motifs including cartoon characters.
	– Once swallowed they take 30–60 minutes to work. The trip will last up to 12 hours and cannot be stopped.
	– LSD is not addictive but is illegal.
Signs and symptoms	▪ Agitated, unusual behaviour, clear mental disturbance.
	▪ The patient may appear distant and display anxious behaviour.
Effects	▪ The alterations in perception may be pleasant or 'nightmarish', or a mix of both, and last for some 12 hours.
	Central nervous system
	▪ Visual hallucinations (distortion and delusions), which can cause dangerous behaviour.
	▪ Nightmarish perceptions ('bad trips') may last for 12 hours.
	▪ Nausea and vomiting.
	▪ Personality changes and psychiatric illness.
	▪ Nightmarish flashbacks that can last for years after drug use stops.
	▪ Delusions – false sensations or visions – may affect taste, hearing and vision.
	▪ Can trigger hidden mental illness in individuals.
	▪ Permanent eye damage can occur.

(continued)

3 Medical Emergencies

SECTION

Overdose and Poisoning in Adults and Children

TABLE 3.95 – Specific Substance Management *(continued)*

▪ Management	**DO NOT** interfere unduly, as the 'trip' will self-limit and communication is easier then. Keep the patient safe, and remember other drugs and alcohol will aggravate the effects of LSD.
	▪ Agitation can be challenging and difficult to manage and there are a number of options, including safe holding techniques or the use of appropriate medications. Advanced/specialist paramedics may have received additional training in this area. Refer to local procedures.

3,4-Methylenedioxymethamphetamine

MDMA, Ecstasy, 'E'. Street names: doves, apples, strawberries and diamonds.

▪ Signs and symptoms	▪ Sweating, dilated pupils and elevated mood.
▪ Description	▪ MDMA is a psychoactive drug with hallucinogenic effects.
	▪ Administration:
	– 'E' tablets may be white embossed 'headache'-sized pills, or coloured capsules.
	– They take 40 minutes to work, lasting for 2–6 hours.
	– 'E' may not be addictive but is illegal.
▪ Effects	Feeling warm, energetic and friendly, rising to a state of euphoria.
	Cardiovascular system
	▪ Tachycardia (refer to **Cardiac Rhythm Disturbance**).
	▪ Capillary rupture, causing red marking on the face in particular.
	Central nervous system
	▪ Some patients develop hyperpyrexia, which can be life-threatening. These patients need urgent transfer to hospital for specialist care. Active cooling measures (refer to **Heat Related Illness**) may be helpful but should not delay transfer to further care.
	▪ Depression, panic and anxiety may also occur.
	Liver and kidney injury
	▪ Liver failure and severe kidney damage may occur.
	Other
	▪ Cystitis and heavy periods may occur in females who use 'E'.
▪ Management	▪ Agitation can be challenging and difficult to manage, and there are a number of options, including safe holding techniques or the use of appropriate medications. Advanced/specialist paramedics may have received additional training in this area. Refer to local procedures.
	▪ Treat convulsions with diazepam (refer to **Diazepam**).
	▪ If the systolic BP >220 and diastolic >140 mmHg in the absence of longstanding hypertension, seek medical advice.
	▪ Correct hypotension by raising the foot of the bed and/or by giving fluids as per medical emergencies (refer to **Intravascular Fluid Therapy in Adults** and **Intravascular Fluid Therapy in Children**).
	▪ Active cooling measures (refer to **Heat Related Illness**) may be helpful but should not delay transfer to further care.

Mephedrone

Street names: MCAT, M-CAT, M kat, M-Cat, MD3, meow, meow meow, meph. Meth, M-Cat, White Magic, Meow Meow.

▪ Signs and symptoms	▪ Agitation.
▪ Description	▪ Amphetamine-based drug of misuse.
	▪ Administration: sniffed or, rarely, injected.

Overdose and Poisoning in Adults and Children

TABLE 3.95 – Specific Substance Management *(continued)*

▪ Effects	Psychoactive stimulant. **Cardiovascular** ▪ Tachycardia can lead to heart failure even in healthy individuals (refer to **Cardiac Rhythm Disturbance**). ▪ Hypertension can produce pinpoint haemorrhages in skin, especially on the face, and even lead to stroke. **Central nervous system** – Agitation, confusion, hyperpyrexia.
▪ Management	▪ **Vital signs** – Monitor pulse, blood pressure, cardiac rhythm. ▪ **Agitation** – Agitation can be challenging and difficult to manage and there are a number of options, including safe holding techniques or the use of appropriate medications. Advanced/specialist paramedics may have received additional training in this area. Refer to local procedures. ▪ **Convulsions** (refer to **Convulsions in Adults** and **Convulsions in Children**). ▪ **Cardiac rhythm disturbance** – Narrow complex tachycardia with cardiac output is best left untreated. ▪ **Hypertension** – If systolic BP >220 and diastolic BP >140 mmHg in the absence of longstanding hypertension, seek medical advice. ▪ **Hypotension** – Correct hypotension by raising the foot of the trolley and/or by the administration of intravascular fluid (refer to **Intravascular Fluid Therapy in Adults** and **Intravascular Fluid Therapy in Children**). ▪ **Hyperthermia** – Rapid transfer to hospital; active cooling measures may be undertaken en-route (refer to **Heat Related Illness**).

Novel Psychoactive Substances (NPSs)[15,16]

Commonly known as 'illegal highs'

	▪ Novel psychoactive substances (NPSs) is the name given to drugs that are newly synthesised or newly available. They include a multitude of substances and a diverse group of chemicals, and have many different effects. ▪ There is often little correlation between the drug a misuser believes they have taken and the actual chemical identity of the substance. NPSs include substances with primarily stimulant effects, those with primarily hallucinogenic effects, as well as some central nervous system depressants and synthetic cannabinoids.

Opioids

Heroin, Diamorphine, Amidone, Dolophine, Methadone, Fentanyl.

▪ Signs and symptoms	▪ Drowsiness, nausea, vomiting, small pupils, respiratory depression, cyanosis, decreased level of consciousness, convulsions, non-cardiac pulmonary oedema.
▪ Description	▪ There are a wide variety of opioids, both naturally derived and synthetic. ▪ Administration: injected, snorted or smoked.
▪ Effects	▪ Central nervous system and respiratory depression associated with pinpoint pupils. ▪ Withdrawal symptoms may also occur: sweating, shivering, muscle cramps, lacrimation. ▪ Reduced physical and psychological pain – relieving anxiety. The effects of methadone are less intense but may be prolonged. **Side effects:** ▪ Cardiovascular system – damage to veins and lungs, infection.

(continued)

3 Medical Emergencies

SECTION

Overdose and Poisoning in Adults and Children

TABLE 3.95 – Specific Substance Management *(continued)*

Management	▪ Ensure the airway is open – administer supplemental oxygen (refer to **Oxygen**).
	▪ Profound respiratory depression can be reversed with naloxone (refer to **Naloxone Hydrochloride**).
	▪ Methadone is extremely dangerous for young children and its effects may take several hours to become apparent.

Orthochlorobenzalmalononitrile

CS gas

Signs and symptoms	▪ Lacrimation, burning sensation of the eyes, excessive mucus production, nausea and vomiting.
Effects	▪ Carried by police forces for defensive purposes. CS spray is aerosolised fine powder, which irritates the eyes ('tear gas') and respiratory tract.
Management	▪ **AVOID** contact with the gas, which is given off from patient's clothing. Where possible keep two metres, **upwind**, from the patient and give them self-care instructions. Symptoms normally resolve in 15 minutes but may potentiate or exacerbate existing respiratory conditions. If symptoms are present: ▪ Remove the patient to a well-ventilated area. ▪ Remove contaminated clothes and place them in a sealed bag. ▪ If possible, remove contact lenses. ▪ **DO NOT** irrigate the eyes as CS gas particles may dissolve and exacerbate irritation. If irrigation is required use copious amounts of saline. ▪ Patients with severe respiratory problems should be immediately transported to hospital (refer to **Airway and Breathing Management**). ▪ Ensure good ventilation of the vehicle during transfer to further care.

Paracetamol and paracetamol-containing compound drugs

Signs and symptoms	▪ Nausea, vomiting, malaise, right upper quadrant abdominal pain, jaundice, confusion, drowsiness – unconsciousness may develop later. **NB** Frequently asymptomatic, symptoms are unreliable.
Effects	▪ Paracetamol, even in modest doses, is **dangerous** and can induce severe liver and kidney damage. Initially there are no clinical features to suggest this, which may lull the patient and ambulance clinicians into a false sense of security. It frequently takes 24–48 hours for the effects of paracetamol damage to become apparent and urgent blood paracetamol levels are required to assess the patient's level of risk. ▪ Patients who are malnourished, have been fasting, take enzyme-inducing drugs or regularly drink alcohol to excess are at higher risk of liver damage.
Management	▪ Codeine and dextropropoxyphene are both derived from opioid drugs. This in overdose, especially if alcohol is involved, may well produce profound respiratory depression. This can be reversed with naloxone (refer to **Naloxone Hydrochloride**). ▪ There are a number of analgesic drugs that contain paracetamol and a combination of codeine or dextropropoxyphene. Patients are not always aware that a medicine contains paracetamol. Always ask what medicines they have taken rather than just focusing on how much paracetamol they have taken. ▪ Consider **Activated Charcoal**.

Synthetic Cannabinoid Receptor Agonists (SCRAs)

Street names: Spice, JWH-015, 5F-ADBICA, 5F-AKB48, X, Hawaiian Haze, Bombay Blue, Black Mamba.

Signs and symptoms	▪ Agitation, confusion, hallucinations, psychosis, syncope, tachycardia, hypertension, hypotension, chest pain, acute kidney injury and muscle rigidity.

Overdose and Poisoning in Adults and Children

TABLE 3.95 – Specific Substance Management *(continued)*

Description	Potent agonists of the cannabinoid-1 (CB₁) receptor, unlike Δ^9-tetrahydrocannabinoid, the active alkaloid found in *Cannabis sativa*, which is a partial agonist at the CB₁ receptor. Administration: the active chemical is usually impregnated onto plant matter and then smoked.
Effects	Disassociative with greater central nervous system and cardiovascular effects compared with cannabis.
Management	Agitation can be challenging and difficult to manage and there are a number of options, including safe holding techniques or the use of appropriate medications. Advanced/specialist paramedics may have received additional training in this area. Refer to local procedures. Treat convulsions with diazepam (refer to **Diazepam**). If the systolic BP >220 and diastolic >140 mmHg in the absence of longstanding hypertension, seek medical advice. Correct hypotension by raising the foot of the bed and/or by giving fluids as per medical emergencies (refer to **Intravascular Fluid Therapy in Adults** and **Intravascular Fluid Therapy in Children**).

Tricyclic antidepressants

Signs and symptoms	Central nervous system: excitability, confusion, blurred vision, dry mouth, fever, pupil dilation, convulsions, decreased level of consciousness, arrhythmias, hypotension, tachycardia, respiratory depression; physical condition can rapidly change.
Effects	Poisoning with tricyclic antidepressants may cause impaired consciousness, profound hypotension and cardiac arrhythmias. They are a common treatment for patients who are already depressed. Newer antidepressants, such as fluoxetine (Prozac) and paroxetine (Seroxat), have different effects. These medicines can be extremely dangerous to young children.
Management	Continuous ECG monitoring. Obtain IV access. Arrhythmias (refer to **Cardiac Rhythm Disturbance**). The likelihood of convulsions is high (refer to **Convulsions in Adults** and **Convulsions in Children**). Monitor closely, as the patient's physical condition can rapidly change. Consider **Activated Charcoal**.

TABLE 3.96 – Signs and Symptoms of Carbon Monoxide Poisoning

Acute low-level exposure	Acute high-level exposure	Chronic low-level exposure
Headache	Headache	Headache
Dizziness	Dizziness	Dizziness
Nausea	Nausea	Nausea
Vomiting	Vomiting	Vomiting
General lethargy	Lethargy	General lethargy
	Muscle ataxia	Flu-like symptoms
	Confusion	Neurological decline
	Chest pains	Visual problems
	Shortness of breath/difficulty in breathing	
	Neurological deficit	
	Coma	

Overdose and Poisoning in Adults and Children

TABLE 3.97 – Questions to be Asked in Cases of Carbon Monoxide Poisoning[17,18]	
Cohabitants/companions	Does anyone else feel unwell? Are any pets behaving abnormally?
Outdoors	Do you feel better if you go outside or when you are away from the property for a prolonged time?
Maintenance	Are any heating appliances properly maintained?
Alarms	Do you have a working CO alarm? Has it activated?

7. Duty of Care

- It is not uncommon to find patients who have or claim to have taken an overdose and subsequently refuse treatment or admission to hospital. An assessment of their mental health state, capacity and suicide risk should be made (refer to **Mental Capacity Act 2005** and **Mental Health Presentation: Crisis, Distress and Disordered Behaviour**). If, despite reasonable persuasion, the patient refuses treatment, it is not acceptable to leave them in a potentially dangerous situation without any access to care.

- Assistance may be obtained from the medical/clinical director or a member of the clinical team and a judgement must be made to seek appropriate advice. Attendance of the police or local mental health team may be required, especially if the safety of the patient or others is at risk.

KEY POINTS!

Overdose and Poisoning in Adults and Children

- **Establish the event, drug or substance involved, the quantity, mode of poisoning and any alcohol consumed.**
- **NEVER induce vomiting.**
- **Bring the substance or substances and any containers for inspection at hospital, if it is safe to do so.**
- **Anyone with deliberate overdose must be transferred to hospital or referred to an appropriate mental health service.**
- **After confirmed exposure to a low toxicity substance, some patients may be considered for home management.**
- **Consider exposure to carbon monoxide.**
- **Agitation can be challenging and difficult to manage and there are a number of options, including safe holding techniques or the use of appropriate medications. Advanced/specialist paramedics may have received additional training in this area. Refer to local procedures.**

Acknowledgements

We would like to gratefully acknowledge the National Poisons Information Service for their contributions, comments and input to this JRCALC guideline.

Bibliography

1. Soar J, Perkins GD, Abbas G, Alfonzo A, Barelli A, Bierens JJLM, et al. European Resuscitation Council Guidelines for Resuscitation 2010 Section 8: Cardiac arrest in special circumstances: electrolyte abnormalities, poisoning, drowning, accidental hypothermia, hyperthermia, asthma, anaphylaxis, cardiac surgery, trauma, pregnancy, electrocution. *Resuscitation* 2010, 81(10): 1400–1433.

2. The British National Formulary for Children. *Emergency Treatment of Poisoning.* Available from: https://www.evidence.nhs.uk/formulary/bnfc/current/emergency-treatment-of-poisoning, 2012–2013.

3. National Institute for Health and Clinical Excellence. *Self-harm in over 8s: short-term management and prevention of recurrence* (CG16). London: NICE, 2004. Available from: http://www.nice.org.uk/CG16.

4. Gunnell D, Bennewith O, Peters TJ, House A, Hawton K. The epidemiology and management of self-harm amongst adults in England. *Journal of Public Health* 2005, 27(1): 67–73.

5. Gwini SM, Shaw D, Iqbal M, Spaight A, Siriwardena AN. Exploratory study of factors associated with adverse clinical features in patients presenting with non-fatal

Overdose and Poisoning in Adults and Children

drug overdose/self-poisoning to the ambulance service. *Emergency Medicine Journal* 2011, 28(10): 892–894.

6. Health Protection Agency, Centre for Radiation, Chemical and Environmental Hazards. *National Poisons Information Service Annual Report 2010/2011.* London: The Stationery Office, 2010.

7. Health Protection Agency, Centre for Radiation, Chemical and Environmental Hazards. *Current Awareness in Clinical Toxicology.* London: The Stationery Office, 2012.

8. Health Protection Agency, Centre for Radiation, Chemical and Environmental Hazards. *Chemicals & Poisons A–Z and Compendium.* London: The Stationery Office, 2012.

9. Health Protection Agency, Centre for Radiation, Chemical and Environmental Hazards. *Chemicals and Poisons.* London: The Stationery Office, 2012.

10. National Poisons Information Service. *TOXBASE.* Available from: http://www.npis.org/toxbase.html, 2012.

11. National Poisons Information Service. Available from: http://www.npis.org/index.html, 2012.

12. The British National Formulary. Emergency treatment of poisoning. *BNF 63.* London: Royal Pharmaceutical Society, 2012.

13. The British National Formulary. Medicines information services. *BNF 63.* London: Royal Pharmaceutical Society, 2012.

14. Coulson JM, Thompson JP. Investigation and management of the poisoned patient. *Clin Med* (Lond) 2008. 8(1): 89–91.

Paediatric Gastroenteritis

1. Introduction

- Every year 10% of the UK's under-5s will have an episode of infective gastroenteritis.

- Characteristically they present with sudden onset of diarrhoea (with or without vomiting), which usually resolves without any specific treatment.

- When severe, dehydration can occur, which can be life-threatening. Younger children are most at risk of dehydration.

- Children should not simply be viewed as 'little adults'. They pose many pitfalls for the unwary and inexperienced, and present healthcare providers with significant challenges whatever the setting.

- Children display important differences in their anatomy, their physiology, their immunity and the illnesses they encounter, as well as the ways in which these conditions present, develop and progress.

- Difficulties verbalising and communicating their condition further add to these challenges.

1.1 'Major' and 'minor' illnesses

- Before considering 'minor' illnesses in children, it is crucial to both appreciate and understand that 'major' childhood illnesses – including life-threatening conditions such as meningococcal disease – rarely present in extremis, but more commonly present with relatively innocent features that can easily be mistaken for minor illnesses.

- Children with advanced major illness (or significant injury) typically have deranged vital signs that are usually readily detected. Earlier in their illness, these children may well have had normal physiology and appeared relatively well – if assessed early in their illness, these children might be misdiagnosed as only having a minor illness.

2. Severity and Outcome

In children with gastroenteritis:

- vomiting usually lasts 1–2 days, and stops within 3 days.

- diarrhoea usually lasts 5–7 days, and stops within 2 weeks.

3. Pathophysiology

- Many viruses, bacteria or other microbes can cause gastroenteritis. However, the most common cause in children is the Rotavirus. This virus can be spread easily through close contact as it is passed out in an infected person's diarrhoea.

- Once exposed to the virus, the incubation period is approximately 48 hours before symptoms start to show. It is thought that almost every child in the UK suffers a rotavirus infection at some point before they turn 5 years old. However, it is most common in children aged 6 months to 2 years old.

- In the UK, 18,000 children each year present at a hospital with a rotavirus infection. Ten percent will need admission due to dehydration.

- Other causes include bacterial infection such as *Escherichia Coli (E. coli)*, Salmonella and Campylobacter bacteria that produce toxins that the food we eat. Once exposed to the virus, normally immunity is developed; hence it is uncommon in adults.

3.1 *Escherichia coli* 0157:H7 infection

- *E. coli* 0157:H7 is a bacterium found in the intestines of healthy cattle that can cause serious human infections, especially in the young and older people.

- It often leads to bloody diarrhoea and occasionally kidney failure (referred to as haemolytic uraemic syndrome or HUS). Outbreaks have occurred following school farm visits or following consumption of undercooked, contaminated beef. (Beef burgers are notorious, as the meat comes from many animals.)

- When *E. coli* 0157:H7 infection is suspected (e.g. contact with a confirmed case), urgent specialist advice must be sought.

4. Assessment

- Gastroenteritis is diagnosed on clinical findings and should be suspected where there is a sudden change in stool consistency to loose or watery stools and/or a sudden onset of vomiting.

History: consider the diagnosis when the child has had:

- recent contact with someone with acute diarrhoea and/or vomiting

- exposure to a known source of enteric infection (farm visits, contaminated water or food – see *Escherichia coli* 0157 infection above)

- recent overseas travel.

4.1 Differential diagnosis

Apart from gastroenteritis, alternative diagnoses must be considered when the following features are found, and a more experienced paediatric assessment should be sought:

- Fever:
  - temp ≥38°C in child <3 months old
  - temp ≥39°C in child ≥3 months old.

- Shortness of breath or tachypnoea.

- Altered consciousness.

- Neck stiffness.

- Bulging fontanelle in infants.

- Non-blanching rash.

Paediatric Gastroenteritis

- Blood and/or mucus in stool.
- Bilious (green) vomit.
- Severe or localised abdominal pain.
- Abdominal distension or rebound tenderness.
- History/suspicion of poisoning.
- History of head injury.
- Appears systemically unwell.

Examination: clinical assessment for dehydration and shock

- Establish whether the child is red, amber or green on the traffic light system in Table 3.98.

TABLE 3.98 – Traffic Light System for Clinical Dehydration and Shock

	Green Low Risk	Amber Intermediate Risk	Red High Risk
Activity	- Responds normally to social cues - Content/smiling - Stays awake/awakens quickly - Strong normal cry/not crying	- Aged less than 1 year old - Altered response to social cues - Decreased activity - No smile	- Not responding normally to or no response to social cues - Appears ill to a healthcare professional - Unable to rouse or if roused does not stay awake - Weak, high-pitched or continuous cry
Skin	- Normal skin colour - Normal turgor	- Warm extremities	- Pale/mottled/ashen/blue - Cold extremities - Reduced skin turgor
Respiratory	- Normal breathing		- Tachypnoeic (refer to **Page for Age**)
Hydration	- CRT≤ 2 secs - Moist mucous membranes - Normal urine	- CRT 2–3 secs - Dry mucous membranes (except after a drink) - Reduced urine output - Clinically dehydrated (refer to Table 3.99)	- CRT >3 seconds - Clinically shocked (refer to Table 3.99)
Pulses/Heart Rate	- Heart rate normal (refer to **Page for Age**) - Peripheral pulses normal		- Tachycardic (refer to **Page for Age**) - Peripheral pulses weak
Blood Pressure	- Normal, refer to **Page for Age**		- Hypotensive (refer to **Page for Age**)
Eyes	- Normal eyes	- Sunken eyes	
Other		- At risk of dehydration	

Children most at risk of dehydration include:

- Infants of low birth weight (i.e. <2.5 kg).
- Children <1 year, especially those aged <6 months.
- >5 diarrhoeal stools in the previous 24 hours.
- >2 vomits in the previous 24 hours.
- Those who have not been offered/not been able to tolerate oral fluids.
- Breastfed infants who have stopped feeding.
- Malnourished children.

Paediatric Gastroenteritis

TABLE 3.99 – Symptoms and Signs of Clinical Dehydration and Shock

Increasing severity of dehydration

→

Symptoms **No clinically detectable dehydration**	**Clinically dehydrated**	**Clinically shocked**
Appears well	Appears to be unwell or deteriorating	–
Alert and responsive	Altered responsiveness (e.g. irritable, lethargic)	Decreased level of consciousness
Normal urine output	Decreased urine output. Output often decreased in those with normal hydration as a compensatory mechanism Unreliable in those in nappies with diarrhoea	–
Skin colour unchanged	Skin colour unchanged	Pale or mottled skin
Warm extremities	Warm extremities	Cold extremities
Signs **No clinically detectable dehydration**	**Clinically dehydrated**	**Clinically shocked**
Alert and responsive	Altered responsiveness (e.g. irritable, lethargic)	Decreased level of consciousness
Skin colour unchanged	Skin colour unchanged	Pale or mottled skin
Warm extremities	Warm extremities	Cold extremities
Eyes not sunken	Sunken eyes	–
Moist mucous membranes (except after a drink)	Dry mucous membranes (except for 'mouth breather')	–
Normal heart rate	Tachycardia	Tachycardia
Normal breathing pattern	Tachypnoea	Tachypnoea
Normal peripheral pulses	Normal peripheral pulses	Weak peripheral pulses
Normal capillary refill time	Normal capillary refill time	Prolonged capillary refill time
Normal skin turgor	Reduced skin turgor	–
Normal blood pressure	Normal blood pressure	Hypotension (decompensated shock)

NB Rectal examinations should never be performed in the pre-hospital assessment of the paediatric acute abdomen.

Consider dehydration risk factors when interpreting symptoms and signs.

Within the category of 'clinical dehydration', there is a spectrum of severity indicated by increasingly numerous and more pronounced symptoms and signs.

Within the category of 'clinical shock', one or more of the symptoms and/or signs listed would be expected to be present.

Dashes (–) indicate that these clinical features do not specifically indicate shock but may still be present. Symptoms and signs with red flags may help to identify children at increased risk of progression to shock.

If uncertain, manage as if the child has those red flag symptoms and/or signs.

5. Management

Most children with gastroenteritis can be managed at home with oral fluids, although dehydrated children require NG or IV fluid replacement and those in shock may require urgent intravenous fluid resuscitation. Fluid losses can be replaced via the oral route, via a nasogastric tube or intravenously.

Paediatric Gastroenteritis

- Oral (and nasogastric) fluids:
  - oral rehydration salt (ORS) solutions are given orally or via a nasogastric (NG) tube.
  - they should be given as small, frequent volumes.
  - response to oral rehydration must be monitored by regular clinical assessment.
  - Over-the-counter (OTC) commercially available ORS solutions include Dioralyte, Dioralyte Relief, Electrolade and Rapolyte.
- Intravenous interventions (IV):
  - IV fluids are required when shock is suspected or confirmed and requires urgent hospital transfer.
  - when intravenous access cannot be established, intraosseous fluids may be required.
- Other treatments:
  - antibiotics, antidiarrhoeals and anti-emetics are not routinely used in the management of gastroenteritis.

Consider the outcome for the child identified by clinical assessment

- In those children who can be managed in the community:
  - fluid intake should be actively encouraged (e.g. milk, water, squash) – under-fives need approximately 10 ml of fluid every 10 minutes.
  - in infants, breastfeeding and other milk feeds should be continued.
  - in older children, fruit juices and fizzy drinks must be stopped.
  - ORS solutions should be offered to those at increased risk of dehydration as supplemental fluids, although toddlers and small children frequently refuse ORS because of the taste!
  - if oral intake is insufficient or if the child is persistently vomiting, they should be transferred to secondary care for NG or IV fluid replacement. (Inpatient management often includes a trial of ORS or NG fluids prior to IV fluid replacement.)
- Any child found to be **in shock** must be taken to hospital (refer to red flag system, ⚑ see Table 3.98). They will need additional fluids to not just **maintain** their normal body water but also to replace their fluid losses.
- **Clinically shocked** children require intravenous fluid resuscitation and urgent hospital transfer:
  - a rapid 20 ml/kg IV of infusion sodium chloride 0.9% may be given but should not delay hospital transfer.
  - clinical response to fluid boluses must be monitored.

- if shock persists, this infusion should be repeated and other causes of shock considered (refer to **Sodium Chloride 0.9%**).
- Stool samples are not normally required but should be obtained in certain situations:
  - Diarrhoea ≥7 days
  - Recent overseas travel
  - Possible septicaemia
  - Blood/mucus in stool
  - Immunocompromise
  - Persisting diagnostic uncertainty
  - Contact the GP or out-of-hours service where this is thought to be necessary.

See Figure 3.38 for a decision support tool.

6. Referral Pathway

Children with gastroenteritis that are not dehydrated or shocked can initially be managed at home; if their condition progresses, seek an additional medical opinion (GP, OOH, emergency department, paediatrician) (see 'Safety netting' below).

- Hospital transfer is required if:
  - Oral intake is insufficient.
  - The child is persistently vomiting.
  - A child is found to be clinically dehydrated.
  - A child is found to be clinically shocked (Emergency Transfer).
  - A child requires intravenous therapy.
  - Suspicion of an alternative cause for the child's symptoms, e.g. UTI, meningococcal disease.
  - Additionally, some children's social circumstances will dictate additional/continued involvement of healthcare professionals.
- Give the following advice for non-dehydrated children managed at home.

6.1 Nutritional considerations

- During rehydration:
  - Continue breastfeeding.
  - Give full-strength milk straight away.
  - Continue the child's usual solid food.
  - Avoid fruit juices and fizzy drinks until the diarrhoea has stopped.
  - Consider giving an extra 5 ml/kg of ORS solution after each large watery stool in children at increased risk of dehydration.
  - If dehydration recurs after rehydration, restart oral rehydration therapy.

'**Safety Netting**' should be provided for children who do not require referral, giving written information to parents and carers on how to:

- Recognise developing red flag symptoms (⚑ refer to Table 3.99), and get immediate help from an appropriate healthcare professional if

Paediatric Gastroenteritis

Child presenting with diarrhoea and vomiting. Assess using the traffic light system for clinical dehydration and shock

If all green features and no amber or red

No clinical dehydration

- Consider management on-scene.
- Follow up by arranging a review by an appropriate health care professional.
- Provide parents/carers with advice.

If any amber features and no red

Consider admission according to clinical and social need. If the child is under one year old, you must discuss the case with a GP or paediatric advice line where they exist. In all other cases, if unsure please contact a specialist Paramedic/Nurse, GP or Paediatric Advice Line where pathways exist

If any red features

Clinical shock suspected or confirmed

- Convey to nearest appropriate ED with ATMIST if indicated.
- Treatment based on clinical presentation.

Figure 3.38 – Decision support tool for the assessment of children with gastroenteritis.

red flag symptoms develop and, if necessary, make arrangements for follow-up at a specified time and place, that is face-to-face assessment.

Information and advice for parents and carers

Advise parents, carers and children that:

- good handwashing is essential to prevent the spread of gastroenteritis to themselves and other family members; use soap (liquid if possible) in warm, running water followed by careful drying.

- hands should be washed after going to the toilet (children) or changing nappies (parents/

carers) and before preparing, serving or eating food.

- infected children should not share towels.

- children should not go to school or other childcare facility while they have diarrhoea or vomiting caused by gastroenteritis and must stay away for at least 48 hours after the last episode of diarrhoea or vomiting.

- children should not swim in swimming pools for 2 weeks after the last episode of diarrhoea.

KEY POINTS!

Paediatric Gastroenteritis

- **Gastroenteritis is common, frequently viral and usually self-limiting.**

- **When severe, shock and life-threatening dehydration can occur.**

- **Clinical assessment determines whether dehydration or shock is present (seek Red Flag (🚩) symptoms and signs).**

- **Non-dehydrated children can frequently be managed at home with oral fluids or ORS.**

- **Failed oral rehydration requires either NG or IV fluid replacement in secondary care.**

- **Shocked children need urgent hospital treatment.**

- **Early meningococcal disease is known to mimic gastroenteritis in small children. An urgent second opinion should be sought if meningococcal disease cannot be excluded.**

- **Provide a 'safety net', with written information, for all children with gastroenteritis not transferred to hospital.**

- **If uncertain, seek advice from the child's GP, an out-of-hours doctor or specialist advice line where available.**

Paediatric Gastroenteritis

Bibliography

1. National Institute for Health and Clinical Excellence. *Diarrhoea and Vomiting in Children: Diarrhoea and vomiting caused by gastroenteritis: Diagnosis, assessment and management in children younger than 5 years* (CG84). Available from: https://www.nice.org.uk/guidance/cg84, 2009.

2. South Western Ambulance Service Trust. *Paediatric Gastroenteritis Clinical Guideline.* 2018.

3. Sandell JM, Charman SC. Can age-based estimates of weight be safely used when resuscitating children? *Emergency Medicine Journal* 2009, 26(1): 43–47.

4. Armon K, Stephenson T, MacFaul R, Eccleston P, Werneke U. An evidence and consensus based guideline for acute diarrhoea management. *Archives of Disease in Childhood* 2001, 85(2): 132–142.

5. Health Protection Agency. *Avoiding Infection on Farm Visits: Advice for the public.* 2011. Available from: http://www.hpa.org.uk/webc/HPAwebFile/HPAweb_C/1270122184581.

SECTION **3** Medical Emergencies

Pulmonary Embolism

1. Introduction

- Pulmonary embolism (PE) is an obstruction of the pulmonary vessels which usually presents as one of four types:

1 **Multiple small pulmonary emboli** – characterised by progressive breathlessness more commonly identified at outpatient appointments than through emergency presentation due to the long standing nature of the problem.

2 **Segmental emboli with pulmonary infarction** – may present with pleuritic pain and/or haemoptysis but with little or no cardiovascular compromise.

3 **Major pulmonary emboli obstruction of the larger branches of the pulmonary tree** – may present with sudden onset of shortness of breath with transient rise in pulse and/or fall in blood pressure. Often a precursor to a massive PE.

4 **Massive pulmonary emboli** – often presenting with loss of consciousness, tachypnoea and intense jugular vein distension, and may prove immediately or rapidly (within 1 hour) fatal or unresponsive to cardiopulmonary resuscitation.

- PE can present with a wide range of symptoms (refer to Table 3.100). The presence of predisposing factors (refer to Table 3.101) increases the index of suspicion of PE. However, in approximately 30% of cases, the presentation is idiopathic.

- Symptoms such as dyspnoea, tachypnoea or chest pain have been found in >90% of cases of patients with PE; pleuritic chest pain is one of the most frequent symptoms of presentation.

- There may be sudden collapse with no obvious physical signs, other than cardiorespiratory arrest.

- Lesser risk factors include air, coach or other travel leading to periods of immobility, especially whilst sitting, oral oestrogen (some contraceptive pills) and central venous catheterisation.

- Over 70% of patients who suffer PE have peripheral vein thrombosis and vigilance is therefore of great importance – it may not initially appear logical to check the legs of a patient with chest pain but can be of great diagnostic value in such cases.

TABLE 3.100 – Signs and Symptoms of PE

Symptoms

- Dyspnoea.
- Pleuritic chest pain.
- Substernal chest pain.
- Apprehension.
- Cough.
- Haemoptysis.
- Syncope.

Signs

- Respiratory rate >20 breaths per minute.
- Pulse rate >100 beats per minute.
- SpO_2 <92%.
- Signs of deep vein thrombosis (DVT).

TABLE 3.101 – Predisposing Factors

Factor

Surgery especially recent

- Abdominal.
- Pelvic.
- Hip or knee surgery.
- Post-operative intensive care.

Obstetrics

- Pregnancy.

Cardiac

- Recent acute myocardial infarction.

Limb problems

- Recent lower limb fractures.
- Varicose veins.
- Lower limb problems secondary to stroke or spinal cord injury.

Malignancy

- Abdominal and/or pelvic in particular advanced metastatic disease.
- Concurrent chemotherapy.

Other

- Risk increases with age.
- ≥60 years of age.
- Previous proven PE/DVT.
- Immobility.
- Thrombotic disorder.
- Neurological disease with extremity paresis.
- Thrombophilia.
- Hormone replacement therapy and oral contraception.
- Prolonged bed rest >3 days.
- Other recent trauma.

Pulmonary Embolism

2. Incidence

- PE is a relatively common cardiovascular condition affecting approximately 21 per 10,000 per annum.

3. Severity and Outcome

- PE can be life-threatening leading to death in approximately 7–11% of cases; however, treatment is effective if given early.
- Patients with a previous episode(s) of PE are three times more likely to experience a recurrence.

4. Pathophysiology

- The development of a PE occurs when a blood clot (thrombus), comprising red cells, platelets and fibrin, forms in a vein, subsequently dislodges (embolism) and travels in the circulation. This is known as venous thromboembolism (VTE). If the embolism is small it may be filtered in the pulmonary capillary bed, but if the embolism is large it may occlude pulmonary blood vessels. The development of a VTE can also lead to DVT.
- The haemodynamic problems occur when >30–50% of the pulmonary arterial bed is occluded.
- The probability of a PE can be assessed using a clinical predication tool such as the Wells Criteria (refer to Table 3.102). However, a low probability cannot rule out PE.

TABLE 3.102 – Wells Criteria for PE

Item	Score
Clinical signs and symptoms of DVT (leg swelling and pain with palpation of the deep veins).	3
An alternative diagnosis is less likely than PE.	3
Pulse rate >100 beats per minute.	1.5
Immobilisation or surgery in the previous 4 weeks.	1.5
Previous DVT/PE.	1.5
Haemoptysys.	1
Malignancy (treatment ongoing or within previous 6 months or palliative).	1

Clinical Probability of PE		Total
High	>6 points	
Moderate	2–6 points	
Low	<2 points	

5. Assessment and Management

For the assessment and management of PE, refer to Table 3.103 and Figure 3.39.

TABLE 3.103 – ASSESSMENT and MANAGEMENT of: Pulmonary Embolism

Assess <C>ABCD

- If any of the following **TIME-CRITICAL** features are present:
  - major **<C>ABCD** problems
  - extreme breathing difficulty
  - cyanosis
  - severe hypoxia (SpO$_2$) <90% – unresponsive to oxygen.
- Start correcting any **<C>ABCD** problems.
- Undertake a **TIME-CRITICAL** transfer to nearest appropriate receiving hospital.
- Continue patient management en-route.
- Provide an ATMIST information call.

Specifically Assess

- Respiratory rate and effort.
- Signs and symptoms combined with predisposing factors.
- Lower limbs for unilateral swelling; may also be warm and red.
- Calf tenderness/pain may be present – extensive leg clots may also lead to femoral tenderness.
- Differential diagnoses include pleurisy, pneumothorax or cardiac chest pain.

Position

- Position patient for comfort and ease of respiration – often sitting forwards – but be aware of potential hypotension.

Respiratory Rate

- Measure and record respiratory rate.

(continued)

Pulmonary Embolism

TABLE 3.103 – ASSESSMENT and MANAGEMENT of: Pulmonary Embolism *(continued)*
Oxygen Saturation
◽ Monitor the patient's SpO$_2$; administer oxygen to achieve saturations of >94% if the patient presents as hypoxaemic on air (refer to **Oxygen**).
Ventilation
◽ Consider assisted ventilation if indicated (refer to **Airway and Breathing Management**).
Pulse
◽ Measure and record pulse.
Blood Pressure and Fluids
◽ Measure and record blood pressure; if required, administer fluids (refer to **Intravascular Fluid Therapy in Adults** and **Intravascular Fluid Therapy in Children**).
Blood Glucose
◽ If appropriate, measure and record blood glucose for hypo/hyperglycaemia (refer to **Glycaemic Emergencies in Adults and Children**).
Temperature
◽ Measure and record temperature.
NEWS2
◽ These observations will enable you to calculate a NEWS2 score (refer to **Sepsis**).
ECG
◽ Monitor and record 12-lead ECG – be aware that the classic S1 Q3 T3 12-lead ECG presentation is often NOT present, even during massive PE. The most common finding is a sinus tachycardia (refer to **Cardiac Rhythm Disturbance**).
Assess the Patient's Pain
◽ Where present, assess the **SOCRATES** of pain and record initial and subsequent pain scores.
◽ Consider analgesia if appropriate (refer to **Pain Management in Adults** and **Pain Management in Children**).
Documentation
◽ Complete documentation to include all clinical findings, advice from other clinicians, onward referral and worsening advice given.
Transfer to Further Care
◽ Transfer rapidly to nearest appropriate hospital.
◽ Provide an alert/information call.
◽ Continue patient management en-route.
ADDITIONAL INFORMATION
Whilst there is no specific pre-hospital treatment available, there may be a window of opportunity to manage massive PE before the patient progresses to cardiac arrest. Other in-hospital treatments may be effective, including: haemodynamic and respiratory support, thrombolysis, surgical pulmonary embolectomy, percutaneous catheter embolectomy and fragmentation and anticoagulation.

Pulmonary Embolism

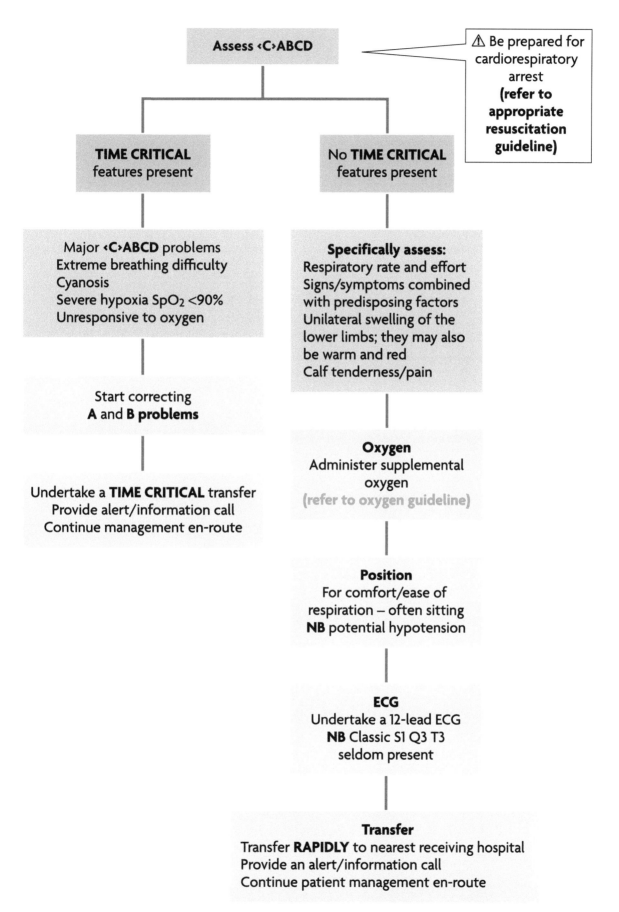

Figure 3.39 — Assessment and management algorithm of pulmonary embolism.

Pulmonary Embolism

Pulmonary Embolism

- Common symptoms of PE are dyspnoea, tachypnoea, pleuritic pain, apprehension, tachycardia, cough, haemoptysis and leg pain/clinical DVT.

- Risk factors may be identifiable from the history.

- Ensure ABCD assessment and apply a pulse oximetry monitor early.

- Patients may present with unilateral swelling of the lower limbs; they may also be warm and red.

- Apply oxygen and if in respiratory distress, transfer to further care as a medical emergency.

Bibliography

1. Soar J, Perkins GD, Abbas G, Alfonzo A, Barelli A, Bierens JJLM, et al. European Resuscitation Council Guidelines for Resuscitation 2010 Section 8: cardiac arrest in special circumstances: electrolyte abnormalities, poisoning, drowning, accidental hypothermia, hyperthermia, asthma, anaphylaxis, cardiac surgery, trauma, pregnancy, electrocution. *Resuscitation* 2010, 81(10): 1400–1433.

2. National Institute for Health and Clinical Excellence. *Venous Thromboembolism: Reducing the risk. Reducing the risk of venous thromboembolism (deep vein thrombosis and pulmonary embolism) in patients admitted to hospital* (CG 92). London: NICE, 2010. Available from: https://www.nice.org.uk/guidance/cg92.

3. Torbicki A, Perrier A, Konstantinides S, Agnelli G, Galie N, Pruszczyk P, et al. Guidelines on the diagnosis and management of acute pulmonary embolism. *European Heart Journal* 2008, 29(18): 2276–315.

4. Wells PS, Anderson DR, Rodger M, Ginsberg JS, Kearon C, Gent M. Derivation of a simple clinical model to categorize patients' probability of pulmonary embolism: increasing the models utility with the SimpliRED D-dimer. *Thrombosis and Haemostasis* 2000, 83: 416–420.

5. Cohen AT, Agnelli G, Anderson FA, Arcelus JI, Bergqvist D, Brecht JG, et al. Venous thromboembolism (VTE) in Europe: the number of VTE events and associated morbidity and mortality. *Thrombosis and Haemostasis* 2007, 98(4): 756–764.

6. Farmer RDT, Lawrenson RA, Todd JC, Williams TJ, MacRae KD, Tyrer F, et al. A comparison of the risks of venous thromboembolic disease in association with different combined oral contraceptives. *British Journal of Clinical Pharmacology* 2000, 49(6): 580–590.

7. Goldhaber SZ, Morrison RB. Pulmonary embolism and deep vein thrombosis. *Circulation* 2002, 106(12): 1436–1438.

8. Meyer G, Roy P-M, Gilberg S, Perrier A. Pulmonary embolism. *British Medical Journal* 2010, 340: c1421.

9. White RH. The epidemiology of venous thromboembolism. *Circulation* 2003, 107: I-4–8.

10. Wolf SJ, McCubbin T, Feldhaus KM, Faragher JP, Adcock DM. Prospective validation of Wells Criteria in the evaluation of patients with suspected pulmonary embolism. *Annals of Emergency Medicine* 2004, 44(5): 503–510.

SECTION **3** Medical Emergencies

Respiratory Illness in Children

1. Introduction

- Children should not be viewed simply as 'little adults'. The assessment and management of paediatric patients may include potential pitfalls for the unwary and inexperienced and present healthcare providers with significant challenges wherever the setting.

- There are many important differences between children and adults in their anatomy, their physiology and their immunity. There may also be differences in the types of illnesses they encounter, as well as the ways in which these conditions present, develop and progress.

- Children may have difficulties verbalising and communicating their condition, presenting an additional challenge to clinicians.

1.1 'Major' and 'Minor' Illnesses

- Before considering 'minor' illnesses in children, it is crucial to both appreciate and understand that 'major' childhood illnesses (including life-threatening conditions such as meningococcal disease) rarely present in extremis, but more commonly present with relatively innocent features that can easily be mistaken for minor illnesses.

- Children with advanced major illness (or significant injury) typically have deranged vital signs that are usually readily detected. Earlier in their illness, these children may well have had normal physiology and appeared relatively well. If they were assessed early in their illness, there is a risk they might be misdiagnosed with only a minor illness.

This guideline on childhood respiratory illnesses includes:

1 Asthma.

2 Bronchiolitis.

3 Croup.

4 URTIs (tonsillitis, otitis media).

5 Pneumonia.

For the management of mild, moderate, severe and life-threatening asthma, refer to **Asthma in Adults and Children**.

Asthma is rare in very young children (under 1 year), and other causes of wheeze (such as bronchiolitis or viral-induced wheeze) should be considered.

2. Bronchiolitis

2.1 Introduction

Bronchiolitis is an acute, self-limiting respiratory infection that is usually caused by respiratory syncytial virus (RSV) and occurs predominantly in the autumn and winter months. It is characterised by inflammation of the bronchioles.

It is more prevalent during the winter months, peaking over a 6–8 week period, and is the most common lower respiratory tract infection during the first year of life.

Most children will recover without intervention. However, some may have difficulty breathing and need more input, especially very young babies.

2.2 Assessment

Bronchiolitis is commonly preceded by coryzal prodrome (upper respiratory infection, characterised by a non-specific cough, rhinorrhea and fever) for 1 to 3 days.

- Clinical presentation: a coryzal baby (peak age 2–5 months) with their first wheezy episode.

- Irregular breathing and apnoeas are frequently reported.

- During the first 72 hours, bronchiolitic infants may deteriorate clinically, before symptomatic improvements are seen.

- The baby's parents and siblings often have concurrent respiratory illnesses and may report sore throats or dry coughs.

Signs and Symptoms
↓Oxygen saturations
↑Respiratory rate
Recession
Fine, bilateral inspiratory crackles
High-pitched expiratory wheezes
Low-grade fever
Rhinorrhoea (runny nose)
Cough
Poor feeding
Vomiting
Pyrexia
Apnoea
Cyanosis

- Consider bronchiolitis as the provisional diagnosis if **all** of the following symptoms are present:
  - persistent cough
  - either tachypnoea or chest recession (or both)
  - either wheeze or crackles on chest auscultation (or both).

- When diagnosing bronchiolitis, take into account that the following symptoms are common in children with this disease:
  - fever (in around 30% of cases, usually of less than 39°C)
  - poor feeding (typically after 3 to 5 days of illness)

Respiratory Illness in Children

– young infants may present with apnoea without other clinical signs.

■ **NB** Consider a diagnosis of pneumonia if the child has high fever (over 39°C) and/or persistently focal crackles.

2.3 Management

■ Give oxygen supplementation to children with bronchiolitis if their oxygen saturation is persistently less than 94%.

■ Treatments aim to provide respiratory support and support feeding/hydration.

■ Antivirals, antibiotics, steroids, nebulisers, physiotherapy, steam treatments, nasal decongestants, homeopathy and complementary therapies have not been shown to be effective.

■ Acute bronchiolitis lasts approximately 2 weeks from its onset, but can last up to 4 weeks.

■ Ongoing cough and persisting wheeze are not uncommon after the initial illness has passed but should prompt further medical assessment.

■ Generally, management of bronchiolitis will be conservative, with oxygen being the only drug administered in the pre-hospital environment. In most cases, medication is not needed to manage bronchiolitis because it is usually self-limiting (i.e. it settles without the need for treatment).

■ Helping parents and carers to understand this can increase their confidence in caring for their child at home. It can also help them understand why medicines are not being administered en-route to hospital.

■ Clinicians should be aware of the increased need for hospital admission in infants fulfilling the following criteria:
– pre-existing lung disease, congenital heart disease, neuromuscular weakness, immunodeficiency
– aged under 3 months
– prematurity
– family anxiety
– re-attendance or re-contact for the same presentation
– duration of illness is less than 3 days.

■ Preterm babies, those with chronic lung disease, children with congenital heart disease, cystic fibrosis, congenital or acquired immune deficiency (HIV) and those either aged <2 months or having apnoeas are at highest risk and must be transferred to further care.

■ Previously well babies with diminished feeding, irregular breathing, hypoxia (O_2 saturations <94% on air), tachypnoea or tachycardia should also be transferred to further care where they will receive respiratory support and help with feeding/hydration.

■ If the patient is managed on scene, robust safety-netting advice should be provided on how to recognise developing red flag symptoms such as:
– worsening work of breathing such as grunting, nasal flaring, marked chest recession
– fluid intake is 50–75% of normal or no wet nappy for 12 hours
– apnoea or cyanosis
– exhaustion (e.g. not responding normally to social cues; wakes only with prolonged stimulation).

■ Safety-netting advice should also include:
– advice that people should not smoke in the child's home because it increases the risk of more severe symptoms in bronchiolitis
– instructions on how to get immediate help from an appropriate professional should any red flag symptoms develop.

■ Salbutamol is not indicated in bronchiolitis. It will not benefit the condition, and the resultant tachycardia may confuse subsequent clinical assessment in hospital.

3. Croup

3.1 Introduction

■ Croup is a common, acute, respiratory illness of gradual onset, characterised by stridor that typically is mild and self-limiting.

■ Viral infections can spread to the larynx and trachea, causing inflammation and therefore compromise of the airway in severe cases.

■ Croup is less common in older children, who are more likely to have epiglottitis, a more serious condition, and need to be admitted.

3.2 Incidence

■ Croup mostly affects children between the ages of 6 months and 3 years, presenting most commonly in the second year of life.[11] However, children up to 15 years of age may be affected.

■ It can occur all year round but peaks are seen in both spring and autumn.

3.3 Pathophysiology

■ Croup results from viral infections, most commonly parainfluenza, but also RSV, influenza A and B, as well as *Mycoplasma pneumoniae*.

■ Stridor, hoarseness and a barking 'seal-like' cough result from inflammation and narrowing around the subglottic region of the larynx. (This is the narrowest point of the paediatric airway).

NB Stridor is also seen in epiglottitis, bacterial tracheitis, retropharyngeal abscesses, foreign-body ingestion, anaphylaxis and angio-oedema, blunt trauma, glandular fever, hot gases inhalation and

Respiratory Illness in Children

diphtheria – all children with any of these conditions should be transferred to further care.

3.4 Assessment

▪ Croup commonly has a gradual onset. Initial symptoms include a mild fever and a runny nose. This progresses to a sore throat and a barking cough, typical of the condition. Young children have smaller air passages and inflammation in the voice box leads to a narrowing of the gap between the vocal cords.

▪ Croup develops over a period of 1 or 2 days; the severity varies over that period but it is normally worse on the second night of the cough.

▪ Stridor associated with croup can also be caused by other conditions. Clinicians should consider differential diagnoses, such as:
 – epiglottitis
 – bacterial tracheitis
 – foreign bodies
 – anaphylaxis
 – angio-oedema
 – glandular fever
 – blunt trauma
 – retropharyngeal abscesses
 – inhalation of hot gases
 – diphtheria.

▪ All children with these conditions should be transferred to further care.

▪ The child with croup may have mild clinical features in keeping with a simple, upper respiratory tract infection, although they can present with more worrying features including respiratory distress, respiratory failure and respiratory arrest.

▪ The features of respiratory distress – increased respiration rate, increased work of breathing, recession, nasal flaring, grunting, use of accessory muscles and stridor – are described in **Medical Emergencies in Children – Overview**.

3.5 Management

▪ Keep the child in a position of comfort, sat upright and supported on a parent's lap – children often 'know' how to maintain their own airways in an optimal position (they often adopt a so-called 'tripod' posture).

▪ A calm approach is to be encouraged at all times. Any intervention likely to upset the child – examining their ears, nose or throat, blood sugar measurement, cannulation and even nebulisation (see below) – must be avoided, as distressing procedures can precipitate acute deterioration and complete airway obstruction. This is of particular importance in the pre-hospital environment where skills for expert airway intervention are not readily available.

Steroids are the mainstay of treatment – usually oral dexamethasone (nebulised budesonide may be used as an alternative but may distress the child, adversely worsening their symptoms) – and work by relieving subglottic inflammation.

▪ Children with mild, moderate or severe croup may benefit from early steroid treatment.

▪ Oral dexamethasone (refer to **Dexamethasone**) is preferred to nebulised budesonide, as nebulisation frequently distresses small children, producing further airway narrowing.

3.6 Referral Pathway

As above, irrespective of whether steroids are given, all children with stridor must still be transferred to further care for subsequent observation, even if clinical improvements are noted at home.

▪ All children under the age of two with croup must be conveyed to hospital

▪ All children with a respiratory rate above 40 breaths/min with croup must be conveyed to hospital.

If the patient is to be discharged on scene, it is important to give parents/guardians appropriate advice:

▪ Explain that croup is self-limiting and that symptoms usually resolve within 48 hours, although occasionally they may last for up to a week. Resolution of croup symptoms is usually followed by symptoms of upper respiratory tract infection.

▪ Advise the use of paracetamol or ibuprofen to control fever and pain/distress.
 – do not over- or under-dress a child with fever
 – tepid sponging is not recommended
 – do not routinely give antipyretic drugs to a child with fever with the sole aim of reducing body temperature.

▪ Explain that cough medicines, decongestants and short-acting beta-agonists are not effective. Croup is usually a viral illness and antibiotics are not needed.

▪ Ensure an adequate fluid intake.

▪ Do not advise humidified air (e.g. steam inhalation).

▪ Arrange for a clinician to review the child within a few hours, either by face-to-face consultation or by telephone. Advise parents to seek urgent medical advice if:
 – There is progression from mild to moderate airways obstruction, such as development of intermittent stridor at rest or increased effort of breathing (chest and suprasternal in-drawing), as the child may need to be observed in hospital.
 – If the child becomes toxic (pale, very high fever, tachycardic) as this may mean the child has an

Respiratory Illness in Children

alternative diagnosis (e.g. bacterial tracheitis or epiglottitis).

- Advise the parents to call 999 or take the patient immediately to the emergency department (ED) if the child:
  - Becomes cyanosed.
  - Is unusually sleepy.
  - Is struggling to breathe and cannot be calmed down quickly.
  - Is restless, agitated or upset.
  - Or if stridor can be heard continually and recession is seen (the skin between the ribs is pulling in with every breath).
  - Is very pale, blue or grey (includes blue lips) for more than a few seconds.
  - Is not responding.
  - Is having a lot of trouble breathing (e.g. the belly is sinking in while breathing, or the skin between the ribs or over the windpipe is pulling in with each breath; the nostrils may also be flaring in and out).
  - Wants to sit instead of lie down.
  - Cannot talk.
  - Is drooling.
  - Is having trouble swallowing.

Ensure that there is a communication to the patient's registered GP to inform them about the episode, the outcomes reached and any treatment given.

4. Upper Respiratory Tract Infections (URTIs), e.g. Tonsillitis (Sore Throat, Acute Pharyngitis, Acute Exudative Tonsillitis), Otitis Media, etc.

4.1 Introduction

Upper respiratory tract infections (URTIs) are one of the commonest reasons for paediatric presentation, especially during the winter months.

4.2 Incidence

25% of all under five year olds will see their GPs each year for tonsillitis.

4.3 Assessment

- Children with URTIs frequently complain of:
  - sore throat
  - cough
  - fever
  - headache
  - earache
  - systemic illness
  - anorexia and lethargy.
- Physical examination may reveal:
  - cervical lymphadenopathy
  - offensive breath

- inflamed, purulent tonsils.

Breathing may also be compromised by either stridor or respiratory distress. In these circumstances, avoid attempts to examine the throat (see croup guidance above) and transfer urgently to further care.

The child's hydration status should be estimated, as fluid intake can be significantly decreased.

4.4 Management

URTIs are usually self-limiting. Parents should be offered simple advice about managing their child's symptoms (rest, extra fluids, analgesia, antipyretics etc.) and informed about the likely duration of their child's illness (refer to Table 3.104).

Antibiotics are not prescribed routinely. Most URTIs are viral and do not respond to antibiotics. Bacteria (e.g. streptococci) also cause URTIs but even in these cases antibiotics are rarely needed; they don't improve the child's symptoms and they can often cause diarrhoea, vomiting and rashes.

TABLE 3.104 – Typical Duration of Acute Respiratory Illnesses

Condition	Duration
Acute otitis media	4 days
Acute sore throat/ pharyngitis/tonsillitis	1 week
Common cold	1½ weeks
Acute rhinosinusitis	2½ weeks
Acute cough/bronchitis	3 weeks

GPs tend to use one of three antibiotic strategies:

1. No antibiotics are needed where the URTI is thought likely to be self-limiting.
2. Delayed antibiotics are useful when symptoms fail to improve or worsen.
3. Immediate antibiotic prescriptions are reserved for the most severe cases, including:
   - Under twos with acute bilateral otitis media.
   - Children with acute otitis media and otorrhoea (ear discharge).
   - Children with acute streptococcal URTIs (no cough but fever, pustular tonsils and tender lymph nodes).

Antibiotics are also prescribed for children who are:
   - Systemically very unwell.
   - At high risk of serious complications because of pre-existing illnesses (heart, lung, renal, liver or neuromuscular disease, diabetes, cystic fibrosis, prematurity, immunosuppression or previous hospitalisations).

Over-the-counter cough and cold preparations often contain sedatives and antihistamines

Respiratory Illness in Children

that are dangerous if taken accidentally by small children in overdose. As a result, these medicines are no longer available for children aged two years or under. Children in this age group with colds and fever should now only be offered paracetamol or ibuprofen to manage their temperature, if needed.

Simple cough syrups containing glycerol, and honey and lemon may still be given, as well as vapour rubs and inhalant decongestants (see individual labelling).

4.5 Referral Pathway

Hospital admission may also be indicated when:

- There is diminished fluid intake (e.g. young child with severe tonsillitis or teenager with glandular fever).

- Where concerns regarding the diagnosis persist (**NB** early meningococcal disease is frequently misdiagnosed as an URTI in small children – where this diagnosis cannot be excluded, arrangements for an urgent medical opinion should be made). Refer to **Febrile Illness in Children**.

- Children with 'muffled' voices – they sound as if they have something hot in their mouths. These children must be transferred to further care to exclude quinsy (peritonsillar abscess).

- Tenderness behind the ear (over their mastoid process) in a child with otitis media, whose ear may or may not be starting to 'stick out', suggests mastoiditis (a dangerous infection of the bone around the ear) and must be transferred to further care.

4.6 Management in the Community

As when managing the febrile child, if a decision not to transfer a child to further care has been reached,

a clinically justifiable reason should be present and properly documented. Refer to **Febrile Illness in Children**.

'Safety netting', with written advice, should again be encouraged and follow-up arrangements should be provided.

Where doubts persist, seek senior advice or review.

5. Pneumonia (Lower Respiratory Tract Infections, 'Chest Infections')

Children with pneumonia are likely to have the following signs and symptoms:

- Fever.
- Cough.
- Tachypnoea.
  - RR > 60 breaths/min, age 0–5 months
  - RR > 50 breaths/min, age 6–12 months
  - RR > 40 breaths/min, age > 12 months
- Nasal flaring.
- Chest indrawing.
- Oxygen saturations <95%.
- Crackles in the chest.
- Cyanosis.

Such children are likely to require antibiotics and additional oxygen and should be seen by either their GP or a paediatrician.

Table 3.105 indicates severity of disease by age of the patient. This should be used to determine whether urgent referral in the community is appropriate or transfer to the Emergency Department. Children with severe symptoms (oxygen saturations <92% or where auscultation demonstrates absent breath sounds or percussion presents as dull) should be transferred to the Emergency Department.

Respiratory Illness in Children

TABLE 3.105 – Severity Assessment

	Mild to moderate	Severe
Infants	Temperature <38.5°C Respiratory rate <50 breaths/min Mild recession Taking full feeds	Temperature >38.5°C Respiratory rate >70 breaths/min Moderate to severe recession Nasal flaring Cyanosis Intermittent apnoea Grunting respiration Not feeding Tachycardia* Capillary refill time ≥2s
Older children	Temperature <38.5°C Respiratory rate <50 breaths/min Mild breathlessness No vomiting	Temperature >38.5°C Respiratory rate >50 breaths/min Severe difficulty in breathing Nasal flaring Cyanosis Grunting respiration Signs of dehydration Tachycardia* Capillary refill time ≥2s

* Values to define tachycardia vary with age and with temperature how to present the citation.

KEY POINTS!

Respiratory Illness in Children

- Childhood respiratory illnesses are common and usually self-limiting.
- Antibiotics are rarely indicated.
- Children with underlying conditions (e.g. prematurity, chronic lung disease, congenital heart disease, cystic fibrosis, congenital or acquired immune deficiency (HIV), cerebral palsy) are especially vulnerable and must be seen either by their GP or a paediatrician in hospital.
- Tachypnoea is a feature in all respiratory illnesses.
- Respiratory distress causes increased respiratory rate, increased work of breathing, recession, nasal flaring, grunting, use of accessory muscles and stridor.
- Exhaustion suggests respiratory failure and respiratory arrest may rapidly follow.
- Stridor can progress rapidly to complete upper airway obstruction and respiratory arrest.
- Approach a child with stridor calmly and gently. Sit them upright in a position of comfort and avoid painful/distressing procedures.
- Transfer all children with stridor for further medical assessment and observation.
- Steroids (dexamethasone) are frequently used to treat croup.
- Children with pneumonia require antibiotics and possibly oxygen therapy. They should be seen by either their GP or a paediatrician.
- Whilst URTIs are very common, early meningococcal disease can easily be misdiagnosed as an URTI. (When unable to exclude this diagnosis, make arrangements for an urgent second opinion.)
- Provide a 'safety net' (with written information) for all children with respiratory illness not transferred to hospital.
- If uncertain, seek advice from either the child's GP or the out-of-hours doctor.
- Asthma is rare in very young children (under 1 year), and other causes of wheeze (such as bronchiolitis or viral-induced wheeze) should be considered.

Respiratory Illness in Children

Bibliography

1. Godden CW, Campbell MJ, Hussey M, Cogswell JJ. Double blind placebo controlled trial of nebulised budesonide for croup. *Archives of Disease in Childhood* 1997, 76(2): 155–158.

2. Russell KF, Liang Y, O'Gorman K, Johnson DW, Klassen TP. Glucocorticoids for croup. *Cochrane Database of Systematic Reviews* 2011(1): CD001955.

3. Scottish Intercollegiate Guidelines Network. *Management of Sore Throat and Indications for Tonsillectomy* (Guideline 117). Edinburgh: SIGN, 2010. Available from: https://www.sign.ac.uk/sign-117-management-of-sore-throat-and-indications-for-tonsillectomy.html.

4. Sparrow A, Geelhoed G. Prednisolone versus dexamethasone in croup: a randomised equivalence trial. *Archives of Disease in Childhood* 2006, 91(7): 580–583.

5. Baumer JH. Glucocorticoid treatment in croup. *Archives of Disease in Childhood Education and Practice Edition* 2006, 91(2): ep58–60.

6. Sandell JM, Charman SC. Can age-based estimates of weight be safely used when resuscitating children? *Emergency Medicine Journal* 2009, 26(1): 43–47.

7. Taussig LM, Castro O, Beaudry PH, Fox WW, Bureau M. Treatment of laryngotracheobronchitis (croup): use of intermittent positive-pressure breathing and racemic epinephrine. *American Journal of Diseases of Children* 1975, 129(7): 790–793.

8. Centre for Clinical Practice at the National Institute for Health and Clinical Excellence. *Acutely Ill Patients in Hospital: Recognition of and response to acute illness in adults in hospital* (CG50). London: NICE, 2007. Available from: https://www.nice.org.uk/guidance/cg50.

9. National Institute for Health and Clinical Excellence. *Respiratory Tract Infections – Antibiotic Prescribing: Prescribing of antibiotics for self-limiting respiratory tract infections in adults and children in primary care* (CG 69). London: NICE, 2008. Available from: https://www.nice.org.uk/guidance/cg69.

10. National Institute for Health and Care Excellence. *Bronchiolitis in Children: Diagnosis and management*. 2015. Available from: https://www.nice.org.uk/guidance/ng9.

11. National Institute for Health and Clinical Excellence. *Croup. NICE Clinical Knowledge Summaries* London: NICE, 2012. Available from: https://cks.nice.org.uk.

SECTION **3** Medical Emergencies

Sepsis

1. Introduction

1.1 Terminology

- Suspected sepsis is not a specific illness but rather a syndrome encompassing a pathophysiology of which understanding is changing on a yearly basis. It is identified by a constellation of clinical signs and symptoms in a sick patient with an infection.

- The final diagnosis of sepsis is usually only confirmed at the end of an admission, when all the evidence becomes available.

- National Early Warning Scores (NEWS) are the best physiological scoring system for assessing sepsis and all causes of deterioration.

- A NEWS2 score greater than or equal to 5 highlights a sick patient who needs urgent clinical review; it does not represent a diagnosis, only a patient at significant risk.

1.2 Clinical Judgement

- Clinical judgement in determining what is or is not suspected sepsis is critical.

- Clinicians can rule out suspected sepsis in mimic conditions (e.g. asthma, diabetic ketoacidosis, mental health crisis), and rule in suspected sepsis when they are concerned.

- Over 70% of cases arise in the community, and ambulance clinicians are often the first point of contact for these patients.

- If left untreated, sepsis can lead to shock, multi-organ failure and death.

- Ambulance clinicians can help improve the outcomes by recognising sepsis early and providing a pre-alert and time-critical transfer to the emergency department (ED). Management should include (if indicated) high-flow oxygen, fluid resuscitation and benzylpenicillin if meningitis or meningococcal septicaemia is suspected.

- **Suspect sepsis in:**
  - anyone that presents with fever/feeling unwell
  - **and** NEWS2 greater than or equal to 5
  - **and/or** looks unwell with a history of infection.

2. Sepsis Definitions

2.1 Surviving Sepsis Campaign (2016)

- Sepsis is defined as life-threatening organ dysfunction caused by a dysregulated host response to infection.[1]

2.2 NICE (2016)

- Sepsis is a clinical syndrome caused by the body's immune and coagulation systems being switched on by an infection. Sepsis with shock is a life-threatening condition that is characterised by low blood pressure despite adequate fluid replacement, and organ dysfunction or failure.

3. Incidence

- There are an estimated 150,000 cases of sepsis each year in the UK, with approximately 44,000 deaths attributed to sepsis. Half of ED sepsis patients arrive by ambulance.[2,3] Sepsis patients arriving at the ED by ambulance are 'sicker' than patients arriving by other means.[4,5,6] Of patients admitted to ITU from the ED, 80–90% will have arrived by ambulance.[7,8]

4. Severity and Outcome

- Sepsis has a high mortality rate and this can be as high as 50% in some patients.[9]

- Sepsis cases are responsible for 27% of all intensive care unit beds in England and Wales, and cost the NHS an estimated £2.5 billion per year.[10]

- Having a high index of suspicion, early recognition and rapid transport to hospital ensures early treatment with antibiotics and access to expert-led care.

- Survivors can suffer from long-term physical and psychological problems, resulting in significantly reduced quality of life.[1]

- Each hour of delay in giving antibiotics to a patient with septic shock has an increased mortality rate of 7.6%.[11] Treatment within 1 hour is considered best practice.

5. Pathophysiology

Sepsis is a multifaceted host response to the invasion of normally sterile tissue by pathogenic, or potentially pathogenic, micro-organisms.[1,12,13] The clinical manifestations of sepsis are highly variable between individuals due to age, underlying comorbidities, the causative pathogen and medications.[1,14] Small amounts of cytokines are released into the circulation, leading to recruitment of inflammatory cells and an acute-phase response normally limited by anti-inflammatory mediators. In sepsis, there is a failure to control the inflammatory cascade, leading to a loss of capillary integrity, maldistribution of microvascular blood flow and stimulation of nitric oxide production, all leading towards organ injury and dysfunction.[12,13]

6. Risk Factors for Sepsis

The following groups of patients are at higher risk of developing sepsis:

- The very young (under 1 year) and older people (over 75 years) or people who are very frail.

- People who have impaired immune systems because of illness or drugs, including those:
  - being treated for cancer with chemotherapy (refer to Section 7 below on Neutropaenic Sepsis)
  - who have impaired immune function (for example, people with diabetes, people who

Sepsis

have had a splenectomy or people with sickle cell disease)
- taking long-term steroids
- taking immunosuppressant drugs to treat non-malignant disorders, such as rheumatoid arthritis.

- People who have had surgery, or other invasive procedures, in the past 6 weeks.

- People with any breach of skin integrity (for example, cuts, burns, blisters or skin infections).

- People who misuse drugs intravenously.

- People with indwelling lines or catheters.

- Pregnant women (refer to Section 8 below on Women and Pregnancy).

Take into account the following risk factors for sepsis in a newborn baby:

- History of maternal fever during labour or in the 24 hours before and after birth or maternal treatment with intravenous antibiotics for suspected infection.

- History of previous baby with sepsis during the newborn period.

- History of ruptured membranes before labour.

- Preterm birth following spontaneous labour (before 37 weeks' gestation).

- Suspected or confirmed sepsis in another baby in the case of a multiple pregnancy.

- Mother with suspected/confirmed sepsis in the puerperium (up to 6 weeks after birth).

7. Neutropaenic Sepsis

- Neutropaenic sepsis is a potentially fatal complication of cancer treatments, such as chemotherapy. Mortality rates as high as 21% have been reported in adults.[15] Patients can have neutropaenia as a result of the cancer therapy, which increases their risk of developing severe infections. Cancer patients can become neutropaenic and not develop severe infections or sepsis. If a patient is neutropaenic and not showing signs of infection but is unwell, this should be taken seriously. Many patients develop this serious complication; therefore, always suspect neutropaenic sepsis in patients having cancer treatment who become unwell.

- Patients may have been given an advice line number to ring by their oncology service. Consider ringing advice lines such as this in line with your local procedures, as it may inform the appropriate destination or care pathway for the patient.

- Any of the following features could indicate that a neutropaenic patient has an infection and is at risk of sepsis:
  - tachypnoea
  - tachycardia

- hypotension
- temperature greater than 37.5°C
- pleuritic chest pain
- shivering episodes
- flu-like symptoms
- catheter site infections.

- Note that neutropaenic patients are unable to produce the pus normally associated with skin infections.

- A neutropaenic patient at risk of sepsis can look deceptively well and can deteriorate rapidly. A high index of suspicion is necessary, particularly if a patient who has recently undergone chemotherapy has an increased temperature. Patients who have received treatment within 6–8 weeks are at risk and at higher risk within the first 10 days after treatment.

- Neutropaenic sepsis is a medical emergency and all patients should be transported to the nearest emergency department or locally agreed pathway (oncology) with a hospital pre-alert.

8. Women and Pregnancy

- Have a very high index of suspicion for pregnant women who are unwell and have signs of infection.

- Take into account that women who are pregnant, have given birth or had a termination of pregnancy or miscarriage in the past 6 weeks are in a high-risk group for sepsis.[10] In particular, women who:
  - have impaired immune systems because of illness or drugs
  - have gestational diabetes, diabetes or other comorbidities
  - needed invasive procedures (for example, caesarean section, forceps delivery, removal of retained products of conception)
  - had prolonged rupture of membranes
  - have or have been in close contact with people with group A streptococcal infection, for example scarlet fever
  - have continued vaginal bleeding or an offensive vaginal discharge.

- Note that the baseline heart rate in pregnancy is 10–15 beats per minute more than normal and there may be a decrease in systolic and diastolic blood pressure by an average of 10–15 mmHg. Therefore, this should be taken into account when considering sepsis, and rapid transport to definitive care is the priority and not extended on-scene times.

- These physiological changes in pregnancy can mask signs of significant sepsis and shock, and so can also 'render the existing NEWS2 inappropriate because the physiological response to acute illness can be modified in children and by pregnancy'.[16] Therefore, a strong

Sepsis

index of suspicion must be maintained and transfer to hospital considered when underlying sepsis is suspected during or after pregnancy, but a **NEWS2 score should NOT be used for pregnant women** (or children under 16 years).

- Refer to **Maternity Care** for other changes in pregnancy.

9. Assessment

- Assess **ABCD** (refer to **Medical Emergencies in Adults – Overview** and **Medical Emergencies in Children – Overview**).

- Take extra care if the patient cannot provide a reliable history.

- Consider sepsis in all patients with non-specific, non-localised presentations, for example feeling very unwell, with a low or high temperature.

- Think about potential infection causing general deterioration, particularly in older patients presenting with new confusion (delirium), falls or new immobility.

- Pay particular attention if concerns are expressed by the patient, or their family/carers, regarding changes in behaviour.

- Examine people with suspected sepsis for mottled or ashen appearance, cyanosis of the skin, lips or tongue, non-blanching rash of the skin, any breach of skin integrity (for example, cuts, burns or skin infections) or other rash indicating potential infection.

- If possible, try to identify a source of infection.

- Be highly suspicious of neutropaenic sepsis in patients having cancer treatment who become unwell.

- Use a structured screening tool and NEWS2 score to stratify risk if sepsis is suspected.

10. Signs of Infection

Look for signs of infection by conducting a systems assessment, with particular regard for the areas covered in Table 3.106.

TABLE 3.106 – Signs of Infection

The review of systems should cover the following areas:

General	Lethargy, fever/rigors.
Neurological system	Severe headaches, new confusion.
	Signs of meningitis or encephalitis (neck stiffness/photophobia).
Cardiovascular	Shortness of breath, shortness of breath on exertion.
Respiratory	Pleurisy, shortness of breath, shortness of breath on exertion, cough, sputum, haemoptysis, increased respiratory rate or effort.
Gastrointestinal	Abdominal pain/distension, diarrhoea/vomiting.
Genito-urinary	UTI symptoms (offensive urine, frequency, dysuria), reduced urine output, abdominal, flank and back pain.
Musculoskeletal	Hot painful joint, non-weight bearing.
Skin	Rapidly progressive cellulitis, diabetic foot and ulcers, burns, purpuric rash/mottling.
Other	Dental problems, foreign travel, exposure to other unwell contacts.

NB This is not an exhaustive list and clinical judgement should be used when considering whether a sign or symptom of a serious bacterial infection is present.

11. Respiratory Rate

- An increased respiratory rate is an early indicator of illness, and can be one of the first clinical observations to become abnormal. Therefore, accurately measuring respiratory rate (e.g. over 30 seconds) is essential. The respiratory rate will increase due to a compensatory mechanism to reduce metabolic acidosis, a consequence of sepsis. Development of sepsis screening tools has demonstrated that respiration rate will be higher in septic patients compared to non-septic patients.[17,18]

- Respiratory rate is particularly important in children, and is a very early sign of illness. It

is recommended that children presenting with signs and symptoms of an infection have an accurate respiration rate measured as it can be an important marker for serious illness.[19]

- Always refer to the relevant '**Page for Age**' for vital signs of normal parameters.

12. Oxygen Saturation in Suspected Sepsis

- Take into account that if peripheral oxygen saturation is difficult to measure in a person with suspected sepsis, this may indicate poor peripheral circulation because of shock.

Sepsis

- In some groups of patients, pulse oximetry may be difficult, for example in children, or those with existing chronic respiratory disease, due to lack of appropriate or suitable equipment, chronic low saturations or patient compliance.

13. Heart Rate in Suspected Sepsis

Interpret the heart rate of a person with suspected sepsis in context, taking into account that:

- Baseline heart rate may be lower in young people and adults who are fit.
- Older people with an infection may not develop an increased heart rate.
- Older people may develop a new arrhythmia in response to infection rather than an increased heart rate.
- Heart rate response may be affected by medicines, such as beta-blockers.

Always refer to the children's '**Page for Age**' for vital signs of normal parameters.

14. Blood Pressure in Suspected Sepsis

- Interpret blood pressure in the context of a person's usual blood pressure, if known.
- Patients may present with a normal BP but still have sepsis, particularly children and young people.

15. Confusion, Mental State and Cognitive State in Suspected Sepsis

- Interpret a person's mental state in the context of their normal function and treat changes as being significant.
- Be aware that changes in cognitive function may be subtle and assessment should include history from the patient and family or carers.
- Changes in cognitive function may present as changes in behaviour or irritability in both children and in adults with dementia.
- Changes in cognitive function in older people may present as acute changes in functional abilities.

16. Temperature in Suspected Sepsis

- Do not use a person's temperature as the sole predictor of sepsis.
- Do not rely on fever or hypothermia to rule sepsis either in or out.
- Ask the person with suspected sepsis and their family or carers about any recent fever or rigors.

- Take into account that some groups of people with sepsis may not develop a raised temperature. These include:
  - people who are older or very frail
  - people having treatment for cancer
  - people deteriorating with sepsis
  - infants or young children.

Do not ignore a high temperature or symptoms of fever/rigors as they are useful in highlighting patients with infection.

17. Prehospital Sepsis Screening Tools

- Exclusion or diagnosis of sepsis is only possible by obtaining complete blood test results from a laboratory or after urine output monitoring.
- Several pre-hospital sepsis screening tools have been proposed/developed; however, none have been validated in pre-hospital clinical practice.
- JRCALC recommends using tools that have been agreed locally in your own organisation, or across a network or region, and use of a NEWS2 score.
- Several additional screening tools have been proposed internationally, the PreSep score, PRESS score and BAS 90-30-90 score have been proposed specifically to identify sepsis in the pre-hospital environment, but none have been validated clinically.[17,20,21] The Critical Illness Score was developed to identify all critically ill patients attended by EMS (not just sepsis patients). Again, this score has not been validated clinically.[22]

18. National Early Warning Score (NEWS2)

- NEWS2 should be undertaken for all patients who are ill, including suspected sepsis. However, NEWS2 should **NOT** be used for pregnant women or children under 16 years.[16]
- NEWS2 is designed as a system to help to identify a seriously ill or deteriorating patient in a standardised way across the NHS. It is not designed to identify the cause of the clinical deterioration. Its strength is its simplicity and pragmatism – using routine physiological measurements.
- NEWS2 allows healthcare workers to communicate in a common language.
- With regard to sepsis, a NEWS2 score of 5 or more predicts at least a twofold increase in the risk of adverse outcomes, **BUT** NEWS2 does not diagnose sepsis – it simply identifies sick patients who need urgent senior medical review and intervention. The nature of the intervention requires confirmation of the diagnosis.

3 SECTION **Medical Emergencies**

Sepsis

Physiological parameter	Score						
	3	2	1	0	1	2	3
Respiration rate (per minute)	≤8		9–11	12–20		21–24	≥25
SpO₂ Scale 1 (%)	≤91	92–93	94–95	≥96			
SpO₂ Scale 2 (%)	≤83	84–85	86–87	88–92 ≥93 on air	93–94 on oxygen	95–96 on oxygen	≥97 on oxygen
Air or oxygen?		Oxygen		Air			
Systolic blood pressure (mmHg)	≤90	91–100	101–110	111–219			≥220
Pulse (per minute)	≤40		41–50	51–90	91–110	111–130	≥131
Consciousness				Alert			CVPU
Temperature (°C)	≤35.0		35.1–36.0	36.1–38.0	38.1–39.0	≥39.1	

Figure 3.40 – NEWS2 chart. Reproduced from: Royal College of Physicians. *National Early Warning Score (NEWS) 2: Standardising the assessment of acute-illness severity in the NHS.* Updated report of a working party. London: RCP, 2017. Available from: https://www.rcplondon.ac.uk/projects/outputs/national-early-warning-score-news-2.

- NEWS2 is the first step in a two-step process: (1) identification of the sick and/or deteriorating patient, and (2) a timely and competent clinical response.
- NEWS2 scores may be masked in patients who are taking beta-blockers and/or steroids.

National Early Warning Score (NEWS2)

Suspect sepsis in:

⚑ anyone that presents with fever/feeling unwell

and

⚑ NEWS2 greater than or equal to 5

⚑ **and/or** looks unwell with history of infection.

TABLE 3.107 – Adult 'Red Flag' Sepsis – Time-Critical Emergency ⚑

The following markers are suggestive of 'red flag' sepsis:

⚑ Responds only to voice or pain/is unresponsive.

⚑ Systolic BP ≤90 mmHg (or drop ≥40 from normal) or mean arterial pressure less than 65 mmHg.

⚑ Heart rate ≥130 per minute.

⚑ Respiratory rate ≥25 per minute.

⚑ Needs oxygen to keep SpO₂ ≥92%.

⚑ Non-blanching rash, mottled/ashen/cyanotic.

⚑ Not passed urine in last 18 hours.

⚑ Recent chemotherapy (in past 6 weeks).

Sepsis

TABLE 3.108 – Adult 'Amber Suspect' Sepsis |🏳

The following are markers to indicate sepsis is likely:

🏳 History from friend/family of new altered mental behaviour/state.

🏳 Impaired immune system.

🏳 Trauma/surgery in past 6 weeks.

🏳 Respiration rate 21–24 per minute or increased work of breathing.

🏳 Heart rate 91–130 per minute.

🏳 Systolic BP 91–100 mmHg.

🏳 Not passed urine in the last 12–18 hours.

🏳 Tympanic temperature <36°C/axillary temperature <35°C.

🏳 Signs of potential infection at wound (increased redness/discharge).

19. Children and Sepsis

Suspect sepsis in:

▪ children <12 years that present with fever/feeling unwell

OR

▪ children with abnormal observations

OR

▪ children with very worried parents/carers.

TABLE 3.109 – Child 'Red Flag' Sepsis – Time-Critical Emergency 🏳

High-risk criteria suspect 'red flag' sepsis:

🏳 Colour	▪ Pale/mottled/ashen/blue.
🏳 Activity	▪ No response to social cues.
	▪ Appears very ill to a healthcare professional.
	▪ Does not wake or, if roused, does not stay awake.
	▪ Weak, high-pitched or continuous cry.
🏳 Respiratory	▪ Grunting.
	▪ Severe tachypnoea.
	▪ Moderate or severe chest indrawing.
	▪ Oxygen saturations ≤90% on air.
🏳 Hydration	▪ Reduced skin turgor.
	▪ Severe tachycardia (see below).
	▪ Bradycardia <60.
	▪ Not passed urine/no wet nappies in last 18 hours.

TABLE 3.109 – Child 'Red Flag' Sepsis – Time-Critical Emergency 🏳 *(continued)*

High risk criteria suspect 'Red flag' sepsis:

🏳 Other	▪ Temperature <36°C.
	▪ Non-blanching rash.
	▪ Bulging fontanelle.
	▪ Neck stiffness.
	▪ Status epilepticus.
	▪ Focal neurological signs.
	▪ Focal seizures.

TABLE 3.110 – Child 'Amber Suspect' Sepsis |🏳

Sepsis likely/intermediate risk for sepsis (if history suggestive of infection):

🏳 Colour	▪ Pallor reported by parent/carer.
🏳 Activity	▪ Not responding normally to social cues/not wanting to play.
	▪ Wakes only with prolonged stimulation.
	▪ Significantly decreased activity.
	▪ No smile.
🏳 Respiratory	▪ Nasal flaring.
	▪ Moderate tachypnoea (see below).
	▪ Oxygen saturations ≤92% on air.
	▪ Crackles.
🏳 Hydration	▪ Dry mucous membranes.
	▪ Moderate tachycardia (see below).
	▪ Poor feeding in infants.
	▪ CRT ≥3 seconds.
	▪ Reduced urine output.
	▪ Cold feet or hands.
🏳 Other	▪ Age 0–3 months ≥38°C.
	▪ Age 3–6 months ≥39°C.
	▪ Fever for ≥5 days.
	▪ Rigors.
	▪ Swelling of a limb or joint.
	▪ Leg pain.
	▪ Non-weight bearing/not using an extremity.

Sepsis

TABLE 3.111 – Child Low Risk for Sepsis

Colour	Normal colour of skin, lips and tongue.
Activity	Responds normally to social cues.
	Content/smiles.
	Stays awake or awakens quickly.
	Strong normal cry/not crying.
Hydration	Normal skin and eyes.
	Moist mucous membranes.
Other	Child >2 years.

Clinical observations in children <12 years with suspected sepsis:

- Assess temperature, heart rate, respiratory rate, level of consciousness, oxygen saturation and capillary refill time.

- Only measure blood pressure in children <12 years in community settings if facilities to measure blood pressure, including a correctly-sized cuff, are available and taking a measurement does not cause a delay in assessment or treatment.

TABLE 3.112 – Sepsis Risk In Children In Relation to Respiratory and Heart Rates

AGE	TACHYPNOEA		TACHYCARDIA	
	Moderate	**Severe**	**Moderate**	**Severe**
1 year	50–59	≥60	150–159	≥160
1–2 years	40–49	≥50	140–149	≥150
3–4 years	35–39	≥40	130–139	≥140
5 years	27–28	≥29	120–129	≥130
6–7 years	24–26	≥27	110–119	≥120
8–11 years	22–24	≥25	105–114	≥115

20. Management

TABLE 3.113 – Management of: Sepsis

Oxygen therapy	Sepsis is categorised as critical illness and requires supplemental oxygen regardless of initial oxygen saturation reading (SpO_2).
	Give oxygen to achieve a target saturation of 94–98% for adult patients or 88–92% for those at risk of hypercapnic respiratory failure (e.g. COPD) where the conscious level or respiratory rates fall at the higher saturation levels.
	Oxygen should be given to children with suspected sepsis who have signs of shock or oxygen saturation (SpO_2) of less than 91% when breathing air. Treatment with oxygen should also be considered for children with an SpO_2 of greater than 92%, as clinically indicated.[14]

Sepsis

TABLE 3.113 – Management of: Sepsis *(continued)*

■ **Fluid therapy**	■ The choice of fluid is crystalloid.
	■ For adults and children aged ≥12 years with suspected sepsis and systolic blood pressure less than 90 mmHg or mean arterial pressure (MAP) less than 65 mmHg, give an intravenous fluid bolus of 500 ml over 15 minutes and monitor response.
	■ Regularly re-assess the patient after completion of the intravenous fluid bolus, and titrate response up to a maximum of 2000 ml if the systolic blood pressure remains below 90 mmHg and MAP below 65.
	■ IV fluids should be given to children if haemodynamically shocked or unresponsive.
	■ Give a bolus of 20 ml/kg over less than 10 minutes up to a maximum of 40 ml/kg. Assess response to fluids. Take into account pre-existing conditions (for example, cardiac disease or kidney disease), because smaller fluid volumes may be needed.
■ **Rapid transport to hospital with pre-alert**	■ Keep on-scene times to a minimum.
	■ Make a **TIME-CRITICAL** transfer.
	■ Provide a pre-alert and NEWS2 score to the receiving hospital – 'patient has suspected sepsis' – in line with local arrangements.
	■ Handover to hospital using local handover tools, such as SBAR, and give a NEWS2 score:
	■ **S** – Situation
	■ **B** – Background
	■ **A** – Assessment
	■ **R** – Recommendation.

20.1 Further Management Considerations

Antibiotic Therapy

■ If meningococcal disease is specifically suspected (fever and purpuric rash), give appropriate doses of parenteral benzylpenicillin and refer to **Meningococcal Meningitis and Septicaemia**.

■ Any organisation considering pre-hospital antibiotic therapy for sepsis, particularly where journey times to hospital are more than 1 hour, should seek agreement from their relevant clinical networks.

■ Early studies suggested significant survival benefit from early antibiotic administration in sepsis.[11] However, more recent studies fail to demonstrate such significant benefit. A recent meta-analysis indicated no survival benefit for antibiotics within the first hour of severe sepsis and septic shock.[23]

■ Very few studies addressing pre-hospital antibiotic therapy have been undertaken. Some studies have also failed to demonstrate any survival benefit.[24] A recent study suggests that each hour of delay in giving antibiotics to a patient with septic shock increases mortality.[25,26,27] At present there is insufficient evidence to make a robust recommendation in favour of, or against, pre-hospital antibiotic therapy.

Paracetamol

■ Paracetamol should not be given solely for reducing a high temperature but may be considered if the patient is in pain or to relieve distressing symptoms such as rigors.

■ Paracetamol should be given intravenously only if the patient is unable to take anything orally or is in severe pain, otherwise oral paracetamol remains the first-line choice.

■ Anti-pyretics such as paracetamol are often used in ICUs to manage fever in critically unwell patients by reducing the physiological stress fever causes; however, there is limited evidence to show any improvement in mortality.[28,29,30] Paracetamol is not part of any agreed sepsis pathway,[31] therefore may not be beneficial and does not improve outcomes in septic patients.[29,32]

■ It should be noted that paracetamol may mask the abnormal physiology and therefore treatment opportunities for sepsis may be missed in hospital due to dampening of the sepsis signs.

■ If paracetamol is used it should be highlighted in the SBAR handover at hospital.

Measurement of Lactate

■ Currently there is insufficient evidence to make a robust recommendation in favour of changing current practice to include pre-hospital lactate measurement.

Sepsis

- NICE have not recommended measuring pre-hospital lactate for suspected sepsis so at this time we do not recommend it for pre-hospital use.

- Lactate itself is not a predictor of sepsis. Lactate may be elevated in a number of clinical conditions, and indeed may be normal in cases of septic shock.

KEY POINTS!

Sepsis

- **Suspect sepsis in:**
  - **anyone that presents with fever/feeling unwell**
  - **and NEWS2 greater than or equal to 5**
  - **and/or looks unwell with a history of infection.**
- **NEWS2 does not diagnose sepsis – it simply identifies sick patients who need urgent senior medical review and intervention.**
- **Keep on-scene times to a minimum.**
- **Provide a pre-alert and NEWS2 score to the receiving hospital – 'patient has suspected sepsis' – in line with local arrangements.**

Further Reading

Further important information and evidence in support of this guideline can be found in the Bibliography.[33,34,35,36] Other useful resources include:

http://sepsistrust.org/

https://www.nice.org.uk/guidance/ng51

Bibliography

1. Singer M, Deutschman CS, Seymour CW, Shankar-Hari M, Annane D, Bauer M, Bellomo R et al. The Third International Consensus definitions for sepsis and septic shock (Sepsis-3). *JAMA* 2016, 315: 801–810.

2. Wang HE, Weaver MD, Shapiro NI, Yealy DM. Opportunities for emergency medical services care of sepsis. *Resuscitation* 2010, 81: 193–197.

3. Guerra WF, Mayfield TR, Meyers MS, Clouatre AE, Riccio JC. Early detection and treatment of patients with severe sepsis by prehospital personnel. *Journal of Emergency Medicine* 2013, 44: 1116–1125.

4. Van der Wekken LC, Alam N, Holleman F, Van Exter P, Kramer MH, Nanayakkara PW. Epidemiology of sepsis and its recognition by emergency medical services personnel in the Netherlands. *Prehosp Emerg Care* 2016, 20(1): 90–96.

5. Groenewoudt M, Roest AA, Leijten FMM, Stassen PM. Septic patients arriving with emergency medical services: A seriously ill population. *European Journal of Emergency* Medicine 2014, 21: 330–335.

6. Roest AA, Stoffers J, Pijpers E, Jansen J, Stassen PM. Ambulance patients with nondocumented sepsis have a high mortality risk: a retrospective study. *Eur J Emerg Med* 2017, 24(1): 36–43.

7. Gray A, Ward K, Lees F, Dewar C, Dickie S, McGuffie C, Committee SS. The epidemiology of adults with severe sepsis and septic shock in Scottish emergency departments. *Emergency Medicine Journal* 2013, 30: 397–401.

8. Ibrahim I, Jacobs IG. Can the characteristics of emergency department attendances predict poor hospital outcomes in patients with sepsis? *Singapore Med J* 2013, 54: 634–638.

9. Martin GS, Mannino DM, Eaton S, Moss M. The epidemiology of sepsis in the United States from 1979 through 2000. *N Engl J Med* 2003, 348(16): 1546–1554.

10. National Institute for Health and Clinical Excellence. *Sepsis: Recognition, Diagnosis and Early Management* (NG51). London: NICE, 2017.

11. Liu VX, Fielding-Singh V, Greene JD, Baker JM, Iwashyna TJ, Bhattacharya J, Escobar GJ. The timing of early antibiotics and hospital mortality in sepsis. *American Journal of Respiratory and Critical Care Medicine*, 2017. Available from: http://atsjournals.org/doi/abs/10.1164/rccm.201609-1848OC.

12. Bone RC, Balk RA, Cerra FB, Dellinger RP, Fein AM, Knaus WA, Schein RM, Sibbald WJ. Definitions for sepsis and organ failure and guidelines for the use of innovative therapies in sepsis. The ACCP/SCCM Consensus Conference Committee. American College of Chest Physicians/Society of Critical Care Medicine. *Chest* 1992, 101: 1644–1655.

13. Bone RC, Sibbald WJ, Sprung CL. The ACCP-SCCM consensus conference on sepsis and organ failure. *Chest* 1992, 101: 1481–1483.

14. Angus DC, Van der Poll T. Severe sepsis and septic shock. *N Engl J Med* 2013, 369: 2063.

15. Herbst C, Naumann F, Kruse EB, Monsef I, Bohlius J, Schulz H, Engert A. Prophylactic antibiotics or G-CSF for the prevention of infections and improvement of survival in cancer patients undergoing chemotherapy, *Cochrane Database Syst Rev* 2009, 21(1): CD007107.

16. NICE. *National Early Warning Score Systems That Alert to Deteriorating Adult Patients in Hospital [MIB205]*. 2020. Available from: https://www.nice.org.uk/advice/mib205.

Sepsis

17. Polito CC, Isakov A, Yancey AH, Wilson DK, Anderson BA, Bloom I, Martin GS, Sevransky JE. Prehospital recognition of severe sepsis: development and validation of a novel emergency medical services screening tool. *Am J Emerg Med* 2015, 33(9): 1119–1125.

18. Goerlich CE, Wade CE, McCarthy JJ, Holcomb JB, Moore LJ. Validation of sepsis screening tool using StO$_2$ in emergency department patients. *J Surg Res* 2014, 190: 270–275.

19. Davis T. NICE guideline: feverish illness in children--assessment and initial management in children younger than 5 years. *Arch Dis Child Educ Pract Ed* 2013, 98: 232–235.

20. Bayer O, Schwarzkopf D, Stumme C, Stacke A, Hartog CS, Hohenstein C, Kabisch B, Reichel J, Reinhart K, Winning J. An early warning scoring system to identify septic patients in the prehospital setting: The PRESEP Score. *Acad Emerg Med* 2015, 22: 868–871.

21. Wallgren UM, Castren M, Svensson AE, Kurland L. Identification of adult septic patients in the prehospital setting: a comparison of two screening tools and clinical judgment. *Eur J Emerg Med* 2014, 21: 260–265.

22. Seymour CW, Kahn JM, Cooke CR, Watkins TR, Heckbert SR, Rea TD. Prediction of critical illness during out-of-hospital emergency care. *JAMA* 2010, 304: 747–754.

23. Sterling SA, Miller WR, Pryor J, Puskarich MA, Jones AE. The impact of timing of antibiotics on outcomes in severe sepsis and septic shock: A systematic review and meta-analysis. *Crit Care Med* 2015, 43: 1907–1915.

24. Band RA, Gaieski DF, Hylton JH, Shofer FS, Goyal M, Meisel ZF. Arriving by emergency medical services improves time to treatment endpoints for patients with severe sepsis or septic shock. *Academic Emergency Medicine* 2011, 18: 934–940.

25. Seymour CW, Gesten F, Prescott HC, Friedrich ME, Iwashyna TJ, Phillips GS et al. Time to treatment and mortality during mandated emergency care for sepsis. *New England Journal of Medicine* 2017. Available from: http://www.nejm.org/doi/full/10.1056/NEJMoa1703058?query=featured_home#t=articleTop.

26. Shaw J, Fothergill RT, Clark S, Moore F. Can the prehospital National Early Warning Score identify patients most at risk from subsequent deterioration? *EMJ Online First*, 13 May 2017.

27. Jarvis S, Kovacs C, Briggs J, Meredith P, Schmidt PE, Featherstone PI et al. Aggregate National Early Warning Score (NEWS) values are more important than high scores for a single vital signs parameter for discriminating the risk of adverse outcomes. *Resuscitation* 2015, 87: 75–80.

28. Anderson HA, Young J, Marrelli D, Black R, Lambreghts K, Twa MD. Training students with patient actors improves communication: a pilot study. *Optom Vis Sci* 2014, 91: 121–128.

29. Lee BH, Inui D, Suh GY, Kim JY, Kwon JY, Park J, Tada K et al. Association of body temperature and antipyretic treatments with mortality of critically ill patients with and without sepsis: multi-centered prospective observational study. *Crit Care* 2012, 16: R33.

30. Janz DR, Bastarache JA, Rice TW, Bernard GR, Warren MA, Wickersham N, Sills G et al. Randomized, placebo-controlled trial of acetaminophen for the reduction of oxidative injury in severe sepsis: the Acetaminophen for the Reduction of Oxidative Injury in Severe Sepsis trial. *Crit Care Med* 2015, 43: 534–541.

31. Daniels R, Nutbeam T, McNamara G, Galvin C. The sepsis six and the severe sepsis resuscitation bundle: a prospective observational cohort study. *Emerg Med J* 2011, 28: 507–512.

32. Young P. Acetaminophen to treat fever in intensive care unit patients with likely infection: a response from the author of the HEAT trial. *J Thorac Dis* 2016, 8: E631–632.

33. Boland LL, Hokanson JS, Fernstrom KM, Kinzy TG, Lick CJ, Satterlee PA, Lacroix BK. Prehospital lactate measurement by emergency medical services in patients meeting sepsis criteria. *West J Emerg Med* 2016, 17: 648–655.

34. Brown AFT, Cadogan MD. *Emergency Medicine: Diagnosis and Management*. London: Hodder Arnold, 2001.

35. Chamberlain D. Prehospital administered intravenous antimicrobial protocol for septic shock: A prospective randomized clinical trial. *Critical Care* 2009, 13: S130–S131.

36. Tobias AZ, Guyette FX, Seymour CW, Suffoletto BP, Martin-Gill C, Quintero J, Kristan J, Callaway CW, Yealy DM. Pre-resuscitation lactate and hospital mortality in prehospital patients. *Prehosp Emerg Care* 2014, 18: 321–327.

SECTION 3 Medical Emergencies

Sickle Cell Disease

1. Introduction

- Sickle cell disease is a hereditary condition affecting the haemoglobin contained within red blood cells. As a result, the patient's red blood cells form an abnormal sickle shape which results in increased risk of blockage of the small blood vessels (vaso-occulsion) and red cell breakdown resulting in anaemia.

- A previous history of sickle cell disease and complications will be present in most cases, with the patient almost always being aware of their condition and how best to manage their health and care. Sickle cell disease is a lifelong condition and patients often suffer chronic complications of their disease. They are often the best source of advice on how to manage their condition.

- The signs and symptoms include, but are not limited to, any of the following:
  - Severe pain, most commonly in the long bones and/or joints of the arms and legs, but also in the back, chest and abdomen
  - Fever/high temperature
  - Difficulty in breathing
  - Reduced oxygen (O_2) saturation
  - Cough
  - Chest pain
  - Pallor or jaundice
  - Tiredness/weakness
  - Inability to move a limb
  - Change in level of consciousness
  - Dehydration
  - Headache
  - Priapism – a prolonged erection of the penis.

2. Incidence

- There are different types of sickle cell disease (HbSS, HbSC, HbS Thalassaemia, HbSD, HbSO) which can vary in severity. Sickle cell disease is found most commonly in people of African or Caribbean origin, but can also affect people of Mediterranean, Middle Eastern and Asian origin. In the United Kingdom it is estimated that 15,000 adults and children suffer from sickle cell disease, with 1 in every 2,000 babies born with the condition.

3. Medical Emergencies

- Painful episodes are the commonest symptom, due to vaso-occlusion from sickled red cells in the small capillaries in the long bones. In the long term, vaso-occlusion also results in damage to the lungs, heart, kidneys, bones and other organs and tissues. Most patients will know what pain relief works best for them and if an ambulance has been called it is because the pain is severe.

- Painful crises are the commonest symptom due to vaso-occlusion of small blood vessels. Patients with sickle cell disease normally manage these episodes at home, however they can be severe and require emergency management and hospitalisation. Patients often understand which pain relief works best for them during these episodes.

- Acute chest syndrome is the leading cause of death amongst sickle cell patients. This is a common and potentially life-threatening complication of painful crises and is often precipitated by a chest infection. Patients present with shortness of breath, hypoxia and tachypnoea and tachycardia. Chest pain is often present, and the hypoxia responds poorly to inhaled oxygen. Crackles are often present in the lung bases and will ascend rapidly to involve the whole lung fields in severe cases. Patients with acute chest syndrome should be managed on intensive care and require exchange transfusion.

- Patients with sickle cell disease are at a high risk of thrombosis. Pulmonary embolus is an important differential diagnosis when patients complain of shortness of breath or chest pain.

- A stroke should be suspected in patients with any change in consciousness, a seizure, severe headache, loss of movement in a limb or loss of speech, and treated accordingly (refer to **Stroke/Transient Ischaemic Attack**). Stroke in children is usually due to a thrombotic event and may not present as a medical emergency.

- Overwhelming infection – sickle cell disease causes splenic atrophy and children, in particular, may die very suddenly due to pneumococcal infection or other bacteria.

- Sepsis and infection – sickle cell disease causes splenic atrophy which reduces the patient's immune response to encapsulated bacteria. In particular, children may quickly develop severe sepsis due to pneumococcal infection or other bacteria. Similarly, osteomyelitis is a common infective complication of sickle cell disease and is associated with fever and bone pain.

4. Pathophysiology

- The red cells of patients with sickle cell disease are prone to assuming an abnormal sickled shape when exposed to a variety of factors including hypoxia, extreme temperatures (cold and hot), dehydration and a variety of other factors that cause physiological and psychological stress. Sickle cells are prone to mechanical damage, hence haemolytic anaemia is common in this group of patients. Sickled cells pass less easily through blood vessels and this can lead to occlusion of the microvasculature resulting in tissue hypoxia, pain and end organ damage. Sickle cell symptoms can therefore occur in all organs of the body.

Sickle Cell Disease

- A crisis may follow as a result of an infection, during pregnancy, following surgery or a variety of other causes including physiological and psychological stress.

5. Assessment and Management

For the assessment and management of patients with sickle cell crisis, refer to Table 3.114 or Figure 3.41.

TABLE 3.114 – ASSESSMENT and MANAGEMENT of: Sickle Cell Disease

Assess <C>ABCD

- If any of the following **TIME-CRITICAL** features present:
  - Major **<C>ABCD** problems (refer to **Medical Emergencies in Adults – Overview** and **Medical Emergencies in Children – Overview**).
  - Acute chest syndrome, then:
    - Start correcting **<C>ABCD** problems.
    - Undertake a **TIME-CRITICAL** transfer to nearest receiving hospital.
    - Continue patient management en-route.
    - Provide an ATMIST information call.

Ask the Patient If They Have an Individualised Treatment Plan

- Be aware that the patient may have a treatment plan and follow this if it is available. Some patients have Coordinate My Care records which are easily accessible to clinicians. Check if the patient has a care record as part of the assessment.
- Patients with long-term conditions will often be able to guide their care.
- Follow **Medical Emergencies in Adults – Overview** and **Medical Emergencies in Children – Overview** in addition to the specific management detailed below.

Pulse

- Measure and record pulse rate.

Respiratory Rate

- Measure and record respiratory rate.

Oxygen

- Measure oxygen saturations.
- Administer supplemental oxygen to **ALL** patients as per **Oxygen** guidelines, including those with chronic sickle lung disease; oxygen helps to counter tissue hypoxia and reduce cell clumping.
- Administer high levels of supplemental oxygen via an appropriate mask/nasal cannula until a reliable SpO_2 measurement is available; then adjust the oxygen flow to aim for target saturation within the range of 94–98%. Refer to **Oxygen**.

NB It is safer to over-oxygenate until a reliable SpO_2 measurement is available.

Blood Glucose

- If appropriate, measure and record blood glucose for hypo/hyperglycaemia (refer to **Glycaemic Emergencies in Adults and Children**).

Temperature

- Measure and record temperature.

NEWS2

- These observations will enable you to calculate a NEWS2 Score (refer to **Sepsis**).

ECG

- If required, monitor and record 12-lead ECG. Assess for abnormality (refer to **Cardiac Rhythm Disturbance**).

Blood Pressure and Fluids

- Patients with a sickle cell crisis will not have acute fluid loss but may present with dehydration if they have been ill for an extended period of time.
- Measure and record blood pressure; if required, administer fluids (refer to **Intravascular Fluid Therapy in Adults** and **Intravascular Fluid Therapy in Children**).

(continued)

Sickle Cell Disease

TABLE 3.114 – ASSESSMENT and MANAGEMENT of: Sickle Cell Disease *(continued)*

Pain Management

- Where present, assess the **SOCRATES** of pain and record initial and subsequent pain scores. Offer ALL patients pain relief. Consider any pain relief the patient may have taken prior to calling the ambulance service. Note that the patient will often understand which pain relief works best for them during a crisis.

- **Entonox** – administer initially but do not administer for extended periods (refer to **Nitrous Oxide (Entonox® or Nitronox™)**).

- **Opiate analgesia** – administer via the oral, subcutaneous or intramuscular route (refer to **Morphine Sulfate**), but not intravenously. The dose should be guided by the patient's individualised treatment plan if available; otherwise refer to **Pain Management in Adults** and **Pain Management in Children**.

- Always assess the effectiveness of any pain relief administered.

Conveyance to Hospital

- Consider conveying direct to specialist unit where the patient is usually treated, as per local pathways.

- Patients should not walk to the ambulance as this will exacerbate the effects of hypoxia in the tissues.

- Consider conveyance to hospital for patients with:
  - A temperature >38°C, as there is a risk of rapid deterioration.
  - Chest symptoms, as acute chest syndrome may develop quickly.
  - Unmanageable pain.
  - Severe vomiting/diarrhoea.

- Consider management in the community or referral to other services for:
  - Adult patients who are well and have only mild or moderate pain and a temperature of <38°C.
  - Paediatric patients who are well, have only mild or moderate pain and do not have an increased temperature. Consider referral in line with local pathways.
  - Admission is not necessarily required if the source of infection is obvious (such as a viral illness) and can be managed in the community.

Appropriate Advice

- Make sure that patients are aware of chest symptoms and/or their parents/carers understand the importance of seeking urgent medical advice if their clinical condition deteriorates, especially if breathing becomes faster or more laboured.

- Advice to be given includes:
  - Increase fluid intake, as dehydration will prolong a painful episode.
  - Avoid other factors that may trigger acute painful crisis, such as cold weather and excessive physical activity.
  - For pain management, use distraction techniques, such as games, computers and television.

- If the patient has no individualised treatment plan for pain, advise over-the-counter analgesia techniques, such as Paracetamol and Ibuprofen. **NB** Avoid Ibuprofen if the patient has renal impairment.

- Advise the patient and/or their parents/carer to seek urgent medical advice or go straight to hospital if they:
  - Become unwell or develop a fever with a temperature greater than 38°C (or any increased temperature in a child).
  - Develop chest symptoms, such as breathlessness or pain.
  - Have severe vomiting or diarrhoea, due to the risk of dehydration.
  - Are unable to control their pain at home.

Documentation

- Complete documentation to include all clinical findings, advice from other clinicians, onward referral and worsening advice given.

Sickle Cell Disease

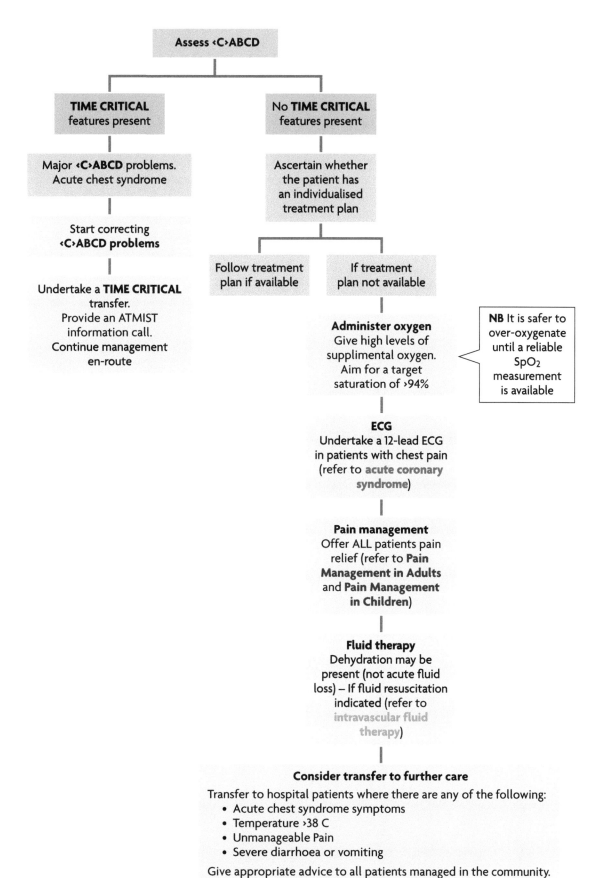

Figure 3.41 – Assessment and management algorithm for sickle cell disease.

Assess ‹C›ABCD

TIME CRITICAL
features present

No **TIME CRITICAL**
features present

Major **‹C›ABCD** problems.
Acute chest syndrome

Ascertain whether
the patient has
an individualised
treatment plan

Start correcting
‹C›ABCD problems

Undertake a **TIME CRITICAL**
transfer.
Provide an ATMIST
information call.
Continue management
en-route

Follow treatment
plan if available

If treatment
plan not available

Administer oxygen
Give high levels of
supplimental oxygen.
Aim for a target
saturation of ›94%

NB It is safer to
over-oxygenate
until a reliable
SpO₂
measurement
is available

ECG
Undertake a 12-lead ECG
in patients with chest pain
(refer to **acute coronary
syndrome**)

Pain management
Offer ALL patients pain
relief (refer to **Pain
Management in Adults**
and **Pain Management
in Children**)

Fluid therapy
Dehydration may be
present (not acute fluid
loss) – If fluid resuscitation
indicated (refer to
intravascular fluid
therapy)

Consider transfer to further care
Transfer to hospital patients where there are any of the following:
- Acute chest syndrome symptoms
- Temperature ›38 C
- Unmanageable Pain
- Severe diarrhoea or vomiting

Give appropriate advice to all patients managed in the community.

Refer to Assessment and Management Table.

Sickle Cell Disease

KEY POINTS!

Sickle Cell Disease

- Sickle cell disease is a hereditary condition affecting the haemoglobin contained within red blood cells; the cells are irregular in shape and occlude the microvasculature, leading to tissue ischaemia.

- The management of pain should be undertaken as early as possible.

- Sickle cell crises can result in damage to the lungs, heart, kidneys, liver, bones and other organs and tissues.

- Sickle cell crises can be very painful and patients should be offered pain relief as soon as possible.

- In sickle cell crisis and acute chest syndrome, aim for an oxygen saturation of 94–98% or the saturation level that is usual for the individual patient.

- Patients with sickle cell disease can be dangerously unwell but in no pain (e.g. aplastic crisis, stroke, hepatic sequestration, PE, etc.).

- Acute chest syndrome is a leading cause of death amongst sickle cell patients and is characterised by hypoxia and tachypnoea.

Acknowledgements

We would like to gratefully acknowledge the Sickle Cell Society for their contributions, comments and input to this JRCALC guideline.

Bibliography

1. Johnson AG. *Report of a Working Party of the Standing Medical Advisory Committee on Sickle Cell, Thalassaemia and other Haemoglobinopathies: Policy in confidence.* London: HMSO, 1993.

2. Maxwell K, Streetly A, Bevan D. Experiences of hospital care and treatment-seeking behavior for pain from sickle cell disease: qualitative study. *Western Journal of Medicine* 1999, 171(5–6): 306–313.

3. Vichinsky EP, Neumayr LD, Earles AN, Williams R, Lennette ET, Dean D, et al. Causes and outcomes of the acute chest syndrome in sickle cell disease. National Acute Chest Syndrome Study Group. *The New England Journal of Medicine* 2000, 342(25): 1855–1865.

4. Yale SH, Nagib N, Guthrie T. Acute chest syndrome in sickle cell disease: crucial considerations in adolescents and adults. *Postgraduate Medicine* 2000, 107(1): 215–222.

5. National Institute for Health and Care Excellence. *Sickle Cell Disease.* Clinical Knowledge Summaries. 2016. Available from: https://cks.nice.org.uk/sickle-cell-disease#!references/1381889.

Steroid-dependent Patients

1. Introduction

- While there are many types of steroids, the two most encountered in the pre-hospital setting are corticosteroids and anabolic-androgenic steroids.

1.1 Corticosteroids

- Corticosteroids are a naturally occurring group of hormones produced by the adrenal glands, which are located just above both kidneys. They help to manage stress, blood pressure and blood glucose, immune function and anti-inflammatory processes. The pituitary gland produces adrenocorticotropic hormone (ACTH) which stimulates the adrenal glands to produce cortisol.

- Synthetic pharmaceutical corticosteroids are commonly prescribed to reduce inflammation and the activity of the immune system throughout the body.

- Common conditions treated with corticosteroids include:
  - Rheumatoid arthritis
  - Asthma
  - Chronic obstructive pulmonary disorder (COPD)
  - Lupus and other autoimmune disorders
  - Multiple sclerosis
  - Inflammatory bowel diseases, e.g. Crohn's disease
  - Rashes and skin conditions, e.g. eczema
  - Endocrine conditions, e.g. adrenal insufficiency and pituitary disorders.

- Synthetic pharmaceutical corticosteroids come in many different forms and are used to treat a wide range of conditions. Common examples of corticosteroids can be found in Table 3.115.

TABLE 3.115 – Common Examples of Corticosteroids

ROUTE	FORM	COMMON EXAMPLES
Oral	Tablets, syrups, liquids	Prednisolone, Dexamethasone, Hydrocortisone, Betamethasone
Inhaled	Inhalers, nasal spray	Beclomethasone, Fluticasone
Injected	Injections (given into joints, muscles or blood vessels)	Methylprednisolone, Hydrocortisone, Triamcinolone
Topical absorption	Creams, lotions, eye drops, gels	Hydrocortisone skin cream, Beclomethasone dipropionate

1.2 Anabolic Steroids

- Anabolic steroids are manufactured drugs that mimic the effects of the male hormone testosterone.

- They may be legitimately prescribed to treat several conditions such as delayed puberty, and growth and weight gain in those with cachexia (secondary to condition such as cancer and AIDS), and to support in producing masculine characteristics in transgender men.

- However, more commonly, anabolic steroids are misused to gain muscle mass and improve athletic performance; misused anabolic steroids may come in tablet or injectable form. Common slang terms for anabolic steroids include 'roids', 'gear' and 'juice'.

- Although physical effects from sudden withdrawal of anabolic steroids are unpleasant, they are rarely dangerous. Withdrawal symptoms may include depression, aggressive behaviour, headache, anxiety, insomnia, nausea, vomiting, abdominal pain and hypotension.

- Symptoms should resolve once the body can restore its normal production of testosterone.

2. Incidence

- Primary adrenal insufficiency (when the adrenal glands cannot produce cortisol) affects around 3,400 people in the UK, and 1 in 20,000 people in western Europe.

- Secondary adrenal insufficiency (when the pituitary gland cannot produce ACTH, and therefore cannot stimulate the adrenal gland to produce cortisol) is more common, with 150–280 people per million affected. It is more common in women than men. The peak age of onset is between 50 and 60 years.

Steroid-dependent Patients

3. Pathophysiology

3.1 Glucocorticoid Steroid-dependent Patients

- The cause of steroid dependency can be broken down into three types: primary, secondary and tertiary.

- Primary adrenal insufficiency occurs in patients who have direct impairment of the adrenal glands such as those with Addison's disease (autoimmune endocrine condition where the adrenal glands cease to function), congenital adrenal hyperplasia (genetic condition) or surgery or trauma to the adrenal glands.

- Secondary adrenal insufficiency is caused by pituitary disease, hypothalamic or pituitary tumours and their treatment (surgery and radiotherapy) or brain injury.

- Tertiary adrenal insufficiency may occur in patients who have taken high doses or multiple courses of steroids, or who have taken steroids for prolonged periods of time or via multiple routes. Prolonged use may lead to a reduction or cessation of naturally occurring cortisol production by the adrenal glands.

- Regardless of type, those with adrenal insufficiency are at risk of adrenal crisis which can be life-threatening.

3.2 Adrenal Crisis

- Adrenal crisis, also termed acute adrenal insufficiency, is a **life-threatening endocrine emergency** due to a lack of production of the adrenal hormone cortisol.

- Adrenal crisis can also occur if existing cortisol replacement does not meet the body's increased need for cortisol due to illness such as fever, persistent vomiting or diarrhoea or trauma. Equally, sudden cessation of corticosteroid medication for conditions listed above will risk adrenal crisis in those with adrenal insufficiency.

- Identifying patients at risk and prompt management can save lives.

- Recently issued national guidance promotes a new patient-held Steroid Emergency Card (see Figure 3.42) to help healthcare staff identify patients with adrenal insufficiency and provide information on emergency treatment if the patient is acutely ill or experiences trauma, surgery or other major stressors.

Steroid-dependent Patients

Steroid Emergency Card (Adult)

IMPORTANT MEDICAL INFORMATION FOR HEALTHCARE STAFF

THIS PATIENT IS PHYSICALLY DEPENDENT ON DAILY STEROID THERAPY as a critical medicine. It must be given/taken as prescribed and never omitted or discontinued. Missed doses, illness or surgery can cause adrenal crisis requiring emergency treatment.

Patients not on daily steroid therapy or with a history of steroid usage may also require emergency treatment.

Name...

Date of Birth .... NHS Number ....

Why steroid prescribed ....

Emergency Contact ....

When calling 999 or 111, emphasise this is a likely adrenal insufficiency/Addison's/Addisonian crisis or emergency AND describe symptoms (vomiting, diarrhoea, dehydration, injury/shock).

Emergency treatment of adrenal crisis

1) **Immediate** 100mg Hydrocortisone i.v. or i.m. injection. **Followed by** 24 hr continuous i.v. infusion of 200mg Hydrocortisone in Glucose 5% **OR** 50mg Hydrocortisone i.v. or i.m. qds (100mg if severely obese).

2) Rapid rehydration with Sodium Chloride 0.9%.

3) Liaise with endocrinology team.

 Scan here for further information or search
https://www.endocrinology.org/adrenal-crisis

Figure 3.42 – NHS Steroid Emergency Card (Adult).

Steroid-dependent Patients

4. Assessment and Management

TABLE 3.116 – ASSESSMENT and MANAGEMENT of: Steroid-Dependent Patients or Patients at Risk of Adrenal Insufficiency

Assess <C>ABCD

- If any of the following **TIME-CRITICAL** features present:
  - Major **<C>ABCD** problems (refer to **Medical Emergencies in Adults – Overview** and **Medical Emergencies in Children – Overview**).
- Start correcting **<C>ABCD** problems.
- Undertake a **TIME-CRITICAL** transfer to nearest receiving hospital.
- Continue patient management en-route.
- Provide an ATMIST information call.

Symptoms and Signs

- Symptoms and signs of adrenal insufficiency include:
  - Severe fatigue, lethargy, drowsiness, confusion, coma
  - Low blood pressure, postural dizziness and hypotension (≥20 mmHg drop in BP from supine to standing position), dizziness, collapse and hypovolaemic shock in severe cases
  - Abdominal pain, tenderness and guarding, anorexia, nausea, vomiting (in particular in primary adrenal insufficiency), diarrhoea
  - Fever
  - Patients may have a history of weight loss and increasing skin pigmentation over weeks to months (primary adrenal insufficiency).
- Assess patient for underlying acute conditions that may have precipitated the adrenal crisis and treat that condition too.
- Follow guidance in **Medical Emergencies in Adults – Overview** and **Medical Emergencies in Children – Overview** in addition to the specific management detailed below.

Pulse

- Measure and record pulse rate.

Respiratory Rate

- Measure and record respiratory rate.

Oxygen

- Measure oxygen saturations.

Blood Glucose

- Measure and record blood glucose for hypoglycaemia.
- Treat hypoglycaemia (refer to **Glycaemic Emergencies in Adults and Children**).

Temperature

- Measure and record temperature.

NEWS2

- These observations, along with a blood pressure, will enable you to calculate a NEWS2 score (refer to **Sepsis**).

ECG

- If required, monitor and record 12-lead ECG and assess for abnormality (refer to **Cardiac Rhythm Disturbance**).

Blood Pressure and Fluids

- Measure and record blood pressure; if required, administer fluids (refer to **Intravascular Fluid Therapy in Adults** and **Intravascular Fluid Therapy in Children**).
- Patients with adrenal crisis may be hypotensive or have postural hypotension. Assess for postural hypotension if normotensive when lying/sitting.
- There may be a profound postural drop in blood pressure when the patient is moved from the lying position to the semi-recumbent or sitting position. It may be necessary to give IV fluids prior to moving the patient if extrication requires a head-up posture.

Steroid-dependent Patients

Administer Hydrocortisone

- Administer hydrocortisone to:
  - Patients in an established adrenal crisis (IV or IM administration). Ensure parenteral hydrocortisone is given prior to transportation.
  - Patients with suspected adrenal insufficiency or on long-term steroid therapy who have become unwell, to prevent them having an adrenal crisis. IM administration is usually sufficient.
- If in doubt about adrenal insufficiency, hydrocortisone should be administered.
- Pregnant women who have Addison's disease who are established in labour should receive hydrocortisone.
- Refer to **Hydrocortisone**.

Conveyance to Hospital

- Convey patients who have required intravenous fluids or management of hypoglycaemia.
- Convey patients if the underlying condition precipitating the adrenal crisis needs hospital assessment/ management.

Consider Management in the Community or Referral to Other Services

- Patients with mild illness/injury where they have followed their treatment plan to increase steroid dose and have normal physiological parameters.

Appropriate Advice

- Patients on replacement steroids (e.g. Addison's disease or hypopituitarism) may have a treatment plan to increase their maintenance steroids in the event of illness/injury. This should be followed but they may require monitoring and higher doses for more significant illness/injury.

Documentation

- Complete documentation to include all clinical findings, advice from other clinicians, onward referral and worsening advice given.

KEY POINTS!

Steroid-dependent Patients

- **Adrenal crisis is a medical emergency requiring prompt treatment with hydrocortisone and IV fluids.**
- **Steroid-dependent patients can have an adrenal crisis triggered when the body's requirement for corticosteroids increases, such as due to infection, as the body is unable to increase its own production.**
- **If extrication requires a head-up posture, IV fluids may be required before moving the patient, to prevent profound postural hypotension.**
- **Look for an underlying cause that may have triggered the episode and treat that condition too.**

Acknowledgements

We would like to gratefully acknowledge the Addison's Disease Self-Help Group for their contributions, comments and input to this JRCALC guideline.

Bibliography

1. NHS. *Steroids*. 2020. Available from: https://www.nhs.uk/conditions/steroids/.

2. Addison's Disease Self-help Group. *What Is Addison's Disease?* n.d. Available from: https://www.addisonsdisease.org.uk/what-is-addisons-disease.

3. Society for Endocrinology. *Adrenal Crisis Information*. n.d. Available from: https://www.endocrinology.org/adrenal-crisis.

Section 3 Medical Emergencies

Stroke and Transient Ischaemic Attack

1. Introduction

- Stroke is a major health problem in the UK. Improving care for patients with stroke and transient ischaemic attack (TIA) is a key national priority. The most recent national clinical guideline for stroke was developed by the Intercollegiate Stroke Guideline Working Party and published by the Royal College of Physicians in 2016, under a process accredited by the National Institute for Health and Care Excellence (NICE). The JRCALC guidelines draw heavily on these. NICE published an updated guideline (NG128) in May 2019.

- The Intercollegiate Stroke Guideline Working Party (2016) and JRCALC acknowledge the paucity of evidence for pre-hospital assessment and management of patients with suspected stroke. Many recommendations are therefore based on expert consensus and accepted practice. Ambulance services are increasingly engaging with stroke specialists and academic partners on high-quality research to help develop the evidence to inform future guidelines and practice.

2. Pathophysiology

2.1 Acute Stroke

- Stroke is defined as a clinical syndrome, of presumed vascular origin, typified by rapidly developing signs of focal or global disturbance of cerebral functions lasting more than 24 hours or leading to death. Cerebrovascular disease is the third leading cause of disability in the UK. Approximately 85% of strokes are caused by cerebral infarction resulting from ischaemic stroke, 10% by primary intracerebral haemorrhage (ICH) and 5% by subarachnoid haemorrhage. The risk of recurrent stroke is 26% within 5 years of a first stroke and 39% by 10 years.

- Acute stroke is a **TIME-CRITICAL** medical emergency. For eligible patients with ischaemic stroke, treatment with thrombolytic therapy with alteplase is highly time dependent. Data from the Sentinel Stroke National Audit Programme (SSNAP) shows that in 2019–20 only 11.7% of all UK stroke patients received thrombolysis and 1.8% underwent thrombectomy. In order to determine suitability for treatment, patients must undergo a CT brain scan; therefore, patients need to be transferred to an appropriate hospital as rapidly as possible once the diagnosis is suspected. As an additional treatment for a specific cohort of selected patients, interventional arterial therapy is available. Mechanical Intra-Arterial Thrombectomy (IAT) is becoming increasingly available in specialist centres (now known as comprehensive stroke centres).

- According to the Intercollegiate Stroke Working Party (2016): 'There is strong evidence that specialised stroke unit care initiated as soon as possible after the onset of stroke provides effective treatments that reduce long-term brain damage, disability and healthcare costs'.

- The vast majority (95%) of people with stroke present in the community setting. Public information campaigns, notably the Stroke Association's FAST campaign, have raised awareness of stroke symptoms and encourage early call for help using the 999 system. Research has helped to inform procedures in ambulance Emergency Operations Centres to recognise stroke symptoms as early and accurately as possible to facilitate an appropriate emergency response. Reducing time from symptom onset by calling for help, and by speeding up pre-hospital assessment and reducing on-scene time, can expedite admission to an appropriate hospital. This reduces overall time to treatment and helps improve patient outcomes. The recently published Utstein recommendation for Emergency Stroke Care describes a 'Chain of Survival' for stroke care.

- The most sensitive features associated with diagnosing stroke in the pre-hospital setting are unilateral facial weakness, arm or leg weakness and speech disturbance.

- It is important to remember that thrombolysis and/or thrombectomy are not the only management proven to benefit stroke patients. Admission to a stroke unit for early specialist care is known to be life saving and to reduce disability.

- Not all stroke symptoms can be identified by using the FAST test in isolation.

- Have a high index of suspicion of acute stroke in patients presenting with new, sudden onset of the signs and symptoms listed in Table 3.117.

TABLE 3.117 – Signs and Symptoms

- Sudden onset numbness or weakness of the face, arm or leg, especially on one side of the body.
- Sudden onset new confusion, trouble speaking, difficulty understanding speech or difficulty swallowing.
- Sudden onset visual disturbance including in one or both eyes, blurred or double vision or loss of visual field.
- Sudden onset trouble walking, changes in gait, loss of balance or lack of coordination.

SECTION **3** Medical Emergencies

Stroke and Transient Ischaemic Attack

TABLE 3.117 – Signs and Symptoms *(continued)*

- Sudden onset severe headache resulting in a blinding pain/photophobia unlike anything experienced before (unlike their usual pattern of headaches).
- Sudden onset of dizziness, nausea or vomiting.
- Reduced level of consciousness, or altered mental status including transient loss of consciousness or behavioural changes.
- Acute onset focal neurological deficit, witnessed acute focal neurological deficit which has since resolved or new onset focal seizures.
- Acute onset neck pain or neck stiffness with no known cause.
- Locked-in syndrome (full body paralysis below the neck).

- Be aware that the following non-specific symptoms may occur in a child presenting with stroke:
  - nausea or vomiting
  - fever
  - neck pain.
- Acute focal neurological signs may be absent, and attention should be given to parental or young person concerns about the presentation of unusual symptoms.
- However, there may be other non-neurological causes for these symptoms, referred to as 'stroke mimics', which are commoner than acute stroke:
  - seizures
  - syncope
  - sepsis
  - hypoglycaemia
  - migraine
  - decompensation of previous stroke
  - functional disorders.
- About 40% of suspected strokes are eventually diagnosed as a stroke 'mimic'. However, it is extremely difficult to distinguish a stroke mimic from a true stroke in the pre-hospital environment.

2.2 Suspected TIA

- TIA is defined as an acute loss of focal cerebral or ocular function with symptoms lasting less than 24 hours. It is thought to be caused by inadequate cerebral or ocular blood supply as a result of low blood flow, thrombosis or embolism associated with diseases of the blood vessels, heart or blood. TIA is associated with a very high risk of stroke in the first month and up to one year after the event. A suspected cerebrovascular event needs to be urgently followed up with investigation and treatment at a timely TIA specialised clinic.
- During the first few hours of a patient's symptoms it is not possible to differentiate between a TIA or stroke. Therefore, patients presenting with any ongoing facial weakness, arm weakness, speech impairment, loss of focal cerebral or ocular function should immediately be taken to hospital and investigated as suspected stroke.

- Patients with a suspected TIA must have completely returned to their normal level of functioning. Any remaining signs or symptoms, however slight, must be treated as ongoing stroke symptoms and be conveyed to definitive care.
- The 2019 update of NICE guidelines states:
  - Immediately refer patients who have had a suspected TIA for specialist assessment and investigation, to be seen within 24 hours of onset of symptoms. Follow local pathways; these may include ensuring that aspirin is administered to patients who are not conveyed to hospital.
- Do not use scoring systems, such as ABCD2, to assess risk of subsequent stroke or to inform urgency of referral for people who have had a suspected or confirmed TIA.

2.3 Intracerebral and Subarachnoid Haemorrhage

- Haemorrhagic strokes are generally more severe and are associated with a considerably higher risk of dying within the first three months and beyond when compared to ischaemic strokes. Around 1 in 10 patients who have a haemorrhagic stroke die before reaching hospital.
- Intracerebral haemorrhage (ICH) is a type of stroke often due to a spontaneous rupture of a vessel, causing bleeding within the brain itself. Uncontrolled hypertension (HTN) is the most common risk factor for spontaneous ICH. Ten to twenty percent of acute ICH occurs in patients taking oral anticoagulants and this brings an association with a high risk of early haematoma expansion. Rapid transportation to normalise coagulation can reduce this risk.
- Subarachnoid haemorrhage (SAH) is a haemorrhage from a cerebral blood vessel, aneurysm or vascular malformation into the subarachnoid space, which is the space surrounding the brain where blood vessels lie between the arachnoid and pia mater. The presentation of SAH is usually different from other types of stroke as it typically presents with the sudden onset of severe headache and vomiting,

Stroke and Transient Ischaemic Attack

and with non-focal neurological signs that may include loss of consciousness and neck stiffness.

- Sudden onset (thunderclap) occipital headache is a common presentation, the significance of which can be all too easily overlooked. Refer to **Headache** guideline.

3. Incidence

3.1 Stroke

- According to the *State of the Nation* report published by the Stroke Association in 2018, there are more than 100,000 strokes in the UK each year. That is calculated at approximately one stroke every 5 minutes. The *Burden of Stroke in Europe* report published by King's College, London using 2015 data highlighted 39.3 strokes per 100,000 inhabitants annually within the UK. There are over 1.2 million stroke survivors residing within the UK. Stroke is the fourth biggest killer in England and Wales, and the third biggest killer in Scotland and Northern Ireland.

3.2 Childhood Stroke

- There are over 400 childhood strokes a year in the UK, which is more than one child every day. Anyone of any age can have a stroke, including babies and children. The causes of stroke in children are very different from those in adults, including cardiovascular malformations and genetic causes (such as clotting disorders). Although the risk of stroke in healthy children is extremely low, the risk of a thrombotic stroke is six times higher following a recent illness, such as cold/flu or chickenpox. For children having had none or only some of their routine vaccinations, the risk of a thrombotic stroke is eight times higher compared to those who have had all of their routine vaccinations. The risk of stroke in children is 19 times higher in children with congenital heart disease. Newborns are the most likely to have a stroke.

3.3 TIA

- The estimated incidence of first-ever TIA in the UK is 50 people per 100,000 population each year. This is likely to be an underestimate. One in twelve people (8%) will have a full stroke within a week of having a TIA.

3.4 Haemorrhage

- SAH incidence is 6–12 people per 100,000 population each year in the UK. Approximately 85% of patients bleed from an intracranial aneurysm, 10% from a non-aneurysmal peri-mesencephalic haemorrhage and 5% from other vascular abnormalities including arteriovenous malformation.

4. Severity and Outcome

- The case fatality of ischaemic stroke in adults aged 45 or older is estimated at 10.4 per

100 discharges, suggesting 53,004 deaths, or 41.5 per 100,000 inhabitants, due to stroke each year.

5. Assessment and Management

- The FAST (Face, Arms, Speech, Time) assessment tool should be used and carried out on **ALL** patients with suspected stroke/TIA. A deficit in any one of the face, arms or speech domains is sufficient for the patient to be identified as 'FAST positive'.

- A suspected acute stroke patient should be considered a **TIME-CRITICAL** patient. Perform a brief secondary survey but do not allow this, or any other non-essential pre-hospital interventions, to delay transport to hospital.

- Clinicians may consider using the PASTA (Paramedic Acute Stroke Treatments Assessments) structured assessment and handover as per local arrangements (see Price et al).

TABLE 3.118 – FAST Test

Facial weakness	Ask the patient to smile or show teeth. Look for **NEW** lack of symmetry.
Arm weakness	Ask the patient to lift their arms together and hold for 5 seconds. Does one arm drift or fall down? The arm with motor weakness will drift downwards compared to the unaffected limb.
Speech	Ask the patient to repeat a phrase. Assess for slurring or difficulty with the words or sentence, hesitation or even an inability to speak at all.
Time	Note the time of onset, if known, and pass this to the hospital as this has been shown to expedite time to CT scan.

- The FAST test is well established in UK practice for both clinicians and the general public. FAST has recognised limitations in that it will not identify all patients with stroke, such as those with sudden-onset visual disturbance/lateralising cerebellar dysfunction. The Intercollegiate Working Party (2016) recommends clinicians continue to treat a person as having a suspected stroke if they are suspicious of the diagnosis despite a negative FAST test.

- The majority of strokes are ischaemic. Distinguishing between ischaemic and haemorrhagic strokes is not currently feasible clinically in the pre-hospital setting.

Stroke and Transient Ischaemic Attack

- Prehospital brain imaging is being evaluated in other countries (and in one UK centre) but the evidence is not sufficient to recommend wider implementation at this time.

- Video-conferencing is currently being evaluated in some parts of the UK to determine whether it assists in the triage and treatment of patients suffering some symptoms of stroke. (See: https://aace.org.uk/initiatives/stroke-video-conferencing/)

- A recent review of prehospital diagnostic technology to assist ambulance clinicians during emergency assessment of suspected stroke concluded that while such technologies are in development there is insufficient evidence of their routine use in the prehospital setting.

TABLE 3.119 – ASSESSMENT and MANAGEMENT of: Stroke/TIA
Assess <C>ABCD
<ul><li>If any of the following **TIME-CRITICAL** features are present:<ul><li>Major **<C>ABCD** problems (refer to **Medical Emergencies in Adults – Overview** and **Medical Emergencies in Children – Overview**).</li><li>Fast positive or suspected stroke.</li><li>May have airway and breathing problems (refer to **Airway and Breathing Management**).</li><li>Level of consciousness may vary (refer to **Altered Level of Consciousness**).</li><li>Assess blood glucose level, as hypoglycaemia may mimic a stroke.</li></ul></li><li>Start correcting any **<C>ABCD** problems.</li><li>Undertake a **TIME-CRITICAL** transfer to a Hyper Acute Stroke Unit (HASU) or a thrombectomy-capable hospital, as per local pathway.</li><li>Continue patient management en-route.</li><li>Provide an ATMIST pre-alert call including time of onset of symptoms, if known.</li></ul>
NB A UK study (Sheppard et al.) reported that providing a hospital pre-alert message is the most influential pre-hospital factor in facilitating timely assessment for acute stroke patients upon arrival in hospital and confirms in a UK setting the findings of previous work elsewhere. However, patients were only pre-alerted where stroke was recognised and symptom onset time recorded.
GCS
<ul><li>Assess Glasgow Coma Scale (GCS) on unaffected side. Eye and motor assessments may be more readily assessed if speech is badly affected.</li></ul>
Respiratory Rate
<ul><li>Measure and record respiratory rate.</li></ul>
Pulse
<ul><li>Measure and record pulse.</li></ul>
Oxygen Saturation
<ul><li>Monitor the patient's SpO$_2$, administer oxygen to achieve saturations of >94% if the patient presents as hypoxaemic on air (refer to **Oxygen**).</li></ul>
NB Among non-hypoxaemic patients with acute stroke, the prophylactic use of low-dose oxygen supplementation does not reduce death or disability at 3 months. Oxygen therapy is not recommended unless the patient is hypoxaemic.
Blood Pressure and Fluids
<ul><li>Measure and record blood pressure; if required, administer fluids (refer to **Intravascular Fluid Therapy in Adults** and **Intravascular Fluid Therapy in Children**).</li></ul>
NB The BP will be used as a baseline in hospital.
<ul><li>Intravenous access is not essential unless the patient requires specific interventions as it may delay transport to hospital.</li></ul>
Blood Glucose
<ul><li>Measure and record blood glucose for hypo/hyperglycaemia (refer to **Glycaemic Emergencies in Adults and Children**).</li></ul>
NB Hypoglycaemia may mimic a stroke.

(continued)

Stroke and Transient Ischaemic Attack

TABLE 3.119 – ASSESSMENT and MANAGEMENT of: Stroke/TIA *(continued)*
Temperature
▪ Measure and record temperature en-route to hospital.
NEWS2
▪ These observations will enable you to calculate a NEWS2 Score (refer to **Sepsis**).
ECG
▪ **Do NOT delay transfer to hospital to record a 12-lead ECG. A 12-lead ECG is not necessary for stroke patients unless there are specific reasons (such as concurrent chest pain).**
▪ The recording of a pre-hospital 12-lead ECG has been associated with delay and worse outcomes in stroke patients.
▪ **Patients should have continuous (e.g. 3-lead) cardiac monitoring en-route to capture arrhythmia**s and specifically AF which increases the risk of stroke fivefold. This valuable information will help during any subsequent specialist assessment.
Assess the Patient's Pain
▪ Where present, assess the **SOCRATES** of pain and record initial and subsequent pain scores.
▪ Consider analgesia if appropriate (refer to **Pain Management in Adults** and **Pain Management in Children**).
Transfer
▪ A suspected acute stroke is a **TIME-CRITICAL** condition. Every effort **MUST** be made to minimise on-scene time.
▪ The destination hospital will depend on local pathways. For example, bypassing local hospitals and taking the patient direct to a HASU or a thrombectomy-capable hospital may be appropriate, as per local pathways.
▪ Pre-alert the receiving hospital for all suspected acute stroke patients within locally agreed treatment windows of care.
▪ Conscious patients should be conveyed in the most comfortable position for them. A large international randomised trial of hospitalised stroke patients reported that outcomes after acute stroke did not differ significantly between patients assigned to a lying-flat position and those assigned to a sitting-up position with the head elevated.
▪ Patients with suspected acute stroke should remain nil by mouth until they have a swallowing assessment in hospital. Have suction available for patients who are aphagic to protect their airway from secretions if necessary.
▪ Where possible, a witness should be asked to accompany the patient to hospital, to assist with further assessment.
Documentation
▪ Complete documentation to include all clinical findings, advice from other clinicians, onward referral and worsening advice given.

6. Audit Information

▪ Ambulance services are required to monitor aspects of stroke care through the National Ambulance Quality Indicators, and all are linking pre-hospital data to SSNAP to capture the entire acute patient journey. Careful documentation of your assessment and management, including accurate timings, is essential to improving care for this group of patients.

▪ SSNAP are currently working with NHS England on an ambulance-linkage project to complement and extend the current dataset, incorporating pre-hospital data.

Stroke and Transient Ischaemic Attack

Bibliography

1. Royal College of Physicians. *Stroke Guidelines.* London: RCP, 2016. Available from: https://www.rcplondon.ac.uk/guidelines-policy/stroke-guidelines.

2. National Institute for Health and Clinical Excellence. *Stroke and Transient Ischaemic Attack in over 16s: Diagnosis and initial management.* NICE guideline [NG128]. 2019. Available from: https://www.nice.org.uk/guidance/ng128.

3. Stroke Audit. Pre-hospital Care Concise Stroke Guide for Stroke 2016. Available from: https://www.strokeaudit.org/SupportFiles/Documents/Guidelines/Profession-Specific-Guides/5-Pre-Hospital.aspx.

4. Kobayashi A, Czlonkowska A, Ford GA, Fonseca AC, Luijckx GJ, Korv J, de la Ossa NP, Price C, Russell D, Tsiskaridze A, Messmer-Wullen M, De Keyser J. European Academy of Neurology and European Stroke Organization consensus statement and practical guidance for pre-hospital management of stroke. Eur J Neurol 2018, 25(3): 425–433. Available from: https://onlinelibrary.wiley.com/doi/epdf/10.1111/ene.13539

5. Stroke Association. *State of the Nation: Stroke statistics 2018.* Available from: https://www.stroke.org.uk/resources/state-nation-stroke-statistics.

6. SAFE. *Burden of Stroke in Europe.* Available from: http://strokeeurope.eu/data-comparison/results/?country1=United+Kingdom&country2=Belgium&criteria=StrokeEpidemilogy.

7. Stroke Audit. *Sentinel Stroke National Audit Programme.* Available from: https://www.strokeaudit.org/.

8. Watkins CL, Jones SP, Leathley MJ, Ford GA, Quinn T, McAdam JJ, Gibson JME, Mackway-Jones KC, Durham S, Britt D, Morris S, O'Donnell M, Emsley HCA, Punekar S, Sharma A, Sutton CJ. *Emergency Stroke Calls: Obtaining Rapid Telephone Triage (ESCORTT) — A programme of research to facilitate recognition of stroke by emergency medical dispatchers.* Southampton: NIHR Journals Library, 2014. Available from: https://www.ncbi.nlm.nih.gov/books/NBK262723/.

9. Nor AM, McAllister C, Louw SJ, Dyker AG, Davis M, Jenkinson D, et al. Agreement between ambulance paramedic- and physician-recorded neurological signs with Face Arm Speech Test (FAST) in acute stroke patients. Stroke: A Journal of Cerebral Circulation 2004, 35(6): 1355–1359.

10. Harbison J, Hossain O, Jenkinson D, Davis J, Louw SJ, Ford GA. Diagnostic accuracy of stroke referrals from primary care, emergency room physicians, and ambulance staff using the face arm speech test. Stroke: A Journal of Cerebral Circulation 2003, 34(1): 71–76.

11. Wilson C, Harley C, Steels S. Systematic review and meta-analysis of pre-hospital diagnostic accuracy studies. Emerg Med J 2018, 35: 757–764. Available from: https://emj.bmj.com/content/35/12/757.long

12. McClelland G, Rodgers H, Flynn D, Price C. The frequency, characteristics and aetiology of stroke mimic presentations: a narrative review. Eur J Emerg Med 2019, 26(1): 2–8. Available from: https://insights.ovid.com/pubmed?pmid=29727304

13. Neves Briard J, Zewude RT, Kate MP, Rowe BH, Buck B, Butcher K, Gioia LC. Stroke mimics transported by emergency medical services to a comprehensive stroke center: the magnitude of the problem. J Stroke Cerebrovasc Dis. 2018, 27(10): 2738–2745. Available from: https://www.strokejournal.org/article/S1052-3057(18)30293-3/fulltext

14. Fothergill RT, Williams J, Edwards MJ, Russell IT, Gompertz P. Does use of the recognition of stroke in the emergency room stroke assessment tool enhance stroke recognition by ambulance clinicians? Stroke 2013, 44(11): 3007–3012.

15. Morris S, Hunter RM, Ramsay AI, Boaden R, McKevitt C, Perry C, Pursani N, Rudd AG, Schwamm LH, Turner SJ, Tyrrell PJ, Wolfe CD, Fulop NJ. Impact of centralising acute stroke services in English metropolitan areas on mortality and length of hospital stay: difference-in-differences analysis. BMJ 2014, 349: g4757.

16. Ramsay AI, Morris S, Hoffman A, Hunter RM, Boaden R, McKevitt C, Perry C, Pursani N, Rudd AG, Turner SJ, Tyrrell PJ, Wolfe CD, Fulop NJ. Effects of centralizing acute stroke services on stroke care provision in two large metropolitan areas in England. Stroke 2015, 46(8): 2244–2251.

17. Rodrigues FB, Neves JB, Caldeira D, Ferro JM, Ferreira JJ, Costa J. Endovascular treatment versus medical care alone for ischaemic stroke: systematic review and meta-analysis. BMJ 2016, 353: i1754.

18. Zerna C, Thomalla G, Campbell BCV, Rha JH, Hill MD. Current practice and future directions in the diagnosis and acute treatment of ischaemic stroke.

Stroke and Transient Ischaemic Attack

Lancet 2018, 392(10154): 1247–1256. Available from: https://www.thelancet.com/journals/lancet/article/PIIS0140-6736(18)31874-9/fulltext

19. Evans BA, Ali K, Bulger J, Ford GA, Jones M, Moore C, Porter A, Pryce AD, Quinn T, Seagrove AC, Snooks H, Whitman S, Rees N; TIER Trial Research Management Group. Referral pathways for patients with TIA avoiding hospital admission: a scoping review. Available from: https://bmjopen.bmj.com/content/7/2/e013443.long.

20. Bulger JK, Ali K, Edwards A, Ford G, Hampton C, Jones C, Moore C, Porter A, Quinn T, Seagrove A, Snooks H, Rees N. Care pathways for low-risk transient ischaemic attack. *Journal of Paramedic Practice* 2018, 10(6).

21. Roffe C Nevatte T, Sim J, Bishop J, Ives N, Ferdinand P, Gray R; Stroke Oxygen Study Investigators and the Stroke OxygenStudy Collaborative Group. Effect of Routine Low-Dose Oxygen Supplementation on Death and Disability in Adults With Acute Stroke: The Stroke Oxygen Study Randomized Clinical Trial. *JAMA* 2017, 318(12): 1125–1135. Available from: https://jamanetwork.com/journals/jama/fullarticle/2654819

22. Munro SF, Cooke D, Kiln-Barfoot V, Quinn T. The use and impact of 12-lead electrocardiograms in acute stroke patients: a systematic review. *Eur Heart J Acute Cardiovasc Care* 2018, 7(3): 257–263. Available from: https://journals.sagepub.com/doi/full/10.1177/2048872615620893?url_ver=Z39.88-2003&rfr_id=ori%3Arid%3Acrossref.org&rfr_dat=cr_pub%3Dpubmed

23. Bobinger T, Kallmünzer B, Kopp M, Kurka N, Arnold M, Heider S, Schwab S, Köhrmann M. Diagnostic value of prehospital ECG in acute stroke patients. *Neurology* 2017, 88(20): 1894–1898. Available from: http://n.neurology.org/content/88/20/1894.long

24. Anderson CS, Arima H, Lavados P, Billot L, Hackett ML, Olavarría VV, Muñoz Venturelli P, Brunser A, Peng B, Cui L, Song L, Rogers K, Middleton S, Lim JY, Forshaw D, Lightbody CE, Woodward M, Pontes-Neto O, De Silva HA, Lin RT, Lee TH, Pandian JD, Mead GE, Robinson T, Watkins C; HeadPoST Investigators and Coordinators. Cluster-Randomized, Crossover Trial of Head Positioning in Acute Stroke. *N Engl J Med* 2017, 376(25): 2437–2447. Available from: https://www.nejm.org/doi/10.1056/NEJMoa1615715?url_ver=Z39.88-2003&rfr_id=ori:rid:crossref.org&rfr_dat=cr_pub%3dwww.ncbi.nlm.nih.gov

25. Royal College of Paediatrics and Child Health. *Stroke in Childhood – Clinical guideline for diagnosis, management and rehabilitation*. London: Royal College of Paediatrics and Child Health, 2017. Available from: https://www.rcpch.ac.uk/resources/stroke-childhood-clinical-guideline-diagnosis-management-rehabilitation.

26. Royal College of Paediatrics and Child Health. *Management of children and young people with an acute decrease in conscious level – Clinical guideline*. London: Royal College of Paediatrics and Child Health, 2016. Available from: https://www.rcpch.ac.uk/resources/management-children-young-people-acute-decrease-conscious-level-clinical-guideline.

27. AACE. *Stroke Video Conferencing*. 2020. Available from: https://aace.org.uk/initiatives/stroke-video-conferencing/.

28. Lumley HA, Flynn D, Shaw L, McClelland G, Ford GA, White PM, Price CI. A scoping review of pre-hospital technology to assist ambulance personnel with patient diagnosis or stratification during the emergency assessment of suspected stroke. *BMC Emergency Medicine* 2020, 20(30). Available from: https://bmcemergmed.biomedcentral.com/articles/10.1186/s12873-020-00323-0

29. Stroke Audit. *The Seventh SSNAP Annual Report: Stroke care received for patients admitted to hospital between April 2019 to March 2020*. Available from: https://www.strokeaudit.org/Documents/National/Clinical/Apr2019Mar2020/Apr2019Mar2020-AnnualReport.aspx.

30. Feldborg Lyckhage L, Hansen ML, Procida K, Wienecke T. Prehospital continuous ECG is valuable for very early detection of atrial fibrillation in patients with acute stroke. *Journal of Stroke and Cerebrovascular Diseases* 2020, 29(9).

31. Fassbender K, Walter S, Grunwald I, Merzou F, Mathur S, Lesmeister M, Liu Y, Bertch T, Grotta J. Prehospital stroke management in the thrombectomy era. *Lancet Neurology* 2020, 19.

32. Li T, Cushman JT, Shah MN, Kelly AG, Rich DQ, Jones CMC. Prehospital time intervals and management of ischemic stroke patients. *American Journal of Emergency Medicine* 2020, 7.

33. Hifumi T, Yamakawa K, Shiba D, Okazaki T, Kobata H, Gotoh J, Unemoto K, Kondo Y, Yokobori S, for the Japan Resuscitation Council (JRC) Neuroresuscitation Task Force and the Guidelines Editorial Committee. Head positioning in suspected patients with acute stroke from prehospital to emergency department settings: a systematic review and meta-analysis. *Acute Medicine & Surgery* 2021, 8(1). DOI: 10.1002/ams2.631.

34. Rudd AG, Bladin C, Carli P, De Silva DA, Field TS, Jauch EC, Kudenchuk P, Kurz MW, Lærdal T, Ong M, Panagos P, Ranta A, Rutan C, Sayre MR, Schonau L, Shin SD, Waters D, Lippert F. Utstein recommendation for emergency stroke care. *International Journal of Stroke* 2020, 15(5).

35. Ashton C, Sammut-Powell C, Birleson E, Mayoh D, Sperrin M, Parry-Jones AR. Implementation of a prealert to improve in-hospital treatment of anticoagulant-associated strokes: analysis of a prehospital pathway change in a large UK centralised acute stroke system. *BMJ Open Quality* 2020, 9: e000883. DOI: 10.1136/bmjoq-2019-000883.

36. Price CI, Shaw L, Islam S, Javanbakht M, Watkins A, McMeekin P, Snooks H, Flynn D, Francis R, Lakey R, Sutcliffe L, McClelland G, Lally J, Exley C, Rodgers H, Russell I, Vale L, Ford GA. Effect of an enhanced paramedic acute stroke treatment assessment on thrombolysis delivery during emergency stroke care: a cluster randomized clinical trial. *JAMA Neurology* 2020. DOI: 10.1001/jamaneurol.2020.0611.

37. Lally J, Vaittinen A, McClelland G, Price CI, Shaw L, Ford GA, Flynn D, Exley C. Paramedic experiences of using an enhanced stroke assessment during a cluster randomised trial: a qualitative thematic analysis. *Emergency Medicine Journal* 2020, 37: 480–485. DOI: 10.1136/emermed-2019-209392.

Vascular Emergencies

1. Introduction

- Vascular services deal with disorders of the arteries, veins and lymphatics.

- In the emergency setting, this includes aortic aneurysm and aortic dissection, except those of the ascending aorta or aortic arch, which are managed by cardiac surgeons.

- Cardiovascular disease (CVD) affects not only the heart but also the aorta and the arteries to the brain (ischaemic stroke), to the gastrointestinal tract (mesenteric ischaemia) and to the legs (peripheral arterial disease, PAD). Acute ischaemia could involve the upper limbs, gut and brain as well as the lower limbs.

- Acute limb ischaemia is a common cause of emergency vascular admissions when it is due to acute arterial occlusion by an embolus, or thrombus.

1.1 Conveyance Destinations

- Many regions have vascular services networks. Vascular emergencies are treated at an arterial centre (AC). Some but **NOT** all of these manage thoracic aortic pathology. Some patients require referral for cardiac/aortic surgery in a regional cardiac centre. Refer to local pathways on destination decisions.

2. Incidence

- The prevalence of CVD is set to rise nationally due to an increasingly older population with rising levels of obesity and diabetes.
  - Over 40% of admitted patients under the vascular team have diabetes.
  - Over 80% of all vascular patients are current or past smokers.

- From 2010 to 2022, the number of people at more than a 20% risk of developing CVD could rise from 3.5 million to 4.2 million nationally (DoH, 2013).[2]

- In England, one in five people over the age of 65 years have peripheral arterial disease; 20% of these will deteriorate to develop critical limb-threatening ischaemia.

- The incidence of aortic aneurysm rupture was decreasing even before the introduction of the NHS abdominal aortic aneurysm (AAA) screening programme for men aged 65 years or older.

- The number of emergency admissions for aortic dissection, acute limb ischaemia and new diabetic foot problems has risen.

- Be aware that AAAs are less likely to be routinely diagnosed in women and therefore no prior diagnosis may have been made before the acute presentation of a rupture.[1]

3. Severity and Outcome

- There are around 3,000 deaths each year from ruptured AAAs in men aged 65 and over in England and Wales, which accounts for 1.7% of all deaths in this age group.

- The national screening programme for AAAs aims to reduce the death rate by 50%.

4. Aortic Aneurysm

- Aneurysms occur within four main areas of the aorta (refer to Table 3.120 and Figure 3.43). However, they are most common in the abdominal aorta, where they are referred to as abdominal aortic aneurysms (AAAs).

4.1 Pathophysiology

- An aneurysm occurs when the artery wall weakens and stretches as a result of atherosclerotic degeneration. As the aneurysm expands, the aorta dilates, increasing the risk of rupture. Overall mortality, including out-of-hospital mortality, is 85%.

- As AAAs expand in size, they may become painful in the chest, lower back, loin or groin. They may also lead to new pulsating sensations in the abdomen. The risk of rupture is high in a symptomatic aneurysm, which is therefore considered an indication for urgent surgery (for assessment and management of rAAAs, refer to Table 3.121 and Figure 3.44).

TABLE 3.120 – Complications of Aortic Aneurysm by Site

AORTIC AREA	PROGNOSIS
Ascending aorta	- Haemopericardium, which leads to syncope, sudden death or both.
	- Right haemothorax, which invariably leads to sudden death.
Arch of aorta	- Mediastinal haematoma.
	- Compression of pulmonary trunk or artery.
Descending thoracic aorta	- Compression of pulmonary trunk or artery.
	- Left haemothorax, which leads to sudden death.
	- Rarely, erosion into the oesophagus, which leads to profuse haematemesis.
Abdominal aorta	- Retroperitoneal haemorrhage, which leads to back pain with shock.
	- Intraperitoneal haemorrhage, which leads to acute abdominal pain and shock. Rarely, erosion into the intestine (small 'herald' or profuse GI bleed).

Vascular Emergencies

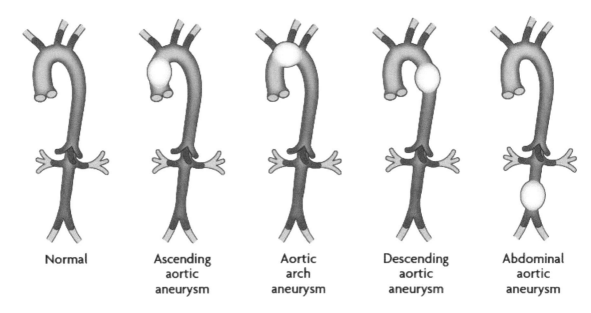

Normal

Ascending
aortic
aneurysm

Aortic
arch
aneurysm

Descending
aortic
aneurysm

Abdominal
aortic
aneurysm

Figure 3.43 – Various aortic aneurysms.

TABLE 3.121 – ASSESSMENT and MANAGEMENT of: Ruptured Aortic Aneurysms
Assess <C>ABCDE
▪ If any of the following **TIME-CRITICAL** features are present:
– major **<C>ABCDE** problems (refer to **Medical Emergencies in Adults – Overview**).
▪ Start correcting any **<C>ABCDE** problems; see blood pressure targets below.
▪ Undertake a **TIME-CRITICAL** transfer to the nearest appropriate receiving arterial centre.
▪ Continue patient management en-route.
▪ Provide an **ATMIST** information call.
History
▪ Patients presenting with a suspected rAAA will commonly present with one of the following:
– back pain
– abdominal pain
– syncope
– groin pain.
Risk Factors
▪ Known AAA.
▪ Cardiovascular disease.
▪ Peripheral arterial disease.
▪ Current or past smoker.
▪ Hypertension.
▪ Family history of AAA.
▪ Marfan syndrome (or other connective tissue disease).
Respiratory Rate
▪ Measure and record respiratory rate.
Pulse
▪ Measure and record pulse.
Oxygen Saturation
▪ Monitor the patient's SpO$_2$, and administer oxygen to achieve saturations of 94–98% if the patient presents as hypoxaemic on air (refer to **Oxygen**).

Vascular Emergencies

TABLE 3.121 – ASSESSMENT and MANAGEMENT of: Ruptured Aortic Aneurysms *(continued)*
Blood Pressure
▪ Measure and record blood pressure.
Blood Glucose
▪ If appropriate, measure and record blood glucose for hypoglycaemia or hyperglycaemia (refer to **Glycaemic Emergencies in Adults and Children**).
Temperature
▪ Measure and record temperature.
NEWS2
▪ These observations will enable you to calculate a NEWS2 score (refer to **Sepsis**).
ECG
▪ If required, monitor and record a 12-lead ECG. Assess for abnormality (refer to **Cardiac Rhythm Disturbance**).
Assess the Patient's Pain
▪ Where present, assess the **SOCRATES** of pain and record initial and subsequent pain scores.
▪ Consider analgesia if appropriate (refer to **Pain Management**), but strong analgesia such as morphine should be avoided as muscle spasm in the abdominal wall muscles can help maintain circulating volume by increasing the intra-abdominal pressure and tamponading the bleeding.
Physical Examination
▪ May be pale or appear unwell.
▪ Tachycardia, possibly weak femoral pulses.
▪ Palpable abdominal pulsating mass may not be present in approximately 50% of cases. If present, this will be in the epigastric area.
▪ Abdominal tenderness.
▪ Hypotension.
Management
▪ Patients presenting with the following symptoms should be conveyed directly to an arterial centre:
– Sudden onset of abdominal, lower back, loin or groin pain with or without collapse or hypotension in a patient with a previously diagnosed AAA which has not been repaired. A collapse may not occur if the rupture is initially into the retroperitoneal area and contained rather than into the abdominal cavity.
– Sudden onset of abdominal, lower back, loin or groin pain and collapse or hypotension in a patient aged 50 years or older with a palpable AAA.
▪ Patients outside of this presentation, even with a known AAA, should be transported to their nearest ED for further assessment.
▪ The following are considered exclusions to ED bypass in the case of a suspected rAAA. In these cases, the patient should be conveyed to the nearest ED or managed at home as per patient-specific pathway:
– Patient has suffered a cardiac arrest or a cardiac arrest is imminent.
– Airway unable to be safely managed.
– Patient was recognised prior to this event as approaching the end of their life, and are on an end of life care pathway.
– Patient has an advanced directive specifically declining surgery even if their life is at risk.
– Patients where it has been previously agreed that they are not for surgical intervention, and are not likely to survive elective or emergency surgery.
– Avoid intravenous fluid therapy where possible, as raising the blood pressure will increase the bleeding. If there are signs of impaired cerebral perfusion such as confusion, cautious administration of Sodium Chloride 0.9% can be given.

(continued)

SECTION **3** Medical Emergencies

        Vascular Emergencies

Vascular Emergencies

TABLE 3.121 – ASSESSMENT and MANAGEMENT of: Ruptured Aortic Aneurysms *(continued)*
Differentials
▪ A common differential is ureteric (renal) colic. Patients who are presenting with ureteric colic pain will not be hypotensive.
Documentation
▪ Complete documentation to include all clinical findings and advice from other clinicians.

5. Aortic Dissection

▪ Aortic dissection is classified into dissection of the ascending aorta, Type A, and dissection of the descending thoracic and/or abdominal aorta, Type B (refer to Table 3.122).

▪ Type A dissection is more common, occurring in 70% of patients, and has a higher rate of early mortality. The mortality increases by 1–2% every hour patients are untreated.

▪ Refer to Table 3.123 for calculating the possibility of an occurrence of an aortic dissection in the patient.

5.1 Pathophysiology

▪ Aortic dissection originates as a **tear** within the intimal layer of the aorta, with blood flow occurring within the outer layer of the tunica media. Blood then flows both through the new channel, the 'false' lumen, and along its original channel, the 'true' lumen. The aorta may dissect down from the aortic root to the bifurcation of the common iliac arteries in a matter of seconds.

▪ The majority of these tears occur within the ascending aorta because of higher stresses on the aortic wall due to being closer to the aortic valve.

▪ Acute dissection causes sudden onset of severe pain, which is often described as '**tearing**' in nature.

▪ The aortic wall can rupture, leading to blood loss within the mediastinum or thoracic cavity and hypotension – patients require **immediate surgery**.

▪ Refer to Table 3.124 for the assessment and management of an aortic dissection.

▪ Pain is typically maximal at onset and then improves.

TABLE 3.122 – Complications of Dissection	
Type A aortic dissection	▪ Cardiac tamponade, which leads to hypotension and/or sudden death.
	▪ Haemothorax, which leads to hypotension and/or sudden death.
	▪ Myocardial infarction.
Type B aortic dissection	▪ Mediastinal haematoma.
	▪ Renal, intestinal or lower limb malperfusion.
	▪ Spinal cord infarction (leg numbness or weakness).

TABLE 3.123 – Aortic Dissection Detection Risk Score (ADD-RS)		
PREDISPOSING CONDITIONS	**PAIN FEATURES**	**EXAMINATION FINDINGS**
▪ Marfan syndrome	▪ Abrupt or rapid onset	▪ Pulse deficit of BP differential
▪ Family history of aortic disease	▪ Severe	▪ Focal neurological deficit and pain
▪ Known aortic valve disease	▪ Ripping or tearing	▪ New aortic regurgitant murmur and pain
▪ Recent aortic surgery		▪ Hypotension or shock
▪ Known aortic aneurysm		
If any positive in any column then add 1 point. Total possible score is 0–3.		
THINK AORTA		

Vascular Emergencies

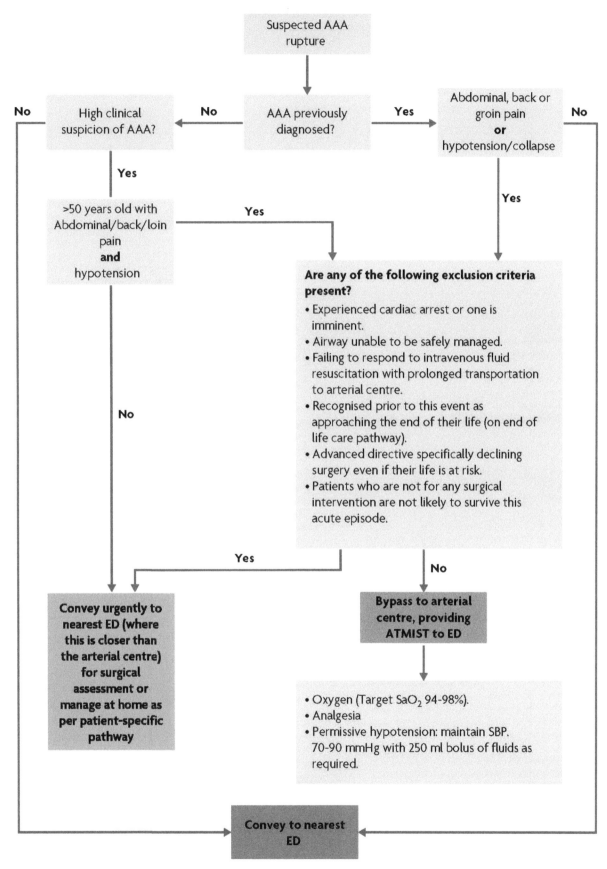

Figure 3.44 – Assessment and management of rAAA.

Vascular Emergencies

TABLE 3.124 – ASSESSMENT and MANAGEMENT of: Aortic Dissection
Assess ABCDE
▪ If any of the following **TIME-CRITICAL** features are present: – Major **ABCDE** problems (refer to **Medical Emergencies in Adults – Overview**). ▪ Start correcting any **ABCDE** problems. ▪ Undertake a **TIME-CRITICAL** transfer to nearest arterial or cardiac centre, as per local pathways. ▪ Continue patient management en-route. ▪ Provide an **ATMIST** information call.
History
▪ Mediastinal haematoma. ▪ Renal, intestinal or lower limb malperfusion. ▪ Spinal cord infarction (leg numbness or weakness).
Risk Factors
▪ Marfan syndrome, or another connective tissue disease. ▪ Family history of aortic disease. ▪ Known aortic valve disease (i.e. bicuspid aortic valve). ▪ Recent aortic surgery. ▪ Known thoracic aortic aneurysm. ▪ Hypertension, which is often poorly controlled. ▪ Age is 60 years or more. ▪ Smoking. ▪ Recent cocaine use. ▪ Can be precipitated by exercise, lifting weights or cycling, and can complicate blunt thoracic trauma.
Respiratory Rate
▪ Measure and record respiratory rate.
Pulse
▪ Measure and record pulse.
Oxygen Saturation
▪ Monitor the patient's SpO$_2$, and administer oxygen to achieve saturations of 94–98% (refer to **Oxygen**).
Blood Pressure
▪ Measure and record blood pressure, which may be high as a consequence of the dissection. ▪ Hypotension is a poor prognostic sign.
▪ Differential blood pressures may be present in around 30% of ascending or descending thoracic aortic dissections. A difference of 20 mmHg or greater between the R arm and a site beyond the dissection (left arm or leg) is considered diagnostic.
Blood Glucose
▪ If appropriate, measure and record blood glucose for hypoglycaemia or hyperglycaemia (refer to **Glycaemic Emergencies in Adults and Children**).
Temperature
▪ Measure and record temperature.
NEWS2
▪ Calculate a NEWS2 score (refer to **Sepsis**).

SECTION **3** Medical Emergencies

Vascular Emergencies

TABLE 3.124 – ASSESSMENT and MANAGEMENT of: Aortic Dissection *(continued)*

ECG

- If indicated, monitor and record 12-lead ECG. Assess for abnormality (refer to **Cardiac Rhythm Disturbance**).

- A 12-lead ECG is not a diagnostic tool to distinguish between aortic dissection and acute coronary syndrome. A patient with dissection may present with a normal ECG, ST depression or ST elevation.

Assess the Patient's Pain

- Where present, assess the **SOCRATES** of pain and record initial and subsequent pain scores.

- Sudden onset of severe chest pain or back pain or both occurs in 80% of patients. This pain is often described as sharp, ripping, tearing or knife-like pain.

- This maximum onset sharp, knife-like pain assists in differentiating between the classic cardiac chest pain that builds up in intensity over a few minutes.

Physical Examination

- Faint or absent heart sounds.

- Distended neck veins.

- Restlessness, feeling of impending doom.

- Signs of clinical shock, including hypotension.

- Chest auscultation for signs of pleural effusion representing a haemothorax.

Management

- Minimise time spent on scene, with rapid transportation to hospital, ideally an arterial/cardiac centre. Refer to local pathways.

- Ensure effective analgesia to minimise pain and reduce the sympathetic nervous response which can worsen the dissection. Where haemodynamically stable, cautious use of opiate and/or alternative analgesia should be considered.

- Do not administer aspirin, clopidogrel or GTN if the features are thought to be more consistent with aortic dissection than STEMI/NSTEMI.

Documentation

- Complete documentation to include all clinical findings, and advice from other clinicians.

6. Ischaemic Limbs

- **Acute limb ischaemia** (ALI) is a vascular emergency that can result in the loss of life or limb if not treated promptly. Ischaemia is considered 'acute' when symptoms have developed over 2 weeks or less.

- ALI is the result of **embolic**, **thrombotic** or **traumatic** arterial occlusion.

- In the most severely ischaemic limbs, treatment within **6 hours** is required to prevent permanent damage or amputation.

- ALI is most common in patients aged 60 years or older but can occur in younger patients due to rare pre-existing conditions such as thrombophilia.

- Refer to Table 3.125 for the assessment and management of ALI.

TABLE 3.125 – ASSESSMENT and MANAGEMENT of: Ruptured Aortic Aneurysms

Assess <C>ABCDE

- If any of the following **TIME-CRITICAL** features are present:
  - major **<C>ABCDE** problems (refer to **Medical Emergencies in Adults – Overview**).

- Start correcting any **<C>ABCDE** problems; see blood pressure targets below.

- Undertake a **TIME-CRITICAL** transfer to the nearest appropriate receiving arterial centre.

- Continue patient management en-route.

- Provide an **ATMIST** information call.

(continued)

Vascular Emergencies

TABLE 3.125 – ASSESSMENT and MANAGEMENT of: Ruptured Aortic Aneurysms *(continued)*
History

▨ Assess the patient for history associated with vascular concerns. Specific history related to ALI includes:
   – sudden onset of limb pain
   – limb going white
   – limb feels cold to touch
   – reduced sensation
   – inability to move limb
   – mottling of skin (severe or late ischaemia) compared to other limb
   – sudden onset or deterioration of pain in the limb of patient who has recently undergone vascular surgery
   – sudden onset of painful, cold, insensate limb, which patient may be unable to move, with absent pulses
   – mottling of a limb with absent pulses.

Risk Factors

▨ The following risk factors are associated with an increased risk of an ALI:
   – peripheral artery disease
   – aortic or popliteal aneurysm
   – recent vascular surgery, previous vascular graft or angioplasty
   – cardiac arrhythmias (AF)
   – valve replacement
   – recent MI
   – malignancy
   – smoking
   – diabetes.

Respiratory Rate
▨ Measure and record respiratory rate.
Pulse
▨ Measure and record pulse.
Oxygen Saturation
▨ Monitor the patient's SpO$_2$, and administer oxygen to achieve saturations of 94–98% if the patient presents as hypoxaemic on air (refer to **Oxygen**).
Blood Pressure
▨ Measure and record blood pressure.
Blood Glucose
▨ If appropriate, measure and record blood glucose for hypoglycaemia or hyperglycaemia (refer to **Glycaemic Emergencies in Adults and Children**).
Temperature
▨ Measure and record temperature.
NEWS2
▨ These observations will enable you to calculate a NEWS2 score (refer to **Sepsis**).
ECG
▨ If required, monitor and record a 12-lead ECG. Assess for abnormality (refer to **Cardiac Rhythm Disturbance**).

Vascular Emergencies

TABLE 3.125 – ASSESSMENT and MANAGEMENT of: Ruptured Aortic Aneurysms *(continued)*

Assess the Patient's Pain

- Where present, assess the **SOCRATES** of pain and record initial and subsequent pain scores.
- Consider analgesia if appropriate (refer to **Pain Management**).

Physical Examination

- The 6 'P's on physical examination are associated with identifying ALI. The patients will always have persistent pain.
  - **P**ain
  - **P**aresthesia, reduced sensation or numbness
  - **P**allor, cyanosis or mottling
  - **P**ulselessness
  - **P**aralysis
  - **P**erishing with cold.

Management

- For patients presenting with any of the following presentations, consider direct conveyance to an arterial centre:
  - sudden onset or deterioration of pain in the limb of patient who has recently undergone vascular surgery or angioplasty
  - sudden onset of painful, cold, numb limb, which patient may be unable to move, with absent pulses
  - mottling of a limb with absent pulses
  - recent onset of rest pain in a patient with known peripheral vascular disease.
- Intravenous access should be gained in limbs that are not affected or suspected to be affected by neurovascular compromise.
- The following are considered exclusions to primary bypass in the case of a suspected ALI:
  - patients recognised prior to the acute event as approaching the end of their life, that is they are on an end of life care pathway.
  - patients with an advanced directive in place specifically declining any vascular intervention even if their life is at risk.

Documentation

- Complete documentation to include all clinical findings, advice from other clinicians and onward referral.

7. Diabetic Foot Problem

- Diabetes is increasingly common in the UK, and a major cause of foot problems leading to lower limb amputation.
- When people with diabetes present with sepsis, both the person's life and limb are at risk if it is not recognised as a matter of urgency that the foot is the source.

7.1 Pathophysiology

- Diabetes is associated with more rapid progression of CVD. Type II diabetes specifically is associated with a high rate of peripheral arterial disease.
- People with diabetes often have reduced sensation in their feet (neuropathy), meaning that ulcers may develop, minor injuries may be missed and sepsis can develop.
- People with diabetes are more prone to infections and less able to fight them.
- Refer to Table 3.126 for a summary of this.

Vascular Emergencies

TABLE 3.126 – ASSESSMENT and MANAGEMENT of: Acute Diabetic Foot Problems

Assess <C>ABCDE
- If any of the following **TIME-CRITICAL** features are present:
  – major **<C>ABCDE** problems (refer to **Medical Emergencies in Adults – Overview**).
- Start correcting any **<C>ABCDE** problems; see blood pressure targets below.
- Undertake a **TIME-CRITICAL** transfer to the nearest appropriate receiving arterial centre.
- Continue patient management en-route.
- Provide an **ATMIST** information call.

History
- New or recurrent foot ulcer.
- Pain or swelling in the foot.

Risk Factors
- Diabetes, especially if blood sugar control has been poor.
- History of foot ulceration.
- Peripheral arterial disease.
- Peripheral neuropathy.

Respiratory Rate
- Measure and record respiratory rate.

Pulse
- Measure and record pulse.

Oxygen Saturation
- Monitor the patient's SpO$_2$, and administer oxygen to achieve saturations of 94–98% (refer to **Oxygen**).

Blood Pressure
- Measure and record blood pressure.

Blood Glucose
- Measure and record blood glucose for hypoglycaemia or hyperglycaemia (refer to **Glycaemic Emergencies in Adults and Children**).

Temperature
- Measure and record temperature.

NEWS2
- These observations will enable you to calculate a NEWS2 score (refer to **Sepsis**).

ECG
- If required, monitor and record a 12-lead ECG. Assess for abnormality (refer to **Cardiac Rhythm Disturbance**).

Assess the Patient's Pain
- Where present, assess the **SOCRATES** of pain and record initial and subsequent pain scores.
- Patients may have little to no pain, as sensation has been lost in the foot.

Physical Examination
- **Examination of the feet of patients with diabetes is essential when a foot problem could be a cause of pain or sepsis:**
  – foot ulceration
  – foot abscess
  – necrosis or dry gangrene
  – local infection or cellulitis or both
  – blistering
  – nail abnormalities with infection or ischaemia

Vascular Emergencies

TABLE 3.126 – ASSESSMENT and MANAGEMENT of: Acute Diabetic Foot Problems *(continued)*

- – painful, hot, swollen foot with break in the skin
- – spreading cellulitis
- – clinical shock.
- Severity of diabetic foot infections is classified as:
  - – Mild – local, superficial infection less than 2 cm from ulcer edge
  - – Moderate – local infection with more than 2 cm erythema or involving deeper structures (such as abscess, osteomyelitis, septic arthritis or fasciitis)
  - – Severe – local infection with signs of a systemic inflammatory response. Refer to **Sepsis**.

Management

- Transfer to hospital immediately if there are limb- or life-threatening problems such as:
  - – Foot ulceration with fever or sepsis
  - – Foot ulceration with limb ischaemia
  - – Suspected deep-seated soft tissue or bone infection, or 'If patient has already been taking antibiotics and symptoms have worsened rapidly or significantly, the person has become systemically very unwell, or if they have severe pain out of proportion to the infection'.
- Ensure effective analgesia to minimise pain.
- For all other active diabetic foot problems, refer to local pathways.

Differentials

- Other sources of sepsis, limb ischaemia, osteomyelitis or necrotising fasciitis.

Documentation

- Complete documentation to include all clinical findings and advice from other clinicians.

8. AV Fistula Bleeds

8.1 What Is an AV Fistula/Graft?

- Arteries and veins do not normally connect; an arteriovenous fistula or arteriovenous graft is a surgically constructed connection of an artery and a vein. When a vein is joined directly to the artery, this is an arteriovenous fistula (also known as an AV fistula, or fistula, or AVF for short). When an artificial tube or conduit (usually made of plastic) is used to bridge the gap between an artery and a vein, this is called an arteriovenous graft (also known as an AV graft, or graft, or AVG for short). They are commonly used in patients that require haemodialysis. When a patient's kidneys fail, dialysis keeps the body in balance by: removing waste, salt and extra water; keeping a safe level of certain chemicals in the blood, e.g. potassium, sodium and bicarbonate; also helping to control blood pressure. In haemodialysis, an artificial kidney machine is used to remove waste and extra chemicals and fluid from the blood. All patients requiring long-term haemodialysis will have an AVF or AVG constructed for this purpose. Haemodialysis can occur in a hospital, in a satellite haemodialysis unit away from a hospital but staffed by trained dialysis nurses or in the patient's own home.

- Both AVFs and AVGs are deliberately sited just a few millimetres below the skin surface and can carry between 500 ml and 4000 ml of blood every minute.

- Patients should have been given first-aid instructions about what to do if bleeding occurs and what the warning signs of bleeding are. They may also have been given a patient information sheet or advice leaflet.

8.2 Where Is an AV Fistula Sited?

- Both AVFs and AVGs are ideally and commonly sited in the forearm (wrist area); however, they can also be sited in the upper arm (above the elbow) or even in the leg, usually the groin or thigh area. Connecting an artery to a vein causes more blood to flow in the vein, which results in the vein growing larger and stronger and the vessel wall becoming thicker. The presence of an AVF or AVG allows the 14-gauge to 16-gauge dialysis needles to be inserted easily and allows blood to be circulated to the dialyser for haemodialysis treatment, and then back to the patient's body.

8.3 Why May an AV Fistula Haemorrhage?

- Over time, repeated needling of the AVF or AVG can result in weakening or thinning of the skin over them and/or the wall of the AVF or AVG itself. The AVF or AVG can also become infected as a result of the repeated needling. These can lead to scabs, ulcers and/or false aneurysms forming. Weakness of the fistula wall can lead to tear or rupture, resulting in arterial blood at high pressure spurting from the opening. If no action is taken, the person can die very quickly from loss of blood.

Vascular Emergencies

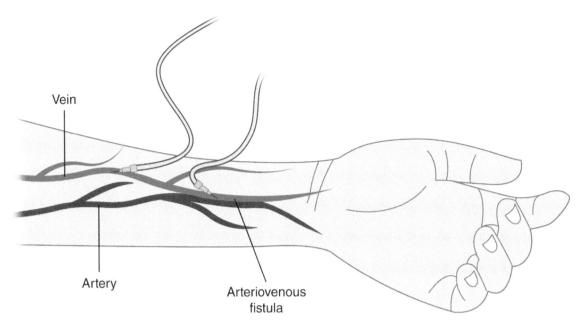

Figure 3.45 – AV fistula site.

8.4 Complications and Increased Risks of Bleeding Associated with AV Fistulas and AV Grafts

1 Infection of the AV fistula/graft site – indicated by redness or painful swelling, discharge or pus. This increases the risk of the fistula/graft rupturing and the patient bleeding catastrophically. An infected fistula/graft needs urgent treatment in hospital.

2 Damage or injury to the AV fistula/graft due to trauma or infection – anything which damages the fistula/graft (direct blow to the AV fistula/graft), increased pressure in the arm (e.g. lying on the arm when asleep or wearing a tight shirt above the fistula) or infection can cause serious damage. If the AV fistula/graft is punctured or cut, it is likely to bleed very heavily.

3 Alteration in the fistula/graft, skin or arm, e.g. damaged skin, any abnormal lumps, a swollen or painful area or altered sensation in the arm, may indicate a serious problem with the AV fistula/graft.

4 Any non-healing scab/wound over the AV fistula/graft.

5 Prolonged bleeding – post haemodialysis or bleeding in between dialysis sessions.

6 Aneurysms that are increasing in size – either at cannulation sites or elsewhere.

7 Shiny, thin skin over the fistula/graft – particularly over aneurysms.

8 Other skin integrity issues in the vicinity of the AV fistula/graft.

8.5 Management of AV Fistulas and AV Grafts Haemorrhage

- Management should be the same as for any external bleeding by applying direct pressure.

- The quickest and simplest first aid measure to control bleeding from an AVG or AVF is to use an inverted plastic bottle top (the concave/inside part of the bottle top applied to the skin) to seal it – sterility is not an issue in an emergency. Direct pressure can also be applied with the limb elevated directly over the artery feeding the fistula. The objective is to stop the bleeding, not to save the fistula/graft.

- Tourniquets are not generally recommended, as incorrect placement can exacerbate the bleeding significantly; therefore, they should only be used if other options have been unsuccessful. If used, a tourniquet should be positioned 'above' the bleeding site and as near to the axilla as possible, i.e. between the heart and the bleeding site. The intention is to occlude the arterial blood flow, which may be challenging due to the calcification of vessels. If applying a tourniquet, failure to occlude arterial flow can result in a venous tourniquet exacerbating haemorrhage.

- The high arterial pressure means that bleeding is profuse and therefore the length of time compression will be required will be longer than for other types of bleed.

- If available, an Olaes dressing is a suitable option, utilising the plastic cup component of the dressing (refer to Figure 3.46). The cup should be applied directly to the skin over the bleeding

Vascular Emergencies

Figure 3.46 – AV fistula bleed.

point and secured in place using the elasticated dressing to seal and tamponade the bleeding. It may be easiest to do this having removed the gauze from the dressing pocket of the dressing to debulk it.

- Do NOT use multiple ambulance absorbent dressings as these do not apply adequate pressure and therefore do not arrest the haemorrhage.

- Advice to first aiders or carers may have been given to control the bleeding using a plastic bottle top (concave/inside of bottle top in contact with the skin) held in position with a secure dressing prior to the arrival of the ambulance service. If this is controlling the haemorrhage, do not take down the bottle top dressing as catastrophic bleeding may recur.

- All patients experiencing a spontaneous bleed from their AV fistula/graft (however minor) and/ or felt to be at immediate risk of a bleed or further bleed MUST be conveyed to hospital for review.

- Consider direct admission to the regional renal transplant centre as per locally agreed care pathways.

- Most patients should be admitted for a period of observation.

- These patients should be discussed with and ideally seen by a surgeon who specialises in vascular access or, if unavailable, the renal team before they leave hospital.

- Those whose bleeding has been severe and uncontrolled will require surgical intervention as an emergency and lifesaving procedure.

8.6 Other Considerations

- If you need to cannulate a patient with an AV fistula/graft, never cannulate the fistula or the arm or limb it is sited on.

- Do not record a blood pressure on the arm with the fistula/graft.

- Patients with a fistula/graft may be prescribed anticoagulant medications during their dialysis treatment, which will increase the bleeding time.

KEY POINTS!

Vascular Emergencies

- **Vascular emergencies require TIME-CRITICAL transfers. Refer to local pathways for destination decisions for the nearest ED, arterial centre or cardiac unit.**

- **Ruptured abdominal aortic aneurysm should be considered in people aged over 50 years with abdominal, back or loin pain and collapse.**

- **Acute aortic dissection causes sudden onset maximum pain, which is often described as 'tearing' in nature.**

- **Acute limb ischaemia is a vascular emergency that can result in the loss of life or limb if not treated promptly. People with diabetes often have reduced sensation in their feet and neuropathy, meaning that ulcers develop, minor injuries are missed and sepsis develops.**

- **To control bleeding from an AV fistula, direct local pressure should be used rather than dressings or a tourniquet.**

- **All patients with a spontaneous bleed from their AV fistula/graft must be conveyed to hospital.**

- **In patients with unexplained severe abdominal or back pain: Think aorta!**

Vascular Emergencies

Bibliography

1. Lo RC, Lu B, Fokkema MTM, Conrad M et al. Relative importance of aneurysm diameter and body size for predicting abdominal aortic aneurysm rupture in men and women. *Journal of Vascular Surgery* 2014 59(5): 1209–1216. DOI: 10.1016/j.jvs.2013.10.104.

2. DoH. Cardiovascular Disease Outcomes Strategy: Improving Outcomes for People with or at risk of Cardiovascular Disease. 2013. Available from: https://www.gov. uk/government/publications/cardiovascular-disease-outcomes-strategy-improving-outcomes-for-people-with-or-at-risk-of-cardiovascular-disease.

3. Royal College of Emergency Medicine. *Best Practice Guidelines for the Management and Transfer of Patients with a diagnosis of Ruptured Abdominal Aortic Aneurysm to a specialist Vascular Centre*. 2012. Available from: www.rcem.ac.uk/docs/.

4. The Vascular Society of Great Britain and Ireland at the Royal College of Surgeons. *The Provision of Services for Patients with Vascular Disease.* 2015. London.

5. Brearley S. Acute leg ischaemia. *BMJ* 2013, 346.

6. Cumberbatch G. *Aortic Dissection*. 2017. Available from: https://www.rcemlearning.co.uk/references/aortic-dissection/.

7. Dr Joseph, TM. *Thoracic Aortic Aneurysm*. 2017. Available from: http://drjosephtm.blogspot.com/2017/04/thoracic-aortic-aneurysms.html#!/2017/04/thoracic-aortic-aneurysms.html.

8. Erbel R, Aboyans V, Boileau C, Bossone E, Di Bartolomeo R, Eggebrecht H et al. ESC Guidelines on the diagnosis and treatment of aortic diseases. *European Heart Journal* 2014, 35: 2873–2926.

9. French C. *CBP: Aortic Aneurysm*. 2016. Available from: http://slideplayer.com/slide/6845630/.

10. Wheatley G. *Acute Aortic Dissections: 'It's complicated'*. 2015. Available from: https://badaorta.com/acute-aortic-dissections-its-complicated/.

11. British Renal Society. Vascular Access Special Interest Group — A multi professional initiative. *Kidney Care* 2016, 1(3): 150–152.

12. Ellingson KD, Palekar RS, Lucero CA et al. Vascular hemorrhages contribute to deaths among hemodialysis patients. *Kidney Int.* 2012, 82(6): 686–692.

13. Inston N, Mistry H, Gilbert J, et al. Aneurysms in vascular access: State of the art and future developments. *J Vasc Access* 2017, 18(6): 464–472.

4

Trauma

Trauma Emergencies in Adults – Overview

1. Introduction

For references, refer to individual trauma guidelines.

- Trauma is a leading cause of death in the UK. The wide range of traumatic injuries encountered in pre-hospital care can present a complex challenge. Research suggests that assessing and managing patients in a systematic way can lead to improved outcomes.

- This overview will outline the process of assessment and management of trauma patients. This guideline supports the following related guidelines:
  - abdominal trauma
  - head trauma
  - limb trauma
  - spinal injury and spinal cord injury
  - major pelvic trauma
  - thoracic trauma
  - trauma in pregnancy
  - traumatic cardiac arrest
  - airway management
  - burns and scalds
  - electrical injuries
  - fluid therapy
  - oxygen therapy
  - pain management.

This guideline uses mechanism of injury (MOI) and primary survey as the basis of care for all trauma patients.

2. Incidence

- In England it is estimated that there are approximately 20,000 cases of major trauma annually. Road traffic collisions (RTC) are the most common cause.

3. Severity and Outcome

- In England major trauma accounts for approximately 5,400 deaths each year, with many more cases leading to significant short- and long-term morbidity. In Scotland (1992–2002) there were 5,847 deaths resulting from trauma. Major trauma is the leading cause of death in patients under 45 years of age.

4. Incident Management

- Overall control of the incident allows paramedics to concentrate on patient assessment and management and it is recommended that a model, such as SCENE, is used to assess the initial trauma scene so that it can be managed effectively (refer to Table 4.1).

TABLE 4.1 – SCENE	
S	**Safety** Perform a dynamic risk assessment: are there any dangers now or will there be any that become apparent during the incident? This needs to be continually re-assessed throughout the incident. Appropriate personal protective equipment should be utilised according to local guidelines.
C	**Cause including MOI** Establish the events leading up to the incident. Is this consistent with your findings?
E	**Environment** Are there any environmental factors that need to be taken into consideration? These can include problems with access or egress, weather conditions or time of day.
N	**Number of patients** Establish exactly how many patients there are during the initial assessment of the scene.
E	**Extra resources needed** Additional resources should be mobilised now. These can include additional ambulances, helicopter or senior medical support. Liaise with the major trauma advisor according to local protocols.

5. Patient Assessment

A primary survey should be undertaken for **ALL** patients as this will rapidly identify patients with actual or potential **TIME-CRITICAL** injuries (refer to Table 4.3).

A secondary survey is a more thorough 'head-to-toe' assessment of the patient. It should be undertaken following completion of the primary survey, where time permits. The secondary survey will usually be undertaken during transfer to further care; however, in some patients with time-critical

Trauma Emergencies in Adults – Overview

trauma, it may not be possible to undertake the secondary survey before arrival at further care (refer to Table 4.4).

5.1 Primary Survey

- The primary survey should take no more than 60–90 seconds and follow the **<C>ABCDE** approach. Document the vital signs and the time they were taken.

- Consider MOI and the possible injury patterns that may result, but be aware that mechanism alone cannot predict or exclude injury and physiological signs should be utilised as well.

- Assessment and management should proceed in a '**stepwise**' manner and life-threatening injuries should be managed as they are encountered, i.e. do not move onto breathing and circulation until the airway is secured. Every time an intervention has been carried out, re-assess the patient.

- As soon as a life-threatening injury is identified and managed, it is recommended that transport should be immediately instigated to the appropriate trauma facility according to local procedures.

- If immediate transfer is not possible, consider mobilising senior clinical support if not already done during the SCENE assessment.

MANAGEMENT OVERVIEW

If the patient has a life-threatening condition, start immediate transfer to an appropriate trauma facility according to local procedures, with treatment undertaken en-route to hospital.

- Provide an alert/information call.

- Continue patient re-assessment and management.

- If a patient requires IV fluids (refer to **Intravascular Fluid Therapy in Adults**) and fulfils the criteria in steps 1 or 2 of the Pre-Hospital Major Trauma Triage Tool (Appendix) then they should receive a bolus of tranexamic acid if available (refer to **Tranexamic Acid**).

- **Pain management** – if analgesia is indicated, refer to **Pain Management in Adults**.

- Handover – it is recommended that the patient is handed over to receiving clinicians using the ATMIST format (refer to Table 4.2).

If the patient is **NON-TIME-CRITICAL**, undertake a secondary survey (refer to Table 4.4).

5.2 Secondary Survey

- A secondary survey should only commence after the primary survey has been completed and in critical patients only during transport.

TABLE 4.2 – ATMIST

A	**A**ge
T	**T**ime of incident
M	**M**echanism
I	**I**njuries
S	**S**igns and symptoms
T	**T**reatment given/immediate needs

TABLE 4.3 – ASSESSMENT and MANAGEMENT of: Trauma Emergencies

- **All stages should be considered but some may be omitted if not considered appropriate.**
- **To reduce clot disruption, avoid unnecessary movements.**
- **When available, consider administration of tranexamic acid to all patients who require TIME-CRITICAL transfer.**

At each stage, consider the need for:

- **TIME-CRITICAL – transfer to nearest appropriate hospital as per local trauma care pathway.**
- **Early senior clinical support.**

<C> – Catastrophic Haemorrhage

- Assess for the presence of **LIFE-THREATENING EXTERNAL BLEEDING**
- Follow the management in Figures 4.1 and 4.2.

A – Airway

- Assess the airway and **AT ALL TIMES** consider C-spine injury and the need to immobilise (refer to **Spinal Injury and Spinal Cord Injury**).
- **Look for** obvious obstructions (e.g. teeth/dentures, foreign bodies, vomit, blood, trauma, soot/burns/oedema in burn patients).
- **Listen for** noisy airflow (e.g. snoring, gurgling or no airflow).
- **Feel for** air movement.

(continued)

Trauma Emergencies in Adults – Overview

TABLE 4.3 – ASSESSMENT and MANAGEMENT of: Trauma Emergencies *(continued)*

Correct any airway problems immediately by:
- jaw thrust, chin lift (no neck extension).
- suction (if appropriate).
- nasopharyngeal airway.
- oropharyngeal airway.
- supraglottic airway (if appropriate).
- endotracheal intubation (only if trained/authorised and waveform capnography available).
- needle cricothyroidotomy.

B – Breathing

Assess rate, depth and quality of respiration.

Grade breathing 1–5:

1 patient not breathing

2 slow <12 per min

3 normal 12–20 but check depth

4 fast 20–30 observe very closely

5 very fast >30.

Feel for depth and equality of chest movement, any instability of chest wall.

Look for obvious chest injuries, wounds, bruising or flail segment.

Auscultate lung fields assessing air entry on each side.

Percuss the chest wall checking the pitch of the percussion note.

In addition, assess the chest and neck for the following using the mnemonic **TWELVE**:
- **T**racheal deviation
- **W**ounds, bruising or swelling
- **E**mphysema (surgical)
- **L**aryngeal crepitus
- **V**enous engorgement
- **E**xcluding open/tension pneumothorax, flail segment, massive haemothorax.

Administer 100% O_2 in all patients with critical trauma to target O_2 sats of 94–98%, even if there are risk factors such as COPD.
- Breathing graded at 1,2 should receive O_2 via BVM, as should grade 5 if clinically appropriate.
- Breathing graded at 3,4 should receive supplemental 100% O_2 but be monitored very closely.
- Apply non-occlusive dressing to sucking chest wounds (refer to **Thoracic Trauma**).
- Decompress a tension pneumothorax (refer to **Thoracic Trauma**).
- Flail segments should not be splinted (refer to **Thoracic Trauma**).

NB Restraint (POSITIONAL) asphyxia – If the patient is required to be physically restrained (e.g. by police officers) in order to prevent them injuring themselves or others, or for the purpose of being detained under the Mental Health Act, then it is paramount that the method of restraint allows both for a patent airway and adequate respiratory volume. **Under these circumstances it is essential to ensure that the patient's airway and breathing are adequate at all times.**

C – Circulation

If massive external haemorrhage was controlled at start of assessment, re-assess this now.

Assess for radial and carotid pulses, noting rate, rhythm and volume, assess central and peripheral capillary refill time, note skin colour, texture and temperature.

Remain alert to the possibility of internal bleeding and assess for signs of blood loss in five places (blood on the floor and four more):

1 External

2 Chest (already done during breathing assessment)

3 Abdomen by palpation and observation of bruising or external marks

TABLE 4.3 – ASSESSMENT and MANAGEMENT of: Trauma Emergencies *(continued)*

4 Pelvis – do not manipulate the pelvis – MOI may suggest a fracture

5 Long bones – assess for but do not be distracted by limb trauma.

- Consider hypovolaemic shock but be aware that blood loss of 1000–1500 ml is required before classical signs start to appear. Signs of hypovolaemic shock include pallor, cool peripheries, anxiety and abnormal behaviour, increased respiratory rate and tachycardia. Signs of shock also appear much later in certain patient groups (e.g. pregnant women, patients on beta-blockers and the physically fit). There may well be little evidence of shock.

- Follow the management for haemorrhage control in Figures 4.1 and 4.2.

- Consider splinting:
  - In the critical patient, **long bone fractures** should be splinted en-route to the trauma facility.
  - **Pelvic fractures** should be stabilised at the earliest possible opportunity, preferably before the patient is moved (refer to **Major Pelvic Trauma**).

Fluid therapy

- If fluid replacement is indicated, refer to **Intravascular Fluid Therapy in Adults**.

TRANEXAMIC ACID

- If a patient requires IV fluids and fulfils the criteria in steps 1 or 2 of the Pre-Hospital Major Trauma Triage Tool (Appendix) then they should receive a bolus of tranexamic acid (refer to **Tranexamic Acid**).

- In cases of internal or uncontrolled haemorrhage, undertake a **TIME-CRITICAL** transfer to appropriate hospital according to local procedures.

- To minimise clot disruption, avoid unnecessary movement in victims of blunt trauma:
  - Log roll should be avoided wherever possible.
  - Patients should be lifted from the ground using a scoop (bivalve) stretcher.
  - Once on a scoop (bivalve) stretcher, patients should be transported on it.
  - A long spinal board is an extrication device and should not be used unless required (refer to **Spinal Injury and Spinal Cord Injury**).
  - A patient with penetrating trauma who has no neurology and no possibility of direct trauma to the spinal column should NOT be immobilised.

D – Disability

- Obtain a full GCS (refer to Table 4.5) for the patient, as this is required for the Pre-Hospital Major Trauma Triage Tool (Appendix).

- Assess and note pupil size, equality and response to light.

- Altered mental status:
  - Check blood glucose level to rule out hypo/hyperglycaemia as the cause (refer to **Glycaemic Emergencies in Adults and Children**).

E – Exposure and Environment

- At this stage, further monitoring may be applied.

- Exposure:
  - Ensure patient does not suffer from exposure to cold/wet conditions.

- Trapped patient:
  - Consider mobilising early senior clinical support.

- The secondary survey is a more thorough 'head-to-toe' survey of the patient; however, it is important to monitor the patient's vital signs during the survey.

- In some patients with critical trauma it may not be possible to undertake a secondary survey before arriving at a trauma facility. However, in patients with altered mental status it is recommended that a blood glucose reading should be taken during transport.

- Consider scoring a patient's level of frailty.[7]
  - The Rockwood Clinical Frailty Scale (CFS) is a judgement-based frailty assessment tool. It is not validated for people under the age of 65 years or those with long-term disabilities. Frailty must be sensed, described and measured: not guessed. If the patient you are assessing is acutely unwell and over 65 years, consider using the CFS, as per local pathways.

Trauma Emergencies in Adults – Overview

— The score is based on the patient's baseline, so use the tool to score how the patient was 2 weeks ago (prior to deterioration) or their usual level of functioning when well, rather than how they present today. If possible, cross-reference what the patient describes to you with a description from relatives/carers.

— Do NOT compare the patient to the pictures (e.g. person using walking aids) alone to make a judgement on the level of frailty.

TABLE 4.4 – Secondary Survey
ASSESSMENT
Head
▪ Re-assess airway.
▪ Check skin colour and temperature.
▪ Palpate for bruising/fractures.
▪ Check pupil size and reactivity.
▪ Examine for loss of cerebrospinal fluid.
▪ Establish Glasgow Coma Scale (refer to Table 4.5).
▪ Assess for other signs of basal skull fracture.
NB For further information, refer to **Head Injury**.
Neck
▪ The collar will need to be loosened for proper examination of the neck.
▪ Re-assess for signs of life-threatening injury using the mnemonic **TWELVE**:
— **T**racheal deviation
— **W**ounds, bruising or swelling
— **E**mphysema (surgical)
— **L**aryngeal crepitus
— **V**enous engorgement (jugular)
— **E**xcluding open/tension pneumothorax, flail segment, massive haemothorax.
▪ Assess and palpate for spinal tenderness; particularly note any bony tenderness.
NB For further information, refer to **Spinal Injury and Spinal Cord Injury**.
Chest
▪ Assess rate, depth and quality of respiration and grade breathing 1–5:
1 patient not breathing
2 slow <12 per min
3 normal 12–20 but check depth
4 fast 20–30 observe very closely
5 very fast >30
▪ Breathing graded at 1,2 should receive O_2 via BVM, as should grade 5 if clinically appropriate.
▪ Breathing graded at 3,4 should receive supplemental 100% O_2 but should be monitored very closely.
▪ Feel for rib fractures, instability and surgical emphysema.
▪ Look for contusions, seat-belt marks and flail segments.
▪ Auscultate lung fields for signs of:
— Pneumothorax
— Tension pneumothorax
— Haemothorax
— Cardiac tamponade
— Assess for signs of pulmonary contusion.
▪ Examine the front and as much of the back as is possible.
NB for further information, refer to **Thoracic Trauma**.

TABLE 4.4 – Secondary Survey *(continued)*

Abdomen

- Examine for open wounds, contusions and seat-belt marks.
- Palpate the entire abdomen for tenderness and guarding.
- Examine the front and as much of the back as is possible.

NB For further information, refer to **Abdominal Trauma**.

Pelvis

- Blood loss may be visible either from the urethra or per vaginum (PV).
- The patient may have the urge to urinate.

NB For further information, refer to **Major Pelvic Trauma**.

Lower/upper limbs

- Examine lower limbs then upper limbs.
- Look for wounds and evidence of fractures.
- Check for MSC in **ALL** four limbs:
  - **MOTOR** – Test for movement.
  - **SENSATION** – Apply light touch to evaluate sensation.
  - **CIRCULATION** – Assess pulse and skin temperature.

NB For further information, refer to **Limb Trauma**.

TABLE 4.5 – Glasgow Coma Scale

Item	Element	Score
Eyes Opening:		
	Spontaneously	4
	To speech	3
	To pain	2
	None	1
Verbal Response:		
	Orientated	5
	Confused	4
	Inappropriate words	3
	Incomprehensible sounds	2
	No verbal response	1
Motor Response:		
	Obeys commands	6
	Localised pain	5
	Withdraws from pain	4
	Abnormal flexion	3
	Extensor response	2
	No response to pain	1

6. The Trapped Patient

Entrapment can be:

- **Relative:** trapped by difficulty in access/egress from the wreckage, including the physical injury stopping normal exit.
- **Absolute:** firmly trapped by a vehicle and its deformity, necessitating specialised cutting techniques to free the patient.

All patients that have an **absolute** entrapment are at high risk of having suffered significant transfer of energy and therefore are at increased risk of severe injury.

6.1 Management

- Conduct a thorough assessment of the incident using SCENE or similar model.
- Consider mobilising senior clinical support at the earliest opportunity.
- Mobilise and liaise with other emergency services.
- Perform primary survey and manage as per Table 4.3.
- Form a rescue plan.
- Provide analgesia (refer to **Pain Management in Adults**).

Trauma Emergencies in Adults – Overview

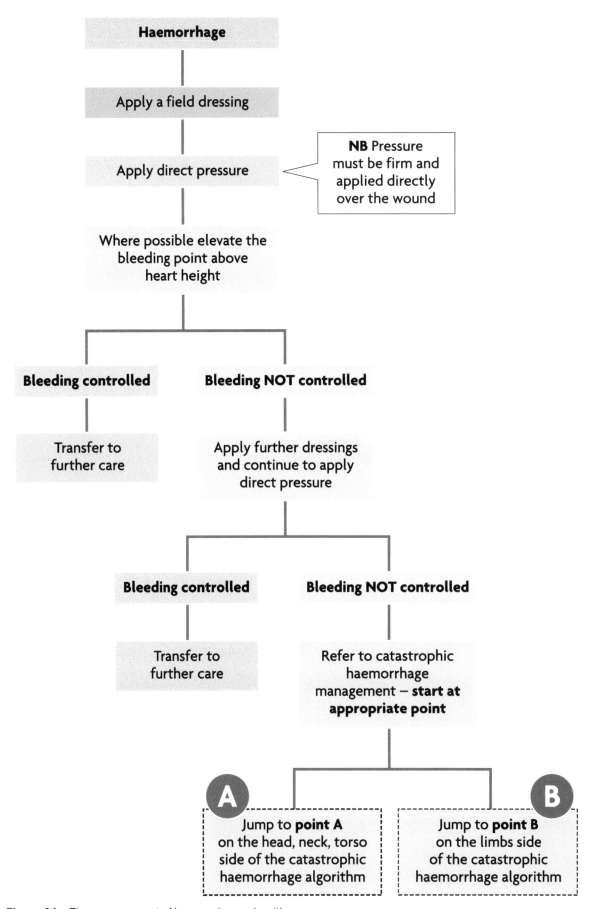

Figure 4.1 – The management of haemorrhage algorithm.

Trauma Emergencies in Adults – Overview

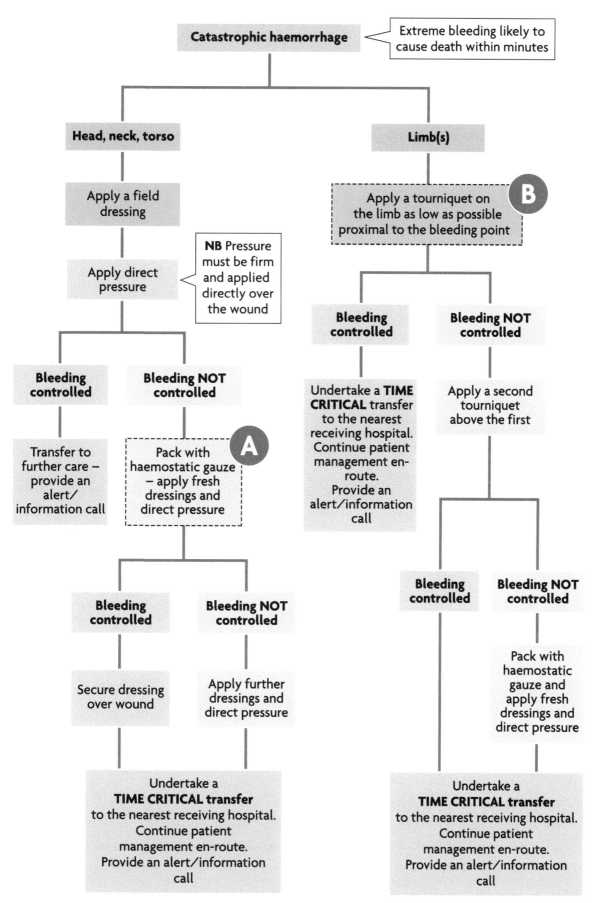

Catastrophic haemorrhage ← Extreme bleeding likely to cause death within minutes

Head, neck, torso

Apply a field dressing

Apply direct pressure
← **NB** Pressure must be firm and applied directly over the wound

Bleeding controlled

Transfer to further care – provide an alert/ information call

Bleeding NOT controlled — **A**

Pack with haemostatic gauze – apply fresh dressings and direct pressure

Bleeding controlled

Secure dressing over wound

Bleeding NOT controlled

Apply further dressings and direct pressure

Undertake a **TIME CRITICAL transfer** to the nearest receiving hospital. Continue patient management en-route. Provide an alert/information call

Limb(s)

Apply a tourniquet on the limb as low as possible proximal to the bleeding point — **B**

Bleeding controlled

Undertake a **TIME CRITICAL** transfer to the nearest receiving hospital. Continue patient management en-route. Provide an alert/information call

Bleeding NOT controlled

Apply a second tourniquet above the first

Bleeding controlled

Bleeding NOT controlled

Pack with haemostatic gauze and apply fresh dressings and direct pressure

Undertake a **TIME CRITICAL transfer** to the nearest receiving hospital. Continue patient management en-route. Provide an alert/information call

Figure 4.2 – The management of catastrophic haemorrhage algorithm.

Trauma Emergencies in Adults – Overview

7. Hanging

7.1 Introduction

- Hanging is the most common method of suicide, accounting for 61% of all suicides in those aged 10 years and above (Apr–Jul 2020). Males outnumber females by roughly 3:1 and ages 45–64 have the highest rate.[1] Hanging may be accidental or deliberate.

7.2 Mechanisms and Definitions

- Hanging may be defined as a short drop or long drop, fully suspended or partially supported (where the entire weight of the body is not supported by the ligature). A long drop can lead to sudden death as a result of a fracture-dislocation of the upper cervical vertebrae. A short drop may lead to death by asphyxia. There is no agreed definition of the height required for a long or short drop; the approximate height of the drop should be handed over to other clinicians and documented.

- In a short-drop or partially supported hanging, the patient may asphyxiate and may not have a cervical spine fracture. The mechanism of death in short drop is compression of the airway and blood vessels of the neck. This can also cause vagal discharge through pressure on the baroreceptors in the carotid sinus and the carotid body.[2]

7.3 Assessment & Management

- Undertake a risk assessment with regards to whether you are able to safely get access to the patient.

- Identify if there are any conditions unequivocally associated with death (refer to **Termination of Resuscitation and Verification of Death in Adults**).

- Identify if there are signs of life or the need for resuscitation.

- Remove (and if necessary, cut) ligatures.

- Consider dispatching or calling for additional specialist teams or critical care resources at an early stage, as per local procedures.

- Consider the need for requesting additional support, particularly for the management of the post-ROSC agitated patient and for advanced airway management.

- Safely move the patient into an appropriate position for further assessment and management, protecting the cervical spine if a cervical spine or serious laryngeal injury is suspected.

- Refer to **Trauma Emergencies in Adults – Overview** and **Trauma Emergencies in Children – Overview** for assessment and management of injuries.

- Airway management should be prioritised over cervical spine management (refer to **Advanced Life Support**).

- Ventilation and/or intubation may be difficult due to the potential for airway injury and laryngeal swelling.

7.4 Hanging and Cardiac Arrest

- Manage as per **Advanced Life Support** and refer to **Termination of Resuscitation and Verification of Death in Adults**.

- If CPR is not commenced, where possible clinicians should not disturb the scene to assist police investigations.

7.5 Post-ROSC Care

- Be aware that patients are likely to be hypoxic and agitated, and may benefit from interventions by specialist or critical care teams.

- Consider the possibility of spinal or spinal cord injury (refer to **Spinal Injury and Spinal Cord Injury**).

7.6 Staff Wellbeing

- All staff may be affected by this type of incident. This could affect them immediately after the incident or in the longer term. Always offer support to all staff that have attended and follow local procedures for this. Undertake post-incident debriefs as per local procedures. Refer to **Staff Health and Wellbeing**.

- Consider the need to signpost bystanders/witnesses/family to support as well.

KEY POINTS!

Trauma Emergencies in Adults – Overview

- **Overall assessment of safety is of prime importance: self, scene, casualties.**
- **The primary survey forms the basis of patient assessment, with due consideration for C-spine immobilisation.**
- **Arrest of external haemorrhage can be life-saving.**
- **Consider seeking senior clinical advice/support at the earliest opportunity.**

Trauma Emergencies in Adults – Overview

Acknowledgements

We would like to gratefully acknowledge the contribution of John JM Black, Paul Gibbs, Graham McClelland, Lee Thompson and Gary Shaw to this JRCALC guideline.

Further Reading

British Renal Society. Vascular Access Special Interest Group – a multi professional initiative. *Kidney Care* 2016, 1(3): 150–152.

Ellingson KD, Palekar RS, Lucero CA et al. Vascular hemorrhages contribute to deaths among hemodialysis patients. *Kidney International* 2012, 82(6): 686–692.

Inston N, Mistry H, Gilbert J, et al. Aneurysms in vascular access: state of the art and future developments. *Journal of Vascular Access* 2017, 18(6): 464–472.

Bibliography

1. Office for National Statistics (ONS). *Deaths from Suicide That Occurred in England and Wales: April to July 2020.* 2021. Available from: https://www.ons.gov.uk/peoplepopulationandcommunity/birthsdeathsandmarriages/deaths/articles/deathsfromsuicidethatoccurredinenglandandwales/aprilandjuly2020.

2. Gubbins K. The hanging/hanged patient and relevance to pre-hospital care. *Journal of Paramedic Practice* 2016, 8(6). DOI: 10.12968/jpar.2016.8.6.290.

3. Alqahtani S, Nehme Z, Williams B, Bernard S, and Smith K. Temporal Trends in the incidence, characteristics, and outcomes of hanging-related out-of-hospital cardiac arrest. *Prehospital Emergency Care* 2020, 24(3): 369–377. DOI: 10.1080/10903127.2019.1666944.

4. Paul SP, Paul R, Heaton PA. Accidental hanging injuries in children: recognition and management. *British Journal of Hospital Medicine* 2017, 78(10): 572–577. DOI: 10.12968/hmed.2017.78.10.572.

5. Shaw G, Thompson L, McClelland G. Hangings attended by emergency medical services: a scoping review. *British Paramedic Journal* 2021, 5(4): 40–48. DOI: 10.29045/14784726.2021.3.5.4.40.

6. Turner J, et al. Out-of-hospital cardiac arrest due to hanging: a retrospective analysis. *Emergency Medicine Journal* 2021. DOI: 10.1136/emermed-2020-210839.

7. Rockwood, K et al. (2005) A global clinical measure of fitness and frailty in elderly people. *Canadian Medical Association Journal* 173(5): 489–495.

SECTION 4 Trauma

Trauma Emergencies in Children – Overview

1. Introduction

- Paediatric trauma is managed following the standard **<C>ABCDE** approach to trauma, taking into account differences in the child's anatomy, relative size and physiological response to injury. These differences are addressed below.

2. Incidence

- 700 children die as a result of accidents in England and Wales each year.

- 50% of child trauma deaths occur in motor vehicle incidents. Children travelling by car should legally be restrained but this law is not always followed and many deaths and serious injuries occur following vehicular ejection. Additionally, child deaths from cycle and pedestrian incidents are also very common.

- 30% of child trauma deaths occur at home, with burns and falls being the leading causes.

- Child death reviews often identify circumstances that could potentially have been avoided had injury prevention methods been rigorously applied.

- Hanging is the most common method of suicide, accounting for 61% of all suicides in those aged 10 years and above (Apr–Jul 2020). Hanging may be accidental or deliberate. Please refer to Section 7 in **Trauma Emergencies in Adults – Overview**.

3. Assessment: The Basic Trauma Approach

3.1 SCENE

Overall control of the incident allows paramedics to concentrate on patient assessment and management and it is recommended that a model, such as SCENE, is used to assess the initial trauma scene so that it can be managed effectively (see below).

3.2 Primary Survey

- Catastrophic haemorrhage (refer to Figure 4.4).
- Airway with cervical spine control (refer to **Spinal Injury and Spinal Cord Injury**).
- Breathing.
- Circulation.
- Disability.
- Exposure.

S	Safety
	Risk assessment. Perform a dynamic risk assessment. Are there any dangers now or will there be any that become apparent during the incident? This needs to be continually re-assessed throughout the incident. Appropriate personal protective equipment should be utilised according to local protocols.
C	Cause including MOI
	Establish the events leading up to the incident. Is this consistent with your findings? Read the scene/wreckage looking for evidence that children were involved (e.g. toys or child seats). These may provide a clue that a child has been ejected from the vehicle or wandered off from the scene but may still require medical attention or other care. Ask if children were involved.
E	Environment
	Are there any environmental factors that need to be taken into consideration? These can include problems with access or egress, weather conditions or time of day.
N	Number of patients
	Establish exactly how many patients there are during the initial assessment of the scene
E	Extra resources needed
	Additional resources should be mobilised now. These can include additional ambulances, helicopter or senior medical support. Liaise with the major trauma advisor according to local protocols.

The management of a child suffering a traumatic injury requires a careful approach, with an emphasis on explanation, reassurance and honesty. Trust of the carer by the child makes management much easier.

If possible, it is helpful to keep the child's parents/carers close by for reassurance, although their distress can exacerbate that of the child.

3.3 Stepwise Primary Survey Assessment

As for all trauma care, a systematic approach, managing problems as they are encountered before moving on, is required.

Trauma Emergencies in Children – Overview

4. Catastrophic Haemorrhage

Catastrophic blood loss must be arrested immediately (refer to Figure 4.4).

5. Airway

- In small children, the relatively large occiput tends to flex the head forward. In order to return the head to the neutral position it may be necessary to insert a small amount of padding under the shoulders.

- Vomit, blood or foreign material may obstruct the airway. Apply gentle suctioning under direct vision. Blind finger sweeps are contra-indicated.

- Head tilt should be avoided in trauma and a chin lift alone or a jaw thrust used to open the airway.

- If an airway adjunct is needed, then an oropharyngeal airway should be inserted under direct vision. If it is necessary to insert a nasopharyngeal airway (e.g. because of trismus), care must be taken in all head-injured children in case there is an underlying skull fracture, causing a risk of misplacement through the cribriform plate into the brain. It is also important to avoid damage to the adenoidal tissue. This can cause considerable bleeding, making the airway even more difficult to manage.

- High concentration oxygen (O_2) (refer to **Oxygen**) should be administered routinely, whatever the oxygen saturation, in children sustaining major trauma or long bone fractures.

- Administer high concentration O_2 via a non-rebreathing mask, to maintain an oxygen saturation of at least 94%. If a high-flow mask is not tolerated, the mask (or just the oxygen tubing) may be held near the child's nose or mouth.

- Airway burns are considered as a 'special case' (refer to **Burns and Scalds**). Examine for soot in the nostrils and mouth, erythema and blistering of the lips and hoarseness of the voice. These suggest potential airway injury. These children require early endotracheal intubation and may deteriorate faster than adults due to the smaller diameter of their airway. Unless there is somebody at the scene who is trained in pre-hospital paediatric anaesthesia and difficult paediatric airway management who can electively intubate the child, it is best to transport the child rapidly (time-critical transfer) and to pre-alert the hospital so they can have suitable experts standing by. If the airway swelling becomes life-threatening, and the airway cannot be controlled any other way, needle cricothyroidotomy may be required. Surgical airways should be avoided for those under the age of 12 years.

6. Cervical Spine

- Cervical spinal immobilisation is essential when an injury to the neck has possibly occurred.

Manual immobilisation is initially used, although the subsequent use of a correctly sized cervical collar, head blocks and forehead/chin tapes and a scoop stretcher or a long board where the child has to be extricated is recommended. If the child is combative, this may not be possible and manual immobilisation may be the only possible method (refer to **Spinal Injury and Spinal Cord Injury**).

7. Breathing

- A child's chest wall is readily deformable and may withstand significant force. As a result, significant intra-thoracic injuries can occur without any apparent external chest wall signs.

- **Auscultate** the chest if practical.

- **Look at** the chest for bruising and record the rate and adequacy of breathing. Chest wall movement and the presence of any wounds should be sought. Poor excursion may suggest an underlying pneumothorax.

- **Feel** for rib fractures, or surgical emphysema.

- This should reveal good, bilateral air entry and the absence of any added sounds. Listen specifically to the following three areas:
  1. above the nipples in the mid-clavicular line
  2. in the mid-axilla under the armpits
  3. at the rear of the chest, below the shoulder blades when it is possible to access this area.

TABLE 4.6 – Normal Respiratory Rates

Age	Respiratory rate
<1 year	40–60 breaths per minute
1–2 years	25–35 breaths per minute
2–5 years	25–30 breaths per minute
5–11 years	20–25 breaths per minute
>12 years	15–20 breaths per minute

- Percuss the chest if possible assessing for hyporesonance or hyperresonance.

- Assess for:
  - Tension pneumothorax.
  - Massive haemothorax.
  - Sucking chest wounds (open pneumothorax).
  - Flail chest.

NB Refer to **Thoracic Trauma** for the management of these conditions.

NB Distended neck veins are very difficult to see in children and in shock may be absent.

7.1 Management

- If ventilation is inadequate (see below) the child's respiratory effort may require support from bag-valve-mask ventilation and high-flow oxygen. Assist ventilation at a rate equivalent to the

Trauma Emergencies in Children – Overview

normal respiratory rate for the age of the child (refer to Table 4.6) if:

- The child is hypoxic (SpO$_2$ <90%) and remains so after 30–60 seconds on high concentration O$_2$.
- Respiratory rate is <50% normal or >3 times normal.

■ Treat life-threatening chest injuries as per appropriate guideline (see above).

8. Circulation

■ Refer to Medical Emergencies – Recognition of Circulatory Failure.

■ Look firstly for evidence of significant external haemorrhage and treat as per haemorrhage guideline (refer to Figures 4.3 and 4.4).

■ Assess the:
- Brachial or carotid pulses; record rate and volume (refer to Table 4.7):
  - tachycardia (with a poor pulse volume) suggests shock
  - bradycardia also occurs in the shocked child but is a **PRE-TERMINAL SIGN**.

■ Respiratory rate: elevated due to compensatory mechanisms in shock.

■ Capillary refill time: measure on the forehead or sternum.

■ Colour.

■ Conscious level.

■ Examine the abdomen for signs of intra-abdominal bleeding (if present, assume a pelvic fracture).

■ Remember cardiac tamponade in a rapidly deteriorating child where chest injury has occurred and where the cause of the deterioration is not clear (refer to **Thoracic Trauma**).

TABLE 4.7 – Normal Heart Rates

Age	Heart rate
<1 year	110–160 beats per minute
1–2 years	100–150 beats per minute
2–5 years	95–140 beats per minute
5–11 years	80–120 beats per minute
>12 years	60–100 beats per minute

■ Significant blood losses are seen in long bone fractures, with even greater losses (double the volume) seen when the fracture is open, when compared to a corresponding closed fracture; for example, in a closed femoral fracture 20% of the circulating blood volume may bleed into the surrounding tissues compared to losses of 40% from an open femoral shaft fracture.

8.1 Management

■ Splintage, traction and full immobilisation can reduce blood loss and pain.

■ Where possible, vascular access can be gained en-route to hospital, reducing the time spent on scene. Use the widest possible cannula for the veins available.

■ In paediatric trauma, **5 ml/kg fluid boluses** are used and repeated as needed to improve clinical signs (e.g. RR, HR, capillary refill, conscious level) **towards normal**. Seek advice to exceed maximum dose in trauma.

NB Hypotensive resuscitation practices (as used in adult trauma) should not be used in children.

■ Due to their physiological reserves, children maintain their systolic blood pressures in the face of major blood loss, with hypotension only occurring at a very late stage. Significant cardiovascular compromise and even cardiac arrest may occur if volume resuscitation were to be delayed until a child had reached such an advanced state of hypovolaemia.

■ Following IV fluid resuscitation, in paediatric major trauma with catastrophic haemorrhage, a bolus of tranexamic acid should be given, if available (refer to **Tranexamic Acid**).

9. Disability – Assessment

■ **Record** the initial level of consciousness using the AVPU Scale (below):

A	Alert
V	Responds to voice
P	Responds to painful stimulus
U	Unresponsive

as well as:

- The time of the AVPU assessment.
- Pupil size, shape, symmetry and response to light.
- Whether the child was moving some or all limbs. If there is no movement, then ask the child to 'wiggle' their fingers and toes, paying particular note to movements peripheral to any injury site.
- Any abnormalities of posture.
- If the child is not **alert** they should be considered time-critical. A formal GCS (see Appendix) en-route may be valuable to the receiving hospital but should only be recorded if it can be accurately done and does not delay transfer.

Trauma Emergencies in Children – Overview

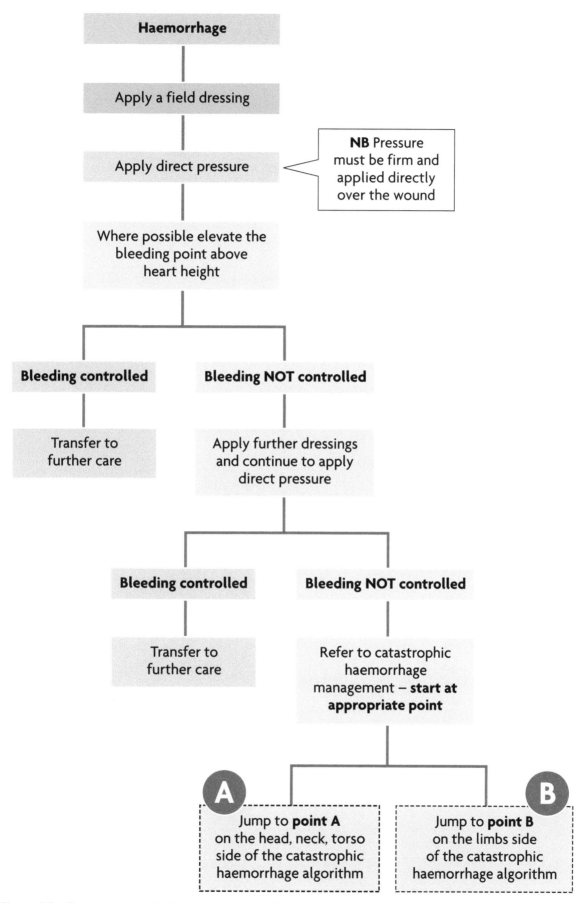

Figure 4.3 – The management of haemorrhage algorithm.

Trauma Emergencies in Children – Overview

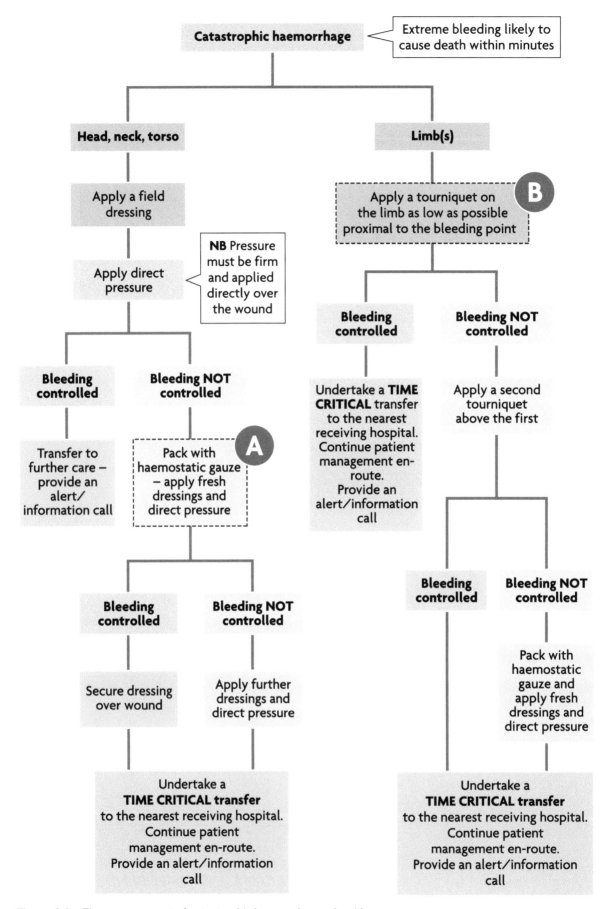

Figure 4.4 – The management of catastrophic haemorrhage algorithm.

Trauma Emergencies in Children – Overview

9.1 Stepwise Disability Management

- Confusion or agitation in an injured child may result directly from a significant head injury, but equally may be secondary to hypoxia from an impaired airway or compromised breathing or else hypoperfusion due to blood loss and shock.

- The management of any child with impaired consciousness is based on ensuring an adequate airway, oxygenation, ventilation and circulation.

- Always measure the blood glucose level in any child with altered consciousness. If hypoglycaemia is detected, refer to **Glycaemic Emergencies in Adults and Children** for treatment.

10. Exposure

- Children will lose heat rapidly when exposed for examination and immobilised during trauma care. Do protect the child from a cold environment during your assessment.

- Expose children 'piecemeal' if possible, replacing a piece of clothing before removing the next, as stripping a child may cause insecurity or embarrassment as well as exposing them to cold.

- If the child is **TIME-CRITICAL** they must be packaged appropriately (with full spinal immobilisation – or improvisation as tolerated – and pelvic splint if pelvic injury suspected) and transported rapidly to hospital.

- An **alert/information call should be given for all TIME-CRITICAL children** en-route.

- If there is no apparent problem with the primary survey, a secondary survey may be commenced en-route. This should not delay the transfer to definitive care.

10.1 Secondary Survey

- This is a systematic and careful review of each part of the injured child looking for non-critical and/or occult injuries. It is rarely possible to complete this before hospital in a seriously injured child.

- Any deterioration in the child's condition mandates an immediate return to the primary survey and the problem sought and treated.

- Dress and immobilise any injuries found as required. Perform a simple **MSC** check of **ALL** four limbs (see below):

M	MOTOR	Test for movement
S	SENSATION	Apply light touch to evaluate sensation
C	CIRCULATION	Assess pulse and skin temperature

11. Analgesia in Trauma

- As would happen for an adult, a child's pain must be addressed once their life-threatening problems have been attended to (refer to **Pain Management in Children**).

- **Note:** Paediatric drug doses are expressed as mg/kg (refer to **specific drug protocols/Page-for-Age** for dosages and information). Drug doses **MUST** be checked prior to **ANY** drug administration, no matter how confident the practitioner may be.

12. Summary

- Read the scene for mechanism of injury and the presence of children.

- Trauma emergencies in childhood are managed using similar priorities and techniques to those used in adult practice. Remember the important anatomical and physiological differences encountered in children whilst performing primary (and/or secondary) surveys.

- Children may **conceal** serious underlying injuries using compensatory mechanisms, so a high index of clinical suspicion is required. Agitation and/or confusion may indicate primary brain injury, but may also be due to inadequate ventilation and/or cerebral perfusion.

SECTION **4** Trauma

Trauma Emergencies in Children – Overview

TABLE 4.8 – Glasgow Coma Scale

Item	Element	Score
Eyes Opening:		
	Spontaneously	4
	To speech	3
	To pain	2
	None	1
Verbal Response:		
	Orientated	5
	Confused	4
	Inappropriate words	3
	Incomprehensible sounds	2
	No verbal response	1
Motor Response:		
	Obeys commands	6
	Localised pain	5
	Withdraws from pain	4
	Abnormal flexion	3
	Extensor response	2
	No response to pain	1

TABLE 4.9 – Modification of Glasgow Coma Scale for Children Aged Under Four Years Old

Item		Score
Eyes Opening:		As per adult scale
Best Verbal Response:	Appropriate words or social smiles, fixes on and follows objects	5
	Cries, but is consolable	4
	Persistently irritable	3
	Restless, agitated	2
	Silent	1
Motor Response:		As per adult scale

Trauma Emergencies in Children – Overview

Trauma Emergencies in Children – Overview

- Important anatomical and physiological differences exist between children and adults – a different approach will often be needed.

- Read the wreckage – toys or child seats may indicate that children have been involved in the incident.

- Assess and continuously re-assess <C>ABCDE.

- Detect time-critical problems as part of the primary survey and transport urgently with a hospital pre-alert.

Bibliography

1. Office for National Statistics (ONS). *Deaths from Suicide That Occurred in England and Wales: April To July 2020*. 2021. Available from: https://www.ons.gov.uk/peoplepopulationandcommunity/birthsdeathsandmarriages/deaths/articles/deathsfromsuicidethatoccurredinenglandandwales/aprilandjuly2020.

Abdominal Trauma

1. Introduction

- Trauma to the abdomen can be extremely difficult to assess even in a hospital setting. In the field, identifying which abdominal structure(s) has been injured is less important than identifying that abdominal trauma itself has occurred.

- It is therefore of major importance to note abnormal signs associated with blood loss and to establish that abdominal injury is the probable cause, rather than being concerned with, for example, whether the source of that abdominal bleeding originates from the spleen or liver.

- There may be significant intra-abdominal injury with very few, if any, initial indications of this at the time the abdomen is examined by the paramedic at the scene.

2. Severity and Outcome

The leading cause of morbidity and mortality is as a result of blunt trauma. Mortality from isolated abdominal stab wounds is approximately 1–2%.

3. Pathophysiology

The abdomen may be described as three anatomical areas:

a **Abdominal cavity**
b **Pelvis**
c **Retro-peritoneal area**

a **Abdominal cavity** – extends from the diaphragm to the pelvis. It contains the stomach, small intestine, large intestine, liver, gall bladder and spleen.
The upper abdominal organs are partly in the lower thorax and lie under the lower ribs; therefore, fractures of lower ribs may damage abdominal structures such as the liver and spleen.

b **Pelvis** – contains the bladder, the lower part of the large intestine and, in the female, the uterus and ovaries. The iliac artery and vein overlie the posterior part of the pelvic ring and may be torn in pelvic fractures, adding to already major bleeding.

c **Retro-peritoneal area** – lies against the posterior abdominal wall, and contains the kidneys and ureters, pancreas, abdominal aorta, vena cava and part of the duodenum. These structures are attached to the posterior abdominal wall, and are often injured by shearing due to rapid deceleration forces.

4. Abdominal Injuries

Blunt trauma – the most common pattern of injury seen; results from direct blows to the abdomen or rapid deceleration. Blunt trauma may also result from all phases of a blast.

- The spleen, liver (hepatic tear) and 'tethered' structures such as the duodenum are the most commonly injured. The small bowel, mesentery and aorta may also sustain injury.

Penetrating trauma – stab wounds, gunshot wounds, blast injuries and other penetrating injuries.

- **Stab wounds** – stab injuries should be assumed to have caused serious damage until proved otherwise. Damage to liver, spleen or major blood vessels may cause massive haemorrhage. **NB** Upper abdominal stab wounds may have caused major intra-thoracic damage if the weapon was directed upwards (refer to **Thoracic Trauma**). Similarly, chest-stabbing injuries may also cause intra-abdominal injury.

- **Gunshot wounds** – tend to cause both direct and indirect injury, due to the forces involved and the chaotic paths that bullets may take. The same rules apply to associated intra-thoracic injuries.

- **Blast injuries** – can lead to both blunt and penetrating injuries. Where an explosion occurs in a confined space, the blast wave can cause injuries to the bowel (perforation and haemorrhage) and penetrating ballistics can lead to organ damage.

5. Assessment and Management

For the assessment and management of abdominal trauma, refer to Table 4.10.

TABLE 4.10 – ASSESSMENT and MANAGEMENT of: Abdominal Trauma

Assess <C>ABCD

- Control any external catastrophic haemorrhage – refer to **Trauma Emergencies in Adults – Overview** and **Trauma Emergencies in Children – Overview**.

- If any of the following **TIME-CRITICAL** features are present:
  - major <C>ABCD problems
  - haemodynamic compromise
  - decreased level of consciousness
  - neck and back injuries – refer to **Spinal Injury and Spinal Cord Injury**, then:

Abdominal Trauma

TABLE 4.10 – ASSESSMENT and MANAGEMENT of: Abdominal Trauma *(continued)*
▪ Start correcting **A** and **B** problems.
▪ Undertake a **TIME-CRITICAL** transfer to nearest appropriate receiving hospital. This may be a major trauma centre; refer to local protocols.
▪ Provide an alert/information call.
▪ Continue patient management en-route.

Assess

▪ Ascertain the mechanism of injury:

▪ **Road traffic collision:** look for impact speed and severity of deceleration; seat-belt and lap-belt use are particularly associated with torn or perforated abdominal structures.

▪ **Stabbing and gunshot wound(s):** consider the length of the weapon used or the type of gun and the range.

▪ **Blast injuries:** blast wave injuries and penetrating ballistics.

Assess the chest and abdomen. **NB** Some abdominal organs (e.g. liver and spleen) are covered by lower ribs/chest margins.

ABDOMEN:

▪ Examine for signs of tenderness.

▪ Examine for external signs of injury (e.g. contusions, seat/lap-belt abrasions).

▪ Examine for evisceration (protruding abdominal organs).

GENTLY palpate the four quadrants of the abdomen for signs of tenderness, guarding and rigidity. Shoulder-tip pain should increase suspicion of injury or internal bleeding.

NB Significant **INTRA-ABDOMINAL TRAUMA** may show little or no evidence in the early stages, therefore DO NOT rule out injury if initial examination is normal.

CHEST:

▪ Fractures of the lower ribs – if confirmed or suspected, refer to **Thoracic Trauma**.

Evisceration

▪ **DO NOT** push protruding abdominal organs back into the abdominal cavity.

▪ Cover protruding abdominal organs with warm moist dressings.

Impaling Objects

▪ Leave impaling objects (e.g. a knife) **IN SITU**.

▪ Secure the object prior to transfer to further care. If the object(s) is pulsating, **DO NOT** completely immobilise it, but allow it to pulsate.

Haemorrhage

▪ In the case of external haemorrhage, apply a field dressing and direct pressure (refer to **Trauma Emergencies in Adults – Overview** and **Trauma Emergencies in Children – Overview**).

Oxygen

▪ Administer high levels of supplemental oxygen (aim for SpO_2 94–98%) (refer to **Oxygen**).

▪ Apply pulse oximeter.

Ventilation

Consider assisted ventilation at a rate of 12–20 respirations per minute if:

▪ Oxygen saturation (SpO_2) is <90% on high levels of supplemental oxygen.

▪ Respiratory rate is <10 or >30 bpm.

▪ Inadequate chest expansion.

Refer to **Airway and Breathing Management**.

Vital Signs

▪ Monitor vital signs.

▪ Monitor ECG.

(continued)

Abdominal Trauma

TABLE 4.10 – ASSESSMENT and MANAGEMENT of: Abdominal Trauma *(continued)*
Pelvic Injuries
■ Consider pelvic injuries – if suspected, refer to **Major Pelvic Trauma**.
Thoracic Injuries
■ If the injury affects the chest, refer to Thoracic Trauma.
Pain Management
■ If pain relief is indicated, refer to **Pain Management in Adults** and **Pain Management in Children**.
Fluid
■ If fluid resuscitation is indicated, refer to **Intravascular Fluid Therapy in Adults** and **Intravascular Fluid Therapy in Children**.
■ **DO NOT** delay on scene for fluid replacement.
Transfer to Further Care
■ Continue patient management en-route.
■ Provide an alert/information call.

KEY POINTS!

Abdominal Trauma

- **Abdominal trauma can be difficult to assess.**
- **Identifying that abdominal trauma has occurred is more important than identifying which structure(s) has been injured, therefore note signs associated with blood loss.**
- **Observe mechanism of injury.**
- **Ensure <C>ABCDs are assessed and managed; consider C-spine immobilisation.**
- **Transport to the nearest appropriate facility, providing an alert/information call en-route. This may be a major trauma centre; refer to local protocols.**

Bibliography

1. Porter A, Snooks H, Youren A, Gaze S, Whitfield R, Rapport F et al. 'Covering our backs': ambulance crews' attitudes towards clinical documentation when emergency (999) patients are not conveyed to hospital. *Emergency Medicine Journal* 2008, 25(5): 292–295.

2. Jorgensen H, Jensen CH, Dirks J. Does pre-hospital ultrasound improve treatment of the trauma patient? A systematic review. *European Journal of Emergency Medicine* 2010, 17(5): 249–253.

3. Best Evidence Topics. Does the 'Seatbelt Sign' predict intra-abdominal injury after motor vehicle trauma in children? *Emergency Medicine Journal* 2012, 29(2): 163–164.

4. Demetriades D, Murray J, Brown C, Velmahos G, Salim A, Alo K, et al. High-level falls: type and severity of injuries and survival outcome according to *age*. *Journal of Trauma and Acute Care Surgery* 2005, 58(2): 342–345.

5. England RJ, Dalton R, Walker J. Penetrating handlebar injury causing bowel evisceration. *Injury Extra* 2004, 35(4): 40–41.

6. Feliciano DV, Burch JM, Spjut-Patrinely V, Mattox KL, Jordan GL Jr. Abdominal gunshot wounds: an urban trauma center's experience with 300 consecutive patients. *Annals of Surgery* 1988, 208(3): 362–370.

7. Hardcastle TC, Coetzee GJN, Wasserman L. Evisceration from blunt trauma in adults: an unusual injury pattern: 3 cases and a literature review. *Scandinavian Journal of Trauma, Resuscitation & Emergency Medicine* 2005, 13: 234–235.

8. Holmes IF, Sokolove PE, Brant WE, Palchak MJ, Vance CW, Owings JT, et al. Identification of children with intra-abdominal injuries after blunt trauma. *Annals of Emergency Medicine* 2002, 39(5): 500–509.

9. Mulholland SA, Cameron PA, Gabbe BJ, Williamson OD, Young K, Smith KL, et al. Pre-hospital prediction of the severity of blunt anatomic injury. *Journal of Trauma and Acute Care Surgery* 2008, 64(3): 754–760. DOI: 10.1097/01.ta.0000244384.85267.c5.

10. Newgard CD, Lewis RJ, Kraus IF. Steering wheel deformity and serious thoracic or abdominal injury among drivers and passengers involved in motor vehicle crashes. *Annals of Emergency Medicine* 2005, 45(1): 43–50.

11. Nishijima DK, Simel DL, Wisner DH, Holmes JF. Does this adult patient have a blunt intra-abdominal injury? *Journal of the American Medical Association* 2012, 307(14): 1517–1527.

12. Owers C, Morgan JL, Garner JP. Abdominal trauma in primary blast injury. *British Journal of Surgery* 2011, 98(2): 168–179.

13. Plurad DS. Blast injury. *Military Medicine* 2011, 176(3): 276–282.

SECTION **4** Trauma

Abdominal Trauma

14. Smith J, Caldwell E, D'Amours S, Jalaludin B, Sugrue M. Abdominal trauma: a disease in evolution. *ANZ Journal of Surgery* 2005, 75(9): 790–794.

15. Sugrue M, Balogh Z, Lynch J, Bardsley J, Sisson G, Weigelt J. Guidelines for the management of haemodynamically stable patients with stab wounds to the anterior abdomen. *ANZ Journal of Surgery* 2007, 77(8): 614–620.

16. Demetriades D, Murray J, Martin M, Velmahos G, Salim A, Alo K, et al. Pedestrians injured by automobiles: relationship of age to injury type and severity. *Journal of the American College of Surgeons* 2004, 199(3): 382–387.

17. Royal College of Emergency Medicine. *Abdominal Trauma*. 2010. Available from: https://www.rcemlearning.co.uk/references/abdominal-trauma/.

SECTION **4** Trauma

Burns and Scalds

1. Introduction

- Burns arise in a number of accident situations, and may have a variety of presentations (refer to Table 4.11), accompanying injuries or pre-existing medical problems associated with the burn injury. Scalds, flame or thermal burns and chemical and electrical burns will all produce a different burn pattern, and inhalation of smoke or toxic chemicals from the fire may cause serious accompanying complications.

- A number of burn patients will also be seriously injured following falls from a height in fires, or injuries sustained as a result of road traffic collision where a vehicle ignites after a collision or crash.

- Explosions will often induce flash burns and other serious injuries due to the effect of the blast wave or flying debris.

- Inhalation of superheated smoke, steam or gases in a fire will induce major airway swelling and respiratory obstruction – refer to Table 4.12 for signs of airway burns. The likelihood of an airway injury increases with the presence of multiple risk factors or signs.

- Non-accidental injury should always be considered when burns have occurred in children and vulnerable adults including older people, in particular where the mechanism of injury described does not match the injury sustained, or there is inconsistency in the history (refer to **Safeguarding Children** and **Safeguarding Adults at Risk**).

TABLE 4.11 – Burns/Scalds

Electrical
Search for entry and exit sites. Assess ECG rhythm. The extent of burn damage in electrical burns is often impossible to assess fully at the time of injury (refer to **Electrical Injuries**).

Thermal
The skin contact time and temperature of the source determine the depth of the burn. Scalds with boiling water are frequently of short duration as the water flows off the skin rapidly. Record the type of clothing (e.g. wool retains the hot water). Those resulting from hot fat and other liquids that remain on the skin may cause significantly deeper and more serious burns. Also the time to cold water and removal of clothing is of significant impact.

TABLE 4.11 – Burns/Scalds *(continued)*

Chemical
It is vital to note the nature of the chemical. Alkalis in particular may cause deep, penetrating burns, sometimes with little initial discomfort. Certain chemicals such as phenol or hydrofluoric acid can cause poisoning by absorption through the skin and therefore must be irrigated with COPIOUS amounts of water for a minimum of 20 minutes (this should be continued until definitive care is available if patient condition and water supply allows) (refer to **CBRN**).

TABLE 4.12 – Signs/Increased Risk of Airway Burns

Signs
- Facial or neck burns.
- Soot in the nasal and oral cavities.
- Coughing up blackened sputum.
- Cough and hoarseness.
- Difficulty with breathing and swallowing.
- Blistering around the mouth and tongue.
- Scorched hair, eyebrows or facial hair.
- Stridor or altered breath sounds such as wheezing.
- Loss of consciousness.
- Fires/blasts in enclosed spaces.

- Preceding long-term illness, especially chronic bronchitis and emphysema, will seriously worsen the outcome from airway burns.

- Remember that a burn injury may be preceded by a medical condition causing a collapse (e.g. elderly patient with a stroke collapsing against a radiator).

- Burns can be very painful (refer to **Pain Management in Adults** and **Pain Management in Children**).

2. Burn Severity

- Refer to Wallace's Rule of Nines or the Lund and Browder chart to assess total body surface area (TBSA).

- For small or large burns (<15% or > 85%), it is acceptable to use the patient's palmar surface including the fingers as a size estimate. This equates to approximately 1% TBSA.

Burns and Scalds

- Be aware of the risk of underestimating the size of burns with patients with large breasts or who are obese. These factors can significantly affect the proportion of TBSA using standardised charts.

- Use all of the burn area, but do not consider areas of erythema as this is often transient in the initial phases of a burn. Do not try to differentiate between levels of burn (superficial, partial thickness, full thickness etc.) as it is impractical to estimate the depth of burns in the initial hours following injury.

- Only a rough estimate is required; an accurate measure is not possible in the early stages. However, the size of a burn may well influence referral and management pathways.

3. Assessment and Management

- For the assessment and management of burns and scalds in adults, refer to Table 4.13.

TABLE 4.13 – ASSESSMENT and MANAGEMENT of: Burns and Scalds
Ensure Scene Safety for Rescuer and Patient   **If safe to do so, stop the burning process:**   ▪ Remove from the burn source.   ▪ Brush off dry chemical.

Assess <C>ABCD
 ▪ If any of the following **TIME-CRITICAL** features present:
   – major **<C>ABCD** problems
   – airway burns (soot or oedema around the mouth and nose)
   – history of hot air or gas inhalation; these patients may initially appear well but can deteriorate very rapidly and need complex airway intervention
   – respiratory distress
   – evidence of circumferential (completely encircling) burns of the chest, neck, limb
   – significant facial burns
   – burns >15% in adults and >10% in children TBSA
   – presence of other major injuries, then:
 ▪ Start correcting A and B and undertake a **TIME-CRITICAL** transfer to nearest appropriate hospital according to local care pathways.
 ▪ Continue patient management en-route.
 ▪ Provide an alert/information call.

Specifically Assess   ▪ Airway patency as early intervention may be required with inhalational burns; if intubation is impossible, needle cricothyroidotomy is the management of choice.   ▪ Waveform capnography should be used whenever intubation is performed.   ▪ Breathing for rate, depth and any breathing difficulty (refer to **Airway and Breathing Management**).   ▪ Evidence of trauma – for neck and back trauma, refer to **Spinal Injury and Spinal Cord Injury**.   ▪ Co-existing or precipitating medical conditions.
Oxygen   ▪ Administer supplemental **oxygen** via a non-rebreathing mask – SpO_2 readings may be false due to carboxyhaemoglobin.
Cool/Irrigate the Burn   ▪ Irrigate with copious amounts of water as soon as is practicable; this can still be effective up to 3 hours after the injury. Irrigate the burn for a maximum of 20 minutes, except for chemical burns (acid, alkalis and other corrosive substances) where the irrigation can be continued up to 1 hour.   ▪ Cut off burning or smouldering clothing, providing it is not adhering to the skin.   ▪ Remove any constricting jewellery, including rings.   ▪ **DO NOT** use ice or ice water, as this can worsen the burn injury and exaggerate hypothermia.   ▪ Use saline if no other irrigant available.

(continued)

Burns and Scalds

Burns and Scalds

TABLE 4.13 – ASSESSMENT and MANAGEMENT of: Burns and Scalds *(continued)*

- Gel-based dressings may be used but water treatment is preferred.
- Alkali burns require prolonged irrigation – continue until definitive care.

Assess Burn Size

- Rule of Nines or Lund and Browder Chart.
- Patient's palmar surface, including adducted fingers.
- Consider obesity and large breasts when estimating burn size.

Dress the Burn

- Use small sheets of clingfilm – do not wrap around limbs but layer the film.
- In the absence of clingfilm, use a clean cotton sheet.

Elevate the affected area if possible, to reduce the risk of oedema.

NB Do not apply creams, ointments, wet gauze or non-adherent dressings; they interfere with the assessment process.

Fluid Resuscitation

- Large burns (>10% in children and >15% in adults) require intravenous fluids (refer to **Intravascular Fluid Therapy in Adults** and **Intravascular Fluid Therapy in Children**).
- If IV access is required, obtain on a non-affected limb where possible.

Wheezing

If the patient is wheezing as a result of smoke inhalation:

- Administer nebulised salbutamol (refer to **Salbutamol**) 6–8 litres of O_2 per minute.

Assess the Need for Analgesia

If indicated (refer to **Pain Management in Adults** and **Pain Management in Children**).

NB Cooling and application of dressings frequently eases pain.

Documentation

- How the patient was burned.
- Time the burn occurred and how long patient was exposed to source of burning.
- Temperature of the source of burning (e.g. boiling water, hot fat etc.).
- Whether first aid was undertaken.
- Time and volume of infusions.

Transfer to Further Care

- The following patients should be conveyed to the nearest Emergency Department (ED), from where transfer to a regional burns unit may be arranged, if necessary, or transfer in accordance with local referral pathways:
  - Any full-thickness burns.
  - Deep dermal burns affecting more than 5% of TBSA in adults, and all deep dermal burns in children.
  - All chemical and electrical burns (including lightning injuries).
  - Any high-pressure steam injury.
  - Any burn associated with suspected non-accidental injury, regardless of the complexity.
  - Burns affecting the face, hands, feet, genitalia perineum or any flexural surface such as the neck, axilla, elbow or knee.
  - Circumferential deep dermal burns.
  - Burns associated with suspected inhalation injury.
  - Burns associated with co-morbidities that may affect wound healing or increase the risk of complications.
  - Burns associated with significant other injuries.
  - Burns associated with sepsis.
  - People who may require admission due to social circumstances or inadequate pain control.
- Complete documentation.

Burns and Scalds

| **TABLE 4.13** – ASSESSMENT and MANAGEMENT of: Burns and Scalds *(continued)* |

Alkali Burns to the Skin and Eye(s)

▪ When irrigating the eyes, ensure that the fluid runs away from the contralateral eye to avoid contamination.

▪ Irrigate with water and continue en-route to hospital – it may take hours of irrigation to neutralise the alkali. This also applies to eyes, which require copious and continual irrigation, ideally with water or saline in the absence of a water source.

Acid/Chemical Burns to the Skin and Eye(s)

▪ When irrigating the eyes, ensure that the fluid runs away from the contralateral eye to avoid contamination.

▪ Irrigate copiously, ideally with water or otherwise with saline if no water source available.

NB Specific treatment agents may be available in industrial settings with on-site medical/first aid.

Chemical Burns

▪ **DO NOT** wrap in clingfilm.

NB Do not attempt to neutralise chemicals, as additional heat will be generated, which may increase tissue damage.

Circumferential Burns

▪ Encircling completely a limb or digit. Full thickness burns may be 'limb threatening', and require early in-hospital incision/release of the burn area along the length of the burnt area of the limb (surgical escharotomy).

Corrosive Substances

▪ Following a significant increase in the frequency of serious criminal assaults using acids and corrosive substances, the National Ambulance Resilience Unit (NARU) has advised:

Personal Safety

- Make a dynamic risk assessment and ensure your own safety.
- Exercise extreme caution if there appear to be multiple patients or an ongoing attack.
- Ensure accurate updates are provided to ensure awareness of the severity of the incident, so this can be escalated if necessary.
- Activate specialist resources early where there appear to be multiple patients or extensive contamination.
- Wear eye protection and double-glove nitrile gloves.
- Protect any exposed skin by wearing a jacket to provide a barrier.
- Do not carry out sniff tests on contaminants or containers.
- If attacked, use hands to protect face; skin may blister and scar, but corrosives in the eyes may cause irreversible loss of vision.
- Corrosive vapours should be considered in terms of ventilation from around any contaminants.

Patient Management

- Irrigate freely with clean water for 20 minutes; this includes utilisation of the fire brigade if required.
- If a shower is available, use this with a mild soap which can be used safely on skin.
- Try to ensure any run-off does not come into contact with other uncontaminated parts of the body.
- Early and thorough irrigation of the face and eyes is important to reduce the risk of long-term damage.
- Eye irrigation can be achieved by using a bag of saline, giving set (maximum half open) and washing with a gentle stream.
- Contaminated clothing should be cut off whenever possible and left on scene. Do not pull contaminated clothing over the head or remove clothing that is adhering to the skin.
- Contaminated jewellery should be removed, rinsed and placed in a bag or wrapped to avoid skin contact and then handed back to the patient.
- If possible, get the patient to do as much as possible with directions; this may not always be possible but will greatly reduce the exposure to the first responders.
- Do not apply any form of dressing or gel until the burn has been adequately irrigated.
- Minimise on-scene duration for patients with large burns or burns on the face, eyes or hands.

Burns and Scalds

KEY POINTS!

Burns and Scalds

- Airway status can deteriorate rapidly and may need complex interventions available at the emergency departments.
- Stopping the burning process is essential.
- The time from burning is an essential piece of information.
- Pain relief is important.
- Consider non-accidental injury in children and vulnerable adults, including older people.
- When irrigating the eyes, ensure that the fluid runs away from the contralateral eye to avoid contamination.

Bibliography

1. The Royal Children's Hospital Melbourne. *Burns/Management of Burn Wounds.* 2018. Available from: https://www.rch.org.au/clinicalguide/guideline_index/Burns/.

2. National Institute for Health and Care Excellence. *Burns and Scalds.* Clinical Knowledge Summaries. 2017. Available from: https://cks.nice.org.uk/burns-and-scalds#!scenario.

3. Porter A, Snooks H, Youren A, Gaze S, Whitfield R, Rapport F et al. 'Covering our backs': ambulance crews' attitudes towards clinical documentation when emergency (999) patients are not conveyed to hospital. *Emergency Medicine Journal* 2008, 25(5): 292–295.

4. Ayers DE, Kay AR. Management of burns in the wilderness. *Travel Medicine and Infectious Disease* 2005, 3(4): 239–248.

5. Boots RJ, Dulhunty JM, Paratz J, Lipman J. Respiratory complications in burns: an evolving spectrum of injury. *Clinical Pulmonary Medicine* 2009, 16(3): 132–138.

6. Cancio LC. Airway management and smoke inhalation injury in the burn patient. *Clinics in Plastic Surgery* 2009, 36(4): 555–567.

7. Enoch S, Roshan A, Shah M. Emergency and early management of burns and scalds. *British Medical Journal* 2009, 338(7700): 937–941.

8. Hassan Z, Wong JK, Bush J, Bayat A, Dunn KW. Assessing the severity of inhalation injuries in adults. *Burns: Journal of the International Society for Burn Injuries* 2010, 36(2): 212–216.

9. Hermans MHE. A general overview of burn care. *International Wound Journal* 2005, 2(3): 206–220, 222–223.

10. Karpelowsky JS, Rode H. Basic principles in the management of thermal injuries. *South African Family Practice* 2008, 50(3): 24–31.

11. Karpelowsky JS, Wallis L, Madaree A, Rode H. South African Burn Society burn stabilisation protocol. *South African Medical Journal* 2007, 97(8): 574–547.

12. Marek K, Piotr W, Stanislaw S, Stefan G, Justyna G, Mariusz N, et al. Fibreoptic bronchoscopy in routine clinical practice in confirming the diagnosis and treatment of inhalation burns. *Burns: Journal of the International Society for Burn Injuries* 2007, 33(5): 554–560.

13. Mlcak RP, Suman OE, Herndon DN. Respiratory management of inhalation injury. *Burns: Journal of the International Society for Burn Injuries* 2007, 33(1): 2–13.

14. Muehlberger T, Ottomann C, Toman N, Daigeler A, Lehnhardt M. Emergency pre-hospital care of burn patients. *The Surgeon: Journal of the Royal Colleges of Surgeons of Edinburgh & Ireland* 2010, 8(2): 101–104.

15. New Zealand Guidelines Group. *Management of Burns and Scalds in Primary Care.* Wellington: Accident Compensation Corporation, 2007. Available from: http://www.moh.govt.nz/notebook/nbbooks.nsf/0/BD251444C120DC0FCC2573210070271D/$file/burns_full.pdf.

16. Palmieri TL. Inhalation injury: research progress and needs. *Journal of Burn Care and Research* 2007, 28(4): 549–554.

17. Pham TN, Gibran NS. Thermal and electrical injuries. *Surgical Clinics of North America* 2007, 87(1): 185–206.

18. Singh S, Handy J. The respiratory insult in burns injury. *Current Anaesthesia and Critical Care* 2008, 19(5–6): 264–268.

19. Spanholtz TA, Theodorou P, Amini P, Spilker G. Severe burn injuries: acute and long-term treatment. *Deutsches Arzteblatt* 2009, 106(38): 607–613.

20. Suzuki M, Aikawa N, Kobayashi K, Higuchi R. Prognostic implications of inhalation injury in burn patients in Tokyo. *Burns: Journal of the International Society for Burn Injuries* 2005, 31(3): 331–336.

21. Walton JJ, Manara AR. Burns and smoke inhalation. *Anaesthesia & Intensive Care Medicine* 2005, 6(9): 317–321.

22. Wasiak J, Cleland H, Campbell F. Dressings for superficial and partial thickness burns. *Cochrane Database of Systematic Reviews* 2007, 3: CD002106.

23. Durrant CAT, Simpson AR, Williams G. Thermal injury: the first 24 h. *Current Anaesthesia and Critical Care* 2008, 19(5–6): 256–263.

24. Freiburg C, Igneri P, Sartorelli K, Rogers F. Effects of differences in percent total body surface area estimation on fluid resuscitation of transferred burn patients. *Journal of Burn Care and Research* 2007, 28(1): 42–48.

25. Hackenschmidt A. Burn trauma priorities for a patient with 80% total body surface area burns. *Journal of Emergency Nursing* 2007, 33(4): 405–408.

26. Hussain S, Ferguson C. Assessing the size of burns: which method works best? *Emergency Medicine Journal* 2009, 26(9): 664–666.

27. Singer AJ, Dagum AB. Current management of acute cutaneous wounds. *New England Journal of Medicine* 2008, 359(10): 1037–1046.

28. Williams C. Successful assessment and management of burn injuries. *Nursing Standard* 2009, 23(32): 53–54.

SECTION 4 Trauma

Burns and Scalds

29. Allison K, Porter K. Consensus on the pre-hospital approach to burns patient management. *Emergency Medicine Journal* 2004, 21(1): 112–114.

30. Williams G, Dziewulski P. Intravascular fluid therapy in burns injury. In Group. TJRCALGD, editor, 2011.

31. Blackhurst H. Estimation of burn surface area using the hand. *BestBets* 2007. Available from: http://www.bestbets.org/bets/bet.php?id=01516.

32. Jose RM, Roy DK, Vidyadharan R, Erdmann M. Burns area estimation: an error perpetuated. *Burns: Journal of the International Society for Burn Injuries* 2004, 30(5): 481–482.

33. Jose RM, Roy DK, Wright PK, Erdmann M. Hand surface area: do racial differences exist? *Burns: Journal of the International Society for Burn Injuries* 2006, 32(2): 216–217.

34. Lee J-Y, Choi J-W, Kim H. Determination of hand surface area by sex and body shape using alginate. *Journal of Physiological Anthropology* 2007, 26(4): 475–483.

35. Liao C-Y, Chen S-L, Chou T-D, Lee T-P, Dai N-T, Chen T-M. Use of two-dimensional projection for estimating hand surface area of Chinese adults. *Burns: Journal of the International Society for Burn Injuries* 2008, 34(4): 556–559.

36. Yu C-Y, Hsu Y-W, Chen C-Y. Determination of hand surface area as a percentage of body surface area by 3D anthropometry. *Burns: Journal of the International Society for Burn Injuries* 2008, 34(8): 1183–1189.

37. Hidvegi N, Nduka C, Myers S, Dziewulski P. Estimation of breast burn size. *Plastic and Reconstructive Surgery* 2004, 113(6): 1591–1597.

38. Ichiki Y, Kato Y, Kitajima Y. Assessment of burn area: most objective method. *Burns: Journal of the International Society for Burn Injuries* 2008, 34(3): 425–426.

39. Singer AJ, Brebbia J, Soroff HH. Management of local burn wounds in the ED. *American Journal of Emergency Medicine* 2007, 25(6): 666–671.

40. Cuttle L, Kravchuk O, Wallis B, Kimble RM. An audit of first-aid treatment of pediatric burns patients and their clinical outcome. *Journal of Burn Care & Research: Official publication of the American Burn Association* 2009, 30(6): 1028–1034.

41. Health Protection Agency. *HPA Compendium of Chemical Hazards.* London: HPA, 2007. Available from: http://www.hpa.org.uk/Topics/ChemicalsAndPoisons/CompendiumOfChemicalHazards.

Electrical Injuries

1. Introduction

- Electrical injury is potentially life-threatening.
- Incidents which occur in the workplace are likely to involve high-voltage electricity (415 volts), whereas incidents which occur in the home are likely to involve lower-voltage electricity (240 volts).
- Electrical injury may also result from a lightning strike, which may deliver up to 300 kV.

2. Incidence

- In the UK, approximately 1,000 people at work are injured following contact with an electrical supply; of these, 25 will die from their injuries.[1]
- Approximately five fatalities from lightning strike are recorded in Britain each year.[2]

3. Severity and Outcome

- Electrical injury can cause serious multi-system damage, leading to morbidity and mortality. This is caused by electric shock and tissue damage from the thermal effects along the current pathway.

The nature and extent of injury depends on:

- The voltage and whether it is alternating (AC) or direct (DC).
- The magnitude of the current.
- Resistance to current flow.
- Duration of exposure to the current.
- The pathway of the current – current traversing the myocardium is more likely to be fatal and hand-to-hand travel is more dangerous than hand-to-foot or foot-to-foot.

4. Pathophysiology

Injury occurs when electricity passes through the body, causing:

- **Cardiac** arrhythmias (e.g. ventricular fibrillation); cardiorespiratory arrest can arise from the direct effects of the current on cell membranes and smooth muscle as it traverses the myocardium. Myocardial ischaemia can occur due to spasm of the coronary artery.
- **Burns** to the skin at the point of contact (entry and exit) and in deeper tissues, including viscera, muscles and nerves as thermal energy traverses the body and tends to follow neurovascular bundles. Unusual burn patterns may be left on the body following a lightning strike.
- **Trauma** including joint dislocation, fractures and compartment syndrome can arise from sustained tetanic muscle contraction, falling or being thrown.
- **Muscular paralysis** may occur from contact with high-voltage electricity affecting the central respiratory control system or respiratory muscles.
- **Pregnancy** can be affected depending on the magnitude and duration of contact with the current.

5. Assessment and Management

For the assessment and management of electrical injuries, refer to Table 4.14 and Figure 4.5.

Electrical Injuries

TABLE 4.14 – ASSESSMENT and MANAGEMENT of: Electrical Injuries
⚠ **Ensure Scene Safety for Rescuer and Patient**
▪ ⚠ **DO NOT** approach the patient until the electricity supply is cut off and you are certain it is safe to approach.
NOTE: Attach defibrillator pad at the earliest opportunity and keep defibrillator with the patient until handover to hospital staff.
Assess <C>ABCD
▪ If any of the following **TIME-CRITICAL** features present: – major **<C>ABCD** problems   – cardiorespiratory arrest (to **Advanced Life Support**)   – facial/airway burns (refer to **Airway and Breathing Management**)   – cardiac arrhythmia (refer to **Cardiac Rhythm Disturbance**)   – significant trauma (refer to appropriate **Trauma** guideline)   – extensive burns (refer to **Burns and Scalds**), then:
▪ Start correcting <C>ABCD and undertake a **TIME-CRITICAL** transfer to nearest receiving hospital or specialist burns unit if appropriate.
▪ Continue patient management en-route.
▪ Provide an alert/information call.
Burn Process
▪ Remove smouldering clothing and shoes to prevent further thermal injury (refer to **Burns and Scalds**).
Specifically Assess
▪ Airway patency, as early intervention may be required.
▪ Breathing for rate, depth and any breathing difficulty (refer to **Airway and Breathing Management**).
▪ Heart rate/rhythm – undertake a 12-lead ECG: – arrhythmias are unlikely to develop in cases of contact with domestic low-voltage sources once the patient is isolated from the current   – in cases of contact with high-voltage sources, arrhythmias may develop later.
▪ Evidence of trauma (e.g. neck and back, burns) (refer to appropriate **Trauma** guideline).
▪ Magnitude of the current, i.e. domestic low voltage (≤240 volts) or industrial high voltage (>480 volts).
Oxygen
▪ Monitor the patient's SpO$_2$, administer oxygen to achieve saturations of >94% if the patient presents as hypoxaemic on air (refer to **Oxygen**).
Fluid
▪ If fluid resuscitation indicated, refer to **Intravascular Fluid Therapy in Adults** and **Intravascular Fluid Therapy in Children**.
Assess the Need for Pain Relief
▪ If pain relief is indicated, refer to **Pain Management in Adults** and **Pain Management in Children**.
Transfer to Further Care
▪ **ALL** patients exposed to high-voltage current.
▪ Patients exposed to a domestic or low-voltage electrical source who are asymptomatic, with no injuries and have normal initial 12-lead ECG may not require hospital assessment.

Electrical Injuries

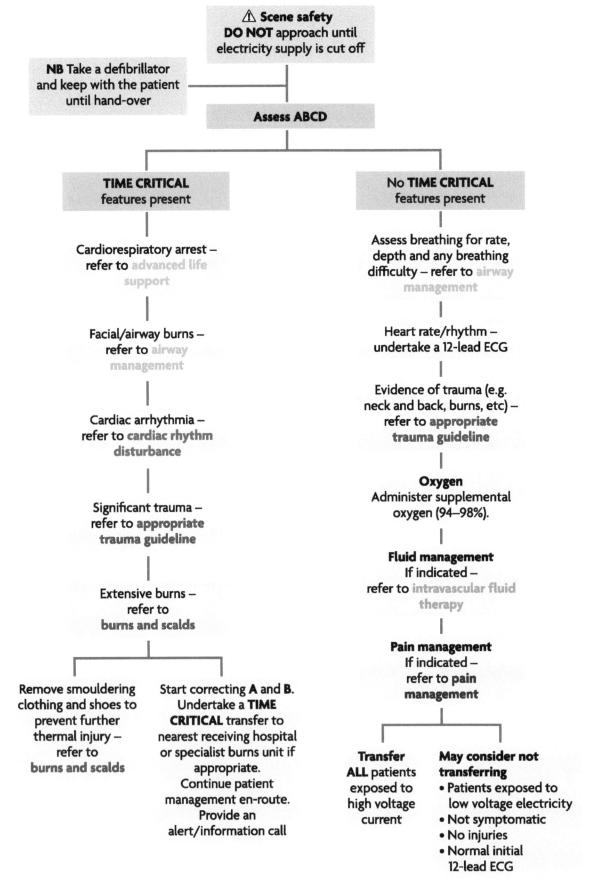

NB Take a defibrillator and keep with the patient until hand-over

⚠ **Scene safety**
DO NOT approach until electricity supply is cut off

Assess ABCD

TIME CRITICAL features present

Cardiorespiratory arrest – refer to advanced life support

Facial/airway burns – refer to airway management

Cardiac arrhythmia – refer to cardiac rhythm disturbance

Significant trauma – refer to appropriate trauma guideline

Extensive burns – refer to burns and scalds

Remove smouldering clothing and shoes to prevent further thermal injury – refer to burns and scalds

Start correcting **A** and **B**. Undertake a **TIME CRITICAL** transfer to nearest receiving hospital or specialist burns unit if appropriate. Continue patient management en-route. Provide an alert/information call

No **TIME CRITICAL** features present

Assess breathing for rate, depth and any breathing difficulty – refer to airway management

Heart rate/rhythm – undertake a 12-lead ECG

Evidence of trauma (e.g. neck and back, burns, etc) – refer to appropriate trauma guideline

Oxygen
Administer supplemental oxygen (94–98%).

Fluid management
If indicated – refer to intravascular fluid therapy

Pain management
If indicated – refer to pain management

Transfer ALL patients exposed to high voltage current

May consider not transferring
- Patients exposed to low voltage electricity
- Not symptomatic
- No injuries
- Normal initial 12-lead ECG

Figure 4.5 – Assessment and management of electrical injuries algorithm.

SECTION **4** Trauma

Electrical Injuries

KEY POINTS!

Electrical Injuries

- Scene safety.
- Manage cardiac/respiratory arrest.
- Consider trauma.
- Severe tissue damage may be present despite apparently minor injury.
- Exposure to domestic voltage may not require hospitalisation.

Further Reading

Further important information and evidence in support of this guideline can be found in the Bibliography.[3,4,5,6,7,8,9,10,11]

Bibliography

1. Health and Safety Executive. *Electrical Injuries*. 2010. Available from: http://www.hse.gov.uk/electricity/injuries.htm.

2. Royal College of Emergency Medicine. *Electrical Injuries – Lightning.* Clinical Knowledge Summaries. 2017. Available from: https://www.rcemlearning.co.uk/references/electrical-injuries-lightning/.

3. Soar J, Perkins GD, Abbas G, Alfonzo A, Barelli A, Bierens JJLM, et al. European Resuscitation Council Guidelines for Resuscitation 2010 Section 8: cardiac arrest in special circumstances: electrolyte abnormalities, poisoning, drowning, accidental hypothermia, hyperthermia, asthma, anaphylaxis, cardiac surgery, trauma, pregnancy, electrocution. *Resuscitation* 2010, 81(10): 1400–1433.

4. Gauglitz GG, Herndon DN, Jeschke MG. Emergency treatment of severely burned pediatric patients: current therapeutic strategies. *Pediatric Health* 2008, 2(6): 761–775.

5. Yarrow J, Moiemen N, Gulhane S. Early management of burns in children. *Paediatrics and Child Health* 2009, 19(11): 509–516.

6. Ritenour AE, Morton MJ, McManus JG, Barillo DJ, Cancio LC. Lightning injury: a review. *Burns: Journal of the International Society for Burn Injuries* 2008, 34(5): 585–594.

7. Dollery W. Cardiac monitoring not needed in household electrical injury if the patient is asymptomatic and has a normal ECG. *BestBets*, 2003. Available from: http://www.bestbets.org/bets/bet.php?id=9.

8. Bailey B, Gaudreault P, Thivierge RL. Cardiac monitoring of high-risk patients after an electrical injury: a prospective multicentre study. *Emergency Medicine Journal* 2007, 24(5): 348–352.

9. Adukauskiene D, Vizgirdaite V, Mazeikiene S. Electrical injuries. [In Lithuanian]. *Medicina (Kaunas)* 2007, 43(3): 259–266. Abstract in English available from: http://www.ncbi.nlm.nih.gov/pubmed/17413256.

10. Spies C, Trohman RG. Narrative review: electrocution and life-threatening electrical injuries. *Annals of Internal Medicine* 2006, 145(7): 531–537.

11. Vierhapper MF, Lumenta DB, Beck H, Keck M, Kamolz LP, Frey M. Electrical injury: a long-term analysis with review of regional differences. *Annals of Plastic Surgery* 2011, 66(1): 43–46. DOI: 10.1097/SAP.0b013e3181f3e60f.

Falls in Older Adults

1. Introduction

- Falls are defined as an unintentional or unexpected loss of balance resulting in coming to rest on the floor, the ground or an object below knee level. The impact of a fall on the individual and their family is not to be underestimated, with falls often leading to a fear of falling and potentially having psychological as well as physical effects. A fall is distinguished from a collapse, which occurs as a result of an acute medical problem such as an acute arrhythmia, a transient ischaemic attack or vertigo.[2] A fall can be precipitated by an acute medical condition, and the actual cause of the fall can be very difficult to establish on initial presentation. This guideline covers falls from a standing height. Falls from above standing height or 2 metres above the ground are not covered in this guideline (refer to **Section 4 – Trauma**).

- The term 'mechanical fall' is **not** an appropriate term to use when describing a fall; it implies that a benign aetiology for an older person's fall exists and it is inaccurate, is inconsistently used, is not associated with a discrete fall evaluation and does not predict outcomes.[3]

- Older people in contact with healthcare professionals for any reason should be asked routinely whether they have fallen in the past year, asked about the frequency, context and characteristics of the falls and referred to appropriate falls prevention pathways as per local arrangements. Recently, the SAFER 2 study (a large multi-centre cluster randomised controlled trial) has shown that a paramedic protocol for assessment of older patients (aged ≥65) who have fallen, with an option to refer direct to a community-based falls service (in place of conveyance to the ED), is safe, inexpensive and reduced subsequent 999 calls in those patients. There was no overall difference in outcomes (whether taken to hospital or managed at home) between the trial arms.

2. Incidence

- Falls are the leading cause of emergency calls in the over 65s and account for 10–25% of emergency ambulance responses each year for adults aged over 65 years.[4] In the London Ambulance Service alone, there were 70,380 incidents of people aged 65 and over who were coded as presenting with a fall in the period for 2015–16.

- Falls represent the second leading cause of accidental injury death worldwide and the leading cause of injury-related mortality in the UK.[5] Every year 1 in 3 people aged over 65 and up to 1 in 2 aged over 80 will fall at least once.[6] By 2025, it is estimated that this will account for over 3.2 million falls in people over the age of 65 in England alone.[7] Up to 14,000 people will die each year as a result of a fall and a subsequent fractured neck or femur.[8]

- A fall of <2 metres is the commonest mechanism of injury in older patients.[9]

3. Severity and Outcome

- As part of the normal ageing process, there are a loss of bone density, loss of muscle tone, skin changes and often increased poly-pharmacy. A simple fall in an older person may result in a much more significant injury than would be seen in a younger person. Clinicians should have a higher index of suspicion of injury in older people. However, falls are not a part of normal ageing and are typically due to pathological changes described earlier.

- The *Silver Book*[10] recommends ways in which emergency admissions for older people can be reduced and emphasises that health and social care services must adapt to meet older people's urgent care needs, including ambulance services.

- Falls can be a marker of frailty, which is associated with common syndromes of ageing including immobility, incontinence, susceptibility to the side effects of medication, delirium and dementia, all of which increase the complexity of the presentation and may indicate a change in normal health status. Frail older people typically suffer falls indoors. For a person with frailty, a relatively small event (e.g. a minor infection, a new medication or constipation) may trigger a sudden and dramatic functional decline. Frailty is a clinically recognised state of increased vulnerability. It results from ageing associated with a decline in the body's physical and psychological reserves. This can cause the person to fall and also to struggle to recover following a fall. It is important to recognise the presence of frailty in weighing the benefits and risks of any intervention or treatment plan. Even if no injury has been sustained, further assessment and support post-fall will enable the provision of the right care and support for the person.

4. Risk Factors for Falls

Refer to Table 4.15.

- Risk factors for falls can be broadly classified into three categories:
  - intrinsic factors – relating to the person
  - extrinsic factors – relating to the person's environment
  - exposure to risk.

- However, it is recognised that falls often result from the dynamic interactions of risks in all categories.

- Intrinsic risk factors include changes in the body caused by the normal ageing process, certain medical conditions, excessive alcohol, being physically inactive or a combination of these.

Falls in Older Adults

- It is important to consider dementia and cognitive impairment in the assessment of a patient who has fallen. As many as 11–26% of patients presenting with a fall will have cognitive impairment, some of which will be undiagnosed.[11,12] Patients with dementia are more likely to fall, to have more falls and to sustain an injury (such as a hip fracture or head injury)

from the fall. If sustaining an injury, the outcomes are worse for the patient, their family, the health service and society at large. It is therefore vital to recognise this as a high-risk group.

- It is important that the cause of the fall is considered so that the correct pathways are chosen or excluded; red flags should always be excluded and modifiable factors considered.

TABLE 4.15 – Intrinsic and Extrinsic Falls Risk Factors[13]

Common intrinsic risks of falls[14]	Common extrinsic risk factors of falls
- lower extremity weakness - previous falls - gait and balance disorders - visual impairment - depression - functional and cognitive impairment - dizziness - low body mass index - urinary incontinence - postural hypotension - female sex - being over age 80. **Other intrinsic causes of falls** - sensory deficit (poor vision, peripheral neuropathy) - musculoskeletal disease (osteoarthritis, proximal muscle weakness, previous joint replacement) - other neurodegenerative conditions - central nervous system disease (cognitive dysfunction, vestibular hypofunction, cerebrovascular disease, cerebral hypoperfusion) - Parkinson's disease and Parkinsonism.	- polypharmacy (use of multiple medications) - psychotropic medications - poor lighting (especially on stairs), glare and shadows - low ambient temperature - wet, slippery or uneven floor surfaces - thresholds at room entrances - obstacles and tripping hazards, including clutter - chairs, toilets or beds being too high, low or unstable - inappropriate or unsafe walking aids - inadequately maintained wheelchairs, for example brakes not locking - improper use of wheelchairs, for example failing to clear foot plates - unsafe or absent equipment, such as handrails - pets, such as cats and dogs - loose-fitting footwear and clothing, such as trailing dressing gowns - access to the property, wheelie bins, the garden, uneven ground.

Many medicines cause postural hypotension and may contribute to over 20% of extrinsic falls. Common causes are:

- cardiac drugs:
  - antiarrhythmics (e.g. digoxin)
  - alpha-blockers (e.g. doxazosin)
  - beta-blockers (e.g. bisoprolol, atenolol)
  - ACE inhibitors (e.g. ramipril, lisinopril)
  - angiotensin 2 blockers (e.g. losartan, candesartan)
  - diuretics (e.g. furosemide, bumetanide, spironolactone, bendroflumethiazide)
  - calcium channel blockers (e.g. amlodipine, diltiazem)
- urological drugs (e.g. oxybutynin)
- neuropsychiatric drugs:

  - Parkinson's drugs (e.g. madopar, sinemet, ropinirole)
  - tricyclic antidepressants (e.g. amitriptyline)
  - antipsychotics (e.g. haloperidol, risperidone)
  - painkillers (e.g. opioids)

- In these patients, a formal medicines optimisation review may be indicated by the GP practice or another clinical lead (following local guidance).

Certain activities can be 'high risk' because of the specific interaction of risk factors involved, for example poor balance combined with standing on a stool to change a light bulb or reach a high shelf. To understand falls risk in the environment fully, it is important to observe a person moving around in their environment; referral for a falls assessment in line with local pathways/guidelines will facilitate this.

Falls in Older Adults

4.1 Risks Related to a 'Long Lie'

- A 'long lie' is usually defined as someone who has been on the floor for over 1 hour and has been unable to get up. However, the estimated time on the floor, and mobility while there, may vary greatly and will influence clinical decision making, i.e. a patient who has been completely immobile on the floor for several hours will be at higher risk than someone who can move across the floor but cannot pull themselves up onto a chair or bed or into a standing position.

- Anyone who has experienced a long lie is at a higher risk of complications, such as pneumonia, pressure areas, rhabdomyolysis, dehydration and hypothermia.

- Increasing age and other co-morbidities will increase the risk of complications from a long lie; each patient will need to be assessed on an individual basis, to plan ongoing management.

5. Psychology of Falling

- Depression, fear of falling and other psychological problems are common effects of falls. Loss of confidence as well as social withdrawal and loneliness can occur, even when there is no injury. A person who is fearful about falls will often avoid physical activity, become weaker and may fall more as a result. Social isolation can also result if the person stops going out.

- Some older people are fearful that a fall may lead to a loss of independence, being admitted to hospital, loss of control over their life or being rehoused. These well-documented fears can lead to patients not reporting falls, masking symptoms or being reluctant to attend an emergency department or be referred to their GP. Clinicians should be aware of these issues and help to promote independence. Positive conversations should emphasise the simple things that can be done to reduce falls risk, regain confidence and maintain independence through referral to other services for further assessment and support.

6. Assessment and Management

6.1 Specific History and Examination Considerations

- A thorough and careful physical examination is required, along with a high index of suspicion, to exclude common but easily missed injuries, such as rib fractures, spinal fractures and delayed presentation of a previous head injury.

- A perceived minor injury, such as a fractured rib, may have more serious long-term consequences for an older person, e.g. pulmonary contusions. Minor injuries can also lead to a temporary loss of independence, which, for a person with frailty, can become permanent without aggressive

management and rehabilitation. Every rib fracture increases the risk of dying by 15% in frail older people.

- The history taken on scene needs to be thorough and well documented in the patient record; where possible it should be corroborated with relatives, carers or associated healthcare professionals.

- Initial assessment should exclude the possibility of syncope. Transient loss of consciousness should be assumed to have occurred unless proven otherwise (refer to **Altered Level of Consciousness**).

- Clinical history should include:
  - details of any previous altered level of consciousness, including number and frequency
  - the person's medical history and family history of cardiac disease (for example, personal history of heart disease and family history of sudden cardiac death)
  - current medication that may have contributed to altered level of consciousness (for example, diuretics)
  - vital signs and NEWS2 score (for example, pulse rate, respiratory rate and temperature) – repeat if clinically indicated
  - lying and standing blood pressure if clinically appropriate
  - other cardiovascular and neurological signs.

- Consider scoring a patient's level of frailty.[1]
  - The Rockwood Clinical Frailty Scale (CFS) is a judgement-based frailty assessment tool. It is not validated for people under the age of 65 years or those with long-term disabilities. Frailty must be sensed, described and measured: not guessed. If the patient you are assessing is acutely unwell and over 65 years, consider using the CFS, as per local pathways.
  - The score is based on the patient's baseline, so use the tool to score how the patient was 2 weeks ago (prior to deterioration) or their usual level of functioning when well, rather than how they present today. If possible, cross-reference what the patient describes to you with a description from relatives/carers.
  - Do NOT compare the patient to the pictures (e.g. person using walking aids) alone to make a judgement on the level of frailty.

- It is important to consider that medications prescribed for co-morbidities may complicate the clinical picture and presentation.

6.2 12-Lead ECG

- Older people who fall should have a 12-lead ECG (with auto-interpretation) recorded. This must be interpreted by the assessing clinician unless they are confident the patient has complete recall of the event and clearly describes an

Falls in Older Adults

extrinsic factor that caused the fall. Transient loss of consciousness (TLoC) should be assumed unless proven otherwise; refer to TLOC and NICE guidance.

> **'Red flags' for syncope seen in a 12-lead ECG include:**
>
> 🚩 conduction abnormality (for example, complete right or left bundle branch block, atrial fibrillation or any degree of heart block)
>
> 🚩 evidence of a long or short QT interval
>
> 🚩 any ST segment or T wave abnormalities.

6.3 Atrial Fibrillation (AF) and Falls

- Ensure that a 12-lead ECG is performed on any patient with an irregular pulse felt on palpation to identify the underlying rhythm.

- It may be difficult to determine if AF is new or not. The patient may know themselves or have been told that they have an irregular heartbeat/AF, or you may be able to contact the patient's health professional/GP or review care plans/medical notes.

- If the patient is asymptomatic and has a heart rate below 120/minute, and an extrinsic cause of the fall has been identified, consider contacting a GP to have a clinical discussion and agree a care plan.

- Consider conveyance to hospital as a priority if the patient is found to be in atrial fibrillation (AF) after a fall and has symptoms such as:
  - altered mental status
  - dizziness
  - chest pain
  - heart rate above 120/minute
  - dyspnoea
  - palpitations
  - hypotension.

- If the patient has AF and has had a potential syncope, refer to local syncope pathways or follow local guidance.

6.4 Postural Hypotension

- Postural hypotension should be checked for if there is no clear extrinsic cause of the fall, if there are no features to suggest an alternative cause, if symptoms are typical such as light-headedness, dizziness or feeling weak and faint on standing and if the patient is being considered for management at home.

- Procedure for checking postural hypotension:

1 Identify if you are going to need assistance to stand the patient and simultaneously record a BP. Use a manual sphygmomanometer if possible and definitely if the automatic machine fails to record.

2 Explain procedure to the patient.

3 The first BP should be taken after lying for at least 5 minutes.

4 The second BP should be taken after standing in the first minute.

5 A third BP should be taken after standing for 3 minutes.

6 This recording can be repeated if the BP is still falling.

7 Symptoms of dizziness, light-headedness, vagueness, pallor, visual disturbance, feelings of weakness and palpitations should be documented.

8 A positive result is: a. A drop in systolic BP of 20 mmHg or more (with or without symptoms) b. A drop to below 90 mmHg on standing even if the drop is less than 20 mmHg (with or without symptoms) c. A drop in diastolic BP of 10 mmHg with symptoms (although clinically much less significant than a drop in systolic BP).

- If the patient is unable to stand, a sitting reading may be taken; however, the sensitivity of the test is reduced in this case.

- Symptomatic postural hypotension is a significant finding that requires further investigation and medication review but rarely requires admission (refer to local guidance for further assessment). Asymptomatic postural hypotension may be managed through primary care.

6.5 Confusion/Delirium

- Confusion is routinely encountered with older adults who have fallen. Often associated with dementia, confusion can also be an indication of an acute pathology presenting as delirium. The patient may be either more (hyperactive delirium) or less (hypoactive delirium) active than normal, although the mixed type is the commonest. However, dementia is characterised by a gradual onset and is not reversible, whereas delirium typically is described as having a rapid onset and is attributed to a reversible cause.

- Be mindful that the confusion may pre-exist and even contribute to the fall, or may occur as a consequence of the fall. This makes gaining a comprehensive and corroborated history very important.

- Where a patient presents with confusion, apply the principles of assessing capacity to consent and be prepared to modify your communication to the needs of the patient. Look for documents such as 'This is me'.[15] Listening to the family, carers or friends who know the patient best may provide clear indications regarding the onset and severity of the confusion, and any changes to it, as this is the most reliable single indicator of delirium, especially in patients who cannot communicate. Where concerns are expressed, you should have

Falls in Older Adults

a high index of suspicion that the confusion is new and requires further investigation or referral.

- New onset confusion can be due to physiological changes resulting from head injury, hypoxia, infection, stroke or transient ischaemic attack (TIA), hypoglycaemia, ketoacidosis, side effects of medications or drugs and the effects of withdrawal from drugs or alcohol. In addition, other causes could include carbon monoxide poisoning, encephalitis or meningitis, electrolyte imbalance, post-seizure and, more rarely, an underactive thyroid gland, tumour, thiamine deficiency, hypo/hyperparathyroidism and Cushing's disease.

6.6 Skin Assessment for Adults

- Consider performing an assessment of the patient's skin after a fall to ensure that the skin is intact. Gain the patient's consent or act in their best interests. Consider patient dignity and body temperature as you examine them. Pay attention to areas of bony prominence that are subject to pressure when lying on a hard surface, such as the back of head and ears, shoulders, elbows, lower back and buttocks, hips, inner knees and heels.

- A skin assessment in adults should take into account:
  - any pain or discomfort reported by the patient
  - skin integrity in areas of pressure
  - colour changes or discoloration
  - variations in heat, firmness and moisture (due to incontinence, oedema or dry or inflamed skin).

- If any concerns are identified, consider referral to community nursing teams in line with local pathways/guidance.

- Refer to Figure 4.6 for an aid to assessing skin breakdown.

6.7 Continence

- Confirm the patient's usual toileting/continence regime. Consider new symptoms, including dysuria, increased frequency of urination, suprapubic tenderness, urgency and polyuria, but do not carry out a urine dipstick in the absence of symptoms of UTI.[16]

- If continent/partially continent, consider if they are likely to be able to locate and physically get to the toilet/commode, rearrange clothes and clean the genital area and hands.

- If incontinent/partially continent, consider if the patient/carer is able to manage pads/catheter care, rearrange clothes, clean the genital area and hands and dispose of waste safely. Community nursing services may be available to provide rapid continence assessment including recatheterisation.

6.8 How to Decide If the Patient Could Be Managed in the Community

- Decisions on whether to manage a patient at home/in the community can be challenging and should be made following a comprehensive history, clinical assessment and examination. Decisions on the best management of an older person who has fallen are made on a risk/benefit basis and may benefit from discussion with locally agreed clinical contacts. These could include ambulance service clinical advice lines or other healthcare professionals clinical advice lines using a shared decision making approach, and should always consider the views of the patient and relatives/carers. The final referral decision will also depend on the availability and responsiveness of local community health and social care services. Well-structured advice on how to assess and make decisions related to choosing an appropriate clinical pathway improves patient safety and outcomes.[17]

- There are also risks in taking an older person to hospital, including institutionalisation and/or deconditioning (the consequence of prolonged bed rest, leading to loss of functional status through reduced muscle mass and strength). The decline in muscle mass and strength has been linked to falls, functional decline, increased frailty, immobility and healthcare-associated infection.[18]

- Some older people who fall may prefer to be managed in the community or at home, and where possible this should be supported, particularly where family/carers can also provide support. Following a comprehensive patient assessment and wider review of the circumstances of the fall (having excluded injuries/acute illness), ambulance clinicians should provide the referral for this to occur in line with local pathways and guidance.

6.9 Ongoing Referral

- All older people who have fallen resulting in an ambulance call/attendance, but who are then managed at home, should be offered referral pathways as per local guidelines. The purpose of referral/re-referral is to prevent further falls and injury.

- Referrals should take into account current care plans and other health and social care organisations already involved in the patient's care.

- Decision making should be a shared process, including the patient and their family/carers/other health and social care professionals/any person holding their lasting power of attorney for health and welfare.

Falls in Older Adults

Early warning sign - blanching erythema

Areas of discoloured tissue that blanch when fingertip pressure is applied and the colour recovers when pressure is released, indicating damage is starting to occur but can be reversed.

On darkly pigmented skin, blanching does not occur and changes to colour, temperature and texture of skin are the main indicators.

Grade 1	Grade 2	Grade 3	Grade 4
Non-blanchable erythema	**Partial thickness skin loss**	**Full thickness skin loss**	**Full thickness tissue loss**
Intact skin with non-blanchable redness, usually over a bony prominence.	Loss of the epidermis/dermis presenting as a shallow open ulcer with a red/pink wound bed without slough or bruising.[1]	Subcutaneous fat may be visible but bone, tendon or muscle is not visible or palpable.	Extensive destruction with exposed or palpable bone, tendon or muscle. Slough may be present but does not obscure the depth of tissue loss.
Darker skin tones may not have visible blanching but the colour may differ from the surrounding area.	May also present as an intact or open/ruptured blister.	Slough may be present but does not obscure the depth of tissue loss. May include undermining or tunnelling.[2]	Often includes undermining or tunnelling.[2]
The affected area may be painful, firmer, softer, warmer or cooler than the surrounding tissue.			

Moisture lesions

Moisture lesions are skin damage due to exposure to urine, faeces or other body fluids.

a) Location:
Located in peri-anal, gluteal, cleft, groin or buttock area. Not usually over a bony prominence.

b) Shape:
Diffuse often multiple lesions. May be 'copy', 'mirror' or 'kissing' lesion on adjacent buttock or anal cleft. Linear.

c) Edges:
Diffuse irregular edges.

d) Necrosis:
No necrosis or slough. May develop slough if infection present.

e) Depth:
Superficial partial thickness skin loss. Can enlarge or deepen if infection present.

f) Colour:
Colour of redness may not be uniform. May have pink or white surrounding skin (maceration). Peri-anal redness may be present.

Where pressure ulcers commonly occur

The shaded points indicate vulnerable areas of the body with regards to pressure ulcers

Head
Back
Knees
Toes
Heels
Elbows
Base of Spine
Bottom

[1] Bruising can indicate deep tissue injury

[2] The depth of a Grade 3 or 4 pressure ulcer varies by anatomical location. Areas such as the bridge of the nose, ears, occiput and malleolus do not have fatty tissue so the depth of these ulcers may be shallow. In contrast areas which have excess fatty tissue can develop deep Grade 3 pressure ulcers where bone, tendon, muscle is not directly visible or palpable.

Figure 4.6 – Grading tool for assessing skin breakdown. Reproduced with kind permission of Healthcare Improvement Scotland.

Falls in Older Adults

- Referral to services via locally agreed pathways may result in:
  - multifactorial falls risk assessment
  - frailty assessment
  - assessment of care needs, including telecare.

6.10 Falls Prevention[5]

- Ambulance clinicians have a role to play in having conversations with people who are at risk of falling, or who have fallen, to try and prevent further falls. The evidence-based Making Every Contact Count (MECC) approach[19] can be applied or other locally agreed methods of ensuring health prevention messages can be given. A MECC interaction takes a matter of minutes and is not intended to add to busy workloads, but should be part of the conversations after a fall or with patients who have been identified as at risk of falling. Evidence suggests that the broad adoption of the MECC approach could potentially have a significant impact on the health of the population.

- Support can be given to older people at risk of falling by routinely asking them about falls and encouraging them to stay active and connected, eat well and reduce alcohol intake, to reduce the risk of falling and to improve outcomes if a fall happens. Consider discussing the measures a person can take to reduce their risk factors for falling, the exercises recommended by falls teams or other healthcare professionals, the preventable nature of some falls and where they can seek further advice and assistance.

- Consider leaving the patient with an information leaflet about falls prevention and suggesting telecare options, such as a pendant-type alarm so help can be summoned for any further falls, or simple solutions to providing a safer physical environment. Conversations can take place with carers/family members if the person has cognitive impairment.

- Older people in contact with healthcare professionals for any reason should be asked **routinely** whether they have fallen in the past year and asked about the frequency, context and characteristics of the falls. Referrals should be made in line with local guidance.

TABLE 4.16 – ASSESSMENT and MANAGEMENT of: Falls in Older People
Primary Survey
▪ Assess <C>ABCD

▪ Are any of the following **TIME-CRITICAL** features present?
  – major <C>ABC problems
  – altered level of consciousness
  – neck and back injuries.

▪ Refer to:
  – **Airway and Breathing Management**
  – **Trauma Emergencies in Adults – Overview**

SECONDARY ASSESSMENT – TRAUMA
Assess for Trauma/Injuries
▪ Make a careful physical assessment, as relatively minor injury can have significant consequences in older people; all should include a pain assessment.
Caution
▪ Older adults can present with major trauma with seemingly minor mechanism of injury and kinetic energy transfer.
▪ Assess specifically for evidence or risk of occult bleeding (intracranial, intrathoracic and intra-abdominal).
▪ Be mindful of apparently minor head injuries in the context of concurrent anticoagulant, clopidogrel or combination anti-platelet therapy and other coagulopathies. Refer to local policies around minor head injuries.

Falls in Older Adults

TABLE 4.16 – ASSESSMENT and MANAGEMENT of: Falls in Older People *(continued)*
Consider Spinal Injuries[20,21,22,23,24,25]
<ul><li>Falls are a more frequent cause of spinal 'cord' injury in the older patient.</li><li>Central Cord Syndrome (CCS) may occur in susceptible older individuals with degenerative spinal disease who sustain hyperextension of the cervical spine during trauma.</li><li>CCS can result from ground height/level surface falls and is also associated with flexion and compression trauma mechanisms.</li></ul>
Specifically Assess
<ul><li>Motor weakness in the upper and lower extremities; any impairment will usually be greater in the upper extremities than in the lower extremities, especially in the muscle of the hands.</li><li>Sensory impairment may be variable and limited to mild sensory impairment in the hands or feet.</li></ul>
Note
<ul><li>In trauma, CCS may present with/without bony spinal injury.</li><li>Assess carefully for fragility fractures.</li></ul> Refer to:<ul><li>**Head Injury**</li><li>**Spinal Injury and Spinal Cord Injury**</li><li>**Thoracic Trauma**</li><li>**Abdominal Trauma**</li><li>**Limb Trauma**.</li></ul> Also consider:<ul><li>skin integrity/turgor (long lies)</li><li>chest injuries, including thorough palpation of the chest to exclude rib fractures</li><li>osteoporosis.</li></ul>
SECONDARY ASSESSMENT – MEDICAL
Intrinsic Factors
<ul><li>Take a detailed history of how the fall is described.</li><li>Can the history be corroborated by a reliable third party?</li><li>Document a NEWS2 score[26,27]</li></ul> Refer to:<ul><li>**Altered Level of Consciousness** (in particular transient loss of consciousness (TLoC))</li><li>**Glycaemic Emergencies in Adults and Children**</li><li>**Cardiac Rhythm Disturbance**</li><li>**Convulsions in Adults**</li><li>**Sepsis** (check for pyrexia or hypothermia as markers of possible infection)</li><li>**Stroke/Transient Ischaemic Attack**</li><li>**Overdose and Poisoning in Adults and Children** (intentional or unintentional).</li></ul> Also consider:<ul><li>possible bleeding – intracranial, intrathoracic, intra-abdominal</li><li>acute kidney injury</li><li>delirium</li><li>frailty, in line with local guidance</li><li>polypharmacy – use of multiple medicines.</li></ul>
REVIEW OF SYSTEMS
<ul><li>Cardiovascular (include postural hypotension assessment and consider 12-lead ECG).</li><li>Respiratory system.</li><li>Gastrointestinal (bowels, bladder, eating/drinking).</li><li>Genitourinary (if a urinary infection is suspected clinically with signs such as increased frequency/dysuria and suprapubic tenderness, follow local guidelines).</li></ul>

(continued)

4 SECTION **Trauma**

Falls in Older Adults

TABLE 4.16 – ASSESSMENT and MANAGEMENT of: Falls in Older People *(continued)*
▪ Neurological (stroke/TIA).
▪ Musculoskeletal.
▪ Hair, skin (look for pressure areas) and nails.
▪ Mental health (anxiety, depression, fear of falling).
HISTORY OF THE FALL

▪ Consider using a mnemonic such as SPLAT:[28]
  – **Symptoms** prior to and at the time of the fall.
  – **Previous** falls, near falls and/or fear of falling.
  – **Location** to identify contributing environmental factors (for example, was there poor lighting, was footing poor, did they trip or were they in a crowd?).
  – **Activity** the person was participating in when they fell (for example, were they turning, changing position or transferring?).
  – **Time** of day the fall occurred (falls in the morning could be due to postural hypotension and later in the day could be due to fatigue).

▪ Ascertain how the fall happened, considering the following:
  – Intrinsic factors (including pathological factors, e.g. collapse).
  – Extrinsic factors (including environment, trips and hazards).
  – Can the patient recall the fall in detail? Words such as 'I must have tripped' suggest no recollection (refer to **Altered Level of Consciousness**, especially transient loss of consciousness (TLoC)).
  – Can the history of the fall be corroborated by a reliable third party?
  – Is there a history of previous falls? When did these occur, with what frequency; were any injurious?
  – Is this fall consistent with previous falls or different?
  – Is there a new onset of confusion?
  – Are alcohol/drugs/medication involved?

FUNCTIONAL ASSESSMENT – MOBILITY

▪ Mobility must be considered to:
  – help exclude injury
  – determine if mobility is a factor contributing to falls risk
  – ascertain a person's ability to function safely at home following the fall.

▪ Observe the person getting up from their chair, balancing on standing, walking round their home (including turning) and sitting down again – using their usual walking aid if applicable.
▪ A formal test may be used as per local guidance, such as the 'get up and go' test or the 'turn 180 degrees' test.[29,30,31]
▪ A mobility assessment should also take into account the use and state of repair of walking aids.
▪ While the person is moving around, check they can weight-bear and consider how steady, safe and confident they are.
▪ Where possible, find out the person's normal mobility status; it may be that a person has limited mobility normally but is managing well with regular visits from family or carers and/or with equipment such as a commode.

▪ Consider whether the person is able to:
  – get to the toilet/commode and transfer on and off it safely
  – access a drink or simple snack
  – manage on the stairs if this is essential to get to the toilet/bed or other rooms
  – take essential medications as prescribed
  – summon help.

▪ If the person receives care, consider the timing of the next visit. Contact the agency if possible. Information may be found in a care plan.
▪ Consider local services that may be available to respond to support the person in remaining at home and avoiding hospital admission.

Falls in Older Adults

TABLE 4.16 – ASSESSMENT and MANAGEMENT of: Falls in Older People *(continued)*

OTHER CONSIDERATIONS

General

- Look/ask for other information about the patient, such as anticipatory care plans that may detail preferences for place of care, clinical management, home care input, nursing/therapy input, including access to electronic care records.
- Ask about lasting power of attorney/end of life and DNACPR/ReSPECT decisions.
- In cases of worsening chronic confusion, consider referral back to GP/local pathway.
- Consider frailty in line with local guidance.
- Consider the need for senior clinical advice/support.

Extrinsic Factors

- Walking aids (consider correct use, state of repair, suitability for the patient).
- Footwear (good fit, not worn out, adequate grip and support).
- Floor surfaces (clear of obstructions, carpets and rugs not frayed or lifted, not slippery or wet/greasy).
- Lighting.
- Temperature.
- Spectacles and hearing aids, telecare alarm (worn, clean and working, regular check-ups).
- Home safety, smoke alarms, clutter and other trip hazards, exit routes, crime risks, ability to self-evacuate, home adaptations.
- Shared decision making with patients and families/carers/other health and social care professionals.
- Respect the autonomy of the individual.

Safeguarding

- Ask the patient if they feel safe.
- Consider the need for additional support, protection or referral for safeguarding.
- Refer to **Safeguarding Adults at Risk**.

Social Context

- Housing type.
- Living alone or with spouse/family/partner.
  - What is the level of support offered by the above?
  - Does the patient have caring responsibilities? What are they and are they affected by the fall?
  - What are the existing support/care packages in place? When is the next planned visit of carers?
  - Are the patient/relatives and carers coping or in denial?
- Is support/care assessment required?
- Does the family and carer burden/need require assessment?
- Does the patient suffer social isolation/loneliness?

Referral and Safety-Netting

- Follow local policies or guidelines.
- Patients who have fallen should be offered referral to a community-based falls service to enable secondary prevention as per local policies.[17]

Prevention

- Self-care and links to the voluntary sector.
- Signposting.
- Local leaflets, contacts and information.
- Written advice for non-injury falls.
- Advice for the patient, their relatives and carers.
- Make Every Contact Count (MECC) opportunities.

Falls in Older Adults

Falls in Older Adults

- The term 'mechanical fall' is not an appropriate term to use when describing a fall.

- Initial assessment should exclude the possibility of syncope.

- A thorough and careful physical examination is required along with a high index of suspicion, to exclude common but easily missed injuries.

- Some older people who fall may prefer to be managed in the community or at home, and where possible this should be supported, particularly where family/carers can also provide support.

- All older people who have fallen resulting in an ambulance call/attendance, but are then managed at home, should be offered referral pathways as per local guidelines.

- Ambulance clinicians have a role to play in talking with people who are at risk of falling, or who have fallen, to try and prevent further falls.

Further Reading

Further important information and evidence in support of this guideline can be found in the Bibliography.[32]

Other useful resources include:

http://www.sciencedirect.com/science/article/pii/S096663621400705X

Bibliography

1. Rockwood K et al. A global clinical measure of fitness and frailty in elderly people. *Canadian Medical Association Journal* 2005, 173(5): 489–495.: https://pubmed.ncbi.nlm.nih.gov/16129869/.

2. National Institute for Health and Clinical Excellence. *Falls in Older People* (QS86). London: NICE, 2017. Available from: https://www.nice.org.uk/guidance/qs86/chapter/Quality-statement-6-Medical-examination-after-an-inpatient-fall.

3. Tirrell GP, Lipsitz LA, Liru SW. Is there such a thing as a mechanical fall? *American Journal of Emergency Medicine* 2016, 34(3): 582–585. DOI: 10.1016/j.ajem.2015.12.009.

4. Ambulance Service Network Community Health Services Forum. Falls prevention: new approaches to integrated falls prevention services. *Briefing* 2012: 234. NHS Confederation. Available from: http://www.nhsconfed.org/~/media/Confederation/Files/Publications/Documents/Falls_prevention_briefing_final_for_website_30_April.pdf.

5. National Institute for Health and Clinical Excellence. *Falls in Older People: Assessing Risk and Prevention* (CG161). London: NICE, 2013.

6. Department of Health. *National Service Framework for Older People*. London: The Stationery Office, 2001.

7. Projecting Older People Population Information Systems. Available from: http://www.poppi.org.uk/index.php?pageNo=315&PHPSESSID=eujokv2jii3d1vj7q70s8eh5c4&sc=1&loc=8640&np=1.

8. Age UK. *Stop Falling: Start Saving Lives and Money*. London: Age UK, 2012.

9. Trauma Audit and Research Network. *Major Trauma in Older People*. Manchester: University of Manchester, 2017.

10. British Geriatrics Society. *Quality Care for Older People with Urgent and Emergency Care Needs: The 'Silver Book'*. London: British Geriatric Society, 2012.

11. Davies AJ, Kenny RA. Falls presenting to the accident and emergency department: types of presentation and risk factor profile. *Age and Ageing*. 1996, 25(5): 362–366.

12. Bloch F, Jegou D, Dhainaut J-F et al. Do ED staffs have a role to play in the prevention of repeat falls in elderly patients? *American Journal of Emergency Medicine* 2009, 27(3): 303–307.

13. College of Occupational Therapists. *Occupational Therapy in the Prevention and Management of Falls in Adults* (Practice Guideline). London: COT, 2015.

14. American Geriatrics Society. *AGS/BGS Clinical Practice Guideline: Prevention of Falls in Older Persons*. 2010. Available from: http://www.medcats.com/FALLS/frameset.htm.

15. Alzheimer's Society. *This Is Me*. Available from: https://www.alzheimers.org.uk/download/downloads/id/3423/this_is_me.pdf.

16. Scottish Intercollegiate Guidelines Network. *Management of Suspected Bacterial Urinary Tract Infection in Adults* (SIGN Guideline 88). Edinburgh: Healthcare Improvement Scotland, 2012.

17. Snooks HA et al. Support and assessment for fall emergency referrals (SAFER) 2. *Health Technol Assess* 2017, 21(13): 1–218. Available from: https://www.ncbi.nlm.nih.gov/pubmed/28397649.

18. Gillis A, McDonald B. Deconditioning in the hospitalised elderly. *Canadian Nurse* 2005, 101(6): 16–20. Available from: https://www.ncbi.nlm.nih.gov/pubmed/16121472.

19. Health Education England. *Making Every Contact Count*. Available from: http://www.makingeverycontactcount.co.uk/.

20. Shadler P, Shue J, Giradi F. Central Cord Syndrome, A review of epidemiology, treatment and prognostic factors. *JSM Neurosurg Spine* 2016, 4(3): 1075.

21. National Association of Emergency Medical Technicians. *Prehospital Trauma Life Support*. Spinal Trauma, Chapter 17 Geriatric Trauma, St Louis, MO: Mosby JEMs Elsevier, 2016. Especially Ch. 11, Spinal trauma and Ch. 17 Geriatric trauma.

Falls in Older Adults

22. McKinley M, Santos K, Meade M et al. Incidence and outcomes of spinal cord injury clinical syndromes. *J Spinal Cord Med* 2007, 30: 215–224.

23. Ryan M, Henderson J. The epidemiology of fractures and fracture-dislocations of the cervical spine. *Injury* 1992, 23: 38–40.

24. Mandavia D, Newton K. Geriatric trauma. *Emerg Med Clin North Am* 1998, 16: 257–274.

25. Wagner R, Jagoda A. Spinal cord syndromes. *Emerg Med Clin North Am* 1997, 15: 699–711.

26. Cei M et al. In-hospital mortality and morbidity of elderly medical patients can be predicted at admission by the modified early warning score: a prospective study. *Int J Clin Pract* 2009, 63(4): 591–595.

27. Romero-Ortunoa R, Wallisa S, Birama R, Keevila V, Clinical frailty adds to acute illness severity in predicting mortality in hospitalized older adults: an observational study. *European Journal of Internal Medicine* 2016, 35: 24–34.

28. Bauman CA, Milligan JD, Patel T et al. Community-based falls prevention: lessons from an Inter-professional Mobility Clinic. *J Can Chiropr* 2014, 58(3): 300–311.

29. Mathias S, Nayak USL, Isaacs B. Balance in elderly patients: the 'get-up and go' test. *Arch Phys Med Rehabil*. 1986, 67: 387–389.

30. Nevitt MC, Cummings SR, Kidd S, Black D. Risk factors for recurrent nonsyncopal falls. A prospective study. *Journal of the American Medical Association* 1989, 261(18): 2663–2668.

31. Simpson JM, Worsfold C, Reilly E, Nye N. A standard procedure for using TURN180: testing dynamic postural stability among elderly people. *Physiotherapy* 2002, 88(6): 342–353.

32. Murdoch I, Turpin S, Johnson B, MacLullich A, Losman E. *Geriatric Emergencies*. London: Wiley-Blackwell, 2015.

Head Injury

1. Introduction

- Head injury is a common presentation to the ambulance service. This can range from a trivial head injury through to severe life-threatening injuries.

- Head injury is defined as any trauma to the head other than superficial injuries to the face. Each year, 1.4 million people attend emergency departments (EDs) in England and Wales with a recent head injury. Between 33% and 50% of these are children aged under 15 years. Annually, about 200,000 people are admitted to hospital with head injury. Of these, 20% have features suggesting skull fracture or have evidence of brain injury. Most patients recover without specific or specialist intervention, but others experience long-term disability or even die from the effects of complications that could potentially be minimised or avoided with early detection and appropriate treatment. While there are a range of patients who require further assessment in hospital, a number of patients may be safely discharged at the scene, providing the patient, family members and carers are given appropriate verbal and written head injury advice.

- The incidence of death from head injury is low, with as few as 0.2% of all patients attending Emergency Departments with a head injury dying as a result of this injury. Ninety-five percent of people who have sustained a head injury present with a normal or minimally impaired conscious level (Glasgow Coma Scale (GCS) greater than 12) but the majority of fatal outcomes are in the moderate (GCS 9–12) or severe (GCS 8 or less) head injury groups, which account for only 5% of attenders at ED.

- It is estimated that 25–30% of children aged under 2 years who are hospitalised with head injury have an abusive head injury (refer to **Safeguarding Children**).

- Ambulance clinicians need to consider early detection and treatment of life-threatening brain injury, where present, but also be able to safely discharge patients with negligible risk of brain injury.

2. Pathophysiology

- Primary brain injury occurs at the time of injury. Prevention strategies include the wearing of motorcycle and cycle helmets, the use of vehicle restraint systems (e.g. seat belts and airbags) and public education.

- Secondary brain injury occurs following the primary event as a result of hypoxia, hypercarbia or hypoperfusion.

- A reduced level of consciousness may lead to airway obstruction or inadequate ventilation, resulting in poor oxygenation, carbon dioxide retention and acidosis.

- Blood loss from other injuries in a patient with multisystem trauma may lead to hypovolaemia, hence a fall in mean arterial pressure (MAP) and consequently cerebral perfusion pressure (CPP).

- CPP needs to be maintained to ensure normal brain physiology and prevent oedema. It is determined by the relationship between the MAP and the intracranial pressure (ICP). This is the mean pressure during the cardiac pumping cycle pushing blood into the brain against the resistance of the ICP (refer to Figures 4.7 and 4.8).

3. Assessment of Patients with Head Injury

- All patients should have an initial A–E assessment, including assessment of:
  - GCS
  - pupils (size and reactivity)
  - focal peripheral neurology (see below).

- Consider full cervical spine immobilisation for patients who have sustained a head injury, where appropriate (refer to **Spinal Injury and Spinal Cord Injury**).

- For patients aged 65 or older, and for older patients that have fallen from a height of greater than 1 metre or 5 stairs, be particularly aware of the potential for more severe brain injury and/or spinal cord injury as well as the increased risk of multiple traumatic injuries in this group (refer to **Falls in Older Adults**).

3.1 Glasgow Coma Scale

- In all communications, documentation and handovers, the individual components of the GCS should be given as well as the total GCS score.

- In some patients (for example, patients with dementia, underlying chronic neurological disorders or learning disabilities), the pre-injury baseline GCS may be less than 15. Establish this where possible and take it into account during assessment.

Figure 4.7 – Cerebral perfusion pressure.

Figure 4.8 – Mean arterial pressure.

Head Injury

- Blood glucose level must be checked as part of initial assessment, as alteration in behaviour or conscious level may be attributed to this.

- History-taking must include assessment of medications (i.e. anticoagulants) and other factors that either place the patient at higher risk of serious underlying injury or may suggest that the patient cannot be safely discharged at the scene.

3.2 Focal Neurological Deficit

- Focal neurological deficit covers problems restricted to a particular part of the body or a particular activity, for example difficulties with understanding, speaking, reading or writing; decreased sensation; loss of balance; general weakness; visual changes; abnormal reflexes; and problems walking.

3.3 Open or Depressed Base of Skull Fracture or Penetrating Head Injury

- Signs include clear fluid running from the ears or nose, black eye with no associated damage around the eyes ('panda eyes'), bleeding from one or both ears, bruising behind one or both ears, penetrating injury signs and visible trauma to the scalp or skull of concern to the clinician.

4. Management of Traumatic Brain Injury in the Pre-Hospital Setting

4.1 Airway with Cervical Spine Control

- It is well recognised that airway obstruction and aspiration are significant and often preventable causes of death in patients with severe traumatic brain injury (TBI). Basic airway manoeuvres are essential to prevent primary airway obstruction and associated brain hypoxia. These should be instigated with consideration for protecting the cervical spine, as it is estimated that up to 10% of TBIs are complicated by a cervical spine injury. However, there is also strong evidence to suggest that, probably due to compression of the jugular veins of the neck, tightly or poorly fitted rigid cervical spinal immobilisation collars create a detrimental rise in ICP. Such ICP rises should be avoided where possible in TBI. Patients should be immobilised using the methods found elsewhere in these practice guidelines.

- Once standard immobilisation has been achieved, with the head and body secured, consideration should be given to loosening or removing the collar. This is to mitigate the effects of the collar on ICP and may help to reduce agitation. The decision to loosen or remove the collar is in no way a decision to clear the C-spine and the reasons for collar removal should be clearly documented and handed over to the receiving hospital team.

- In addition to maintaining C-spine immobilisation, evidence suggests that placing the patient in a 30° head-up position reduces the effects of a raised ICP in patients with TBI, and this is traditionally employed once the cervical collar is removed in the intensive care unit. The logistical challenges of elevating a patient to 30° while immobilised in the pre-hospital setting probably render this process all but redundant. However, clinicians should remain aware of the effect of positioning, and ensure that the patient's head remains above, or at least level with, the feet throughout extrication and transfer.

- For patients with a severe head injury (GCS <8) or who are unable to maintain their own airway, to prevent a worsening secondary brain injury they need to have their airway secured and ventilation optimised, preferably at scene or while they are transferred to definitive care. Consideration should be given to whether an appropriately skilled and trained clinician is available to provide rapid sequence intubation or whether immediate transfer should take place. The distance and journey time from an appropriate receiving unit should be considered in line with local procedures and pathways. Advice may be sought via senior advice systems within your employing service. The level of pre-hospital enhanced care available in any one area and at any time of the day is variable. Diverting to a trauma unit should only be for immediate airway compromise that cannot be managed in the pre-hospital setting.

4.2 Breathing and Ventilation

- Adequate ventilation is essential to the management of TBI through the avoidance of hypoxia and maintenance of 'normocapnia'. Numerous studies have demonstrated the correlation between arterial hypoxaemia and poor prognosis following TBI, with some even demonstrating increased mortality of up to 50% following only brief episodes of desaturation. Current evidence suggests that oxygen should initially be administered at 10–15 l/min via a non-rebreathing mask, with a target saturation of 94–98%.

- Evidence also demonstrates that those patients who remain normocapnic (4.6 and 6.0 kPa) following a TBI have significantly better outcomes. Hyperventilation reduces arterial carbon dioxide concentrations, and leads to a consequent vasoconstriction within the cerebral vasculature, worsening both cerebral hypoxia and oedema. Hypercapnia, associated with hypoventilation, increases the vasodilatation of the cerebral blood vessels, which increases intracranial volumes and therefore ICP.

Head Injury

4.3 Circulation

- It has been estimated that between 8 and 13% of patients with severe traumatic head injuries are hypotensive either at the scene of the injury or in the ED. In addition, a wealth of evidence demonstrates a strong correlation between hypotension and poor outcome in TBI, with some highlighting that a single episode of hypotension (SBP < 90 mmHg) is independently linked to a 100% increase in mortality rate.

- MAP is considered to be a better guide to CCP than systolic blood pressure alone, but ICP measurement is required to established the optimum MAP. This leads to the obvious conclusion that effective management of hypotension in the pre-hospital setting improves the outcomes of patients with TBI.

- Haemorrhage control (especially from the highly vascular scalp) should be established early to avoid the unnecessary consumption of coagulation products, and where hypotension is identified intravenous fluid resuscitation should be commenced. Unfortunately, there still remains a lack of clear research evidence to demonstrate the most appropriate fluid for resuscitation in TBI when blood products are unavailable, and in most cases it will be dictated by local service interpretations and current formulary restrictions.

- Patients with significant head injury, hypotension and evidence of other blunt injury should have intravenous fluids titrated to maintain a palpable radial pulse **OR** systolic BP of >90 mmHg. Patients with significant head injury, hypotension and evidence of penetrating injury to the torso should have intravenous fluids titrated to maintain a good volume central pulse **OR** systolic BP >60 mmHg. In patients with evidence of severe TBI but with no other objective signs of injury (i.e. apparent isolated head injury), the therapeutic goal should be to maintain a systolic BP of 110 mmHg. Refer to **Intravascular Fluid Therapy in Adults**.

- Following the results of the CRASH 3 trial, Tranexamic Acid should be administered to any patient aged 18 years and over who has a known or suspected head injury, with a GCS of 12 or less, where the injury has occurred within the last 3 hours.

4.4 Disability

- The patient's GCS should be calculated, as this can be an important prognostic indicator and is useful for monitoring injury progression over time.

- Pupils should be examined for size, reaction and whether they are equal.

- Acute cerebral herniation, often referred to as 'coning', represents a serious neurosurgical emergency. Clinicians should be vigilant for the clinical signs:

  – Hypertension
  – Bradycardia
  – Reduced level of consciousness
  – Unilateral or bilateral pupil dilatation, non-reactive to light.

- Patients demonstrating signs of cerebral herniation require **TIME-CRITICAL** transfer to a neurosurgical centre. Management of cerebral herniation in the pre-hospital setting is challenging. Clinicians should ensure that they are taking all reasonable steps to manage oxygenation, ventilation and circulation/perfusion. Osmotic diuretic fluid therapy (using hypertonic saline) should be considered as a temporising measure in accordance with locally agreed clinical guidelines, and clinicians should consider seeking senior clinical advice and support.

4.5 Exposure/Environment/Extricate

- There is a high incidence of associated injuries found in patients with TBI, and an attempt to identify these during the secondary survey should be made, while remaining aware of the severe impacts of prolonged scene delays.

- Over recent years, there has been a growing interest in the potential benefits of therapeutic hypothermia in TBI, although to date, research has failed to demonstrate any statistical benefit in long-term outcome. The key message therefore is that the patient should be maintained within a 'normothermic' range.

- Time on scene should be kept to a minimum.

4.6 Pain and Agitation

- Agitation in TBI has a number of potential causes. One commonly overlooked cause of agitation in patients with a TBI is pain, either from the head injury itself or from associated injuries sustained at the time of the TBI. Managing pain in TBI poses a challenge for the pre-hospital clinician; a patient in pain will be agitated and more difficult to manage, and may place themselves at risk of further cerebral hypoxia.

- The administration of opiates in severe TBI can be considered but there is a need to be aware of the potential for exaggerated respiratory depression, hypoventilation, hypercapnia and increased ICP. The decision whether to use opiates in those with a TBI is therefore a clinical one, underpinned by careful assessment and close monitoring for adverse effects.

- Clinicians might consider requesting more senior assistance for patients whose TBI is complicated by agitation associated with acute pain. Midazolam can be considered as an adjunct to help settle an agitated patient (refer to Section 5 below).

Head Injury

4.7 Evacuation Considerations

- The underlying principles of effective pre-hospital management of TBI are rapid assessment; swift and appropriate management; and timely transportation to a receiving centre with sufficient expertise to manage the patient. This will be dependent upon local resources and operational plans for those sustaining significant trauma, but clinicians should consider the most appropriate mode of evacuation early in the incident, to reduce on-scene time as much as possible.

- Helicopter emergency medical services (HEMS) may be able to facilitate more rapid transfer and evacuation but the decision to wait for HEMS arrival should be a balanced decision based on journey time to receiving unit and the need for additional transfer to HEMS at both incident and hospital end.

- A pre-alert call and a detailed clinical handover using ATMIST to the receiving unit is imperative for all patients with a significant TBI.

4.8 Special Considerations

Head Injuries in the Older Person

- Although significant head injury is predominantly a condition seen in the younger generation, a second peak in incidence occurs in those > 65 years. A number of age-related structural changes in the cerebral architecture leave older people with increased susceptibility to intracranial haemorrhage following what may be an apparently minor head injury. In addition, older people are at increased risk of intracranial bleeding following head injury due to co-morbidities such as clotting derangements or polypharmacy. Older patients may present to healthcare services in an atypical way following a head injury, due to altered intracranial anatomy or pre-existing cognitive decline. Clinicians should suspect TBI in all older patients identified to have sustained trauma of any significance, and ensure that they maintain a high index of suspicion when assessing and treating older patients with traumatic injuries.

5. Midazolam in Traumatic Brain Injury

- Patients with TBI can pose a challenge for management in the pre-hospital setting, and any associated hypoxia, hypercapnia and intracranial hypertension can contribute significantly to a poorer prognosis. Although not robust, the evidence suggests that the therapeutic benefits of midazolam for these patients can include amnesia, anxiolysis and, most critically, an ability to effectively provide oxygenation and ventilation, which may help reduce the detrimental secondary brain injury they incur. However, sedating agents will reduce systemic blood pressure, leading to a decrease in CPP, in addition to further jeopardising the patient's airway. Therefore, the decision to use midazolam to facilitate safe patient management needs to be carefully considered. Such interventions should only be undertaken after additional training and confirmation of ability to deal with the complications of midazolam use. Remember – Midazolam is a sedating agent with an unpredictable dose response relationship in a head-injured patient and may cause a patient to rapidly become deeply sedated requiring immediate enhanced care intervention. Any practitioner considering the use of midazolam in head injuries should be specifically trained in and capable of undertaking the additional interventions required.

6. Assessment and Management of Mild to Moderate Head Injury

- Ambulance clinicians need to consider early detection and treatment of life-threatening brain injury, where present, but also be able to safely discharge patients with negligible risk of brain injury. Ninety-five percent of people who have sustained a head injury present with a normal or minimally impaired conscious level (GCS greater than 12).

- Additional care should be taken when assessing children, older people and other patient groups such as those with dementia, underlying chronic neurological disorders or learning disabilities. These can be more difficult to accurately assess and have a higher rate of additional and non-accidental injuries. In some patients, the pre-injury baseline GCS may be less than 15. Establish this where possible, and take it into account during assessment. History-taking must include assessment of medications (e.g. anticoagulants) and other factors that either place the patient at higher risk of serious underlying injury or may suggest that the patient cannot be safely discharged at the scene.

- The following guidance is written to highlight key features of head injuries that require hospital attendance and those patients who can be safely cared for in the community. The list is not exhaustive – a holistic assessment of the patient, mechanism of injury, symptoms, observations and the scene in general must be made. Where any doubt exists regarding the suitability of a patient for discharge, they should be referred to the emergency department.

Head Injury

TABLE 4.17 – Conveyance Decision Tool
Red criteria
Refer to the local major trauma triage tool and consider the need for immediate transfer to a major trauma centre and/or for a pre-alert call.
Immediately transport to hospital if any one of the following is found:
⬚ GCS score of less than 15 on initial assessment.
⬚ Any loss of consciousness as a result of the injury.
⬚ Any focal neurological deficit since the injury.
⬚ Any suspicion of a skull fracture or penetrating head injury since the injury.
⬚ Amnesia for events before or after the injury.
⬚ Persistent headache since the injury.
⬚ Any vomiting episodes since the injury (clinical judgement should be used regarding the cause of vomiting in those aged 12 years or younger and the need for referral).
⬚ Any seizure since the injury.
⬚ Any previous brain surgery.
⬚ A high-energy head injury.
⬚ Any history of bleeding or clotting disorders.
⬚ Current anticoagulant therapy such as warfarin (see further detail below).
⬚ Current drug or alcohol intoxication.
⬚ Any safeguarding concerns (for example, possible non-accidental injury or a vulnerable person is affected).
⬚ Continuing concern by the ambulance clinician about the diagnosis.
⬚ Irritability or altered behaviour, particularly in infants and children aged under five years.
⬚ No visible trauma to the head but still of concern to the clinician.
⬚ No one is able to observe the injured person at home.
⬚ Continuing concern by the injured person or their family or carer about the diagnosis.
Green criteria
Consider discharge where all of the following can be met:
⬚ No Red criteria are identified.
⬚ Able to appropriately safety-net the patient in the community with suitable supervision arrangements. If the patient has no carer at home or lives alone, only discharge them if suitable supervision arrangements have been organised (e.g. arranging for a relative, friend or neighbour to visit regularly) or when the risk of late complications is deemed negligible.
⬚ Verbal and written advice can be given to the patient and those supervising.
⬚ Patient, carers and clinician have no ongoing concerns.
Additional considerations
Patients currently undergoing anticoagulant therapy should be assessed in hospital. Common anticoagulants include:
⬚ Warfarin
⬚ Rivaroxaban
⬚ Apixaban
⬚ Dabigatran
⬚ Edoxaban
⬚ Heparin
⬚ Dalteparin
⬚ Enoxaparin
⬚ Tinzaparin

Head Injury

TABLE 4.17 – Conveyance Decision Tool *(continued)*

Patients undergoing anti-platelet therapy do not automatically require assessment in hospital. Have a lower threshold for conveyance of patients on dual anti-platelets and refer to local procedures. Common anti-platelets include:

- Aspirin
- Clopidogrel
- Ticagrelor

Assessment	**Management**
C – Catastrophic haemorrhage manage catastrophic haemorrhage (see management of catastrophic haemorrhage algorithm)	• See guidelines for management of catastrophic haemorrhage
A – Airway and C-Spine Establish current or impending airway loss. Consider C-Spine status	• Establish and maintain a patent airway • Protect cervical spine to prevent secondary spinal cord injury
B – Breathing Assess rate, pattern and effectiveness of respiration. Obtain oxygen saturations and CRT	• Maintain O₂ saturations with supplemental O₂ as required (See target values) • Instigate capnographic monitoring if available • Avoid hyper / hypoventilation of mechanically ventilated patients (See target values)
C – Circulation Assess pulse rate, rhythm and volume. Assess BP. Confirm control of significant haemorrhage	• Instigate and maintain haemorrhage control • Avoid any episodes of unmanaged hypotension (See target values) • Obtain IV access • Adult: use 250ml boluses of selected fluid to ensure BP remains in target range (See target values) • Children: avoid hypotension (see age specific systolic BP targets) • Avoid excessive dilution of clotting factors through excessive fluid therapy
D – Disability Assess GCS Measure temperature and blood glucose Identify associated injuries taking account of mechanism and injury patterns Check pupil reaction	• Cover patients to prevent heat loss during extrication and evacuation • Avoid using cool or cold infusions • Correct abnormalities of blood glucose • Manage pain in accordance with local or national guidelines • Monitor level of consciousness and be prepared for impending management challenges in those with a diminishing GCS • Treat seizures according to established JRCALC guidelines
Evacuation considerations	• Early referral to specialist neurosurgical centre • Monitor for deterioration Consider 30° head up tilt • Early pre-alert call to receiving unit

Treatment goals (adults):
SpO₂: >94%
Blunt trauma: systolic BP >90 mmHg
Penetrating torso trauma: systolic BP >60 mmHg
Severe TBI: systolic BP >110 mmHg
ETCO₂: 35–40 mmHg, kPa 4.6–6.0

Treatment goals (children):
SpO₂ : 95%
ETCO₂: 35–40 mmHg, kPa 4.6–6.0
Blood Pressure: see age-specific systolic BP targets

Age-specific systolic Blood Pressure targets (children)	
< 1 year	> 80 mmHg
1–5 years	> 90 mmHg
5–14 years	> 100 mmHg
> 14 years	> 110 mmHg

Figure 4.9 – Assessment and management of head injury.

Head Injury

6.1 Discharge at the Scene

- Not all patients who have sustained a head injury will require further assessment in a hospital. Where no red features are present and where all green conditions can be met, patients may be discharged from the scene.

- Complications from head injuries can develop over a number of hours or days, and as such any decision to discharge a patient from the scene needs to be supported by appropriate safety-netting. At a minimum this should include a period of time, for example up to 24 hours, in which the patient can be supervised by a suitable adult who is able to call for help should there be any deterioration. Verbal and written advice that is age appropriate should be given in line with NICE Guideline CG176 (2014). Guidance should refer, at a minimum, to any potential for a developing head injury that would require further assessment, common symptoms that do not require further treatment and guidance around what the patient can or cannot do while recovering from the injury.

Bibliography

1. National Institute for Health and Clinical Excellence. *Head Injury: Assessment and early management.* London: NICE, 2017. Available from: https://www.nice.org.uk/guidance/cg176.

2. Bayless P, Ray VG. Incidence of cervical spine injuries in association with blunt head trauma. *Am J Emerg Med* 1989, 7: 139–142.

3. Boer C, Franschman G, Loer S. Prehospital management of severe traumatic brain injury: conecpts and ongoing controversies. *Curr Opin Anesthesio* l 2012, 25: 556–562.

4. Chestnut R, Marshall L, Klauber M et al. Early and late systemic hypotension as a frequent and fundamental source of cerebral ischaemia following severe brain injry in the Traumatic Coma Data Bank. *Acta Neurochir Suppl* 1993, 59: 121–1253.

5. Clifton G, Valadka A, Zygun D et al. Very early hypothermia induction in patients with severe brain injury (The National Acute Brain Injury Study: hypothermia II): a randomized trial. *Lancet Neurol* 2011, 10: 131–139.

6. Dubick MA, Shek P, Wade CE. ROC trials update on prehospital hypertonic saline resuscitation in the aftermath of the US-Canadian trials. *Clinics* 2013, 68(6): 883–886.

7. Dumont T, Visioni A, Rughani A et al. Inappropriate pre-hospital ventilation in severe traumatic injuries increases in-hospital mortality. *J Neurotrauma* 27: 1223–1241

8. Ferguson J, Mardel SN, Beattie TF, Wytch R. Cervical collars: a potential risk to the head-injured patient. *Injury* 1993, 24(7): 454–456.

9. Flanagan S, Hibbard M, Riordan B. Traumatic Brain Injury in the Elderly: Diagnostic and Treatment Challenges. Clin Geriatr Med 2006, 22: 449–468.

10. Gu J, Yang T, Kuang Y et al. Comparison of the safety and efficacy of propofol with midazolam for sedation of patients with severe traumatic brain injury: A meta-analysis. *Journal of Critical Care* 2014, 29: 287–290.

11. Ho AM, Fung KY, Joynt GM, Karmakar MK, Peng Z. Rigid cervical collar and intracranial pressure of patients with severe head injury. *J Trauma* 2002, 53: 1185–1188.

12. Holly LT, Kelly DF, Counelis GJ, Blinman T, McArthur DL, Cryer HG. Cervical spine trauma associated with moderate and severe head injury: Incidence, risk factors, and injury characteristics. *J Neurosurg* 2002, 96 (Suppl 3): 285–291.

13. Hunt K, Hallworth S, Smith M. The effects of rigid collar placement on intracranial and cerebral perfusion pressures. *Anaesthesia* 2001, 56: 511–513.

14. Langlois JA, Kegler SR, Butler JA, et al. Traumatic brain injury-related hospital discharges: results from a 14-state surveillance system, 1997. MMWR CDC Surveill Summ 2003, 52: 1–20.

15. Ng I, Lim J, Wong H. Effects of head posture on cerebral hemodynamics: its influences on intracranial pressure, cerebral perfusion pressure, and cerebral oxygenation. Neurosurgery 2004, 54(3): 593–597.

16. O'Driscoll B, Howard L, Davison A (On behalf of the British Thoracic Society Emergency Oxygen Guideline Development Group). Guidelines for Emergency Oxygen Use in Adult Patients. *Thorax* 2008, 63 (Suppl VI). DOI: 10.1136/thx.2008.102947.

17. Peterson K, Carson S, Carney N. Hypothermia treatment for traumatic brain injury: a systematic review and meta-analysis. *J Neurotrauma* 2008, 25: 62–71.

18. Piatt JH Jr Detected and overlooked cervical spine injury among comatose trauma patients: from the Pennsylvania trauma outcomes study. *Neurosurg Focus* 2005, 19: E6.

19. Piek J, Chesnut R, Marshall L et al. Extracranial complications of severe head injury. *J Neurosurg* 1992, 77: 901–907.

20. Stiver S, Manley G. Prehospital management of traumatic brain injury. *Neurosurg Focus* 2008, 25(4): E5.

21. Stocchetti N, Furlan A, Volta F. Hypoxemia and arterial hypotension at the accident scene in head injury. *J Trauma* 1996, 40: 764–767.

22. Tian HL, Guo Y, Hu J, Rong BY, Wang G, Gao WW, et al. Clinical characterization of comatose patients with cervical spine injury and traumatic brain injury. *J Trauma* 2009, 67: 1305–1310.

23. Trunkey D. Towards optimal trauma care. *Arch Emerg Med* 1985, 2: 181–195.

24. Urwin SC, Menon DK. Comparative tolerability of sedative agents in head-injured adults. *Drug Saf* 2004, 27: 107–133.

25. Carney N, Totten AM, O'reilly C, Ullman JS et. al. Brain Trauma Guidelines: Guidelines for the Management of Severe Traumatic Brain Injury, Fourth Edition. *Neurosurgery* 2016, 80(1).

Immersion and Drowning

1. Introduction

- Drowning is a common cause of accidental death.
- **Drowning** refers to the 'process resulting in primary respiratory impairment from submersion/immersion in a liquid medium'. Thus the person is prevented from breathing air due to liquid medium at the entrance of the airway. **NB** Drowning does not infer that the patient has died.
- **Immersion** refers to being covered in a liquid medium and the main problems will be hypothermia and cardiovascular collapse from the removal of hydrostatic pressure of the surrounding water on the lower limbs.
- **Submersion** refers to the entire body, including the airway, being under the liquid medium and the main problems are asphyxia and hypoxia.
- **Exacerbating factors** – intoxication from alcohol or drugs may often accompany incidents. Occasionally, an immersion incident may be precipitated by a medical cause such as a convulsion.

2. Incidence

- Worldwide there are approximately 450,000 deaths from accidental drowning per year, with 205 in England and Wales in 2009, and there are with many more near-drownings. A high percentage of deaths involve young males and children.

3. Severity and Outcome

- The extent of hypoxia and hypothermia, resulting from duration of immersion and/or submersion and/or the temperature of the liquid medium, will determine severity and outcome.
- Concomitant trauma may result; for example, <0.5% of patients may suffer neck and/or head injury; diving into shallow water is a common cause.

4. Pathophysiology

- Following submersion, the patient will initially try to hold their breath. They may develop laryngospasm as water irritates the vocal cords or may aspirate large quantities of water. Both processes result in rapid hypoxia and hypercapnia.
- If rescue is not made, the patient will aspirate water into their lungs, exacerbating hypoxia. The patient will become bradycardic and sustain a cardiac arrest; thus correction of hypoxaemia is critical to obtaining a return of spontaneous circulation. In 10–15% of cases, the laryngeal spasm is so intense that none of the liquid medium enters the lungs.
- Changes in haemodynamics after immersion (the 'hydrostatic squeeze effect') make positional hypotension likely. If the patient is raised vertically from the water, their blood pressure will fall – 'after-drop' – which may lead to cardiovascular collapse. Therefore it is recommended that rescuers always attempt to maintain the patient flat and avoid vertical removal from water.

5. Rescue and Resuscitation

⚠ Safety first – **DO NOT** put yourself in danger. Carry out a dynamic risk assessment and undertake measures to preserve your own safety and that of other rescuers.

- Establish the number of patients involved.
- History is often incomplete at the scene, both relating to the incident and the patient.

5.1 Aquatic rescue

- When the patient is rescued, attempt to maintain the patient flat and avoid vertical removal from water.
- If neck and back trauma is suspected, wait until the patient has been rescued before attempting to apply spinal immobilisation, but limit neck flexion and extension.

5.2 Airway and breathing

- Alleviate hypoxaemia as soon as possible, as adequate ventilation and oxygenation may restore cardiac activity.
- In patients in cardiac arrest, clear airway, provide ventilations and commence CPR as soon as the patient is rescued (refer to **Advanced Life Support**).
- Administer supplemental oxygen, preferably via bag-valve-mask. Apply pulse oximeter. If the patient does not respond to oxygen therapy, consider assisted ventilation.
- Mechanical drainage of water from the lungs should not be carried out. The lungs can be ventilated even with large volumes of water inside them, although ventilation may be difficult due to reduced lung compliance.
- Approximately 80% of patients will aspirate water into their stomach. There is a high risk of regurgitation of the stomach contents, especially if the patient has ingested alcohol/drugs – have suction at hand. Tilting to drain aspirated water simply empties water from the stomach into the pharynx, risking further airway contamination.

5.3 For the management of cardiac arrest following drowning

- Refer to **Advanced Life Support**: Drowning.

Immersion and Drowning

5.4 For the management of hypothermia

- Refer to **Hypothermia** and **Advanced Life Support**: Hypothermia.

- If the patient is hypothermic, the heart rate may be extremely slow and external cardiac compression may be required – refer to **Cardiac Rhythm Disturbance**. **NB** Bradycardia often responds to improved ventilation.

5.5 Intravascular fluid therapy

- Following prolonged immersion, patients may become hypovolaemic – if fluid resuscitation indicated, refer to **Intravascular Fluid Therapy in Adults** and **Intravascular Fluid Therapy in Children**.

5.6 Survival and submersion

Research has shown that there is little accurate data on which factors predict survival following submersion. Submersion time may be one significant factor. In order to obtain more accurate data on the factors associated with good outcomes following submersion, data will be collected on a number of parameters, such as:

- Time of the incident.
- Time the patient was rescued.
- Time of first effective CPR.
- Duration of submersion.
- Water temperature.
- Type (salt, fresh, contaminated).
- Precipitating factors (e.g. intoxication from alcohol or drugs, convulsion etc).

As it is often difficult to obtain accurate time information from witnesses, for the purpose of deciding whether to commence resuscitation the submersion time is measured from the time of initial call to the ambulance control centre.

6. Assessment and Management

For the assessment and management of the immersion incident, refer to Table 4.18.

TABLE 4.18 – ASSESSMENT and MANAGEMENT of: Immersion Incident

⚠ **Safety First – DO NOT put yourself in danger – carry out a dynamic risk assessment and undertake measures to preserve your own safety, and where possible that of the patient, bystanders and other rescuers.**

- **Take a defibrillator at the earliest opportunity.**
- **Ascertain how many patients are involved.**
- **NB Information may be incomplete at the scene.**
- **Note the environment – in certain circumstances hair may become entangled in a drain/filter (e.g. pools/hot tubs).**

NB The duration of hypoxia is the most important factor in determining outcome. Oxygenate and restore circulation at the earliest opportunity.

Assess <C>ABCDE

- If any of the following **TIME-CRITICAL** features present:
  - major **<C>ABCDE** problems (refer to **Trauma Emergencies in Adults – Overview** and **Trauma Emergencies in Children – Overview**).
  - pulseless and apnoeic (refer to relevant **Resuscitation** guidelines).
  - major life-threatening trauma (refer to relevant **Trauma** guidelines).
  - neck and back injuries (refer to **Spinal Injury and Spinal Cord Injury**), then:
- Start correcting any <C>ABCD problems.
- Undertake a TIME-CRITICAL transfer to nearest appropriate receiving hospital.
- Continue patient management en-route.
- Provide an ATMIST information call.
- Administer high levels of supplemental oxygen (refer to **Oxygen**).
- Prevent further heat loss/consider warming the patient (refer to **Hypothermia**).

Airway

- Clear airway.
- There is a high risk of regurgitation of the stomach contents, especially if the patient has ingested alcohol/drugs – have suction at hand.

Immersion and Drowning

TABLE 4.18 – ASSESSMENT and MANAGEMENT of: Immersion Incident *(continued)*
Respiratory Rate
▪ Measure and record respiratory rate.
Ventilation
▪ Adequate ventilation and oxygenation may restore cardiac activity. Consider assisted ventilation if: – SpO$_2$ is <90% with oxygen therapy   – respiratory rate is <10 or >30 breaths per minute   – expansion is inadequate.   **NB** Ventilation may be difficult due to reduced lung compliance if water has been inhaled (refer to **Airway and Breathing Management**).
Oxygen
▪ Administer supplemental oxygen (refer to **Oxygen**).   ▪ Apply pulse oximeter. **NB** The measurement may be unreliable in patients with cold peripheries.   – **children** – administer high levels of supplemental oxygen   – **adults** – aim for a target saturation within the range of 94–98%.
Pulse
▪ Measure and record pulse.
Heart Rate
▪ In the presence of hypothermia, the heart rate may be extremely slow and external cardiac compression may be required (refer to **Cardiac Rhythm Disturbance**).   **NB** Bradycardia often responds to improved ventilation and oxygenation.
Concomitant Injuries
▪ Consider concomitant injuries.   ▪ Consider neck and back injuries (refer to **Spinal Injury and Spinal Cord Injury**).   ▪ Treat associated injuries (refer to specific guideline(s)).
ECG
▪ Monitor and record 12-Lead ECG. Assess for abnormality (refer to **Cardiac Rhythm Disturbance**).
Blood Pressure and Fluids
▪ Measure and record blood pressure.   ▪ In cases of prolonged immersion, patients may become hypovolaemic – if fluid resuscitation is indicated, refer to **Intravascular Fluid Therapy in Adults** and **Intravascular Fluid Therapy in Children**.
Blood Glucose
▪ If appropriate, measure and record blood glucose for hypo/hyperglycaemia (refer to **Glycaemic Emergencies in Adults and Children**).
Temperature
▪ Measure and record temperature.
Position
▪ If possible, the patient should be removed from the water and managed in a horizontal position, especially in rescue involving a helicopter or large vessel, where the patient is lifted more than a few metres – however, in **TIME-CRITICAL** conditions speed of removal from the water takes precedence over method of removal.
Assess the Patient's Pain
▪ Where present, assess the **SOCRATES** of pain and record initial and subsequent pain scores.   ▪ Consider analgesia if appropriate (refer to **Pain Management in Adults** and **Pain Management in Children**).

(continued)

Immersion and Drowning

TABLE 4.18 – ASSESSMENT and MANAGEMENT of: Immersion Incident *(continued)*
Transfer to Further Care
▪ Transfer all patients to further care.
▪ If neck and back injury not suspected, transfer in the recovery position.
▪ If the patient is immobilised, prepare for side-tilt.
▪ Prevent further heat loss/consider warming the patient (refer to **Hypothermia**).
▪ Provide an ATMIST information call.
▪ Continue patient management en-route.
Discontinuation of Resuscitative Efforts
▪ Refer to **Advanced Life Support**.
Documentation
▪ Complete documentation to include all clinical findings, advice from other clinicians, onward referral and worsening advice given.

KEY POINTS!

Immersion and Drowning

- **Ensure own personal safety.**
- **Successful resuscitations have occurred after prolonged submersion/immersion.**
- **Hypothermia is a condition often associated with the immersion incident.**
- **There are special considerations in cardiac arrest treatment in the presence of hypothermia.**
- **Severe complications may develop several hours after submersion/immersion.**

Bibliography

1. Soar J, Perkins GD, Abbas G, Alfonzo A, Barelli A, Bierens JJLM, et al. European Resuscitation Council Guidelines for Resuscitation 2010 Section 8: cardiac arrest in special circumstances: electrolyte abnormalities, poisoning, drowning, accidental hypothermia, hyperthermia, asthma, anaphylaxis, cardiac surgery, trauma, pregnancy, electrocution. *Resuscitation* 2010, 81(10): 1400–1433.

2. Brenner RA, Taneja GS, Haynie DL, Trumble AC, Qian C, Klinger RM, et al. Association between swimming lessons and drowning in childhood: a case-control study. *Archives of Pediatrics & Adolescent Medicine* 2009, 163(3): 203–210.

3. Durchholz C, Peters J, Staudt F, Pontz B. Childhood drowning: a retrospective analysis. *Notarzt* 2004, 20(5): 168–172.

4. Ross FI, Elliott EJ, Lam LT, Cass DT. Children under 5 years presenting to paediatricians with near-drowning. *Journal of Paediatrics and Child Health* 2003, 39(6): 446–450.

5. Bierens JJLM, Knape JTA, Gelissen HPMM. Drowning. *Current Opinion in Critical Care* 2002, 8(6): 578–586.

6. Kemp A, Sibert JR. Drowning and near drowning in children in the United Kingdom: lessons for prevention. *British Medical Journal* 1992, 304(6835): 1143–1146.

7. Cummings P, Quan L. Trends in unintentional drowning: the role of alcohol and medical care. *Journal of the American Medical Association* 1999, 281(23): 2198–2202.

8. Franklin RC, Scarr JP, Pearn JH. Reducing drowning deaths: the continued challenge of immersion fatalities in Australia. *Medical Journal of Australia* 2010, 192(3): 123–126.

9. Youn CS, Choi SP, Yim HW, Park KN. Out-of-hospital cardiac arrest due to drowning: an Utstein Style report of 10 years of experience from St Mary's Hospital. *Resuscitation* 2009, 80(7): 778–783.

10. Barbieri S, Feltracco P, Delantone M, Spagna A, Michieletto E, Bortolato A, et al. Helicopter rescue and pre-hospital care for drowning children: two summer season case studies. *Minerva Anestesiologica* 2008, 74(12): 703–707.

11. Hyder AA, Borse NN, Blum L, Khan R, El Arifeen S, Baqui AH. Childhood drowning in low- and middle-income countries: urgent need for intervention trials. *Journal of Paediatrics and Child Health* 2008, 44(4): 221– 227.

12. Salomez F, Vincent J-L. Drowning: a review of epidemiology, pathophysiology, treatment and prevention. *Resuscitation* 2004, 63(3): 261–268.

13. Peden MM, McGee K. The epidemiology of drowning worldwide. *International Journal of Injury Control and Safety Promotion* 2003, 10(4): 195–199.

14. Franklin RC, Scarr JP, Pearn JH. Reducing drowning deaths: the continued challenge of immersion fatalities in Australia. *Medical Journal of Australia* 2011, 192(3): 123–126.

15. al-Talafieh A, al-Majali R, al-Dehayat G. Clinical, laboratory and X-ray findings of drowning and near-drowning in the Gulf of Aqaba. *Eastern Mediterranean Health Journal* 1999, 5(4): 706–709.

16. Papa L, Hoelle R, Idris A. Systematic review of definitions for drowning incidents. *Resuscitation* 2005, 65(3): 255–264.

17. Diplock S, Jamrozik K. Legislative and regulatory measures for preventing alcohol-related drownings and near-drownings. *Australian & New Zealand Journal of Public Health* 2006, 30(4): 314–317.

18. Driscoll TR, Harrison JA, Steenkamp M. Review of the role of alcohol in drowning associated with recreational aquatic activity. *Injury Prevention* 2004, 10(2): 107–113.

19. Eksborg S, Rajs J. Causes and manners of death among users of heroin, methadone, amphetamine, and cannabis in relation to postmortem chemical tests for illegal drugs. *Substance Use and Misuse* 2008, 43(10): 1326–1339.

20. Lossius R, Nakken KO. Epilepsy and sudden death. *Tidsskrift for Den norske legeforening* 2002, 122(11): 1114–1117.

21. Office for National Statistics. *Deaths Registered in England and Wales in 2010, By Cause.* 2010. Available from: http://www.ons.gov.uk.

22. Watson RS, Cummings P, Quan L, Bratton S, Weiss NS. Cervical spine injuries among submersion victims. *Journal of Trauma* 2001, 51(4): 658–662.

23. Hwang V, Shofer FS, Durbin DR, Baren M. Prevalence of traumatic injuries in drowning and near drowning in children and adolescents. *Archives of Pediatrics & Adolescent Medicine* 2003, 157(1): 50–53.

24. Faddy S. Drowning and near-drowning: the physiology and pathology. *Australian Journal of Medical Science* 2001, 22(1): 4–13.

25. Layon AJ, Modell JH. Drowning: update 2009. *Anaesthesiology* 2009, 110(6): 1390–1401.

26. Ouanes-Besbes L, Dachraoui F, Ouanes I, Abroug F. Drowning: pathophysiology and treatment. *Reanimation* 2009, 18(8): 702–707.

27. Claesson A, Svensson L, Silfverstolpe J, Herlitz J. Characteristics and outcome among patients suffering out-of-hospital cardiac arrest due to drowning. *Resuscitation* 2008, 76(3): 381–387.

28. Edwards ND, Timmins AC, Randalls B, Morgan GA, Simcock AD. Survival in adults after cardiac arrest due to drowning. *Intensive Care Medicine* 1990, 16(5): 336–337.

29. Lee LK, Mao C, Thompson KM. Demographic factors and their association with outcomes in pediatric submersion injury. *Academic Emergency Medicine* 2006, 13(3): 308–313.

30. Modell JH, Graves SA, Ketover A. Clinical course of 91 consecutive neardrowning victims. *Chest* 1976, 70(2): 231–238.

31. Modell JH, Idris AH, Pineda JA, Silverstein JH. Survival after prolonged submersion in freshwater in Florida. *Chest* 2004, 125(5): 1948–1951.

32. Nussbaum E, Maggi JC. Pentobarbital therapy does not improve neurologic outcome in nearly drowned, flaccid-comatose children. *Pediatrics* 1988, 81(5): 630–634.

33. Suominen P, Baillie C, Korpela R, Rautanen S, Ranta S, Olkkola KT. Impact of age, submersion time and water temperature on outcome in near-drowning. *Resuscitation* 2002, 52(3): 247–254.

34. Wollenek G, Honarwar N, Golej J, Marx M. Cold water submersion and cardiac arrest in treatment of severe hypothermia with cardiopulmonary bypass. *Resuscitation* 2002, 52(3): 255–263.

35. Wyatt JP, Tomlinson GS, Busuttil A. Resuscitation of drowning victims in south-east Scotland. *Resuscitation* 1999, 41(2): 101–104.

SECTION 4 Trauma

Limb Trauma

1. Introduction

- There is one fundamental rule to apply to limb trauma cases and that is NOT to let limb injuries, however dramatic in appearance, distract the clinician from less visible but life-threatening problems, such as airway obstruction, compromised breathing, poor perfusion and spinal injury.

- Patients with limb trauma are likely to be in considerable pain and distress; therefore consider pain management as soon as clinically possible after arriving on scene (refer to **Pain Management in Adults** and **Pain Management in Children**).

2. Pathophysiology

- The pathophysiology differs depending on the nature of the injury (refer to Table 4.19).

- Blood loss from femoral shaft fractures can be considerable, involving loss of 500–2000 millilitres in volume. If the fracture is open, blood loss is increased.

- Nerves and blood vessels are placed at risk from sharp bony fragments, especially in very displaced fractures, hence the need to return fractured limbs to normal alignment as rapidly as possible. Fractures around the elbow and knee are especially likely to injure arteries and nerves.

- The six 'P's of ischaemia are shown in Table 4.20.

TABLE 4.19 – Types of Limb Injury

Compound fracture (open)

A fracture in which the bone protrudes through an open wound.

Closed fracture

A fracture that is contained, the skin is unbroken.

Dislocation

Where the articular surface of the joint is not in continuity. Commonly affecting the digits, elbow, shoulder, patella and occasionally the hip (high energy).

Compartment syndrome

A complication of limb fractures arising from increased pressure in muscular compartments due to contained haemorrhage or swelling. This can lead to ischaemia, with potentially catastrophic consequences for the limb.

Degloving

Degloving can accompany limb fractures and be to the superficial fascia or full depth down to the bone.

Amputations/partial amputations

Amputations most frequently involve digits, but can involve part or whole limbs. Partial amputations may still result in a viable limb, providing there is minimal crushing damage and survival of some vascular and nerve structures.

Neck of femur fractures

Such fractures commonly occur in older people and are one of the most common limb injuries encountered in the pre-hospital environment. Typical patients present with shortening and external rotation of the leg on the injured side, with pain in the hip and referred pain in the knee. The circumstances of the injury must be taken into account – often the older person has been on the floor for some time, which increases the possibility of hypothermia, dehydration, pressure ulcers and chest infection, so careful monitoring of vital signs is essential.

TABLE 4.20 – Six 'P's of Ischaemia

SIGN	SYMPTOM
Pain	Out of proportion to the apparent injury; often in the muscle, which may not ease with splinting/analgesia.
Pallor	Due to compromised blood flow to limb.
Paralysis	Loss of movement.
Paraesthesia	Changes in sensation.

Limb Trauma

TABLE 4.20 – Six 'P's of Ischaemia *(continued)*	
Pulselessness	The loss of peripheral pulses is a grave late sign caused by swelling, which can lead to the complete occlusion of circulation.
Perishing cold	The limb is cold to the touch.

3. Incidence

- Limb trauma is a common injury in high-energy impacts. Causes can include but are not limited to falls, sports, traffic accidents and occupational and intentional causes, and can occur at any age.
- In older people, injuries can occur from relatively minor trauma (e.g. falls from a standing height can lead to femoral fractures).

4. Severity and Outcome

- Severity and outcome differ depending on the nature of the injury. However, limb trauma can have serious consequences; for example, infection following an open fracture can affect the future viability and long-term function of the limb.

4.1. Splinting

- Splinting will contribute to 'circulation' care by reducing further blood loss and pain en-route to hospital.

- Traction splint – a device for applying longitudinal traction to the femur, using the pelvis and the ankle as static points. Correct splintage technique using a traction splint reduces:
  - pain
  - haemorrhage and damage to blood vessels and nerves
  - bone fragment movement and the risk of a closed fracture becoming an open fracture
  - the risk of fat embolisation (brain and lungs)
  - muscle spasm by pulling the thigh to a natural cylindrical shape
  - blood loss by compression of bleeding sites.
- Traction splints such as the Sager, Trac 3, Donway and Kendrick are easy to apply and some now have quantifiable traction, measured on a scale in pounds. The correct amount of traction is best judged by observing that the injured leg is the same length as the uninjured leg.

TABLE 4.21 – Splinting	
INJURY	**SPLINTAGE TYPE**
Fractured neck of femur	Padding between legs. Figure-of-eight bandage around ankles. Broad bandage: two above, two below the knee.
Fractured shaft of femur	Traction splint or adjacent leg as a splint if the suspected fracture is above the knee. **NB** Fractures of the ankle, tibia, fibula, knee or pelvis on the same side as the femoral fracture may limit use of a traction splint; Trust guidelines should be followed.
Fracture or fracture dislocation around the knee	Vacuum splint. Box splint. Traction splint without the application of traction.
Patella dislocation	Companion strapping (one leg to the other). Support on pillow. Contoured vacuum splint. If the leg is gently straightened, the patella often spontaneously relocates; if resistance is felt, the leg should be splinted in the position of comfort.
Tibia/fibula shaft fracture	Vacuum splint. Box splint.
Ankle fracture	Vacuum splint. Box splint.
Foot fracture	Vacuum splint. Box splint.

(continued)

Limb Trauma

TABLE 4.21 – Splinting *(continued)*	
Clavicle	Self-splintage may be adequate and less painful than a sling.
Humerus	Sling.
Radius Ulna	Vacuum splints may be well suited to immobilising forearm fractures, or a box splint.

5. Crush Injury and Crush Syndrome

- Crush injury is a term used to describe the injury directly resulting from crush and crush syndrome. It relates to the systemic manifestation of muscle cell damage resulting from pressure or crushing. Crush syndrome is relatively rare in the UK and the severity of the condition is related to the degree of force, duration of crush and bulk of tissue/muscle affected. Clinicians should be aware of the risks of crush syndrome in less obvious patient groups such as the elderly or bariatric faller with a prolonged lay in the same position.

- Crush injuries without the risk of crush syndrome should be managed in accordance with the guidance for the injury as it presents: haemorrhage controlled, wounds dressed and fractures splinted. Intravenous fluid should only be administered if the patient is hypotensive (refer to **Intravascular Fluid Therapy in Adults** and **Intravascular Fluid Therapy in Children**).

- Crush syndrome occurs as a result of traumatic rhabdomyolysis. Metabolic acidosis combined with the release of nephrotoxic substances (such as myoglobin, urate and phosphate) leads to the development shock, cardiac arrhythmias and may result in acute kidney injury.

6. Assessment and Management

For the assessment and management of limb trauma, refer to Table 4.22.

TABLE 4.22 – ASSESSMENT and MANAGEMENT of: Limb Trauma
Assess <C>ABCDE
<ul><li>Control any external catastrophic haemorrhage (refer to **Trauma Emergencies in Adults – Overview**).</li><li>If any of the following **TIME-CRITICAL** features are present:<ul><li>major **<C>ABC** complications</li><li>haemodynamic instability (refer to **Intravascular Fluid Therapy in Adults**)</li><li>altered level of consciousness (refer to **Altered Level of Consciousness**)</li><li>neck and back injuries (refer to **Spinal Injury and Spinal Cord Injury**)</li><li>threatened limb – loss of neurovascular function (e.g. resulting from a dislocation that requires prompt realignment), then:</li></ul></li><li>Correct **<C>ABC** complications.</li><li>Mid-shaft femoral fracture – apply a traction splint if this can be done quickly without delaying transfer, otherwise apply manual traction where sufficient personnel are available – once applied it should not be released.</li><li>Undertake a **TIME-CRITICAL** transfer to a major trauma centre, unless the patient needs an immediate lifesaving intervention, in which case transfer to nearest trauma unit.</li><li>Provide a pre-alert using ATMIST.</li><li>Continue patient management en-route.</li></ul>
Specifically Assess
<ul><li>Ascertain the mechanism of injury and any factors indicating the forces involved (e.g. the pattern of fractures may indicate mechanism of injury):<ul><li>fractures of the heel in a fall from a height may be accompanied by pelvic and spinal crush fractures (refer to **Major Pelvic Trauma** and **Spinal Injury and Spinal Cord Injury**)</li><li>'dashboard' injury to the knee may be accompanied by a fracture or dislocation of the hip</li><li>humeral fractures from a side impact are associated with chest injuries (refer to **Thoracic Trauma**)</li><li>tibial fractures are rarely isolated injuries and are often associated with high-energy trauma and other life-threatening injuries.</li></ul></li></ul>

Limb Trauma

TABLE 4.22 – ASSESSMENT and MANAGEMENT of: Limb Trauma *(continued)*
▪ Assess all four limbs for injury to long bones and joints – in suspected fracture, expose site(s) to assess swelling and deformity.
▪ Assess neurovascular function – MSC × 4: motor, sensation and circulation, distal to the fracture site. Assess foot pulses; palpate dorsalis pedis, as capillary refill time can be misleading.
▪ Assess general skin colour.
▪ Assess age of patient – consider greenstick fractures in children, and fractures of wrist and hip in older people.
▪ For accompanying illnesses: – some cancers can involve bones (e.g. breast, lung and prostate) and result in fractures from minor injuries – osteoporosis in older women makes fractures more likely.
NB Where possible, avoid unnecessary pain stimulus.
Oxygen
▪ Administer high levels of supplemental oxygen (aim for SpO$_2$ 94–98%) (refer to **Oxygen**).
Splintage
In pre-hospital care it is difficult to differentiate between ligament sprain and a fracture; therefore, ASSUME a fracture and immobilise.
▪ Remove and document jewellery from the affected limbs before swelling occurs.
▪ Check and record the presence/absence of pulses, and muscle function distal to injury.
▪ Consider realignment of grossly deformed limbs to a position as close to normal anatomic alignment as possible. Where deformity is minor and both distal sensation and circulation are intact, then realignment may not be necessary.
▪ Apply splintage (refer to Table 4.21).
▪ Guidance on alignment: deformed fracture dislocation of the ankle is the most common deformity that may benefit from manipulation in the pre-hospital environment. Indications to attempt manipulation are: – vascular impairment – absent or very weak distal pulse – significantly prolonged capillary refill – critical skin over the fracture site (blanching or discolouration).
▪ Manipulation into alignment as close to normal should be considered when any of these features are present and transfer to an appropriate ED cannot be managed in a suitable time frame.
Compound Fracture
▪ Gross contamination can be removed from wounds but do not irrigate open fractures of the long bones, hindfoot or midfoot in pre-hospital settings as it may force contamination deeper into the bone or tissue.
▪ Apply a saline-soaked dressing and cover with an occlusive layer.
▪ Any gross displacement from normal alignment must, where possible, be corrected, and splints applied (refer to Table 4.21).
NB Document the nature of the contamination, as contaminates may be drawn inside following realignment.
Amputations, Partial Amputations and Degloving
▪ Do not irrigate grossly contaminated wounds with saline.
▪ Immobilise a partially amputated limb in a position of normal anatomical alignment.
▪ Where possible, dress the injured limb to prevent further contamination.
▪ Apply a saline-soaked dressing covered with an occlusive layer.

(continued)

Limb Trauma

TABLE 4.22 – ASSESSMENT and MANAGEMENT of: Limb Trauma *(continued)*
NB Reimplantation following amputation or reconstruction following partial amputation may be possible. In order that the amputated parts are maintained and transported in the best condition possible: ▪ remove any gross contamination ▪ cover the part(s) with a moist field dressing ▪ secure in a sealed plastic bag ▪ place the bag on ice – do not place body parts in direct contact with ice as this can cause tissue damage; the aim is to keep the temperature low but not freezing.
Neck of Femur Fractures ▪ Assess for shortening and external rotation of the leg on the injured side, with pain in the hip and referred pain in the knee. ▪ Ascertain whether the patient has been on the floor for some time, assess for signs of hypothermia, dehydration, pressure ulcers and chest infection. ▪ Monitor vital signs. ▪ Immobilise by strapping the injured leg to the normal one with foam padding between the limbs – extra padding with blankets and strapping around the hips and pelvis can be used to provide additional support while moving the patient (refer to Table 4.21).
Compartment Syndrome ▪ Consider the need for rapid transfer to nearest appropriate hospital as per local trauma care pathway, as the patient may require immediate surgery; elevate limb and consider pain relief en-route.
Pain Management ▪ Pain management is an important intervention; if indicated, refer to **Pain Management in Adults** and **Pain Management in Children**.
Fluid ▪ If fluid resuscitation is indicated, refer to **Intravascular Fluid Therapy in Adults** and **Intravascular Fluid Therapy in Children**. ▪ **DO NOT** delay on scene for fluid replacement if peripheral pulses are present.
Antibiotic ▪ Administer prophylactic intravenous antibiotic co-amoxiclav (in line with local guidance) as soon as possible and preferably within 1 hour of injury to patients with open fractures, without delaying transport to hospital. For patients that are allergic to penicillin, where no alternative antibiotic is available, convey to hospital and inform ED on arrival so that an antibiotic can be administered as soon as possible.
Non-accidental Injury ▪ When assessing an injury in a child, consider the possibility of non-accidental injury (refer to **Safeguarding Children**).

Transfer to Further Care
 	
▪ Transfer suspected open fractures of the long bone, hindfoot or midfoot directly to a major trauma centre or specialist centre for orthoplastic care.
 	
▪ Transfer suspected open fractures of the hand, wrist or toes to nearest trauma unit, unless there are pre-hospital triage indications for direct transport to a major trauma centre.
 	
▪ Continue patient management en-route.
 	
▪ Provide a pre-alert using ATMIST.
 	
▪ At the hospital, inform staff of:
  – any skin wound relating to a fracture
  – any underlying fracture(s) that was initially open.
 	
▪ Complete documentation.

Limb Trauma

KEY POINTS!

Limb Trauma

- Ensure <C>ABCDEs are assessed and managed; consider C-spine immobilisation.
- DO NOT become distracted by the appearance of limb trauma from assessing less visible but life-threatening problems, such as airway obstruction, compromised breathing, poor perfusion and spinal injury.
- Do not irrigate open fractures of the long bones, hindfoot or midfoot.
- Limb trauma can cause life-threatening haemorrhage.
- Assess for intact circulation and nerve function distal to the fracture site.
- Any dislocation that threatens the neurovascular status of a limb must be treated with urgency.
- Splintage is fundamental to prevention of further blood loss and can reduce pain.
- Limb trauma can cause considerable pain and distress – consider pain management as soon as clinically possible after arriving on scene.
- In cases of life-threatening trauma, commence a TIME-CRITICAL transfer and perform any splinting en-route if possible.

Bibliography

1. National Institute for Health and Clinical Excellence. *Fractures (Complex): Assessment and Management (NG37)*. London: NICE, 2016. Available from: https://www.nice.org.uk/guidance/ng37.

2. National Institute for Health and Clinical Excellence. *Fractures (Non-complex): Assessment and Management (NG38)*. London: NICE, 2016. Available from: https://www.nice.org.uk/guidance/ng38.

3. National Institute for Health and Clinical Excellence. *Major Trauma: Assessment and Initial Management (NG39)*. London: NICE, 2016. Available from: https://www.nice.org.uk/guidance/ng39.

4. National Institute for Health and Clinical Excellence. *Major Trauma: Service Delivery (NG40)*. London: NICE, 2016. Available from: https://www.nice.org.uk/guidance/ng40.

5. National Institute for Health and Clinical Excellence. *Spinal Injury: Assessment and Initial Management (NG41)*. London: NICE, 2016. Available from: https://www.nice.org.uk/guidance/ng41.

6. National Institute for Health and Clinical Excellence. *When to Suspect Child Maltreatment (CG89)*. London: NICE, 2009. Available from: https://www.nice.org.uk/guidance/cg89.

7. Porter A, Snooks H, Youren A, Gaze S, Whitfield R, Rapport F et al. 'Covering our backs': ambulance crews' attitudes towards clinical documentation when emergency (999) patients are not conveyed to hospital. *Emergency Medicine Journal* 2008, 25(5): 292–295.

8. Antoniou D, Kyriakidis A, Zaharopoulos A, Moskoklaidis S. Degloving injury. *European Journal of Trauma* 2005, 31(6): 593–596.

9. Arnez ZM, Khan U, Tyler MPH. Classification of soft-tissue degloving in limb trauma. *Journal of Plastic, Reconstructive and Aesthetic Surgery* 2010, 63(11): 1865–1869.

10. Beekley AC, Sebesta JA, Blackbourne LH, Herbert GS, Kauvar DS, Baer DG, et al. Pre-hospital tourniquet use in Operation Iraqi Freedom: effect on hemorrhage control and outcomes. *Journal of Trauma* 2008, 64 (suppl. 2): S28–37; discussion S37.

11. Burns BJ, Sproule J, Smyth H. Acute compartment syndrome of the anterior thigh following quadriceps strain in a footballer. *British Journal of Sports Medicine* 2004, 38(2): 218–220.

12. Cooper C, Dennison FM, Leufkens HGM, Bishop N, van Staa TP. Epidemiology of childhood fractures in Britain: a study using the General Practice Research Database. *Journal of Bone and Mineral Research* 2004, 19(12): 976–981.

13. Daniels JM, Zook EG, Lynch JM. Hand and wrist injuries. Part II: Emergent evaluation. *American Family Physician* 2004, 69(8): 1949–1956.

14. Griffiths R, Alper J, Beckingsale A, Goldhill D, Heyburn G, Holloway J et al. Management of proximal femoral fractures 2011. *Anaesthesia* 2012, 67(1): 85–98.

15. Hodgetts TJ, Mahoney PF, Russell MQ, Byers M. ABC to <C>ABC: redefining the military trauma paradigm. *Emergency Medical Journal* 2006, 23(10): 745–746.

16. Jagdeep N, Durai N, Umraz K, Christopher M, Stephen B, Frances S et al. *Standards for the Management of Open Fractures of the Lower Limb*. London: British Association of Plastic Reconstructive and Aesthetic Surgeons, British Orthopaedic Association, 2009. Available from: http://www.bapras.org.uk/professionals/clinical-guidance/open-fractures-of-the-lower-limb.

17. Kaye JA, Jick H. Epidemiology of lower limb fractures in general practice in the United Kingdom. *Injury Prevention* 2004, 10(6): 368–374.

18. Klos K, Muckley T, Gras F, Hofmann GO, Schmidt R. Early posttraumatic rotationplasty after severe degloving and soft tissue avulsion injury: a case report. *Journal of Orthopaedic Trauma* 2010, 24(2): el–5.

19. Kragh JF Jr, Walters TJ, Baer DG, Fox CJ, Wade CE, Salinas J et al. Practical use of emergency tourniquets to stop bleeding in major limb trauma. *Journal of Trauma* 2008, 64 (suppl. 2): S38–49; discussion S49–50.

20. Lee C, Porter KM. Pre-hospital management of lower limb fractures. *Emergency Medicine Journal* 2005, 22(9): 660–663.

21. Lee C, Porter KM, Hodgetts TJ. Tourniquet use in the civilian pre-hospital setting. *Emergency Medicine Journal* 2007, 24(8): 584–587.

SECTION **4** Trauma

Limb Trauma

22. Lisle DA, Shepherd GJ, Cowderoy GA, O'Connell PT. MR imaging of traumatic and overuse injuries of the wrist and hand in athletes. *Magnetic Resonance Imaging Clinics of North America* 2009, 17(4): 639–654.

23. National Library of Medicine. *Fractures.* 2011. Available from: http://www.nlm.nih.gov/medlineplus/fractures.html.

24. Pearse MF, Harry L, Nanchahal J. Acute compartment syndrome of the leg. *British Medical Journal* 2002, 325(7364): 557–558.

25. Taxter AJ, Konstantakos EK, Ames DW. Lateral compartment syndrome of the lower extremity in a recreational athlete: a case report. *American Journal of Emergency Medicine* 2008, 26(8): 973.el–2.

26. van Staa TP, Dennison EM, Leufkens HGM, Cooper C. Epidemiology of fractures in England and Wales. *Bone* 2001, 29(6): 517–522.

27. Weinmann M. Compartment syndrome. *Emergency Medical Services* 2003, 32(9): 36.

28. Wood SP, Vrahas M, Wedel SK. Femur fracture immobilization with traction splints in multisystem trauma patients. *Pre-hospital Emergency Care* 2003, 7(2): 241–243.

29. British Orthopaedic Association, British Association of Plastic Reconstructive and Aesthetic Surgeons. *The Management of Severe Open Lower Limb Fractures.* 2009. Available from: http://www.boa.ac.uk.

30. Melamed E, Blumenfeld A, Kalmovich B, Kosashvili Y, Lin G, Israel Defense Forces Medical Corps Consensus Group on Pre-hospital Care of Orthopedic Injuries. Pre-hospital care of orthopedic injuries. *Pre-hospital Disaster Medicine* 2007, 22(1): 22–25.

31. Bragg S. Avulsion amputation of the hand. *Journal of Emergency Nursing* 2005, 31(3): 282.

32. Bragg S. The boxers' fracture. *Journal of Emergency Nursing* 2005, 31(5): 473.

33. Bragg S. Vertical deceleration: falls from height. *Journal of Emergency Nursing* 2007, 33(4): 377–378.

34. Greaves I, Porter K, Smith JE. Consensus statement on the early management of crush injury and prevention of crush syndrome. *J R Army Meds Corps* 2003, 149: 255–259. DOI: 10.1136/jramc-149-04-02.

Major Pelvic Trauma

1. Introduction

- Major pelvic injuries are predominantly observed where there is a high-energy transfer to the patient such as might occur following road traffic collision, pedestrian accident, fall from height or crush injury.

- Less-serious pelvic injuries may also occur following low-energy transfer events, particularly in the elderly (such as a simple fall), amongst patients with degenerative bone disease or receiving radiotherapy and rarely as a direct consequence of seizure activity.

- The majority of pelvic injuries do not result in major disruption of the pelvic ring, but rather involve fractures of the pubic ramus or acetabulum. Presentation of these injuries is very similar to neck of femur fractures.

- Mechanism of injury:
  - High-energy transfer
  - Fall from height
  - Crush injury,

- Risk factors:
  - Advancing age
  - Degenerative bone disease
  - Radiotherapy.

2. Incidence

- Pelvic fractures represent 3–6% of all fractures in adults and occur in up to 20% of all polytrauma cases. They display a bimodal distribution of age, with most injuries occurring in the age ranges 15–30 and over 60 years; up to 75% of all pelvic injuries occur in men.

- Unstable pelvic fracture is estimated to occur in up to 20% of pelvic fractures; a further 22% of pelvic fractures will remain stable despite significant damage to the pelvic ring. The remaining 58% of pelvic fractures are less serious, retaining both haemodynamic and structural stability.

- The incidence of pelvic fracture resulting from blunt trauma ranges from 5% to 11.9%, with obese patients more likely to sustain a pelvic fracture from blunt trauma than non-obese patients. Pelvic fracture associated with penetrating trauma is far less frequent. Open pelvic fractures are rare and account for only 2.7–4% of all pelvic fractures.

3. Severity and Outcome

- Major pelvic injuries can be devastating and are often associated with a number of complications that may require extensive rehabilitation. Pelvic trauma deaths frequently occur as a result of associated injuries and complications rather than the pelvic injury itself.

- Haemorrhage is the cause of death in 40% of all pelvic trauma victims and the leading cause of death (60% of fatal cases) in unstable pelvic fracture. Bleeding is usually retroperitoneal; the volume of blood loss correlates with the degree and type of pelvic disruption.

- Reported mortality rates range from 6.4% to 30% depending on the type of pelvic fracture, haemodynamic status and nature of concomitant injuries and their complications.

- The mortality rate among haemodynamically stable patients is around 10%, whereas the mortality rate amongst haemodynamically unstable patients approaches 20–30% but has been reported to be as high as 50% in cases of unstable open fracture; combined mortality approaches 16%.

4. Pathophysiology

4.1 Skeletal Anatomy

- Increasing pelvic volume allows for increased haemorrhage; conversely, reducing pelvic volume reduces potential for bleeding by realignment of broken bone ends.

4.2 Classification of Injury

- As with other fractures, pelvic fractures may be classified as open or closed, and benefit from being further described as either haemodynamically stable or unstable. Patients who are haemodynamically unstable are at greater risk of death and would benefit greatly from a suitable pre-hospital alert message.

- Pelvic ring disruptions (as identified by in-hospital imaging) can be subdivided into four classes by mechanism of injury: antero-posterior compression (APC), lateral compression (LC), vertical shear (VS) and combined mechanical injury (CMI), a combination of the aforementioned classes.

4.3 Vascular Injury

- The arteries most frequently injured are the iliolumbar arteries, the superior gluteal and the internal pudendal because of their proximity to the bone, the sacro-iliac joint and the inferior ligaments of the pelvis. Bleeding from the venous network after a pelvic fracture is more frequent than arterial bleeding because the walls of the veins are more fragile than arteries. Blood may pool in the retroperitoneal space and haemostasis may occur spontaneously in closed fractures, especially if there is no concomitant arterial haemorrhage.

4.4 Other Injuries

- The incidence of urogenital injury ranges from 23% to 57%. Urethral and vaginal injuries are the most common injuries. Vaginal lacerations result from either penetration of a bony fragment or from indirect forces from diastasis of the symphysis pubis. Injuries to the cervix, uterus and ovaries are rare. Bladder rupture occurs in up to 10% of pelvic fractures.

Major Pelvic Trauma

- The incidence of rectal injury ranges from 17% to 64% dependent upon type of fracture. Bowel entrapment is rare.

- Pelvic injury is commonly associated with concomitant intra-thoracic and/or intra-abdominal injury.

TABLE 4.23 – ASSESSMENT and MANAGEMENT of: Major Pelvic Trauma
Assess: <C>ABCD
- Control any external catastrophic haemorrhage (refer to **Trauma Emergencies in Adults – Overview** and **Trauma Emergencies in Children – Overview**).
- Evaluate whether patient is **TIME-CRITICAL** or **NON-TIME-CRITICAL** following criteria as per trauma emergencies guideline. If patient is **TIME-CRITICAL, correct A and B problems, stabilise the pelvis on scene and rapidly transport to nearest suitable receiving hospital. Provide an alert/information call.** En-route, continue patient management of pelvic trauma (see below).
- In **NON-TIME-CRITICAL** patients, perform a more thorough patient assessment with a brief secondary survey.
Specifically Consider
- Pelvic fracture should be considered based upon the mechanism of injury.
- Clinical assessment of the pelvis includes observation for physical injury such as bruising, bleeding, deformity or swelling to the pelvis. Shortening of a lower limb may be present (see also **Limb Trauma**).
- Assessment by compression or distraction (e.g. springing) of the pelvis is unreliable and may both dislodge clots and exacerbate any injury and should not be performed. Any patient with a relevant mechanism of injury and concomitant hypotension **MUST** be managed as having a **time-critical pelvic injury** until proven otherwise.
Oxygen Therapy
- Major pelvic injury falls into the category of critical illness and requires high levels of supplemental oxygen regardless of initial oxygen saturation reading (SpO$_2$). Maintain high-flow oxygen (15 litres per minute) until vital signs are normal; thereafter, reduce flow rate, titrating to maintain oxygen saturations (SpO$_2$) in the 94–98% range (refer to **Oxygen**).
Pelvic Stabilisation
There is currently no evidence to suggest that any particular pelvic immobilisation device or approach is superior in terms of outcome in pelvic trauma, and a number of methods have been reported. Effective stabilisation of the pelvic ring should be instigated at the earliest possible opportunity for patients with suspected major pelvic injury, preferably before moving the patient, and may be achieved by:
- Use of an appropriate pelvic splint.
- Apply the pelvic splint directly to skin, if this can be done easily with minimal handling.
- Expert consensus suggests the use of an appropriate pelvic splint is preferable to improvised immobilisation techniques. In all methods, circumferential pressure is applied over the greater trochanters and not the iliac crests. Care must be exercised so as to ensure that the pelvis is not reduced beyond its normal anatomical position.
- Pressure sores and soft tissue injuries may occur when immobilisation devices are incorrectly fitted.
- Reduction and stabilisation of the pelvic ring should occur as soon as is practicable whilst still on scene, as stabilisation helps to reduce blood loss by realigning fracture surfaces, thereby limiting active bleeding and additionally helping to stabilise clots. Reduction of the pelvis may have a tamponade effect, particularly for venous bleeding; however, there is little evidence to support this belief.
- Log rolling of the patient with possible pelvic fracture should be avoided as this may exacerbate any pelvic injury; where possible, utilise an orthopaedic scoop stretcher to lift patients off the ground and limit movement to a 15° tilt.
Fluid Therapy
- There is little evidence to support the routine use of IV fluids in adult trauma patients (refer to **Intravascular Fluid Therapy in Adults** and **Intravascular Fluid Therapy in Children**).

Major Pelvic Trauma

TABLE 4.23 – ASSESSMENT and MANAGEMENT of: Major Pelvic Trauma *(continued)*

Pain Management

- Patients' pain should be managed appropriately (refer to **Pain Management in Adults** and **Pain Management in Children**); analgesia in the form of Entonox (refer to **Nitrous Oxide (Entonox®)** for administration and information) or morphine sulfate may be appropriate (refer to **Morphine Sulfate** for dosages and information).

5. Referral Pathway

The following cases should ALWAYS be transferred to further care:

- Any patient with hypotension and potential pelvic injury **MUST** be treated as a **TIME-CRITICAL** pelvic injury until proven otherwise.

- Any patient with sufficient mechanism of injury to cause a pelvic injury.

The following cases MAY be considered suitable/safe to be left at home:

- None.

6. Special Considerations for Children

- Pelvic fractures represent 1–3% of all fractures in children, thus there is a lower incidence compared with adults.

- In children, pelvic injuries have a lower mortality, accounting for 3.6–5.7% of trauma deaths, with fewer deaths occurring as a direct result of pelvic haemorrhage; blood loss is more likely to be from solid visceral injury than the pelvis.

- Different injury patterns – multi-system injuries in 60%; greater incidence of diaphragmatic injury.

- Principles of management are the same, with the exception of fluid and oxygen therapy (refer to **Intravascular Fluid Therapy in Children** and **Oxygen**).

- Clinical findings in small children can be unreliable.

7. Audit Information

- Incidence of suspected/actual pelvic fracture.

- Incidence of concomitant hypotension.

- Frequency of pelvic immobilisation when pelvic fracture suspected.

- Method of pelvic immobilisation.

KEY POINTS!

Major Pelvic Trauma

- **Pelvic fracture should be considered based upon mechanism of injury.**

- **The majority of pelvic fractures are stable pubic ramus or acetabular fractures.**

- **Any patient with hypotension and relevant mechanism of injury MUST be considered to have a TIME-CRITICAL pelvic injury.**

- **'Springing' or distraction of the pelvis must not be undertaken.**

- **Pelvic stabilisation should be implemented as soon as is practicable whilst still on scene.**

- **Consider appropriate pain management.**

- **The use of a scoop stretcher is recommended to avoid log rolling the patient unless extrication is required.**

Bibliography

1. Brown JK, Jing Y, Wang S, Ehrlich PF. Patterns of severe injury in pediatric car crash victims: Crash Injury Research Engineering Network database. *Journal of Pediatric Surgery* 2006, 41(2): 362–367.

2. O'Brien DP, Luchette FA, Pereira SJ, Lim E, Seeskin CS, James L, et al. Pelvic fracture in the elderly is associated with increased mortality. *Surgery* 2002, 132(4): 710–714.

3. Stein DM, O'Connor JV, Kufera JA, Ho SM, Dischinger PC, Copeland CE et al. Risk factors associated with pelvic fractures sustained in motor vehicle collisions involving newer vehicles. *Journal of Trauma* 2006, 61(1): 21–30.

4. Dalai SA, Burgess AR, Siegel JH, Young JW, Brumback RJ, Poka A, et al. Pelvic fracture in multiple trauma: classification by mechanism is key to pattern of organ injury, resuscitative requirements, and outcome. *Journal of Trauma* 1989, 29(7): 981–1000; discussion 1000–1002.

5. Demetriades D, Karaiskakis M, Toutouzas K, Alo K, Velmahos G, Chan L. Pelvic fractures: epidemiology and predictors of associated abdominal injuries and outcomes. *Journal of the American College of Surgeons* 2002, 195(1): 1–10.

6. Demetriades D, Murray J, Brown C, Velmahos G, Salim A, Alo K et al. High-level falls: type and severity of

injuries and survival outcome according to age. *Journal of Trauma* 2005, 58(2): 342–345.

7. Ferrera PC, Hill DA. Good outcomes of open pelvic fractures. *Injury* 1999, 30(3): 187–190.

8. Gustavo Parreira J, Coimbra R, Rasslan S, Oliveira A, Fregoneze M, Mercadante M. The role of associated injuries on outcome of blunt trauma patients sustaining pelvic fractures. *Injury* 2000, 31(9): 677–682.

9. Inaba K, Sharkey PW, Stephen DJG, Redelmeier DA, Brenneman FD. The increasing incidence of severe pelvic injury in motor vehicle collisions. *Injury* 2004, 35(8): 759–765.

10. Kimbrell BJ, Velmahos GC, Chan LS, Demetriades D. Angiographic embolization for pelvic fractures in older patients. *Archives of Surgery* 2004, 139(7): 728–732.

11. Tarman GJ, Kaplan GW, Lerman SL, McAleer IM, Losasso BE. Lower genitourinary injury and pelvic fractures in pediatric patients. *Urology* 2002, 59(1): 123–126.

12. Demetriades D, Murray J, Martin M, Velmahos G, Salim A, Alo K et al. Pedestrians injured by automobiles: relationship of age to injury type and severity. *Journal of the American College of Surgeons* 2004, 199(3): 382–387.

13. Hill RMF, Robinson CM, Keating JF. Fractures of the pubic rami. *Journal of Bone & Joint Surgery, British Volume* 2001, 83-B(8): 1141–1144.

14. Baxter NN, Habermann EB, Tepper JE, Durham SB, Virnig BA. Risk of pelvic fractures in older women following pelvic irradiation. Journal *of the American Medical Association* 2005, 294(20): 2587–2593.

15. Boufous S, Finch C, Lord S, Close J. The increasing burden of pelvic fractures in older people, New South Wales, Australia. *Injury* 2005, 36(11): 1323–1329.

16. Hauschild O, Strohm PC, Culemann U, Pohlemann T, Suedkamp NP, Koestler W et al. Mortality in patients with pelvic fractures: results from the German pelvic injury register. *Journal of Trauma* 2008, 64(2): 449–455.

17. Gansslen A, Pohlemann T, Paul C, Lobenhoffer P, Tscherne H. Epidemiology of pelvic ring injuries. *Injury* 1996, 27(1001): S/A13–20, S/A51.

18. Moreno C, Moore EE, Rosenberger A, Cleveland HC. Hemorrhage associated with major pelvic fracture: a multispecialty challenge. *Journal of Trauma* 1986, 26(11): 987–994.

19. Mucha P Jr, Farnell MB. Analysis of pelvic fracture management. *Journal of Trauma* 1984, 24(5): 379–386.

20. Siegel JH, Mason-Gonzalez S, Dischinger P, Cushing B, Read K, Robinson R, et al. Safety belt restraints and compartment intrusions in frontal and lateral motor vehicle crashes: mechanisms of injuries, complications, and acute care costs. *Journal of Trauma* 1993, 34(5): 736–758.

21. Brenneman FD, Katyal D, Boulanger BR, Tile M, Redelmeier DA. Long-term outcomes in open pelvic fractures. *Journal of Trauma and Acute Care Surgery* 1997, 42(5): 773–777.

22. Poole GV, Ward EF, Muakkassa FF, Hsu HSH, Griswold JA, Rhodes RS. Pelvic fracture from major blunt trauma: outcome is determined by associated injuries. *Annals of Surgery* 1991, 213(6): 532–539.

23. Croce MA, Magnotti LJ, Savage SA, Wood IGW, Fabian TC. Emergent pelvic fixation in patients with exsanguinating pelvic fractures. *Journal of the American College of Surgeons* 2007, 204(5): 935–939.

24. Duane TM, Tan BB, Golay D, Cole FJ Jr, Weireter LJ Jr, Britt LD. Blunt trauma and the role of routine pelvic radiographs: a prospective analysis. *Journal of Trauma* 2002, 53(3): 463–468.

25. Gonzalez RP, Fried PQ, Bukhalo M. The utility of clinical examination in screening for pelvic fractures in blunt trauma. *Journal of the American College of Surgeons* 2002, 194(2): 121–125.

26. Ham SJ, Van Walsum ADP, Vierhout PAM. Predictive value of the hip flexion test for fractures of the pelvis. *Injury Prevention* 1996, 27(8): 543–544.

27. Heath FR, Blum F, Rockwell S. Physical examination as a screening test for pelvic fractures in blunt trauma patients. *West Virginia Medical Journal* 1997, 93(5): 267–269.

28. Kaneriya PP, Schweitzer ME, Spettell C, Cohen MJ, Karasick D. The cost effectiveness of routine pelvic radiography in the evaluation of blunt trauma patients. *Skeletal Radiology* 1999, 28(5): 271– 273.

29. Khoury G, Sfeir R, Khalifeh M, Khoury SJ, Nabbout G. Penetrating trauma to the abdominal vessels. *Cardiovascular Surgery* 1996, 4(3): 405–407.

30. Salvino CK, Esposito TJ, Smith D, Dries D, Marshall W, Flisak M, et al. Routine pelvic x-ray studies in awake blunt trauma patients: a sensible policy? *Journal of Trauma* 1992, 33(3): 413–416.

31. Tien IY, Dufel SE. Does ethanol affect the reliability of pelvic bone examination in blunt trauma? *Annals of Emergency Medicine* 2000, 36(5): 451–455.

32. Yugueros P, Sarmiento JM, Garcia AF, Ferrada R. Unnecessary use of pelvic x-ray in blunt trauma. *Journal of Trauma* 1995, 39(4): 722–725.

33. Boulanger BR, Milzman D, Mitchell K, Rodriguez A. Body habitus as a predictor of injury pattern after blunt trauma. *Journal of Trauma* 1992, 33(2): 228–232.

34. Hanson PB, Milne JC, Chapman MW. Open fractures of the pelvis: review of 43 cases. *Journal of Bone & Joint Surgery, British Volume* 1991, 73(2): 325–329.

35. Malangoni MA, Miller FB, Cryer HM, Mullins RJ, Richardson JD. The management of penetrating pelvic trauma. *American Surgeon* 1990, 56(2): 61–65.

36. Perry IF Jr. Pelvic open fractures. *Clinical Orthopaedics* 1980, 151: 41–45.

37. Chong KH, DeCoster T, Osler T, Robinson B. Pelvic fractures and mortality. *Iowa Orthopaedic Journal* 1997, 17: 110–114.

38. Cryer HM, Miller FB, Evers BM, Rouben LR, Seligson DL. Pelvic fracture classification: correlation with hemorrhage. *Journal of Trauma* 1988, 28(7): 973–980.

39. Evers BM, Cryer HM, Miller FB. Pelvic fracture hemorrhage: priorities in management. *Archives of Surgery* 1989, 124(4): 422–424.

40. Heetveld MJ, Harris I, Schlaphoff G, Balogh Z, D'Amours SK, Sugrue M. Hemodynamically unstable pelvic fractures: recent care and new guidelines. *Journal of Surgery* 2004, 28(9): 904–909.

41. Heetveld MJ, Harris I, Schlaphoff G, Sugrue M. Guidelines for the management of haemodynamically unstable pelvic fracture patients. *ANZ Journal of Surgery* 2004, 74(7): 520–529.

42. Poole GV, Ward EF. Causes of mortality in patients with pelvic fractures. *Orthopedics* 1994, 17(8): 691–696.

43. Burgess AR, Eastridge BJ, Young JW, Ellison TS, Ellison PSJ, Poka A, et al. Pelvic ring disruptions: effective

classification system and treatment protocols. *Journal of Trauma* 1990, 30(7): 848–856.

44. Failinger MS, McGanity PLJ. Unstable fractures of the pelvic ring. *Journal of Bone & Joint Surgery, American Volume* 1992, 74(5): 781–791.

45. Henry SM, Tometta IP, Scalea TM. Damage control for devastating pelvic and extremity injuries. *Surgical Clinics of North America* 1997, 77(4): 879–895.

46. Richardson JD, Harty J, Amin M, Flint LM. Open pelvic fractures. *Journal of Trauma* 1982, 22(7): 533–538.

47. Rothenberger DA, Fischer RP, Perry JF Jr. Major vascular injuries secondary to pelvic fractures: an unsolved clinical problem. *American Journal of Surgery* 1978, 136(6): 660–662.

48. Grotz MRW, Gummerson NW, Gansslen A, Petrowsky H, Keel M, Allami MK et al. Staged management and outcome of combined pelvic and liver trauma: an international experience of the deadly duo. *Injury* 2006, 37(7): 642–651.

49. Wubben RC. Mortality rate of pelvic fracture patients. *Wisconsin Medical Journal* 1996, 95(10): 702–704.

50. Starr AJ, Griffen, MA. Pelvic ring disruptions: mechanisms, fracture pattern, morbidity and mortality. An analysis of 325 patients. OTA Annual Meeting, Texas, USA, 2000.

51. Koury HI, Peschiera JL, Welling RE. Selective use of pelvic roentgenograms in blunt trauma patients. *Journal of Trauma, Injury, Infection, & Critical Care* 1993, 34(2): 236–237.

52. Sriussadaporn S. Abdominopelvic vascular injuries. *Journal of the Medical Association of Thailand* 2000, 83(1): 13–20.

53. Moss MC, Bircher MD. Volume changes within the true pelvis during disruption of the pelvic ring: where does the haemorrhage go? *Injury* 1996, 27(suppl. 1): S-A21–3.

54. Rowe SA, Sochor MS, Staples KS, Wahl WL, Wang SC. Pelvic ring fractures: implications of vehicle design, crash type, and occupant characteristics. *Surgery* 2004, 136(4): 842–847.

55. Ben-Menachem Y, Coldwell DM, Young JWR, Burgess AR. Hemorrhage associated with pelvic fractures: causes, diagnosis, and emergent management. *American Journal of Roentgenology* 1991, 157(5): 1005–1014.

56. Dyer GSM, Vrahas MS. Review of the pathophysiology and acute management of haemorrhage in pelvic fracture. *Injury* 2006, 37(7): 602–613.

57. Fleming WH, Bowen JC III. Control of hemorrhage in pelvic crush injuries. *Journal of Trauma* 1973, 13(6): 567–570.

58. Davidson BS, Simmons GT, Williamson PR, Buerk CA. Pelvic fractures associated with open perineal wounds: a survivable injury. *Journal of Trauma* 1993, 35(1): 36–39.

59. Govender S, Sham A, Singh B. Open pelvic fractures. *Injury* 1990, 21(6): 373–376.

60. Sinnott R, Rhodes M, Brader A. Open pelvic fracture: an injury for trauma centers. *American Journal of Surgery* 1992, 163(3): 283–287.

61. Barach E, Martin G, Tomlanovich M. Blunt pelvic trauma with urethral injury in the female: a case report and review of the literature. *Journal of Emergency Medicine* 1984, 2(2): 101–105.

62. Bottlang M, Simpson T, Sigg J, Krieg JC, Madey SM, Long WB. Noninvasive reduction of open-book pelvic fractures by circumferential compression. *Journal of Orthopaedic Trauma* 2002, 16(6): 367–373.

63. Smith RJ. Avulsion of the nongravid uterus due to pelvic fracture. *Southern Medical Journal* 1989, 82(1): 70–73.

64. Sandler CM, Hall JT, Rodriguez MB, Corriere JN Jr. Bladder injury in blunt pelvic trauma. *Radiology* 1985, 158(3): 633–638.

65. Lunt HR. Entrapment of bowel within fractures of the pelvis. *Injury* 1970, 2(2): 121–126.

66. Reiff DA, McGwin G Jr, Metzger J, Windham ST, Doss M, Rue LW III. Identifying injuries and motor vehicle collision characteristics that together are suggestive of diaphragmatic rupture. *Journal of Trauma* 2002, 53(6): 1139–1145.

67. Waydhas C, Nast-Kolb D, Ruchholtz S. Pelvic ring fractures: utility of clinical examination in patients with impaired consciousness or tracheal intubation. *European Journal of Trauma and Emergency Surgery* 2007, 33(2): 170–175.

68. Fox MA, Mangiante EC, Fabian TC, Voeller GR, Kudsk KA. Pelvic fractures: an analysis of factors affecting pre-hospital triage and patient outcome. *Southern Medical Journal* 1990, 83(7): 785–788.

69. MacLeod M, Powell JN. Evaluation of pelvic fractures: clinical and radiologic. *Orthopedic Clinics of North America* 1997, 28(3): 299–319.

70. Sauerland S, Bouillon B, Rixen D, Raum MR, Koy T, Neugebauer EAM. The reliability of clinical examination in detecting pelvic fractures in blunt trauma patients: a meta-analysis. *Archives of Orthopaedic and Trauma Surgery* 2004, 124(2): 123–128.

71. Lee C, Porter K. The pre-hospital management of pelvic fractures. *Emergency Medicine Journal* 2007, 24(2): 130–133.

72. Waikakul S, Harnroongroj T, Vanadurongwan V. Immediate stabilization of unstable pelvic fractures versus delayed stabilization. *Journal of the Medical Association of Thailand* 1999, 82(7): 637–642.

73. Grimm MR, Vrahas MS, Thomas KA. Pressure-volume characteristics of the intact and disrupted pelvic retroperitoneum. *Journal of Trauma* 1998, 44(3): 454–459.

74. Bottlang M, Krieg JC, Mohr M, Simpson TS, Madey SM. Emergent management of pelvic ring fractures with use of circumferential compression. *Journal of Orthopaedic Trauma* 2002, 16(6): 367–373.

75. Brunette DD, Fifield G, Ruiz E. Use of pneumatic antishock trousers in the management of pediatric pelvic hemorrhage. *Pediatric Emergency Care* 1987, 3(2): 86–90.

76. Connolly B, Gerlinger T, Pitcher JD. Complete masking of a severe open-book pelvic fracture by a pneumatic antishock garment. *Journal of Trauma* 1999, 46(2): 340–342.

77. Friese G, LaMay G. Emergency stabilization of unstable pelvic fractures. *Emergency Medical Services* 2005, 34(5): 65.

78. Jowett AJL, Bowyer GW. Pressure characteristics of pelvic binders. *Injury* 2007, 38(1): 118–121.

79. Katsoulis E, Drakoulakis E, Giannoudis PV. (iii) Management of open pelvic fractures. *Current Orthopaedics* 2005, 19(5): 345–353.

80. Krieg JC, Mohr M, Ellis TJ, Simpson TS, Madey SM, Bottlang M. Emergent stabilization of pelvic ring injuries by controlled circumferential compression: a clinical

SECTION **4** Trauma

Major Pelvic Trauma

trial. *Journal of Trauma, Injury, Infection, & Critical Care* 2005, 59(3): 659–664.

81. Routt MLC Jr, Simonian PT, Swiontkowski MF. Stabilization of pelvic ring disruptions. *Orthopedic Clinics of North America* 1997, 28(3): 369–388.

82. Salomone JP, Ustin JS, McSwain NE Jr, Feliciano DV. Opinions of trauma practitioners regarding pre-hospital interventions for critically injured patients. *Journal of Trauma* 2005, 58(3): 509–515; discussion 515–517.

83. Scurr JH, Cutting P. Tight jeans as a compression garment after major trauma. *British Medical Journal (Clinical Research Edition)* 1984, 288(6420): 828.

84. Simpson T, Krieg JC, Heuer F, Bottlang M. Stabilization of pelvic ring disruptions with a circumferential sheet. *Journal of Trauma, Injury, Infection, & Critical Care* 2002, 52(1): 158–161.

85. Vermeulen B, Peter R, Hoffmeyer P, Unger PF. Prehospital stabilization of pelvic dislocations: a new strap belt to provide temporary hemodynamic stabilization. *Swiss Surgery* 1999, 5(2): 43–46.

86. Nunn T, Cosker TDA, Bose D, Pallister I. Immediate application of improvised pelvic binder as first step in extended resuscitation from life-threatening hypovolaemic shock in conscious patients with unstable pelvic injuries. *Injury* 2007, 38(1): 125–128.

87. Krieg JC, Mohr M, Mirza AJ, Bottlang M. Pelvic circumferential compression in the presence of soft-tissue injuries: a case report. *Journal of Trauma, Injury, Infection, & Critical Care* 2005, 59(2): 470–472.

88. Ismail N, Bellemare JF, Mollitt DL, DiScala C, Koeppel B, Tepas IJJ. Death from pelvic fracture: children are different. *Journal of Pediatric Surgery* 1996, 31(1): 82–85.

89. Junkins EPJ, Nelson DS, Carroll KL, Hansen K, Furnival RA. A prospective evaluation of the clinical presentation of pediatric pelvic fractures. *Journal of Trauma* 2001, 51(1): 64–68.

90. Silber JS, Flynn JM, Koffler KM, Dormans JP, Drummond DS. Analysis of the cause, classification, and associated injuries of 166 consecutive pediatric pelvic fractures. *Journal of Pediatric Orthopaedics* 2001, 21(4): 446–450.

91. Junkins EP, Furnival RA, Bake RG. The clinical presentation of pediatric pelvic fractures. *Pediatric Emergency Care* 2001, 17(1): 15–18.

Spinal Injury and Spinal Cord Injury

1. Introduction

- In the major trauma patient, spinal injuries are common. The majority are stable; some are unstable, risking spinal cord damage, and a small number are associated with spinal cord injury (SCI) at the outset. Differentiation between stable and unstable injuries requires specific imaging in the ED.

- Effective management from the time of injury is important to ensure optimal outcomes. This guideline provides guidance for the assessment and initial management of cervical spine and spinal trauma, including indicators to guidance for related conditions.

2. Pathophysiology

- The spinal cord runs in the spinal canal down to the level of the second lumbar vertebra in adults.

- The amount of space in the spinal canal in the upper neck is relatively large, and risk of secondary injury in this area can be reduced if adequate immobilisation is applied. In the thoracic area the cord is wide and the spinal canal relatively narrow; injury in this area is more likely to completely disrupt and damage the spinal cord.

- Spinal shock is a state of complete loss of motor function and often sensory function found sometimes after SCI. This immediate reaction may go on for some considerable time, but some recovery may well be possible. Complete and incomplete cord injury cannot be distinguished in the presence of spinal shock.

- Neurogenic shock is the state of poor tissue perfusion caused by sympathetic tone loss after spinal cord injury.

3. Incidence

- Falls are a frequent cause of SCI in the older person. Maintain a high index of suspicion in cases of older people who have had low-energy falls.

- SCI affects young and fit people and will continue to affect them to a varying degree for the rest of their lives.

- Road traffic collisions (RTCs), falls and sporting injuries are the most common causes of SCI – as a group, motorcyclists occupy more spinal injury unit beds than any other group involved in road traffic collisions. Rollover road traffic collisions where occupants are not wearing seat belts, and the head comes into contact with the vehicle body, and pedestrians struck by vehicles are likely to suffer SCI. Ejection from a vehicle increases the risk of injury significantly.

- UK Trauma Audit Research Network (TARN) data has shown that, in the presence of a cervical bony injury, 13.4% of patients have associated injuries elsewhere in the thoracic and lumbar spine.

3.1. Risk Factors

- RTCs:
  - rollover RTCs
  - non-wearing of seat belts
  - ejection from vehicle
  - struck by a vehicle.
- Sporting injuries:
  - diving into shallow water
  - horse riding
  - rugby
  - gymnastics and trampolining.
- Falls:
  - older people.
  - rheumatoid arthritis.
- Violent attacks and domestic incidents.

- Certain sporting accidents, especially diving into shallow water, horse riding, rugby, gymnastics and trampolining, have a higher than average risk of SCI. Rapid deceleration injury such as gliding and light aircraft accidents also increases the risk of SCI.

- Older people and those with rheumatoid arthritis are prone to odontoid peg fractures that may be difficult to detect clinically. Such injuries can occur from relatively minor trauma (e.g. falls from a standing height).

3.2. Cauda Equina Syndrome (CES)

- Cauda equina syndrome (CES) is caused by compression of the nerves in the spinal canal below the end of the spinal cord (at L2 vertebra level). It can occur in patients with trauma, a herniated disc, chronic or acute low back pain, tumours or infection.

- Clinical diagnosis of CES is not easy. Most cases are of sudden onset and progress rapidly within hours or days. However, CES can evolve slowly and patients do not always complain of pain. Roughly 50–70% of patients have urinary retention on presentation.

- CES is an acute surgical emergency; early diagnosis is essential and the patient requires immediate conveyance to hospital for investigation if CES is suspected. Early surgical decompression is crucial to prevent permanent neurological damage.

Red flag signs and symptoms of CES

⚑ Loss of bladder and/or bowel dysfunction control, causing incontinence.

⚑ Reduced sensation in the saddle (perineal) area.

⚑ New onset sexual dysfunction.

⚑ Neurological deficit in the lower limb (motor/sensory loss, reflex changes).

Spinal Injury and Spinal Cord Injury

4. Severity and Outcome

- Injury most frequently occurs at the junctions of mobile and fixed sections of the spine. Hence fractures are more commonly seen in the lower cervical vertebrae, where the cervical and thoracic spine meets (C5, 6, 7/T1 area), and the thoracolumbar junction. Of patients with one identified spinal fracture, 10–15% will be found to have another.
- In the extreme, SCI may prove immediately fatal where the upper cervical cord is damaged, paralysing the diaphragm and respiratory muscles.
- Partial cord damage, however, may solely affect individual sensory or motor nerve tracts, producing varying long-term disability. It is important to note that there is an increasing percentage of cases where the cord damage is only partial and quality recovery is possible, providing the condition is recognised and managed appropriately.

5. Immobilisation

- All patients with the possibility of spinal injury should have manual immobilisation commenced at the earliest time, while initial assessment is undertaken.
- If immobilisation is indicated then the whole spine must be immobilised. There are differences between the types of semi-rigid collar; acceptable methods of immobilisation are:
  - manual immobilisation while the spine is supported
  - collar, head blocks and spinal support.

The following techniques may be used:

- Patient lying supine:
  - Use a scoop stretcher and cervical spine immobilisation. To minimise movement of the spine, utilise a 10-degree tilt to the left and right.
  - Patients should be transported on the scoop stretcher unless there is a prolonged journey time, when a vacuum mattress should be utilised.
  - To utilise the vacuum mattress, lift the patient using the scoop stretcher, then insert the mattress underneath and remove the scoop stretcher.
- Patient lying prone:
  - Log roll the patient with manual immobilisation of the cervical spine to enable a scoop stretcher to be used.
  - Perform a two-stage log roll onto a vacuum mattress.
- Patient requiring extrication:
  - Extrication devices should be used if there is any risk of rotational movement.
  - Rearward extrication on an extrication board.
  - Side extrication invariably involves some rotational component and therefore has higher risks in many circumstances.

NB The longboard should only be used as an extrication device. Do not transport patients to hospital on a longboard.

5.1. Extrication

- Consider asking a patient who is not physically trapped to self-extricate, providing they have none of the following:
  - significant distracting injuries
  - abnormal neurological symptoms (paraesthesia or weakness or numbness)
  - spinal pain or tenderness.
- Explain to a patient who is self-extricating that they should stop moving and wait to be moved if they develop any spinal pain, numbness, tingling or weakness.
- When a patient has self-extricated:
  - ask them to lay supine on a stretcher positioned adjacent to the vehicle or incident
  - assess them further for any signs of spinal injury, spinal tenderness or abnormal neurology in the ambulance.
- **Inviting a patient to self-extricate is not clearing the cervical spine.**
- Any patient who has not had a cervical spine clearance documented in the ambulance clinician's notes should be treated as an uncleared spine whether immobilised or not, and that information must be specifically relayed to staff on handover.

Emergency Extrication

- If there is an immediate threat to a patient's life and rapid extrication is needed, make all efforts to limit spinal movement without delaying treatment.

5.2. Cautions/Precautions

Vomiting

- Vomiting and consequent aspiration are serious consequences of immobilisation. Ambulance clinicians must always have a plan of action in case vomiting should occur.
- The collar will usually need to be removed and manual in-line immobilisation instituted. This may include:
  - suction
  - head-down tilt of the immobilisation device
  - rolling the patient onto one side on the immobilisation device.

Restless/Combative Patients

- There are many reasons for the patient to be restless and it is important to rule out reversible causes (e.g. hypoxia, pain, fear).

Spinal Injury and Spinal Cord Injury

- If, despite appropriate measures, the patient remains restless, the use of spinal immobilisation devices may be difficult and could be counterproductive. A struggling patient is more likely to increase any injury, so think about letting them find a position where they are comfortable with manual in-line spinal immobilisation.

- The use of restraint can increase forces on the injured spine and therefore a 'best possible' approach should be adopted.

Head Injury

- Patients with a head injury may have raised intracranial pressure, which restraint can increase; therefore a 'best possible' approach should be adopted.

Special Cases

- Some older patients, and those with known spinal deformities (e.g. ankylosing spondylitis), may not be able to tolerate a collar or breathe adequately when positioned absolutely flat. Therefore a 'best possible' approach should be adopted, which may include manual in-line immobilisation or maintenance of the pre-existing spinal deformity where putting the patient in the in-line neutral position is unsafe.

Immobilisation of Spinal Injuries

- Soft collars do not limit movement and should not be used.

- There is variable difference between the various types of semi-rigid collars.

- The addition of head blocks and tape increases immobilisation.

- The application of devices is more important than the variation of devices.

- To achieve neutral position in an adult, the occiput should be raised by 2cm.

- Extrication devices are better than extrication boards at reducing rotational movement.

- Vacuum mattresses are more comfortable, and give better immobilisation.

- Vacuum mattresses cannot be used for extrication and are vulnerable to damage.

- Long extrication/spinal boards should only be used as an extrication device. Patients should be immobilised using a scoop stretcher. Once on a scoop stretcher they should remain on it unless they are placed on a vacuum mattress when there is a prolonged journey time.

5.3. When Not to Apply Immobilisation

- Not all patients require immobilisation (refer to Figure 4.10). When assessing for spinal injury, it is important to consider whether the patient:
  - is under the influence of drugs or alcohol
  - is uncooperative or confused

  - has any bony spinal pain anywhere along the spine
  - has any significant distracting injuries
  - has a reduced level of consciousness
  - has a priapism (unconscious or exposed male)
  - has any foot or hand weakness (motor assessment)
  - has any absent or altered sensation in the limbs (sensory assessment)
  - has a history of past spinal problems, including previous spinal surgery or conditions that predispose to instability of the spine.

- If the assessment cannot be completed or **any of the above factors are present**, carry out full in-line immobilisation.

- Penetrating injury to the head has not been shown to be an indication for spinal immobilisation, and even penetrating injuries of the neck only rarely need selective immobilisation.

- The few patients missed with SCI are often at the extremes of age. Such criteria can be reproducibly used in the pre-hospital environment. Mechanism of injury was not shown to be an independent predictor of injury.

- Use of such guidelines can significantly reduce the use of unnecessary immobilisation.

- Some patients may sustain thoracic or lumbar injuries in addition to, or in isolation from, cervical spine injuries. If you suspect thoracic or lumbar injuries, whether the cervical spine has been cleared, then full spinal immobilisation should be undertaken whenever possible.

5.4. Hazards of Immobilisation

- The value of routine pre-hospital spinal immobilisation remains uncertain and any benefits may be outweighed by the risks of rigid collar immobilisation, including:
  - compromised airway
  - increased intracranial pressure
  - increased risk of aspiration
  - restricted ventilation
  - dysphagia
  - skin ulceration
  - inducement of pain, even in those with no injury
  - known spinal deformities.

5.5. Sequence for Immobilisation

- All patients should be initially immobilised if the mechanism of injury suggests the possibility of SCI.

Blunt Trauma

- Following assessment, it is possible to remove the immobilisation if ALL the criteria are met (refer to Figure 4.10).

Spinal Injury and Spinal Cord Injury

- Spinal pain does not include tenderness isolated to the muscles of the side of the neck.

Penetrating Trauma

- Those with isolated penetrating injuries to limbs or the head do not require immobilisation.

- Those with truncal or neck trauma should be immobilised if there is new neurology and/or the trajectory of the penetrating wound could pass near or through the spinal column.

5.6. Immobilisation of Children

- When carrying out in-line spinal immobilisation in children, manually stabilise the head with the spine in-line and consider the following:

- – If appropriate, involve family members and carers.
- – If possible, keep infants in their car seats.
- – Use a scoop stretcher with blanket rolls, vacuum mattress, vacuum limb splints or Kendrick extrication device.

6. Assessment and Management

For assessment and management of the cervical spine and spine, refer to Table 4.24 and Figure 4.10.

TABLE 4.24 – ASSESSMENT and MANAGEMENT of: Cervical Spine and Spinal Trauma
Assess <C>ABCDE while controlling the spine
⬜ Control any external catastrophic haemorrhage (refer to **Trauma Emergencies in Adults – Overview** and **Trauma Emergencies in Children – Overview**).   ⬜ At all stages of the assessment, protect the patient's cervical spine with manual in-line immobilisation and avoid moving the remainder of the spine.
TIME-CRITICAL Patient

⬜ Follow criteria in **Trauma Emergencies Overview**.
 ⬜ If the patient is **TIME-CRITICAL**:
   – Manage the airway.
   – Immobilise the spine.
   – Transfer to a major trauma centre; unless the patient needs an immediate lifesaving intervention, transfer to nearest trauma unit.
   – Provide a pre-alert using ATMIST.
   – Continue patient management en-route (see below).

Assess Oxygen Saturation
(Refer to **Oxygen**)   ⬜ Adults – administer high levels of supplemental oxygen and aim for target saturation within the range of 94–98% – except for patients with COPD.   ⬜ Children – administer high levels of supplemental oxygen.
Determine mechanism of injury

⬜ Forces causing injury include:
   – hyperflexion
   – hyperextension
   – rotation
   – compression
   – one or more of these.

Specific Symptoms of SCI

⬜ The patient may complain of:
   – cervical and/or spinal pain
   – loss of sensory function in the limbs
   – loss of motor function in the limbs
   – sensation of burning in the trunk or limbs
   – sensation of electric shock in the trunk or limbs.

Spinal Injury and Spinal Cord Injury

TABLE 4.24 – ASSESSMENT and MANAGEMENT of: Cervical Spine and Spinal Trauma (continued)

Rapidly Assess to Determine the Presence and Estimate the Level of Spinal Cord Injury

- The following signs may indicate injury:
  - diaphragmatic or abdominal breathing
  - hypotension (BP often <80–90 mmHg) with bradycardia
  - warm peripheries or vasodilatation in the presence of low blood pressure
  - flaccid (floppy) muscles with absent reflexes
  - priapism – partial or full erection of the penis.
- In a conscious patient – assess sensory and motor function:
  - use light touch and response to pain
  - examine upper limbs and hands
  - examine lower limbs and feet
  - examine both sides
  - undertake the examination in the MID-AXILLARY line, NOT the MID-CLAVICULAR line, as C2, C3 and C4 all supply sensation to the nipple line; use the forehead as the reference point to guide what is normal sensation.

NB Always presume a SCI in the unconscious trauma patient.

Non-TIME-CRITICAL Patient

- Perform a more thorough assessment with a brief secondary survey

Assess for Neurogenic Shock

- Diagnosis is difficult in pre-hospital care – the aim is to:
  - maintain blood pressure of approximately 90 mmHg systolic
  - obtain IV access
  - determine the need for fluid replacement but DO NOT delay on scene (refer to **Intravascular Fluid Therapy in Adults** and **Intravascular Fluid Therapy in Children**).
- In neurogenic shock, a few degrees of head-down tilt may improve the circulation, but remember that in cases of abdominal breathing, this manoeuvre may further worsen respiration and ventilation. This position is also unsuitable for a patient who has, or may have, a head injury.
- If bradycardia is present, consider atropine (refer to **Atropine Sulfate**) – but it is important to rule out other causes (e.g. hypoxia, severe hypovolaemia).

Assess the Need for Assisted Ventilation

- Refer to **Airway and Breathing Management**.

Steroids

- Steroids have no part to play in the pre-hospital management of acute spinal cord injuries.

At Hospital

- The patient should be on a scoop stretcher.
- Complete documentation and, if possible, record information whether the assessments show that the patient's condition is improving or deteriorating.

Additional Information

- Transportation of spinal patients:
  - Driving should balance the advantages of smooth driving and time to arrival at hospital. No immobilisation technique eliminates movement from vehicle swaying and jarring.
  - There is no evidence to show advantage of direct transport to a spinal injury centre.
  - Patients should be transported on the scoop stretcher unless there is a prolonged journey time, when a vacuum mattress should be utilised.
  - As half of all cases of spinal injuries have other serious injuries, any unnecessary delay at the scene or in transit should be avoided.

Spinal Injury and Spinal Cord Injury

Patients with a history of trauma
Is there a potential for spinal injury in an adult >16 years old?

Yes ↓

- Under the influence of drugs or alcohol?
- Is confused or uncooperative?
- Has a reduced level of consciousness?
- Has any spinal pain (or pain elicited on coughing)?
- Any motor weakness in hands or feet?
- Any history of past spinal problems, including previous spinal surgery, severe osteoarthritis, ankylosing spondylitis?
- Any priapism?

→ Yes →

No ↓

High Risk?
- Dangerous mechanism of injury (fall from a height of >1 metre or five steps, axial load to the head - e.g. diving, high-speed motor vehicle collision, rollover motor accident, ejection from a motor vehicle, accident involving motorised recreational vehicles, bicycle collision, horse riding accidents)

→ Yes →

No ↓

Upon Examination:
- Any abnormal neurology (loss of sensation; numbness; 'pins and needles'; burning pain)?
- Any bony spinal pain anywhere along the spine (at rest or on coughing)?
- Any distracting injury?

→ Yes →

No ↓

Low Risk?
- Was involved in a minor rear-end motor vehicle collision
- Is comfortable in a sitting position
- Has been ambulatory at any time since the injury
- Has no midline cervical spine tenderness (answer 'no' if patient has pain)
- Delayed onset of neck pain

Yes ↓

Is the patient able to actively rotate their head 45° to the left and right?
and
Is the patient able to mobilise without pain or abnormal neurology?

→ No →

Yes ↓

> **Spine Cleared**

Use of spinal immobilisation devices may be difficult (e.g. in people with short/wide necks, or people with a pre-existing deformity) and could be counterproductive (i.e. increasing pain, worsening neurological signs and symptoms). In uncooperative, agitated or distressed people, think about letting them find a position where they are comfortable with manual in-line spinal immobilisation.

IMMOBILISE

Immobilise the entire spine.
If the patient is ambulatory or has been ambulatory at the scene, they can self-extricate if appropriate and may be guided to lie down onto the scoop stretcher to be immobilised.
The scoop should be placed on the trolley and located as close as practicable to the patient. Patients MUST NOT be encouraged to walk up any steps (causes potential axial loading).

Patients with suspected spinal injury with abnormal neurology must be transferred to a Major Trauma Centre

Figure 4.10 – Immobilisation algorithm. Republished with permission of Yorkshire Ambulance Service.

SECTION **4** Trauma

Spinal Injury and Spinal Cord Injury

KEY POINTS!

Spinal Injury

- Immobilise the whole spine until it is positively cleared.
- Immobilise the whole spine in all unconscious blunt trauma patients.
- If the cervical spine is immobilised, the thoracic and lumbar spine also need immobilisation.
- Asking a patient to self-extricate is acceptable, but does not clear the cervical spine.
- Standard immobilisation is by means of collar (unless contra-indicated or counterproductive), head blocks, tape and scoop.
- The longboard is solely used as an extrication device, and not for transporting patients to hospital.
- Aspiration of vomit, pressure sores and raised intracranial pressure are major complications of immobilisation.

Bibliography

1. National Institute for Health and Clinical Excellence. Fractures (Complex): Assessment and Management (NG37). London: NICE, 2016. Available from: https://www.nice.org.uk/guidance/ng37.

2. National Institute for Health and Clinical Excellence. Fractures (Non-complex): Assessment and Management (NG38). London: NICE, 2016. Available from: https://www.nice.org.uk/guidance/ng38.

3. National Institute for Health and Clinical Excellence. Major Trauma: Assessment and Initial Management (NG39). London: NICE, 2016. Available from: https://www.nice.org.uk/guidance/ng39.

4. National Institute for Health and Clinical Excellence. Major Trauma: Service Delivery (NG40). London: NICE, 2016. Available from: https://www.nice.org.uk/guidance/ng40.

5. National Institute for Health and Clinical Excellence. *Spinal Injury: Assessment and Initial Management* (NG41). London: NICE, 2016. Available from: https://www.nice.org.uk/guidance/ng41.

6. Hoffman JR, Wolfson AB, Todd K, Mower WR. Selective cervical spine radiography in blunt trauma: methodology of the National Emergency X-Radiography Utilization Study (NEXUS). *Ann Emerg Med*. 1998, 32(4): 461–469.

7. Canadian CT Head and C-Spine (CCC) Study Group. Canadian C-Spine Rule study for alert and stable trauma patients: I. Background and rationale. *CJEM*. 2004, 4(2): 84–90.

8. Trauma Audit and Research Network. *Major Trauma in Older People*. Manchester: University of Manchester, 2017.

SECTION **4** Trauma

Thoracic Trauma

1. Introduction

- In pre-hospital care, the most common problem associated with severe thoracic injuries is hypoxia, either from impaired ventilation or secondary to hypovolaemia from massive bleeding into the chest (haemothorax) or major vessel disruption (e.g. ruptured thoracic aorta).

2. Incidence

- Severe thoracic injuries are one of the most common causes of death from trauma, accounting for approximately 25% of such deaths.

3. Severity and Outcome

- Despite the very high percentage of serious thoracic injuries, the vast majority of them can be managed in hospital with chest drainage and resuscitation, and only 10–15% require surgical intervention.

4. Pathophysiology

- The mechanism of injury is an important guide to the likelihood of significant thoracic injuries. Injuries to the chest wall usually arise from direct contact, for example intrusion of wreckage in a road traffic collision or blunt trauma arising from a direct blow. Seat-belt injuries fall into this category and may cause fractures of the sternum, ribs and clavicle.

- If the force is sufficient, the deformity and the damage to the chest wall structures may induce tearing and contusion to the underlying lung and other structures. This may produce a combination of severe pain on breathing (pleuritic pain) and a damaged lung, both of which will significantly reduce the ability to ventilate adequately. This combination is a common cause of hypoxia.

- Blunt trauma to the sternum may cause myocardial contusion, which may result in cardiac rhythm disturbances.

- Penetrating trauma may well damage the heart, lungs and great vessels, either in isolation or in combination. It must be remembered that penetrating wounds to the upper abdomen and neck may well have caused injuries within the chest remote from the entry wound. Conversely, penetrating wounds to the chest may well involve the liver, kidneys and spleen.

- The lung may be damaged, with bleeding causing a haemothorax or an air leak causing a pneumothorax. Penetrating or occasionally a blunt injury may result in cardiac injuries. Blood can leak into the non-elastic surrounding pericardial sac and build up pressure to an extent that the heart is incapable of refilling to pump blood into circulation. This is known as cardiac tamponade and can be fatal if not rapidly relieved at hospital (see additional information in Table 4.26).

- Rapid deceleration injuries may result in sheering forces sufficient to rupture great vessels such as the aorta, caused by compressing the vessels between the sternum and the spine.

- The five major thoracic injuries encountered in the pre-hospital setting are:

1 tension pneumothorax
2 massive haemothorax (following uncontrolled haemorrhage into the chest cavity)
3 open chest wounds
4 flail chest
5 cardiac tamponade.

5. Assessment and Management

For the assessment and management of thoracic trauma, refer to Tables 4.25 and 4.26.

TABLE 4.25 – ASSESSMENT and MANAGEMENT of: Thoracic Trauma

Assess <C>ABCDE

- Control any external catastrophic haemorrhage (refer to **Trauma Emergencies in Adults – Overview** and **Trauma Emergencies in Children – Overview**).
- If any of the following **TIME-CRITICAL** features are present:
  - major **<C>ABCD** complications
  - penetrating chest injury
  - flail chest
  - tension pneumothorax
  - cardiac tamponade
  - surgical emphysema
  - blast injury to the lungs.
- Correct **<C>ABC** problems.

Thoracic Trauma

TABLE 4.25 – ASSESSMENT and MANAGEMENT of: Thoracic Trauma *(continued)*
▪ Undertake a **TIME-CRITICAL** transfer to a major trauma centre.[1]
▪ Major unmanageable **A** and **B** problems should be transferred to the nearest trauma unit.
▪ Provide a pre-alert using ATMIST.
▪ Continue patient management en-route.
Specifically Consider

– tension pneumothorax
   – open chest wounds
   – flail chest
   – surgical emphysema
   – cardiac tamponade
   – impaling objects.

▪ Refer to Table 4.26 for the assessment and management of these conditions/situations.
Non-time-critical Patient
▪ Undertake a secondary survey
▪ A load-and-go approach is particularly important with penetrating injuries, unless enhanced care support is likely to arrive before the patient can reach an appropriate hospital.
Monitor SpO$_2$ and Assess for Signs of Hypoxia
▪ Administer high levels of supplemental oxygen until the vital signs are normal, then aim for a target saturation within the range of 94–98% (refer to **Oxygen**).
Assess Breathing Adequacy, Respiratory Rate, Effort and Volume and Equality of Air Entry

▪ Consider assisted ventilation at a rate of 12–20 respirations per minute if any of the following are present:
   – SpO$_2$ <90% on high levels of supplemental oxygen.
   – Respiratory rate is <10 or >30 breaths per minute.
   – Inadequate chest expansion.

NB Exercise caution, as any positive pressure ventilation may increase the size of a pneumothorax.
Monitor Nasal EtCO$_2$
▪ EtCO$_2$ presents an immediate picture of the patient's condition.
Monitor Heart Rate and Rhythm
▪ Attach ECG monitor.
Consider IV Fluids
▪ Obtain IV access.
▪ Refer to **Intravascular Fluid Therapy in Adults** and **Intravascular Fluid Therapy in Children** – **DO NOT** delay on scene.
Assess Patient's Level of Pain
▪ Refer to **Pain Management in Adults** and **Pain Management in Children**.
NB Avoid Entonox in a patient with a suspected pneumothorax as there is a significant risk of enlarging a pneumothorax.
NB Adequate morphine analgesia may improve ventilation by allowing better chest wall movement, but high doses may induce respiratory depression. Careful titration of doses is therefore required (refer to **Morphine Sulfate**).

(continued)

---

1   Patients should normally be transported in a semi-recumbent or upright posture; however, this may often not be possible due to other injuries present or suspected.

Thoracic Trauma

TABLE 4.25 – ASSESSMENT and MANAGEMENT of: Thoracic Trauma *(continued)*

Management (Children)

Assessment:

- Assess as above.

Manage as above but consider:

- Children can have severe internal chest injuries with minimal or no external evidence of chest injuries.
- Children show signs of shock late due to good compensatory mechanisms.
- Always consider multiple injuries in children with rib fractures, as this suggests a significant mechanism of injury and isolated chest injuries are rare in children.
- Consider non-accidental injury.

Additional Information

- Chest trauma is treated with difficulty in the field, and prolonged treatment before transportation is **NOT** indicated if significant chest injury is suspected.
- Open chest wounds – seal the wound with a proprietary dressing with a valve, but if none are available use a three-sided dressing.
- Specifically consider the need for thoracic surgery intervention.
- Impaling objects – handle carefully, secure the object with a dressing and if the object is pulsating do not completely immobilise it but allow it to pulsate. **NB** Be vigilant – the patient may try to remove the object and this could be used as a weapon.
- Remember any stab or bullet wound to the chest, abdomen or back may penetrate the heart.
- Patients with significant chest trauma may often insist on sitting upright and this is especially common in patients with diaphragmatic injury who may get extremely breathless when lying down. In this instance, the patient is best managed sitting upright or at 30–45 degrees, and it must be documented that the spine has not been cleared.
- In the rare incident of gunshot/stab injury to personnel wearing protection vests (e.g. ballistic and stab), these may protect from penetrating injury. However, serious underlying blunt trauma (e.g. pulmonary contusion) may be caused to the thorax.
- **NEVER UNDERESTIMATE THESE INJURIES.** There is a strong link between serious blunt chest wall injury and thoracic spine injury. Maintain a high index of suspicion.

TABLE 4.26 – ASSESSMENT and MANAGEMENT of: Specific Thoracic Trauma

FLAIL CHEST

Flail chest is usually the result of a significant blunt chest injury, causing two or more rib fractures in two or more places. A sternal flail can also occur where the ribs or costal cartilages are fractured on both sides of the chest. This results in a flail segment that moves independently of the rest of the chest during respiration, leading to inadequate ventilation. The ensuing pulmonary insufficiency is caused by three pathophysiological processes:

1. The negative pressure required for effective ventilation is disrupted due to the paradoxical motion of the flail segment.
2. The underlying pulmonary contusion, which causes haemorrhage and oedema of the lung.
3. The pain associated with the multiple rib fractures will result in a degree of hypoventilation.
   - Small flail segments may not be detectable.
   - Large flail segments may impair ventilation considerably as a result of pain.

Thoracic Trauma

TABLE 4.26 – ASSESSMENT and MANAGEMENT of: Specific Thoracic Trauma *(continued)*
Assess for Signs of a Flail Chest
▪ Flail segments should not be immobilised and efforts to maintain ventilation are the priority.
▪ Allow the patient to sit supported at 30–45 degrees rather than trying to make them stay on a scoop stretcher.
NB Traditionally, the patient has been turned onto the affected side for transportation, but this CANNOT be achieved on a scoop stretcher.
Assess the Patient's Level of Pain
▪ Consider the need for analgesia (if indicated, refer to **Pain Management in Adults** and **Pain Management in Children**).
Transfer
▪ Undertake a **TIME-CRITICAL** transfer to a major trauma centre, unless the patient needs an immediate lifesaving intervention, in which case transfer to nearest trauma unit.
▪ Provide a pre-alert using ATMIST.
▪ Continue patient management en-route.
TENSION PNEUMOTHORAX
▪ This is a rare respiratory emergency which may require immediate action at the scene or en-route to further care. A tension pneumothorax occurs when a damaged area of lung leaks air out into the pleural space on each inspiration but does not permit the air to exit from the chest via the lung on expiration.
▪ This progressively builds up air under tension on the affected side, collapsing that lung and putting increasing pressure on the heart and great vessels and the opposite lung. Decreased venous return is significantly affected by the kinking of the vessels, especially the inferior vena cava, as the mediastinum is pushed towards the contralateral side. Coughing and shouting can make a situation worse. If this air is not released externally, the heart will be unable to fill and the other lung will no longer be able to ventilate, inducing cardiac arrest.
▪ Tension pneumothorax is most often related to penetrating trauma, but can arise spontaneously from blunt or crushing injuries to the chest and as the result of a blast wave. This will present rapidly with an increase in breathlessness and extreme respiratory distress (respiratory rate often >30 breaths per minute). Subsequently the patient may deteriorate and the breathing rate may rapidly slow to <10 breaths per minute before the patient arrests.
▪ Signs and symptoms: – The chest on the affected side may appear to be moving poorly or not at all.   – At the same time, the affected chest wall may appear to be over-expanded (hyperexpansion).   – Air entry will be greatly reduced or absent on the affected side.   – In the absence of shock, the neck veins may become distended.   – Later, the trachea and apex beat of the heart may become displaced away from the side of the pneumothorax, and cyanosis and breathlessness may appear.   – Hyperresonance may be present.   – Occasionally, the patient will only present with rapidly deteriorating respiratory distress.   – The patient may appear shocked as a result of decreased cardiac output.   – Patients are usually tachycardic and hypotensive.
▪ Ventilation of a patient with a chest injury is a common cause of tension pneumothorax in the pre-hospital setting. Forcing oxygenated air down into the lung under positive pressure will progressively expand a small, undetected simple pneumothorax into a tension pneumothorax. This will take some minutes and may well be several minutes after ventilation has commenced. It is usually noticed by increasing back pressure during ventilation; either by the bag becoming harder to squeeze or the ventilator alarms sounding.

(continued)

Thoracic Trauma

TABLE 4.26 – ASSESSMENT and MANAGEMENT of: Specific Thoracic Trauma *(continued)*
Assess Breathing Adequacy, Respiratory Rate, Volume and Equality of Air Entry
▪ FEEL, LOOK, AUSCULTATE and PERCUSS.
▪ View both sides of the chest and check they are moving; auscultate to ensure air entry is present and percuss on both sides.
▪ **Only perform needle thoracocentesis in a patient if there is haemodynamic instability, hypotension or increasing respiratory compromise.**
▪ If a tension pneumothorax is likely, decompress rapidly by needle thoracocentesis.
▪ If the patient requires positive pressure ventilation, an open thoracostomy should be performed if an appropriately skilled practitioner is available.
Observe the Patient for Signs of Recurrence of the Tension Pneumothorax
▪ If the procedure was unsuccessful, repeat the thoracocentesis.
▪ Consider the use of a thicker needle in patients with a thicker chest wall, following your organisation's guidelines.
Transfer
▪ Undertake a **TIME-CRITICAL** transfer to a major trauma centre, unless the patient needs an immediate lifesaving intervention, in which case transfer to nearest trauma unit.
▪ Provide a pre-alert using ATMIST.
NB Needle thoracocentesis may not always decompress pneumothoraces in large patients. In such cases, a thoracostomy with or without a chest drain may need to be performed. This needs to be done either in hospital or by appropriately skilled practitioners.
CARDIAC TAMPONADE
The heart is enclosed in a tough, non-elastic membrane called the pericardium. A potential space exists between the pericardium and the heart itself. If a penetrating wound injures the heart, the blood may flow under pressure into the pericardial space. As the pericardium cannot expand, a leak of as little as 20–30 ml of blood can cause compression of the heart. This decreases cardiac output and causes tachycardia and hypotension. Further compression reduces cardiac output and cardiac arrest may occur.
Assess for Signs of Cardiac Tamponade
▪ Signs of hypovolaemic shock, tachycardia and hypotension, accompanied by blunt or penetrating chest trauma, may be an indication of cardiac tamponade.
▪ Note the presence of distended neck veins and muffled heart sounds when listening with a stethoscope.
▪ Cardiac tamponade is a **TIME-CRITICAL**, **LIFE-THREATENING** condition that requires rapid surgical intervention, resulting in an open chest operation to evacuate the compressing blood.
▪ DO NOT delay on scene inserting cannulae or commencing fluid therapy.
Transfer
▪ Undertake a **TIME-CRITICAL** transfer to a major trauma centre, unless the patient needs an immediate lifesaving intervention, in which case transfer to nearest trauma unit.
▪ Provide a pre-alert using ATMIST.
▪ Re-assess **ABC** en-route to hospital.
NB Pericardiocentesis is not recommended in the pre-hospital setting, as it is rarely successful, has significant complications and delays definitive care.

Thoracic Trauma

TABLE 4.26 – ASSESSMENT and MANAGEMENT of: Specific Thoracic Trauma *(continued)*
SURGICAL EMPHYSEMA
▪ Surgical emphysema produces swelling of the chest wall, neck and face, with a cracking feeling under the fingers when the skin is pressed. This indicates an air leak from within the chest as a result of a pneumothorax, a ruptured large airway or a fractured larynx.
▪ Normally it requires no specific treatment, but it does indicate potentially SERIOUS underlying chest trauma. Sometimes the surgical emphysema might be extensive and cause the patient to swell up. Where the emphysema is progressively increasing, look for a possible underlying tension pneumothorax.
▪ In some cases, surgical emphysema may become so severe as to tighten the overlying skin and restrict chest movement. A tension pneumothorax must be excluded as above. If there is no improvement, the patient must be transferred to hospital as soon as possible.
Assess for Signs of Surgical Emphysema
▪ Assess for swelling of the chest wall, neck and face, with a cracking feeling under the fingers when the skin is pressed.
Consider Possible Underlying Tension Pneumothorax
▪ Refer to tension pneumothorax guidance above.
BLAST INJURY
▪ Blast injury is caused by three mechanisms:
1 Rupture of air-filled organs.
2 Missiled debris.
3 Contact injury.
▪ Although rare in survivors, strongly suspect a blast lung injury if the patient is suffering from tympanic injury. However, the absence of a tympanic injury DOES NOT exclude lung injury.
NB Being shielded from blast debris DOES NOT exclude lung injury.
Assess for Blast Injury
▪ Pre-hospital management is supportive.

KEY POINTS!

Thoracic Trauma

- **Thoracic injury is commonly associated with hypoxia, either from impaired ventilation or secondary to hypovolaemia from massive bleeding into the chest (haemathorax) or major vessel disruption.**

- **Count the respiratory rate and look for asymmetrical chest movement.**

- **Pulse oximetry must be used as this will assist in recognising hypoxia.**

- **The mechanism of injury is an important guide to the likelihood of significant thoracic injury.**

- **Blunt trauma to the sternum may induce myocardial contusion, which may result in ECG rhythm disturbances.**

- **ECG monitoring.**

- **Impaling objects should be adequately secured. If the object is pulsating, do not completely immobilise but allow it to pulsate.**

- **Do not probe or explore penetrating injuries.**

Bibliography

1. National Institute for Health and Clinical Excellence. *Fractures (Complex): Assessment and Management (NG37)*. London: NICE, 2016. Available from: https://www.nice.org.uk/guidance/ng37.

2. National Institute for Health and Clinical Excellence. *Fractures (Non-complex): Assessment and Management (NG38)*. London: NICE, 2016. Available from: https://www.nice.org.uk/guidance/ng38.

3. National Institute for Health and Clinical Excellence. *Major Trauma: Assessment and Initial Management (NG39)*. London: NICE, 2016. Available from: https://www.nice.org.uk/guidance/ng39.

Thoracic Trauma

4. National Institute for Health and Clinical Excellence. *Major Trauma: Service Delivery (NG40)*. London: NICE, 2016. Available from: https://www.nice.org.uk/guidance/ng40.

5. National Institute for Health and Clinical Excellence. *Spinal Injury: Assessment and Initial Management (NG41)*. London: NICE, 2016. Available from: https://www.nice.org.uk/guidance/ng41.

6. National Institute for Health and Clinical Excellence. *When to Suspect Child Maltreatment* (CG89). London: NICE, 2009. Available from: https://www.nice.org.uk/guidance/cg89.

7. Revell M, Porter K, Greaves I. Fluid resuscitation in pre-hospital trauma care: a consensus view. *Emergency Medicine Journal* 2002, 19(6): 494–498.

8. Lee C, Revell M, Porter K, Steyn R. The pre-hospital management of chest injuries: a consensus statement. Faculty of Pre-hospital Care, Royal College of Surgeons of Edinburgh. *Emergency Medicine Journal* 2007, 24(3): 220–224.

9. Warner KJ, Copass MK, Bulger EM. Paramedic use of needle thoracostomy in the pre-hospital environment. *Prehospital Emergency Care* 2008, 12(2): 162–168.

10. Waydhas C, Sauerland S. Pre-hospital pleural decompression and chest tube placement after blunt trauma: a systematic review. *Resuscitation* 2007, 72(1): 11–25.

11. Dretzke J, Sandercock J, Bayliss S, Burls A. Clinical effectiveness and cost effectiveness of pre-hospital intravenous fluids in trauma patients. *Health Technology Assessment* 2004, 8(23).

12. Turner J, Nicholl J, Webber L, Cox H, Dixon S, Yates D. A randomised controlled trial of prehospital intravenous fluid replacement therapy in serious trauma. *Health Technology Assessment* 2000, 4(31).

13. Stern SA. Low-volume fluid resuscitation for presumed hemorrhagic shock: helpful or harmful? *Current Opinion in Critical Care* 2001, 7(6): 422–430.

14. Pepe PE, Mosesso VNJ, Falk JL. Pre-hospital fluid resuscitation of the patient with major trauma. *Prehospital Emergency Care* 2002, 6(1): 81–91.

15. Borman JB, Aharonson-Daniel L, Savitsky B, Peleg K. Unilateral flail chest is seldom a lethal injury. *Emergency Medicine Journal* 2006, 23(12): 903–905.

16. BMJ Evidence Centre. Best Practice: Cardiac tamponade. 2012. Available from: http://bestpractice.bmj.com/best-practice/monograph/459.html.

17. Fitzgerald M, Spencer J, Johnson F, Marasco S, Atkin C, Kossmann T. Definitive management of acute cardiac tamponade secondary to blunt trauma. *Emergency Medicine Australasia* 2005, 17(5–6): 494–499.

18. Friend KD. Prehospital recognition of tension pneumothorax. *Prehospital Emergency Care* 2000, 4(1): 75–77.

19. Massarutti D, Trillo G, Berlot G, Tomasini A, Bacer B, D'Orlando L et al. Simple thoracostomy in pre-hospital trauma management is safe and effective: a 2-year experience by helicopter emergency medical crews. *European Journal of Emergency Medicine* 2006, 13(5): 276–280.

20. Wanek S, Mayberry JC. Blunt thoracic trauma: flail chest, pulmonary contusion, and blast injury. *Critical Care Clinics* 2004, 20(1): 71–81.

21. Blaivas M. Inadequate needle thoracostomy rate in the pre-hospital setting for presumed pneumothorax. *Journal of Ultrasound in Medicine* 2010, 29(9): 1285–1289.

5

Maternity Care

Maternity Care (including Obstetric Emergencies Overview)

1. Introduction

- Any woman of childbearing age may be pregnant and, unless there is a history of hysterectomy, there must be a high index of suspicion that any abdominal pain or vaginal bleeding may be pregnancy related.

- There are three fundamental rules which must be followed at all times when dealing with a pregnant woman:
  a Resuscitation of the mother must always be the priority.
  b Manual uterine displacement must be employed to support resuscitation measures beyond 20 weeks gestation (refer to Figure 5.1).
  c Hypotension is a late sign of shock. Any signs of hypovolaemia during pregnancy are likely to indicate a 35% (class III) blood loss and must be treated aggressively.

- In cases of maternal cardiac arrest requiring ongoing cardiopulmonary resuscitation, pre-alert the nearest emergency department with an obstetric unit when transferring a pregnant woman in order to ensure preparedness for an emergency perimortem caesarean section (resuscitative hysterotomy), as delivering the fetus may be required to help facilitate maternal resuscitation. **NB Effective resuscitation of the mother will provide effective resuscitation of the fetus.**

- When ambulance clinicians attend an obstetric emergency, they should work as a team, with the paramedics responsible and accountable for the care of the woman or newborn baby and delegating tasks accordingly.

- When a midwife is present, paramedics and midwife must work together to act in the best interests of the woman and the newborn baby. If both mother and newborn baby are clinically well, the midwife is the responsible and accountable clinician. The midwife can either discharge the ambulance clinicians, and arrange for ongoing community midwifery care, or arrange conveyance of the mother and baby together to the most appropriate facility.

- In the event of a newborn requiring conveyance to hospital ahead of the mother, it may be preferable that the midwife remains on scene with the mother to manage the third stage of labour, assess for perineal trauma and manage any ongoing postpartum bleeding. Ambulance clinicians can manage ongoing care of the newborn, utilise the established communication channels and pre-alert the nearest emergency department (ED) where the baby can be assessed. The mother should be repatriated with the baby as soon as reasonably possible at the same location.

- The MBRRACE-UK annual report, *Saving Lives, Improving Mothers' Care,* reviews maternal deaths in the UK and produces recommendations relating to care provision. The report continues to show an overall decrease in the maternal death rate, which is currently 8.5 women per 100,000 maternities.
  - Maternal deaths from direct causes – complication from the pregnancy itself such as bleeding, blood clots, pre-eclampsia or infection – continue to decrease.
  - Maternal deaths from indirect causes – pre-existing conditions that are not direct pregnancy complications such as heart disease, epilepsy, mental health problems or cancer – remain high.
  - Deaths from mental health problems contribute to around a quarter of maternal deaths occurring between 6 weeks and 1 year after the end of pregnancy.
  - The focus of care must be upon establishing appropriate resuscitative measures, placing a pre-alert to the nearest emergency department with an obstetric unit attached, conveying the woman, with manual uterine displacement in place, and preparation for further assessment and treatment, including a perimortem caesarean section if necessary.
  - Effective communication is therefore essential to ensure clinical information being passed on is complete and relevant, utilising a structured communication tool.

- There is a three- to fourfold increased risk of myocardial infarction in pregnancy and the postpartum period.

- Pulmonary embolism is more common throughout pregnancy and the postpartum period.

2. Communication, Information-sharing and Consent

All women who are booked for maternity care should have access to their handheld maternity records. These will provide key information regarding medical history, previous and current pregnancies, obstetric problems as well as emergency contact details for care providers, including next of kin. Information within these notes may aid assessment during the primary and/or secondary survey. Maternity units may also have their own unique set of handheld records or, in some cases, these may be electronic.

2.1 Human Factors and 'SBAR'

- Clinical performance and safe practice can be enhanced through an understanding of the effects of teamwork, tasks, equipment, workspace, culture and organisation on human behaviour and abilities, and application of that knowledge within a clinical setting.

- Increasing situational awareness and the utilisation of communication tools (such as Situation, Background, Assessment,

Maternity Care (including Obstetric Emergencies Overview)

Recommendation, or SBAR) help to promote a safer environment and enhance clinical outcome. Awareness of what is happening around us can be reduced during emergency situations, and this can lead to near misses and/or adverse outcomes. It is therefore essential that enhanced communication skills, and an environment in which open and honest lines of communication are encouraged, are maintained.

- The use of the SBAR communication tool is recommended in order to optimise transfer of information between members of the multi-disciplinary team. The purpose of SBAR is to promote the accurate and unambiguous handover of clinically relevant information regarding care of the mother from one healthcare professional to another. The use of SBAR has the potential to improve the speed at which care is delivered and the quality of care that is ultimately provided.

2.2 Consent

- Consent to treatment is the principle that a person must give permission before they receive any type of medical treatment, investigation or examination. Consent from a woman is needed regardless of the procedure. For consent to be valid it must be voluntary and informed, and the person consenting must have the capacity to make the decision. If an adult has the capacity to make a voluntary and informed decision to consent to or refuse a particular treatment, their decision must be respected. This is still the case even if refusing treatment would result in their death, or the death of their unborn child.

- The provision of adequate information should include the benefits and risks of the proposed treatments, and alternative treatments. If the woman is not offered as much information as they reasonably need to make their decision, and in a format that they can understand, their consent will not be valid.

- Consent can be given verbally or in writing and should be given to the healthcare professional directly responsible for the person's current treatment.

- Consent may not be necessary if a person requires emergency treatment that is believed to be in their best interests or to save their life and they are unable to give consent due to a lack of capacity caused by either mental or physical complications.

- During obstetrics emergencies, it may be necessary to perform intimate examination in order to perform lifesaving treatment. Practitioners must, where possible, obtain informed consent and offer the woman a chaperone. All examinations must be carried out sensitively, with respect for the woman's dignity, cultural beliefs and confidentiality.

3. Physiological Changes in Pregnancy

Pregnancy is timed from the FIRST day of the last period and may last up to or in excess of 42 weeks. The pregnancy is divided into three trimesters (1–12 weeks +6 days, 13–25 weeks +6 days and 26 weeks+). These terms are used with the maternity handheld records; they will also detail the lead clinician, i.e. the midwife or the obstetrician who is responsible for the provision of maternity care with the woman.

There are a multitude of physiological and anatomical changes during pregnancy that may influence the management of the pregnant woman. These changes include:

- Cardiovascular system:
  - An increase in cardiac output by 20–30% in the first 10 weeks of pregnancy.
  - An increase in average maternal heart rate by 10–15 beats per minute.
  - A decrease in systolic and diastolic blood pressure by an average of 10–15 mmHg due to a reduction in peripheral resistance caused by an increase in the release of the progesterone hormone.
  - The weight of the gravid uterus, from 20 weeks gestation onwards, may cause compression of the inferior vena cava (IVC), reducing venous return and lowering cardiac output by up to 40% for women in the supine position; this in turn can reduce blood pressure. The combined effects of the gravid uterus on the IVC and a reduction in peripheral vascular resistance can result in the woman feeling faint or having an episode of syncope, resolved by repositioning her onto her side or into the lateral position.
  - An increase in blood volume through haemodilution (increasing by 45%) occurs together with a small increase in the numbers of red blood cells. The disproportionate increase of plasma volume relative to the increase in red cell mass can lead to a 'physiological' anaemia in the mother from around 27 weeks' gestation. Due to the increase in blood volume, a pregnant woman is able to tolerate greater blood loss before showing signs of hypovolaemia. This compensation is at the expense of shunting blood away from the uterus and placenta, and therefore the fetus.

- Respiratory system:
  - An increase in breathing rate and effort and a decrease in vital capacity, as the gravid uterus enlarges and the diaphragm becomes splinted. Some shortness of breath is common during pregnancy but early consideration should be given to the need for increased oxygen requirements.

Maternity Care (including Obstetric Emergencies Overview)

- Oedema of the larynx may compromise airway management, and a collapsed pregnant woman requires the airway to be secured as soon as possible.
- Placement of an advanced airway (supraglottic airway or endotracheal intubation) should be secured in all maternal cardiac arrests (refer to **Maternal Resuscitation**).

■ Gastrointestinal system:
- An increase in the acidity of the stomach contents, due to a delay in gastric emptying, caused by progesterone-like effects of the placental hormones.
- Relaxation of the cardiac sphincter makes regurgitation of the stomach contents more likely (refer to **Maternal Resuscitation**).
- Nausea and vomiting can occur around 4–8 weeks' gestation and continue until around 14–16 weeks. Some severe cases may continue for a longer period of time and can result in rapid dehydration (hyperemesis gravidarum) requiring hospital assessment/admission.

4. Appropriate Destination for Conveyance

■ The choice of destination to convey mother and baby should be carefully considered and in line with local procedures. Ideally, mother and baby should be conveyed to the same destination. There are units, commonly called birth/birthing centres (or 'standalone' maternity units), that are solely midwifery-led. Be aware that there are no resident obstetricians, anaesthetists or neonatologists with the capability of performing advanced obstetric or neonatal interventions at these sites. There are no specialist neonatal facilities.

■ The mother may choose to book for delivery at a particular unit and request to be conveyed there; however, in an emergency situation this may have to be overridden:
- The nearest emergency department (ED) will be the appropriate destination when there is cardiac arrest, major airway problems, ongoing eclamptic convulsions and severe uncontrollable bleeding.

- In other obstetric emergencies (e.g. shoulder dystocia, mild to moderate bleeding etc.), transfer to the nearest full obstetric unit (i.e. not a birthing centre or 'standalone' midwifery unit) will be appropriate. Remember that in many cases a full obstetric unit will be co-located with an ED but this may not always be the case.

■ Careful consideration should always be given to the most appropriate destination in each case. Also consider carefully the accessibility of a unit (e.g. out-of-hours, locked doors, corridors and lifts). In line with local procedures, pre-alert arrangements and telephone numbers should be agreed and readily available to clinicians.

5. Assessment

■ Critical assessment of the mother is vital in all situations, while fetal assessment may be indirect based on reported movements etc. Refer to Table 5.1.

■ Neonatal assessment is also important, with particular reference to respiratory effort and maintaining body temperature. Refer to Table 5.3.

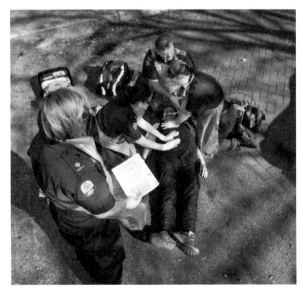

Figure 5.1 – Manual uterine displacement.

Maternity Care (including Obstetric Emergencies Overview)

TABLE 5.1 – Assessment

▪ Quickly assess the woman and scene as you approach	
▪ Primary survey	▪ It is important to remember that a woman and, if born, a newborn baby will require assessment.
	▪ The aim of the primary survey is to identify any life-threatening problems, to enable management to be commenced as rapidly as possible and to reach an early determination of the priority for transportation. The primary survey should be modified in the presence of actual or suspected trauma (refer to **Trauma in Pregnancy**).
▪ Massive external haemorrhage	▪ Is there a significant volume of blood visible without the need to disturb the woman's clothing?
	– Is the woman's clothing soaked?
	– Is there blood on the floor?
	– Are there a number of blood-soaked sanitary pads visible?
▪ Airway	▪ Is the woman able to talk? (Yes = airway open.) If the woman is unresponsive, refer to **Maternal Resuscitation**.
	▪ Is the woman making unusual sounds? (Gurgling = fluid in the airway.)
	▪ Is suction required? (Snoring = tongue/swelling/foreign body obstruction.)
	▪ If the woman is unresponsive, open the airway and look in – suction for fluids, manually remove solid obstructions.
▪ Breathing	▪ Document respiratory rate and effort. (Are accessory muscles being used?)
	▪ Obtain oxygen saturations as soon as possible.
	▪ Auscultate for added sounds. (Wheeze = bronchospasm; coarse sounds = pulmonary oedema.)
	▪ Assess for the presence of cyanosis.
	▪ Give oxygen based on clinical findings (not routinely).
▪ Circulation	▪ Document radial pulse rate and volume. (Capillary refill time (CRT) may be used if neither the radial nor carotid pulses can be palpated.)
	▪ Assess skin colour and temperature (to touch). (Pallor, or cold or damp skin = an adrenergic reaction to shock.)
	▪ Record blood pressure – the systolic is most valuable if you suspect shock.
	▪ Visually inspect the abdominal area and gently palpate for evidence of internal bleeding (indicated by tenderness, guarding, firm woody uterus).
▪ Disability	▪ Perform an AVPU assessment of consciousness level (is the woman Alert, responding only to Voice, responding only to Pain or Unresponsive?).
	▪ Document the woman's posture (normal, convulsing (state whether focal or generalised), abnormal flexion, abnormal extension).
	▪ Document pupil size and reaction (PEaRL – pupils equal and reacting to light).

(continued)

TABLE 5.1 – Assessment *(continued)*

▪ Expose/environment/evaluate	▪ Ensuring consent is obtained, expose and visually inspect the vaginal opening: – Is there any evidence of bleeding? – Can you see a presenting part of the baby? – Is there a prolapsed loop of cord? – Have the waters broken (and if so, is the amniotic fluid clear, blood stained or meconium stained)? – Does the perineum bulge with each contraction? – If the baby has been born, is there a significant perineal tear? Can you see any part of the uterus? ▪ Assess the environment: – Is the woman or baby at risk of hypothermia? – Are the surroundings as clean as you can make them if the birth is imminent? – Are there other children present (this may indicate a previous pregnancy with live birth)? ▪ Evaluate how time-critical the woman's condition is. – If it is time-critical, decide immediately whether you need to transport the woman urgently to the nearest hospital with an obstetric unit, placing a pre-alert as early as reasonably possible. (The nearest hospital with an obstetric unit may not be the booked unit; however, it is critical the woman has rapid obstetric or appropriate assessment at the nearest facility.) – If the birth is imminent, remember to call for additional clinical resource. This may include midwifery assistance, which may be deployed from the nearest maternity unit to the location of the woman (follow local guidelines).
▪ Fundus	▪ Make a quick assessment of fundal height: a fundus at the level of the umbilicus equates to a gestation of approximately 22 weeks. By definition, if fundal height is below the umbilicus, this suggests that if the fetus is delivered, it is unlikely to survive.
▪ Fetal activity	▪ Ask the mother when she last felt her baby move.
▪ Secondary survey	▪ If any critical problems are identified during the primary survey, the secondary survey should only be undertaken when any **ABCDE** problems have been addressed and transportation to definitive care has commenced (if this is possible). In many cases where critical problems are identified, it will not be possible or appropriate to undertake a secondary survey in the pre-hospital phase of care.

6. At-risk Ethnic Groups

6.1 At-risk Ethnic Groups and Maternal Deaths[6]

▪ The Mother and Babies: Reducing Risk through Audits and Confidential Enquiries across the UK (MBRRACE-UK) *Saving Lives, Improving Mothers' Care* report was released in 2020.[7] The data was produced from looking at maternal deaths from 2016 to 2018. This confidential enquiry found that Black women are four times more likely to die during pregnancy than White women. Mixed ethnicity women are three times more likely and Asian women are twice as likely as White women to die during childbirth.

▪ Due to ongoing globalisation and migration patterns, clinicians are increasingly attending patients from diverse cultural and/or ethnic minority backgrounds. According to the Office for National Statistics, approximately a quarter of women giving birth in the UK are from ethnic minority groups.

▪ Despite the publication of a number of national policy documents and local initiatives to improve childbirth experiences, previous work streams have highlighted disparities within ethnic minority

Black and Asian women have a higher risk of dying in pregnancy

White women		8/100,000
Asian women	2x	15/100,000
Mixed ethnicity women	3x	25/100,000
Black women	4x	34/100,000

Figure 5.2 – Maternal deaths.

groups which indicate this group of women have worse pregnancy and birth outcomes than White women.[8]

- Whilst it is not known what causes the increased risk of mortality, it is important that we are aware as out-of-hospital clinicians of the increased risk to patients from ethnic minority groups.

- Communication is an important part of clinical assessment and history-taking. It is important that as clinicians we remember to remove barriers to communication; this may mean using simplified language. Translation services should also be utilised if English is not the patient's first language; family members translating can inadvertently lead to misinformation being given to the clinician. For example, women may struggle to describe in full their symptoms, extent of bleeding or mental health issues, due to cultural beliefs associated with those conditions, especially if partners or family members are acting as translators.

- As clinicians, it is important to recognise that in some cultures there may not be specific psychological terms directly associated with stress/anxiety/depression, or the patient may not be familiar with these terms, and so the patient will often describe having physical symptoms such as palpitations or shortness of breath.

- Once you have provided clinical advice, it is important to check the patient and family have fully understood the information provided. It is important to document specific condition worsening advice and potential consequences to the patient if they choose not to adhere to the advice provided.

- Women unfamiliar with the NHS, even if English-speaking, may not be familiar with the systems and processes in place to support their pregnancy, especially as other countries will often have very different healthcare models. For instance, there may be a cultural expectation from the woman or partner that an all-female ambulance crew attend their emergency. It is important that clinicians respect the patient's wishes and explore the reason for this request. It is important to emphasise that delaying accessing definitive care or further assessment could directly impact the heath of baby and mother. However, in some situations it may be considered appropriate to request a second resource for a woman to attend.

6.2 Pain Management

- Pain management is a particularly important consideration in ethnic minority women, as 'the interpretation of pain behaviours is heavily dependent on the social and cultural learnings and understandings of both the person in pain and the observer'.[9]

- Women may present pain symptoms differently; some women may choose to be quiet, and others more vocal and expressive. As clinicians it is important that we recognise that people do respond differently to pain and it is equally important to remember our own responses to pain are not the only way pain can be expressed.

Maternity Care (including Obstetric Emergencies Overview)

Therefore, it is important to assess pain and manage it in accordance with what the patient is telling you. Refer to **Pain Management in Adults**.

7. Special Cases

7.1 Concealment, Denial and Unknown Pregnancy

Occasionally, pregnancy may be concealed or denied until labour commences. In both situations there may have been no antenatal care. There may be mental health, drug and alcohol abuse issues and safeguarding concerns (refer to **Safeguarding Adults at Risk** and **Safeguarding Children**). Some concealed pregnancies may result in the birth occurring in secret. Ambulance clinicians must be aware that the consequences of concealment and denial can have a fatal outcome for both mother and baby.

- Always consider the possibility of pregnancy in any woman of reproductive age. Ask the woman if she could be pregnant. Be aware that a young teenage girl may not want to answer such a question in the presence of a parent or carer.

- It may be necessary to visually inspect and palpate the abdomen for evidence of a pregnant uterus.

- If labour is confirmed and birth is not imminent, determine if there is any relevant medical history. Transfer the woman to the nearest obstetric unit.

- Determine how many weeks pregnant the woman is if known, or by visual inspection of the abdomen; where the uterine fundus is at the level of the umbilicus the pregnancy may be more than 22 weeks.

- If birth is in progress or occurs en-route, request a midwife from the nearest maternity unit, if this service is available, and additional resources and prepare for birth (see Table 5.1).

- Once the baby has been born and assessed, transfer mother and baby to the nearest obstetric unit.

- If the woman is unaware of pregnancy, consider birth/miscarriage in any significant per vaginum (PV) bleed that cannot be explained.

- Pre-alert the nearest obstetric unit or nearest ED with an obstetric unit, dependent upon considered gestation.

- Discuss at handover any safeguarding concerns identified when attending the home environment (refer to **Safeguarding Adults at Risk** and **Safeguarding Children**).

7.2 Female Genital Mutilation (FGM)

Overview

- Female Genital Mutilation (FGM), also known as 'female genital cutting', 'female genital mutilation/cutting' or 'cutting', refers to all procedures involving partial or total removal of the external female genitalia or other injury to the female genital organs for non-medical reasons.

- FGM is predominately practised in Africa, Yemen, Iraqi Kurdistan and parts of Malaysia and Indonesia.

- The World Health Organization classifies FGM into four categories (see Table 5.2).

TABLE 5.2 – Four Categories of Female Genital Mutilation (FGM) and Management	
Type 1	Partial or total removal of the clitoris and/or the prepuce (clitoridectomy).
Type 2	Partial or total removal of the clitoris and labia minora, with or without excision of the labia majora (excision).
Type 3	Narrowing of the vaginal orifice with creation of a covering seal by cutting and appositioning the labia minora and/or the labia majora, with or without excision of the clitoris (infibulation).
Type 4	All other harmful procedures to the female genitalia for non-medical purposes, for example: pricking, piercing, incising, scraping and cauterisation.

- FGM is practised for a variety of complex reasons. FGM has no health benefits but does increase health risks. FGM is a human rights violation and a form of child abuse. Refer to **Safeguarding Adults at Risk** and **Safeguarding Children** for guidance regarding when, as healthcare professionals, we are legally required to report and raise safeguarding under the Female Genital Mutilation Act 2003.[10]

FGM and Pregnancy

- Women with FGM are more prone to complications in pregnancy. Clinicians should be aware of the increased likelihood of urinary tract infections and other infections. During childbirth, women may also encounter additional complications; the more severe the type of FGM, the higher the risk. Infibulated (Type 3) cannot give birth unassisted; the scar tissue covering the

Maternity Care (including Obstetric Emergencies Overview)

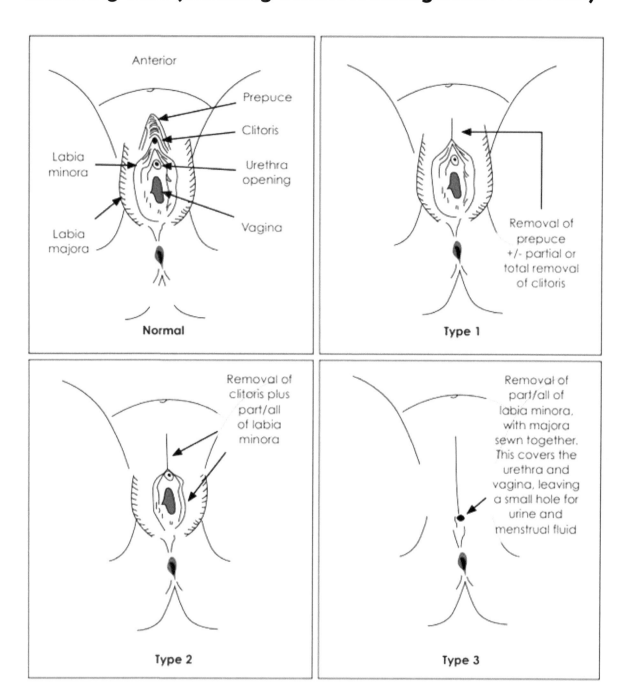

Figure 5.3 – The four FGM categories.

introitus does not allow for the passage of the baby without de-fibulation.

- FGM can cause prolonged labour, increase the risk of a newborn requiring resuscitation and additional support and can cause significant vaginal and perineal tearing resulting in a postpartum haemorrhage.

- As clinicians, it is important to recognise a woman who has had FGM. Women may not know FGM has taken place, therefore clear communication and history-taking are important. Women who have been identified as having had FGM, if known to maternity services, will have their hospital care booked with a consultant obstetrician and a specialist midwife team. If de-fibulation is required,

this may have been undertaken antenatally or be planned for once labour begins.

- If the woman has not received antenatal care and evidence of FGM is present, early recognition and early conveyance of these women is required. If birth is imminent, where possible rapid conveyance to the nearest obstetric unit must be undertaken. Further resources should be considered, but do not delay transportation. An information call should be placed to the identified obstetric unit informing them of the concerns and the estimated arrival time.

Obstetric Problems

- The narrowed vaginal opening in FGM types 3 and 4 is likely to cause obstetric problems.

- These include:
  - prolonged and obstructed labour
  - an increase in the number of episiotomies and perineal tears
  - a high caesarean section rate caused by the difficulty in fetal monitoring and lack of adequately trained obstetric staff
  - an increased incidence of postpartum haemorrhage
  - an increased incidence of postnatal wound infection
  - maternal death from obstructed labour and postpartum haemorrhage
  - increased stillbirth and early neonatal death rates
  - increased neonatal morbidity from hypoxia and brain damage.

7.3 Waterbirths

- This guidance is for use when attending a pregnant woman who is in a birthing pool or bath.
- The woman may want to continue to give birth in the water, there may be no midwife present and there may be other people in attendance who support the wishes of the mother to give birth in the water.
- Attending and managing planned births in water is outside the scope of ambulance clinicians.
- You are responsible for the mother and baby unless there is a qualified midwife or other appropriately trained and qualified healthcare professional on scene with responsibility for the patient.
- The management of the temperature of the water is critical to the safety of the baby at birth.

Actions to Take

- In the first instance, ask the woman to leave the water and assist her in doing so.
- If the woman declines to leave the water, you must explain the risks to her and to the baby, and that you are not trained to manage a waterbirth. Involve birth partner if present.
- Contact senior clinical/medical advice and request a midwife to attend as per local procedures.
- Request additional resources to scene, anticipating the need to extricate the woman in an emergency.

Birth in Water Imminent

- Prepare for the birth:
  - Use sleeve protectors (if available) and gloves over the top on both hands (see Figure 5.4), wear eye protection and an apron (be aware of local guidance).

Figure 5.4 – Sleeve protector with glove over the top.

  - Turn on lights, and prepare an area for resuscitation of the baby.
  - Warm the room and obtain several dry towels.
- The birth:
  - **If the baby is born under the water**, ask the woman to bring the baby's head above the water level.
  - **If the woman cannot bring the baby to the surface of the water**, you must put your hands in the water, lift the baby up and ensure the baby's head is above the water. This ensures that the baby can breathe spontaneously without inhaling the water.
  - Assess the baby at birth as per **Newborn Life Support**. If newborn resuscitation is required, clamp and cut the umbilical cord and transfer the baby to the prepared area for assessment and ongoing management.
  - Once the baby is born, clamp and cut the umbilical cord in preparation for assisting the woman out of the water to a prepared area where a full assessment of the mother and the baby can be undertaken, preferably by two separate clinicians.
  - Manage the third stage of labour outside of the pool as per JRCALC guidance.
  - Ensure the baby is thoroughly dried off and wrapped in dry and warm towels.
  - Remove PPE and perform hand-washing up to and including the forearms.
  - Replace PPE as appropriate and in line with local protocol.
  - Report the incident as per local processes, to facilitate debriefing and welfare follow-up.
  - Document all discussions and care on the care record.

8. Glossary of Terms

Table 5.3 provides a glossary of abbreviations specific to maternity and commonly used in handheld maternity records.

Maternity Care (including Obstetric Emergencies Overview)

TABLE 5.3 – Glossary

ABBREVIATION	TERM
LMP	Last menstrual period.
EDD	Estimated date of delivery – the timing of the pregnancy is written in the notes in the format e.g. 12/40, i.e. 12 weeks have elapsed out of the 40-week pregnancy.
T or D	Term or expected date of delivery/pregnancy, therefore T+3 or D+3 in the notes is 3 days over the EDD.
CEPH	Cephalic (head).
BR	Breech.
G	Gravida, the number of times a woman has been pregnant (including the present pregnancy), e.g. G3.
P	Parity, the number of times a woman has given birth to a liveborn or stillborn baby, e.g. P3. A second figure implies previous miscarriages or terminations, e.g. P3+2.

KEY POINTS!

Maternity Care (including Obstetric Emergencies Overview)

- Any woman of childbearing age MAY be pregnant.

- Due to the increase in blood volume, the pregnant woman is able to tolerate greater blood or plasma loss before showing signs of hypovolaemia; establish large bore (16G) IV cannulation early.

- A pregnant woman in cardiac arrest must ideally be conveyed with left manual uterine displacement after 20 weeks' gestation (maintaining left lateral tilt is an alternative but may be more difficult to use effectively in the pre-hospital care environment).

- The use of SBAR to communicate between ambulance clinicians and maternity clinicians can optimise transfer of information.

- Black women are four times more likely to die during pregnancy than White women. Women with a mixed ethnic background are three times more likely than White women to die in childbirth, and Asian women are twice as likely.

Bibliography

1. Knight M, Tuffnell D, Kenyon S, Shakespeare J, Gray R, Kurinczuk JJ (eds) on behalf of MBRRACE-UK. *Saving Lives, Improving Mothers' Care – Surveillance of maternal deaths in the UK 2011–13 and lessons learned to inform maternity care from the UK and Ireland Confidential Enquiries into Maternal Deaths and Morbidity 2009–13.* Oxford: National Perinatal Epidemiology Unit, University of Oxford, 2015.

2. Catchpole (2010), cited in Department of Health. *Human Factors Reference Group Interim Report, 1 March 2012.* National Quality Board, 2012. Available from: http://www.england.nhs.uk/ourwork/part-rel/nqb/ag-min/.

3. Woollard M, Hinshaw K, Simpson H, Wieteska S (eds). *Pre-hospital Obstetric Emergency Training.* Oxford: Wiley-Blackwell, 2009.

4. Centre for Maternal and Child Enquiries. Saving mothers'lives: reviewing maternal deaths to make motherhood safer: 2006–2008. *BJOG: An International Journal of Obstetrics & Gynaecology* 2011, 118 (suppl. 1).

5. Bourjeily G, Paidas M, Khalil H, Rosene-Montella K, Rodger M. Pulmonary embolism in pregnancy. *The Lancet* 2010, 375(9713): 500–512.

6. Race Disparity Unit, UK Government. *Writing About Ethnicity.* Available from: https://www.ethnicity-facts-figures.service.gov.uk/style-guide/writing-about-ethnicity.

7. Knight M, Bunch K, Tuffnell D, Shakespeare J et al. (eds). MBRRACE (2020) *Saving Lives, Improving Mothers' Care: Lessons learned to inform maternity care from the UK and Ireland Confidential Enquiries into Maternal Deaths and Morbidity 2016–18.* Available from: https://www.npeu.ox.ac.uk/assets/downloads/mbrrace-uk/reports/maternal-report-2020/MBRRACE-UK_Maternal_Report_Dec_2020_v10_ONLINE_VERSION_1404.pdf.

8. Henderson J, Gao H, Redshaw M (2013) Experiencing maternity care: the care received and perceptions of women from different ethnic groups. *BMC Pregnancy and Childbirth* 13. DOI: 10.1186/1471-2393-13-196.

9. Whitburn LY, Jones LE, Davey M, McDonald S (2019) The nature of labour pain: an updated review of the literature. *Women and Birth: Journal of The Australian College of Midwives* 32(1). DOI: 10.1016/j.wombi.2018.03.004.

10. Royal College of Obstetricians & Gynaecologists (2015) *Female Genital Mutilation and Its Management.* Available from: https://www.rcog.org.uk/globalassets/documents/guidelines/gtg-53-fgm.pdf.

Maternity Care (including Obstetric Emergencies Overview)

> **UNDERTAKE PRIMARY SURVEY**
> Establish gestation and frequency of contractions

BIRTH IMMINENT	**BIRTH NOT IMMINENT**

BIRTH IMMINENT

Request midwife if available
Prepare for newborn life support
Reassure the woman and support her in a
comfortable position, avoiding the supine position
Provide Entonox for pain relief

↓

Support the birth of the baby's head by
applying gentle pressure as head advances

↓

Support the baby during the birth and
place on the maternal abdomen

↓

Thoroughly dry the baby with a warm
towel and wrap with a dry towel

↓

If the baby is crying provide
'skin-to-skin' contact with the mother

↓

Allow the umbilical cord to stop
pulsating prior to clamping and cutting

↓

The placenta may take 15–20 mins to birth – **DO NOT**
pull on the cord – encourage the mother to pass urine

Deliver the placenta into a plastic bag for the midwife
to inspect and check for completeness

Assess and record estimated blood loss

If the placenta remains undelivered with minimal
bleeding, plan to transfer to the nearest appropriate
destination as agreed locally

Maternal safety is the prime consideration

Consider the specific clinical situation **and which
interventions may be required for the woman
and baby on arrival**

Refer to 'Appropriate Destination for Conveyance'
in **Maternity Care**

If the placenta remains undelivered and bleeding
refer to Figure 5.8

BIRTH NOT IMMINENT

Contact booked unit for
advice if no time-critical
features present
(The woman may travel by car
or taxi to booked unit if
ambulance is not required)

> If the baby is not crying
> refer to
> **Newborn Life Support**

Figure 5.5 – Pre-hospital maternity emergency management – normal birth.

Birth Imminent: Normal Birth and Birth Complications

1. Introduction

- The best clinical management for a woman who is experiencing an abnormal labour or complications with the birth is to be transferred to the **NEAREST** appropriate unit without delay. This will usually be the nearest obstetric unit but in certain circumstances may involve transfer to the nearest emergency department (ED) (refer to 'Appropriate Destination for Conveyance' in **Maternity Care (including Obstetric Emergencies Overview))**.

- When there is a midwife on scene, it is their responsibility to manage the labour and birth, and ambulance clinicians should work under their direction, while working together as a team. If the midwife is not present, the decision on whether to convey the woman should be based on the principle that any situation that deviates from a normal uncomplicated labour should result in the woman being transported immediately to the nearest hospital with an obstetric unit once the appropriate number of conveying resources are available.

- In this situation, the ambulance clinicians must alert the hospital either directly or via the emergency operations centre (EOC). An early assessment of the need for additional resources may be necessary, including the request for a second ambulance where a newborn baby is required to be conveyed separately from the woman. Ensure that the request is made as soon as possible.

- The most important feature of attending a pregnant woman is to complete a rapid assessment, to ascertain whether there is anything abnormal taking place.

- The maternal assessment process outlined in Table 5.4 MUST be followed in order to decide whether to:
  - STAY ON SCENE AND REQUEST A MIDWIFE (if not already present and available within the locality).
  - TRANSFER TO FURTHER CARE IMMEDIATELY.

- In maternity cases where birth is not imminent and there are no complications, it may be appropriate to contact the midwife in the booked maternity unit for advice regarding the transport arrangements. This may involve the woman making her own way to her planned place of birth if there are no immediately time-critical features, or conveying her to the nearest maternity unit for assessment.

- The assessment should be repeated en-route and, if any complications occur, the condition should be treated appropriately and destination changed if a nearer facility is available. If the woman is booked into a unit that is not within a reasonable distance or travelling time, ambulance clinicians should base their judgements on the maternal assessment, and take her to the nearest appropriate unit.

TABLE 5.4 – ASSESSMENT and MANAGEMENT of: Normal Birth

Assess <C>ABCDE

- Quickly assess the woman and scene as you approach.

- If any **TIME-CRITICAL** features are present, correct **<C>ABC** problems and transport to the nearest ED with an obstetric unit (refer to **Medical Emergencies in Adults – Overview** and **Medical Emergencies in Children – Overview**).

- Ascertain the period of gestation by asking the woman, and also by reviewing the woman's maternity records. Refer to antenatal pages for assessment of any obstetric risk factors or complications.

- Provide a pre-alert.

Primary Survey

- Assess for:
  - operculum (show)
  - ruptured amniotic fluid sac (waters broken)
  - contractions
  - and/or bleeding.

- (See Figure 5.5. For additional information, refer to **Maternity Care (including Obstetric Emergencies Overview).**)

- If **NONE** of these indications is present **AND** there is no other medical/traumatic condition, discuss the woman's management with the **BOOKED OBSTETRIC UNIT**, informing of:
  - woman's name
  - woman's age and date of birth
  - woman's hospital registration number
  - name of lead clinician (midwifery or obstetric-led care)

(continued)

Maternity Care

SECTION 5

TABLE 5.4 – ASSESSMENT and MANAGEMENT of: **Normal Birth** *(continued)*

- history of this pregnancy
- estimated date of delivery (EDD)
- period of gestation (number of weeks pregnant)
- previous obstetric history.

▪ If ANY of the above indications are present, assess:
  - contraction interval
  - the urge to push or bear down
  - crowning/top of the baby's head/breech presentation visible at the vulva.

▪ Undertake a visual inspection of the vaginal entrance if there are regular contractions (1–2-minute intervals) and an urge to push or bear down.

▪ If the amniotic membranes are visible during birth, DO NOT artificially rupture the amniotic sac while the baby is in utero (i.e. before the baby is born).

▪ In the majority of births, the amniotic sac will rupture during labour, before the baby is born. However, occasionally, the amniotic sac will not rupture, particularly in preterm births. The bulging sac may be visible at the vaginal entrance during the second stage of labour, and may be visible for quite some time as the woman pushes before the baby is born.

▪ The decision to artificially rupture the membranes prior to delivery should only be made by a midwife or obstetrician. In some cases of early preterm labour, leaving the amniotic membranes intact may slow the delivery, allowing for steroids to be administered by the midwife or obstetrician which can improve the outcome for the preterm neonate. When the membranes are artificially ruptured, there is a danger that the labour can progress rapidly, leading to birth sooner than expected. More rarely, rupturing membranes can lead to significant complications that can only be managed in hospital, e.g. umbilical cord prolapse.

▪ Rarely, the baby and placenta may be born with the amniotic sac intact and the baby within. This is called an 'en caul' birth. If the membranes do not rupture spontaneously, they should be ruptured away from the baby, the cord and the placenta. 'Pinch' an area of the membranes firmly between index finger and thumb and attempt to tear the membranes open. In the rare circumstance that the membranes are tough, use the tips of a pair of scissors to very carefully make a small 1 to 2 cm incision in the membranes close to your pinched finger and thumb. Once ruptured, the amniotic fluid will rapidly drain away. You may need to carefully peel the remaining membranes away from the baby's mouth and nose in order to ensure the airway is clear. Note in the clinical record the colour of the amniotic fluid — clear, blood stained, meconium present or malodour.

▪ Watch this video with more information about the amniotic sac.

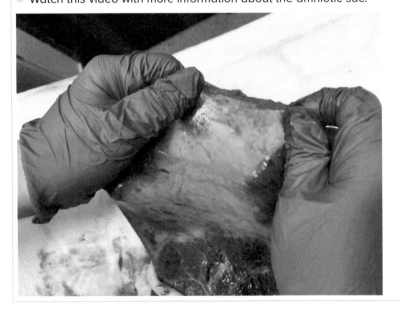

TABLE 5.4 – ASSESSMENT and MANAGEMENT of: **Normal Birth** *(continued)*

(continued)

TABLE 5.4 – ASSESSMENT and MANAGEMENT of: Normal Birth *(continued)*

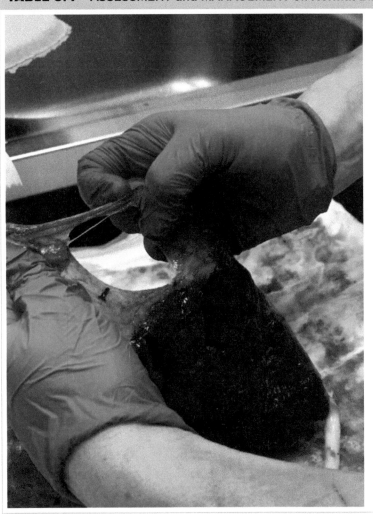

Birth Imminent

- If birth is imminent, that is regular contractions (1–2-minute intervals) and an urge to push or bear down and/or crowning top of the baby's head breech presentation visible at the vulva, remain on scene, request a midwife if available in the locality and an additional ambulance with a paramedic if not already present and prepare for the birth of the baby (see below).

Second Stage of Labour

(From full dilatation of the cervix until complete birth of the baby)

- Continue assessing the woman's level of pain.
- Reassure the woman, tell her what you are doing and include her birth partner if present.
- Ensure the environment is safe and secure for the birth of the baby, with particular attention to the temperature of the room:
  - incontinence pads – cover the ambulance stretcher or birthing area
  - maternity pack – open and set out
  - towels (warm towels if possible) – enough to dry and wrap the baby
  - blanket(s) – cover the mother for warmth and modesty
  - heat – turn the heat up in the birth area (aim for 25°C).

TABLE 5.4 – ASSESSMENT and MANAGEMENT of: **Normal Birth** *(continued)*

Contents of the maternity pack.

- Support the woman in any position she finds comfortable – discourage her from lying flat on her back because of the risk of supine hypotension.
- Encourage the woman to continue taking Entonox to relieve pain/discomfort if necessary.
- **CAUTION** – at this stage, morphine should only be administered in exceptional circumstances due to the risk of neonatal respiratory depression.
- To allow for the baby's head to be born slowly, encourage the woman to concentrate on panting or breathing out during the birth. The use of Entonox can assist here.
- Consider applying gentle pressure to the top of the baby's head as it advances through the vaginal entrance to prevent very rapid birth of the head. Pressure may also assist in keeping the head flexed to allow the smallest diameter of the fetal skull to be born. This may reduce perineal trauma.
- The umbilical cord may be around the baby's neck and does not require removal, as the baby can be born with the cord left in place.
- Hold the baby as it is born and lift it towards the woman's abdomen.
- Wipe any obvious large collections of mucous from the baby's mouth and nose.

ABCD Assessment of the Baby

(Include head, trunk, axilla and groin)

- Newborns are at risk of hypothermia.
- **CAUTION** – preterm babies lose heat faster than full-term babies (refer to **Care of the Newborn**).
- Quickly and thoroughly dry the baby using a warm towel while you make your initial assessment.
- Remove the now-wet towel and wrap the baby in a dry towel to minimise heat losses.

Assess the Baby's Airway

- If the baby is crying, it has a clear airway.
- If the baby is not breathing, confirm that the airway is open – the head is ideally placed in the 'neutral' position, i.e. not the extended 'sniffing position'.

(continued)

Birth Imminent: Normal Birth and Birth Complications

TABLE 5.4 – ASSESSMENT and MANAGEMENT of: **Normal Birth** *(continued)*

Figure reproduced with the kind permission of the Resuscitation Council (UK).

- **SUCTION IS NOT USUALLY NECESSARY** – if required, use the suction unit on low power (around 75 mmHg) with a CH12–14 catheter and then only within the oral cavity. **ONLY** use suction to remove **VISIBLE** thick particulate lumps of meconium. During suctioning, the tip of the catheter should be visible to the operator. **DO NOT** probe blindly with the catheter as this can cause a vagal response and depress respiration.

- If the baby is not breathing, refer to **Newborn Life Support**.

- Once the baby is breathing adequately, cyanosis will gradually improve over several minutes – if the cyanosis is not clearing, enrich the atmosphere near the baby's face with a low flow of oxygen at 2 litres.

- Where available, oxygen saturation probes should be used. Refer to **Care of the Newborn**.

Cutting the Cord

- Assess whether the cord has stopped pulsating.

- Wait until the cord has stopped pulsating; apply two cord clamps securely 3 cm apart and about 15 cm from the umbilicus. Cut the cord between the two clamps. **CAUTION** – ensure the newborn's fingers and genitals are clear of the scissors.

TABLE 5.4 – ASSESSMENT and MANAGEMENT of: **Normal Birth** *(continued)*

- Ensure the baby remains warm; keep the baby wrapped and ensure the head is covered.
- Place the baby with its mother in a position where the mother can breastfeed if she wants to (breastfeeding will also encourage birth of the placenta).
- Reassure the mother, and birth partner if present.
- Await the midwife and third stage (birth of the placenta and membranes).
- If birth has occurred en-route, proceed to the nearest obstetric unit. It is not necessary to await birth of the placenta before continuing with the transfer.
- Provide an alert/information call, including the detail of whether mother and baby are being conveyed together or not.

Third Stage of Labour

(Birth of the placenta and membranes – may take 15–20 minutes)

- Assist the mother in expelling the placenta naturally by encouraging her to adopt a squatting, upright position, but only if there has been no delay in delivery of the placenta and **NOT IF THERE IS ANY SIGNIFICANT BLEEDING**.
- Encourage the woman to empty her bladder to facilitate uterine contraction.
- Do not pull the cord during birth of the placenta, as this could rupture the cord, making birth of the placenta difficult and cause excessive bleeding or inversion of the uterus.
- Allow the placenta to be born straight into a bowl or plastic bag. Keep it, together with any blood and membranes, for inspection by a midwife.

NB If the placenta has not been born within 20 minutes following birth, insert a LARGE BORE (16G) cannula, as there is an increased risk of haemorrhage and intravenous fluid and further intervention (oxytoxics) may be required.

Blood Loss

- Assess how much blood has accompanied the delivery of the placenta and membranes – this should not exceed 200–300 ml.
- If bleeding continues after birth of the placenta, palpate the mother's abdomen and feel for the top of the uterus (fundus), usually at the level of the umbilicus, and massage firmly with a cupped hand in a circular motion.
- The fundus will become firm as massage is applied and this may be quite uncomfortable, so Entonox should be offered (refer to **Nitrous Oxide (Entonox® or Nitronox™)** for administration and information).
- Be aware that the uterus may relax again and bleeding recommence. 'Rubbing up a contraction' may need to be repeated.

Severe Bleeding

- Assess blood loss if bleeding is severe.
- Obtain IV access – insert two LARGE BORE (16G) cannulae.
- Administer an oxytocic drug (refer to **Intravascular Fluid Therapy in Adults** and **Intravascular Fluid Therapy in Children**).
- Administer Syntometrine intramuscularly if available (refer to **Syntometrine**).
- If Syntometrine is **NOT** available, or where systolic BP is 140/90 mmHg or more (or where systolic BP alone is 150 mmHg or more), administer misoprostol 800 micrograms (four tablets) sublingually (refer to **Misoprostol**).
- Tranexamic acid can be given additionally.
- Refer to Post-partum Haemorrhage section within this guideline.

(continued)

Birth Imminent: Normal Birth and Birth Complications

TABLE 5.4 – ASSESSMENT and MANAGEMENT of: Normal Birth *(continued)*

Assess and Monitor Respiration Rate, Pulse and Blood Pressure

- Administer O_2 to aim for target saturation within the range of 94–98% (refer to **Oxygen**).

A number of complications may arise during pregnancy and/or labour. Refer to Table 5.5 for the assessment and management of:

1. preterm birth
2. maternal convulsions (eclampsia)
3. prolapsed umbilical cord
4. post-partum haemorrhage
5. continuous severe/sudden abdominal/back pain/placental abruption
6. multiple births – delayed birth of second or subsequent baby
7. malpresentation
8. shoulder dystocia.

TABLE 5.5 – ASSESSMENT and MANAGEMENT of: Birth Complications

1. Preterm Birth – Birth Before the Completion of 37 Weeks

Ascertain the Period of Gestation

- Less than 20 weeks' gestation – transfer the woman to the nearest ED with an obstetric unit.
- 20–37 weeks' gestation – transfer the woman to the nearest obstetric unit or ED with an obstetric unit dependent on local policy, as the baby will require specialist assessment by the neonatal team once born.

Reassess the Mother Constantly En-route

- Should birth take place en-route, assess both the mother and the baby and take appropriate action.
- Keeping the baby warm is a priority in the preterm newborn (refer to **Newborn Life Support**).
- Convey mother and baby to the **NEAREST** obstetric unit or ED with an obstetric unit dependent on local policy.
- Provide a pre-alert to enable a midwifery and neonatal team to receive the mother and newborn baby upon your arrival.
- In some circumstances, it may be necessary to convey the baby separately from the mother, dependent upon the clinical condition of either newborn or mother. In this instance, mother and baby should be conveyed to the same ED with an ID bracelet placed on each of them.
- If transfer to further care is not possible because the birth is imminent, request a midwife plus an additional ambulance and inform the EOC.
- Once the baby is born, utilise the additional ambulance to transport the baby **IMMEDIATELY** to the **NEAREST** appropriate destination as agreed locally.
- The baby should be transported once appropriate resource is available, even if the midwife has not yet arrived.
- Provide a pre-alert to the hospital (it will be necessary to identify the nearest, most appropriate ED with an obstetric unit, with the necessary neonatal facilities).
- The mother should be transferred to the same location as the baby; where no complications are identified, a courtesy call should be placed ahead of her arrival.

If the Amniotic Membranes Are Visible During Birth

- **DO NOT** artificially rupture the amniotic sac while the baby is in utero (i.e. before the baby is born).
- In the majority of births, the amniotic sac will rupture during labour, before the baby is born. However, occasionally, the amniotic sac will not rupture, particularly in preterm births. The bulging sac may be visible at the vaginal entrance during the second stage of labour, and may be visible for quite some time as the woman pushes before the baby is born.

TABLE 5.5 – ASSESSMENT and MANAGEMENT of: Birth Complications *(continued)*

- The decision to artificially rupture the membranes prior to delivery should only be made by a midwife or obstetrician. In some cases of early preterm labour, leaving the amniotic membranes intact may slow the delivery, allowing for steroids to be administered by the midwife or obstetrician which can improve the outcome for the preterm neonate. When the membranes are artificially ruptured, there is a danger that the labour can progress rapidly, leading to birth sooner than expected. More rarely, rupturing membranes can lead to significant complications that can only be managed in hospital, e.g. umbilical cord prolapse.

- Rarely, the baby and placenta may be born with the amniotic sac intact and the baby within. This is called an 'en caul' delivery. The membranes should be ruptured away from the baby and placenta: 'pinch' an area of the membranes firmly and cut carefully with scissors or a scalpel, ensuring that the umbilical cord within the sac is not damaged. Once ruptured, the amniotic fluid will rapidly drain away. You may need to carefully peel the remaining membranes away from the baby's mouth and nose in order to ensure the airway is clear.

2. Maternal Convulsions (Eclampsia) (see Figure 5.6)

Assess the Woman and Scene

- Refer to **Pregnancy-induced Hypertension (including Eclampsia)**.

- If ≥20 weeks, **ALL** generalised tonic/clonic type convulsions should be regarded as eclampsia until proved otherwise, **EVEN IF THERE IS A HISTORY OF EPILEPSY**.

- If the woman is convulsing, refer to **Convulsions in Adults** and **Convulsions in Children**.

Undertake a Primary Survey <C>ABCDEF

- Assess for **TIME-CRITICAL** features.

- Correct A and B problems and transfer to the nearest ED with an obstetric unit.

3. Prolapsed Umbilical Cord (see Figure 5.7)

Descent of the Umbilical Cord into the Lower Uterine Segment

- This is a **TIME-CRITICAL EMERGENCY** requiring immediate intervention, rapid removal and transfer to the nearest obstetric unit.

- Avoid handling the umbilical cord. Using a dry pad, replace the cord GENTLY within the opening of the vulva to keep it warm and prevent spasm, and use the pad to prevent further prolapse. (Do not use moist/wet pads as this will make the cord cold). If available, use underwear to hold the pad in position.

- If attending as a solo responding clinician, position the woman in the knee/chest position while awaiting an ambulance.

- To enable rapid transfer to the ambulance, the woman can be walked, avoiding the use of the carry chair where possible.

(continued)

SECTION **5** Maternity Care

TABLE 5.5 – ASSESSMENT and MANAGEMENT of: Birth Complications *(continued)*

- Once in the ambulance, position the mother on her side with padding placed under her hips to raise the pelvis and reduce pressure on the cord.

- Administer Entonox if the mother experiences pain or the urge to push.

- Provide ongoing assessment of the woman to ensure that birth is not imminent (if birth is imminent, refer to the normal birth section of this guideline).

- It is not safe to convey the woman in the all-fours position in the ambulance.
  - Transfer to the nearest obstetric unit.
  - Place an early pre-alert stating the obstetric emergency of cord prolapse.
  - It may be necessary to request maternity staff to meet the ambulance clinicians at a suitable entrance to avoid any delays due to accessing lifts or entry to buildings.

4. Post-partum Haemorrhage (PPH)

This is the commonest cause of severe haemorrhage immediately after delivery is uterine atony (i.e. poor uterine contraction) (see Figure 5.8).

- Primary PPH: blood loss of 500 ml or more within 24 hours of birth.

- Massive PPH: blood loss of 50% of the blood volume within 3 hours of birth.

- NOTE – If severe haemorrhage occurs following birth of the baby (post-partum) follow one of the two treatment regimens below en-route to further care if possible.

Maternity pad with 500 W blood and sanitary pad with 50 ml blood.

SECTION 5 Maternity Care

Birth Imminent: Normal Birth and Birth Complications

TABLE 5.5 – ASSESSMENT and MANAGEMENT of: Birth Complications *(continued)*

IF THE PLACENTA HAS DELIVERED:

- Palpate the abdomen and feel for the top of the uterus (fundus), usually at the level of the umbilicus, and massage with a cupped hand in a circular motion.

- The fundus will become firm as massage is applied. This may be quite uncomfortable and Entonox can be offered (refer to **Nitrous Oxide (Entonox® or Nitronox™)** for administration and information).

- Administer **Syntometrine intramuscularly** (refer to **Syntometrine**).

- If Syntometrine or other oxytocics are unavailable, have been ineffective at reducing haemorrhage after 15 minutes or where systolic BP is 140/90 mmHg or more (or where systolic BP alone is 150 mmHg or more), administer misoprostol 800 micrograms sublingually (refer to **Misoprostol**).

- Administer **Tranexamic Acid**.

- Establish IV access (ideally with two large bore (16G) cannulae).

- Convey to the nearest obstetric unit or, where there is ongoing bleeding with evidence of maternal collapse, convey to the nearest appropriate destination as agreed locally.

- In the presence of catastrophic haemorrhage, the first line of management in the pre-hospital setting should be to apply *fundal massage* (known as 'rubbing up' a uterine contraction) and administer first-line drugs such as Syntometrine or Syntocinon.

- The use of 'bimanual uterine compression' is an invasive procedure requiring intimate internal manoeuvres and may be considered only by those paramedics that have received appropriate training to undertake this life-saving intervention.

IF THE PLACENTA HAS NOT DELIVERED:

- In the presence of haemorrhage, **DO NOT** massage the top of the uterus (fundus) when the placenta is undelivered. This may provoke partial separation of the placenta and cause further haemorrhage. (However, in the event of life-threatening haemorrhage, massaging the uterus while transferring to hospital may be considered.)

- Administer a bolus of Syntometrine intramuscularly (refer to **Syntometrine**) – if Syntometrine or other oxytocics are unavailable, have been ineffective at reducing haemorrhage after 15 minutes or where systolic BP is 140/90 mmHg or more (or where systolic BP alone is 150 mmHg or more), administer misoprostol (refer to **Misoprostol**).

- Administer **Tranexamic Acid**.

- **NB** Administration of Syntometrine or misoprostol may cause the placenta to separate and deliver. If the placenta delivers, ensure there is no further bleeding. If bleeding continues after the placenta is delivered, commence massage of uterine fundus.

Assess Blood Loss – Bleeding >500 ml

- Reassess prior to further fluid replacement.

- If bleeding continues, check for bleeding from tears at the vaginal entrance.

- Obtain IV access – insert a **LARGE BORE (16G)** cannula.

- Administer fluid replacement (refer to **Intravascular Fluid Therapy in Adults** and **Intravascular Fluid Therapy in Children**).

- Apply external pressure to a tear using a gauze or maternity pad.

- Transfer the mother and baby to the **NEAREST OBSTETRIC UNIT** immediately.

- Provide a pre-alert stating an obstetric emergency of post-partum haemorrhage.

- During conveyance, provide ongoing assessment and, where necessary, uterine massage.

- Administer **Tranexamic Acid**.

5. Multiple Births – Delayed Birth of Second or Subsequent Baby

NOTE – with a twin birth, the mother is at increased risk of immediate post-partum haemorrhage due to poor uterine tone (refer to 4 above).

It is now very unusual for a mother expecting a multiple birth to give birth outside hospital. However, twin pregnancies are at much higher risk of delivering preterm (i.e. before 37 weeks) – the babies may therefore need resuscitation.

(continued)

Birth Imminent: Normal Birth and Birth Complications

TABLE 5.5 – ASSESSMENT and MANAGEMENT of: Birth Complications *(continued)*

- If birth is **NOT** in progress:
  - Transfer mother to the nearest obstetric unit without delay.
  - Constantly reassess en-route and take appropriate action if the circumstances change.
  - Place an information call informing the hospital of a woman expecting a twin birth.
- If birth is in progress or occurs en-route:
  - Request a second ambulance and, where available, midwifery support.
  - Follow normal birth guidance and refer to **Care of the Newborn**.
- When the first baby has been born and assessed, if birth of the second baby is not imminent, transfer the mother and baby to the **NEAREST OBSTETRIC UNIT IMMEDIATELY** (it is not necessary to await the arrival of the midwife).
- Provide a pre-alert to the hospital. It may be necessary to request maternity staff meet the ambulance clinicians at a suitable entrance to avoid any delays due to accessing lifts or entry to buildings.
- If the birth of the second baby occurs en-route, request via the EOC an **ADDITIONAL AMBULANCE**.
- When the second baby is born, utilise both vehicles to transfer mother and babies to the nearest obstetric unit.
- Provide a pre-alert, including the number of babies due to arrive with one mother (this is particularly relevant with higher birth multiples, although uncommon).
- Assess if any/either baby requires resuscitation. Refer to **Newborn Life Support**.

6. Malpresentation – Including Vaginal Breech Birth (see Figure 5.9)

- Vaginal breech birth is where the feet or buttocks of the baby present first rather than the baby's head.
- **NB** Cord prolapse is more common with a breech presentation (refer to 3 above); follow local guidelines.

Vaginal breech birth – if birth is **NOT** in progress:

- Recognise breech presentation (may be documented in the woman's antenatal notes, thick meconium may be seen at vaginal opening, fetal buttocks or feet visible at vaginal opening).
- Transfer mother to the nearest obstetric unit without delay.
- Constantly reassess en-route and take appropriate action if the circumstances change.

Vaginal breech birth – if birth **IS** in progress:

- Request a midwife (if available locally) and additional resources.
- Prepare for newborn resuscitation (refer to **Newborn Life Support**).
- Encourage the woman to adopt a position to enable gravity to help the birth of the baby, for example the edge of the bed, the edge of a sofa or the 'all-fours' position.

Breech delivery with mother semi-recumbent. Note – the fetal back should be upwards.

Birth Imminent: Normal Birth and Birth Complications

TABLE 5.5 – ASSESSMENT and MANAGEMENT of: Birth Complications *(continued)*

Breech delivery in 'all-fours' position. Note – the fetal abdomen should face upwards (i.e. the fetal back faces the maternal abdomen).

- Allow breech to descend spontaneously with maternal pushing, and maintain a 'hands-off' position. It is not necessary to touch the baby or handle the umbilical cord during the birth.

- The baby's legs and arms will spontaneously birth and do not require any assistance.

- Only assist to ensure the baby's back remains facing towards the woman's abdomen.

- If the baby's back rotates away from the woman's abdomen, handle the baby over the hips (the bony pelvis) and gently rotate the baby's back to face towards the woman's abdomen.

- In the semi-recumbent position, once the baby's body is born to the nape of the neck, allow slow spontaneous birth of the head by supporting the baby's body on your forearm and gently lift the baby to facilitate birth of the baby's head. In the all-fours position, as the head delivers the baby's body will deliver onto the bed/trolley.

- Once the birth is complete, if the baby does not require any resuscitation, management of the umbilical cord should be as per normal birth guidelines, and it should be left to stop pulsating.

- Breech babies are more likely to be covered in meconium and may require resuscitation (refer to **Newborn Life Support**).

- If delays occur during the birth:
  - **Legs.** If the legs delay birth of the body, apply gentle pressure to the back of the baby's knee (popliteal fossa), enabling birth of each individual leg.
  - **Arms.** If the arms are extended, gently rotate baby's pelvis 180 degrees to bring the posterior arm anterior (i.e. uppermost) and deliver that arm first, then rotate the baby in the opposite direction 180 degrees and release the other arm.
  - **Head.** If the head does not deliver in the semi-recumbent position (with the baby's body supported on your forearm), apply pressure to the back of the baby's head with the fingers of your other hand, to aid flexion while the head delivers.

- Where ambulance clinicians have received appropriate training in management of breech birth, additional manoeuvres can be undertaken as detailed above for management of the legs, arms and head where delays in birth are identified.

- Where the ambulance clinician has not received appropriate training, the nearest obstetric unit can be contacted to provide guidance on the ongoing management of the birth.

- For any presenting body part other than the head, buttocks or feet (e.g. one foot or a hand/arm), transfer the mother immediately to the nearest obstetric unit.

- Provide a pre-alert. It may be necessary to request maternity staff meet the ambulance clinicians at a suitable entrance to avoid any delays due to accessing lifts.

(continued)

5 Maternity Care — SECTION

TABLE 5.5 – ASSESSMENT and MANAGEMENT of: Birth Complications *(continued)*

7. Shoulder Dystocia (see Figure 5.10)

- An arrest of spontaneous birth; when birth of the baby's shoulders is delayed because the baby's anterior shoulder is stuck behind the symphysis pubis.
- Request a midwife (if available locally) and additional resources.
- Prepare for newborn resuscitation (refer to **Newborn Life Support**).
- An attempt must be made to deliver the shoulders using the McRoberts manoeuvre if:
  - the shoulders are not born within two contractions following the birth of the head
  - there is difficulty with delivery of the face and chin
  - the head remains tightly applied to the vulva or retracts ('turtle-neck' sign)
  - there is failure of the fetal head to fully rotate to face towards the mother's inner thigh once born.

McRoberts Manoeuvre (Alters the Angle of the Pelvis)

- Ask the woman to lie flat and bring her bottom to the end of the bed.
- Bring the woman's knees up onto her abdomen (the legs will naturally abduct due to the pregnant uterus). If available, use an assistant to support each leg or ask the woman to hold them. Ask the woman to push with the next contraction, as the shoulders may now be released.

- If the shoulders do not release, attempt to deliver the baby's shoulders with gentle 'axial' traction applied to the baby's head (this is outward traction keeping the baby's head in line with its own spine, and is angled just below the horizontal); the mother is encouraged to push. **AVOID** pulling on the baby's head downwards or laterally towards the floor and avoid twisting the baby's neck at any time (this can damage the brachial plexus nerves).
- If undelivered after 30 seconds, move on to applying suprapubic pressure while maintaining the McRoberts position.

Suprapubic Pressure

- Identify where the fetal back is facing.
- With the mother still in McRoberts position, ask the assistant to:

  a Stand on the maternal side where the baby's back is (if the baby's back is facing left, stand on the woman's left or vice versa).

  b Place hands in CPR grip with the heel of the hand two finger breadths above the maternal symphysis pubis.

  c Apply moderate pressure in a downwards and lateral direction **continuously** for 30 seconds.

  d Encourage the mother to push or attempt gentle **AXIAL** traction to deliver the baby.

SECTION **5** Maternity Care

Birth Imminent: Normal Birth and Birth Complications

TABLE 5.5 – ASSESSMENT and MANAGEMENT of: Birth Complications *(continued)*

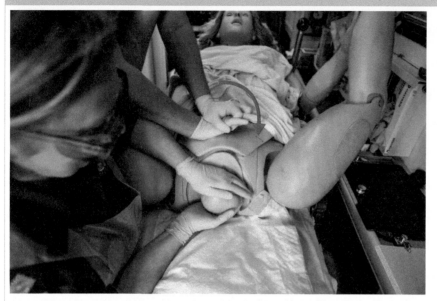

- If the shoulders do not release, attempt **intermittent pressure** on the shoulder for 30 seconds:
  a Ask the assistant to apply intermittent pressure on the shoulder by rocking gently backwards and forwards.
  b Encourage the mother to push or attempt gentle **AXIAL** traction to deliver the baby.
- If unsuccessful, change the woman's position to 'all fours'.

'All-Fours' Position

(For the lone clinician, this is an ideal first position to use as it provides a very effective McRoberts manoeuvre)

- Position the woman on her hands and knees with her hips well flexed (any movement of the pelvis may help release the shoulders).

- Encourage the woman to push to release shoulders or apply gentle **AXIAL** traction to release the shoulder nearest to the maternal back first.
- If unsuccessful, transfer the woman to the ambulance; she may be walked, as this may also encourage the birth. Ambulance clinicians should be prepared to anticipate the birth during transfer and/or conveyance.

(continued)

SECTION **5** Maternity Care

Birth Imminent: Normal Birth and Birth Complications

TABLE 5.5 – ASSESSMENT and MANAGEMENT of: Birth Complications *(continued)*

- Convey the woman to the nearest obstetric unit positioned in a lateral position, using a pillow to separate the woman's legs and avoid pressure on the baby's head. Offer Entonox to provide analgesia if required. Do not delay to await arrival of the midwife.

- Place a pre-alert stating the obstetric emergency of shoulder dystocia. It may be necessary to request maternity staff meet the ambulance clinicians at a suitable entrance to avoid any delays due to accessing lifts or buildings.

The Use of Internal Manoeuvres by Ambulance Clinicians

- Where McRoberts manoeuvre, suprapubic pressure and all-fours position have been attempted to expedite the birth, the use of specific internal manoeuvres may be appropriate where a registered paramedic has received additional training to undertake them.

- In a pre-hospital setting where a lone attending clinician is first on scene, the use of the all-fours position may facilitate the removal of the posterior arm, notably when awaiting an ambulance to the scene.

KEY POINTS!

Birth Imminent: Normal Birth and Birth Complications

- **For a woman experiencing an abnormal labour or birth, transfer immediately to the nearest obstetric unit. This includes:**
    - **severe vaginal bleeding**
    - **preterm or multiple births**
    - **prolapsed umbilical cord**
    - **continuous severe abdominal/epigastric pain**
    - **maternal convulsions (eclampsia)**
    - **presentation of the baby other than the head (e.g. arm or leg or buttocks)**
    - **shoulder dystocia.**

- **If the woman presents with an obvious medical or traumatic condition that puts her life in imminent danger, transfer to the nearest ED with an obstetric unit.**

- **The period of gestation is important in informing the appropriate course of action, including the most appropriate location for conveyance, namely an ED, an early pregnancy unit or an obstetric unit.**

- **In the event of an obstetric emergency, detailing the exact emergency via a pre-alert call will assist the ED or maternity unit to summon the appropriate staff.**

- **Maintaining normothermia in the newborn is critical while on scene and during conveyance. The optimum body temperature of the baby should be between 36.5 and 37.5 degrees.**

Birth Imminent: Normal Birth and Birth Complications

Management of Eclampsia

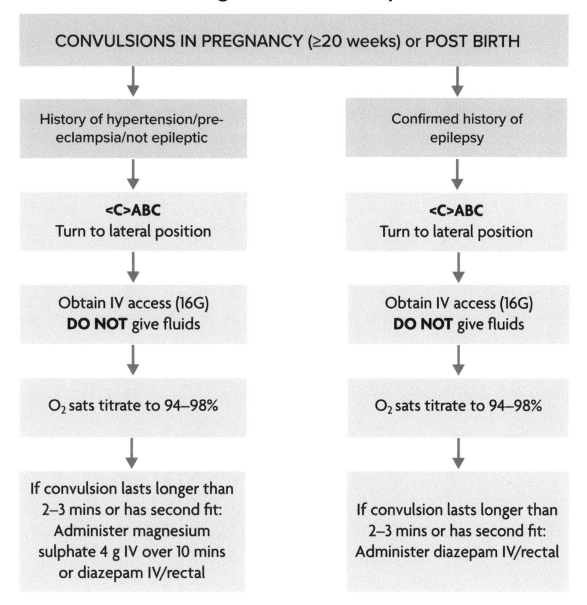

CONVULSIONS IN PREGNANCY (≥20 weeks) or POST BIRTH

History of hypertension/pre-eclampsia/not epileptic	Confirmed history of epilepsy
<C>ABC Turn to lateral position	**<C>ABC** Turn to lateral position
Obtain IV access (16G) **DO NOT** give fluids	Obtain IV access (16G) **DO NOT** give fluids
O₂ sats titrate to 94–98%	O₂ sats titrate to 94–98%
If convulsion lasts longer than 2–3 mins or has second fit: Administer magnesium sulphate 4 g IV over 10 mins or diazepam IV/rectal	If convulsion lasts longer than 2–3 mins or has second fit: Administer diazepam IV/rectal

Transfer to nearest appropriate destination as agreed locally
Maternal safety is the prime consideration
Consider the specific clinical situation **and which interventions may be required for the woman and baby on arrival**
Refer to 'Appropriate Destination for Conveyance'
in **Maternity Care**
Pre-alert stating obstetric emergency eclampsia
Take maternity notes if available

Figure 5.6 – Pre-hospital maternity emergency – management of eclampsia.

SECTION **5** Maternity Care

Birth Imminent: Normal Birth and Birth Complications

Management of Cord Prolapse

Gently replace the umbilical cord within the opening of the vagina using a dry pad

↓

Position the woman in the knee chest position while awaiting the ambulance

↓

Walk the woman to the ambulance

↓

Position the woman in the lateral position
Elevate the pelvis using a blanket below the right hip

↓

Assess for imminent birth en-route
Administer Entonox if required

Transfer to nearest appropriate destination as agreed locally
Maternal safety is the prime consideration
Consider the specific clinical situation **and which interventions may be required for the woman and baby on arrival**
Refer to 'Appropriate Destination for Conveyance' in **Maternity Care**
Pre-alert stating obstetric emergency of cord prolapse
Take maternity notes if available

Figure 5.7 – Pre-hospital maternity emergency – management of cord prolapse.

Birth Imminent: Normal Birth and Birth Complications

Management of Post-partum Haemorrhage

Administer oxygen to maintain O₂ saturations at 94–98%

UTERINE ATONY:
Placenta delivered

UTERINE ATONY:
Placenta not delivered

Firmly rub up a uterine contraction

IF BP **less than** 140/90 administer Syntometrine 1 ml IM

If BP is **140/90 or more** (or if **systolic BP alone is 150 or more**),
give misoprostol 800 mcg sublingual
(If airway is compromised, administer misoprostol rectally)

Obtain IV access (16G) and commence IV fluids

For ongoing bleeding administer Tranexamic acid
en-route to hospital

If uterus is well contracted, check for perineal trauma:
Apply external direct pressure gauze/maternity pad
Obtain IV access (16G) and commence IV fluids
For ongoing bleeding administer Tranexamic acid
en-route to hospital

Transfer to nearest appropriate destination as agreed locally
Maternal safety is the prime consideration
Consider the specific clinical situation **and which interventions may be required for the woman and baby on arrival**
Refer to 'Appropriate Destination for Conveyance' in Maternity Care
Pre-alert stating obstetric emergency PPH
Perform ongoing assessment of uterine contraction
and/or perineal trauma/maternal observations

Figure 5.8 – Pre-hospital maternity emergency – management of post-partum haemorrhage.

Birth Imminent: Normal Birth and Birth Complications

Management of Breech Birth

Breech position noted in maternal notes or thick meconium seen at vaginal opening

BREECH BIRTH IMMINENT	**BREECH BIRTH NOT IMMINENT OR ANY OTHER PRESENTING PART (i.e. hand/arm)**

BREECH BIRTH IMMINENT:

Request midwife if available
Prepare for newborn life support

↓

Position on edge of bed/trolley
or on all fours

↓

HANDS OFF
Allow breech to descend spontaneously
with maternal pushing
DO NOT touch baby or handle
umbilical cord

↓

In either position, ensure the baby's
back is always facing towards the
maternal abdomen

↓

Support baby as head births

↓

Treat as normal birth or
refer to Newborn Life Support

BREECH BIRTH NOT IMMINENT OR ANY OTHER PRESENTING PART:

Transfer to nearest appropriate
destination as agreed locally
Maternal safety is the prime consideration
Consider the specific clinical situation
**and which interventions may be required
for the woman and baby on arrival**
Refer to 'Appropriate Destination for
Conveyance' in **Maternity Care**
Continuously assess for birth imminent en-route

IF DELAY OCCURS DURING THE BIRTH:

LEGS: apply gentle pressure behind the baby's knee
ARMS: gently rotate the baby's pelvis 90 degrees to aid birth of the first arm – rotate
the baby's body in the opposite direction if required to birth the second arm – allow
the baby's body to hang unassisted
HEAD: support the baby with one arm and use the other hand to aid flexion of the
back of the baby's head while delivering baby

DO NOT PULL ON THE BABY
DO NOT CLAMP AND CUT THE UMBILICAL CORD DURING THE BIRTH

Figure 5.9 – Pre-hospital maternity emergency – management of breech birth.

Birth Imminent: Normal Birth and Birth Complications

Management of Shoulder Dystocia

REQUEST A MIDWIFE IF AVAILABLE AND PREPARE FOR NEWBORN LIFE SUPPORT
Position the woman in the McRoberts position
For a solo clinician – ask the woman to hold her legs and push with her next contraction

If shoulders do not release:
Attempt to deliver the baby
- With your hands on the baby's head apply gentle 'axial' traction, keeping the baby's head in line with its spine for up to 30 seconds

Undelivered?

Apply suprapubic pressure with the woman in the McRoberts position
- Identify the position of the fetal back and place assistant on that maternal side
- Using a CPR grip, apply continuous pressure downwards and lateral for 30 seconds (2 fingers above symphysis pubis)
- Encourage the woman to push **OR** attempt gentle 'axial' traction to deliver baby

Undelivered?

- Attempt intermittent 'rocking' suprapubic pressure for 30 seconds and encourage woman to push
- Or attempt gentle 'axial' traction to deliver baby

Undelivered?

- Change the woman's position to 'all fours' and encourage her to push
- Or attempt gentle 'axial' traction to deliver baby

Undelivered?

- Walk the woman to the ambulance and anticipate the birth during transfer
- Convey in a lateral position with legs separated by a blanket to protect the baby's head
- Reassure the woman and provide Entonox as required.

Baby born
Refer to **Care of the Newborn**

Transfer to the nearest appropriate destination as agreed locally
Maternal safety is the prime consideration
Consider the specific clinical situation **and which interventions may be required for the woman and baby on arrival**
Refer to 'Appropriate Destination for Conveyance' in **Maternity Care**
Pre-alert stating the obstetric emergency shoulder dystocia
Keep a log of the time each intervention is attempted

Figure 5.10 – Pre-hospital maternity emergency – management of shoulder dystocia.

Birth Imminent: Normal Birth and Birth Complications

Bibliography

1. Woollard M, Hinshaw K, Simpson H, Wieteska S. Normal delivery. In *Pre-hospital Obstetric Emergency Training*. Oxford: Wiley-Blackwell, 2009: 28–37.

2. Woollard M, Hinshaw K, Simpson H, Wieteska S. Structured approach to the obstetric patient. In *Pre-hospital Obstetric Emergency Training*. Oxford: Wiley-Blackwell, 2009: 38–52.

3. Woollard M, Hinshaw K, Simpson H, Wieteska S. Emergencies in late pregnancy. In *Pre-Hospital Obstetric Emergency Training*. Oxford: Wiley-Blackwell, 2009: 62–110.

4. Woollard M, Hinshaw K, Simpson H, Wieteska S. Emergencies after delivery. In *Pre-hospital Obstetric Emergency Training*. Oxford: Wiley-Blackwell, 2009: 111–124.

5. Woollard M, Hinshaw K, Simpson H, Wieteska S. Care of the baby at birth. In *Pre-hospital Obstetric Emergency Training*. Oxford: Wiley-Blackwell, 2009: 125–135.

6. Royal College of Obstetricians and Gynaecologists. *The Management of Breech Presentation* (Green-top Guideline 20b). London: RCOG, 2006.

7. Royal College of Obstetricians and Gynaecologists. *Placenta Praevia, Placenta Praevia Accreta and Vasa Praevia: Diagnosis and Management* (Green-top Guideline 27). London: RCOG, 2011.

8. Royal College of Obstetricians and Gynaecologists. *Shoulder Dystocia* (Green-top Guideline 42). London RCOG, 2012.

9. Royal College of Obstetricians and Gynaecologists. *Umbilical Cord Prolapse* (Green-top Guideline 50). London: RCOG, 2008.

10. Royal College of Obstetricians and Gynaecologists. *Prevention and Management of Postpartum Haemorrhage* (Green-top guideline 52). London: RCOG, 2016.

11. Mousa HA, Alfirevic Z. Treatment for primary postpartum haemorrhage. *Cochrane Database of Systematic Reviews* 2007, 1: CD003249.

12. Starrs A, Winikoff B. Misoprostol for postpartum hemorrhage: moving from evidence to practice. *International Journal of Gynaecology and Obstetrics* 2012, 116(1): 1–3.

13. Health and Care Professions Council. *Standards of Conduct, Performance and Ethics: Your Duties as a Registrant*. London: Health Professions Council, 2003.

14. Crofts JF, Lenguerrand E, Bentham GL, Tawfik S, Claireaux HA, Odd D, Fox R, Draycott TJ. Prevention of brachial plexus injury – 12 years of shoulder dystocia training: an interrupted time-series study. *BJOG* 2016, 123(1): 111–118.

15. Griffin C. Re: Prevention of brachial plexus injury – 12 years of shoulder dystocia training: an interrupted time-series study: posterior arm delivery at the time of caesarean section. *BJOG* 2016, 123(1): 144.

16. Menticoglou S. Delivering shoulders and dealing with shoulder dystocia: should the standard of care change? *JOGC* 2016, 38(7): 655–658.

17. Gherman RB. Shoulder dystocia. *Clinical Obstetrics and Gynecology* 2016, 59(4): 789–790.

Care of the Newborn

1. Introduction

- The physiology of the fetus is fundamentally different from that of the newborn baby, with both structural and functional distinctions. The transition from intra- to extrauterine life is characterised by changes in circulatory pathways, initiation of ventilation and oxygenation via the lungs instead of the placenta and many changes in metabolism.

- The majority of term newborn babies complete this process in a rapid, smooth and organised fashion in the first few moments after birth. However, circulatory and pulmonary changes continue for up to 6 weeks after birth. Preterm babies or those with underlying disease may experience a delay in transition.

- Regular assessment is required to ensure that the baby who is experiencing problems with transition is recognised and appropriate interventions are initiated.

2. Thermal Care

- Thermoregulation is a crucial aspect of newborn care. Heat loss occurs by radiation, convection and conduction. A wet baby will also lose heat by evaporation. Babies have a large surface area relative to weight, so losses are proportionately greater. Preterm babies are at particular risk as their surface area to volume ratio is even larger. A cold baby has increased oxygen consumption and is at risk of hypoglycaemia and acidosis. For each degree below 36.5°C, the risk of mortality increases by 28%.

- Exclude any draughts, and heat the environment as much as possible. Babies should be thoroughly dried, a hat applied and be wrapped in towels or placed skin to skin. Use a pod or foil wrap if available. The ambulance should be kept well heated to prevent cooling during the transfer to hospital. Time with doors open or with the baby outside of a warm building/ambulance should be kept to a minimum (refer to **Newborn Life Support**).

- Normal newborn temperature is 36.5 to 37.5°C. Temperature recordings should be taken with an appropriately calibrated thermometer as soon as practical after birth, ideally at least once during transport and then on arrival at destination.

2.1 Skin to Skin

- Skin to skin (Figure 5.11) should be facilitated in line with the mother's wishes as long as mother and baby are well and the mother is able to hold the baby securely. If the mother is unwell, cold, shocked or does not want to do skin to skin, it can be done with a partner or other family member. Alternatively, the baby can be wrapped in towels.

- When skin to skin, the baby should be placed in a prone position with their head turned to one side so that the face is easily visible to the mother. The baby should have a hat on.

Figure 5.11 – Skin-to-skin care.

Note: The baby has a hat on and is covered with towel/blanket to keep warm. The position allows observation of airway and breathing efforts and may, if the situation permits, allow early breast feeding.

- Vigilant observation of the mother and baby should continue, with prompt removal of the baby if the health of mother or baby gives concern.

- Staff should have a conversation with the mother and family about recognising any changes in the baby's condition while the baby is skin to skin.

- The mother and baby will need regular observation by caregivers.

- Follow local guidance for any transport of the baby and mother to hospital.

3. Newborn Pathophysiology

3.1 Perinatal Hypoxia

- Perinatal hypoxia can occur for various reasons, including cord compression, cord prolapse, significant placental or umbilical bleeding. The presence of thick meconium may indicate an episode of perinatal hypoxia. Babies can cope with a degree of hypoxia at birth. However, severe perinatal hypoxia has a poor prognosis and is often associated with neurological deficit and cerebral palsy. A low APGAR score at 10 minutes suggests a risk of long-term neurological complications.

- Therapeutic hypothermia is used by neonatal teams in a hospital environment to reduce the risk of neurodevelopment impairment or death. It is not within the scope of pre-hospital clinicians to initiate therapeutic hypothermia. Unless carrying out an intra-facility transport and you have been specifically instructed to keep the ambulance cold, always heat the ambulance and follow the thermoregulation guidance above.

3.2 Hypoglycaemia

- Following birth, the baby undergoes a process of metabolic adaptation. Keeping the baby warm reduces metabolic stress and energy use to help maintain blood sugar. Breast milk is an ideal source of energy after birth, so if the baby is well

Care of the Newborn

and not requiring any support, women should be encouraged to breastfeed as soon as possible (within the first hour if possible/appropriate).

- The newborn baby has a relatively immature liver with limited glycogen stores. Therefore, hypoglycaemia must not be treated using intramuscular glucagon (glucagon works by stimulating the liver to convert glycogen into glucose). Buccal glucose 40% oral gel can be used (refer to **Glucose 40% Oral Gel**).

- Many hypoglycaemic babies are asymptomatic, so babies at risk of hypoglycaemia undergo blood sugar checks in the hospital setting.

- **Those at risk of hypoglycaemia include babies who are:**
  - preterm (<37 weeks)
  - small for gestational age
  - <2.5 kg at birth
  - in need of resuscitation at birth
  - born to diabetic mothers
  - born to mothers using beta-blockers (labetalol)
  - suffering from perinatal hypoxia
  - suffering from hypothermia
  - suffering from infection/sepsis.

- **Signs and symptoms of hypoglycaemia can be non-specific and include:**
  - jitteriness
  - irritability
  - lethargy
  - apnoeic episodes
  - convulsions
  - high-pitched cry
  - suspected or confirmed sepsis
  - hypotonia
  - cyanosis
  - altered level of consciousness
  - abnormal feeding behaviour (e.g. not waking for feeds after a period of feeding well).

- **Severe and prolonged hypoglycaemia can lead to convulsions and brain injury. Any baby at risk of hypoglycaemia or who has signs/symptoms of hypoglycaemia must be transported to hospital as soon as possible for further investigation and management. Seek advice/inform the receiving centre where the clinical situation is of concern.**

- While pre-hospital clinicians would not usually be expected to take blood glucose samples from a newborn baby, if the clinical situation or signs suggest possible hypoglycaemia or if advised to treat potential low blood sugar (despite feeding, or where feeds are not possible), then buccal glucose gel can be administered as per JRCALC guidance.

3.3 Neonatal Jaundice

- Jaundice refers to the yellow colouration of the skin, sclera and mucous membranes caused by a raised bilirubin level.

- Jaundice can be physiological or pathological. It is not possible to measure the level of bilirubin or to decipher between physiological or pathological causes in the pre-hospital environment.

- Babies at risk of pathological jaundice include:
  - those <38 weeks
  - those with a previous sibling with neonatal jaundice requiring phototherapy where there may be a familial predisposition, such as a blood group incompatibility
  - babies born by instrumental or caesarean birth where bruising has occurred
  - babies born to a diabetic mother.

- The following jaundiced babies justify transfer to hospital, as the cause may be pathological and the baby will require urgent investigation:
  - ≤ 24 hours of age
  - lethargic or sleepy
  - babies with chalky stools and/or dark urine
  - babies at risk of pathological jaundice
  - babies showing any other sign of being unwell
  - jaundice after 14 days.

- Jaundiced babies that do not meet the categories above still require a review by a midwife, GP, neonatal doctor or health visitor within the next 4 hours either in the community or in ED.

3.4 Preterm Birth

- Prematurity is defined as <37 weeks' gestation. Preterm infants are more likely to need increased assistance with thermoregulation, airway support and breathing, as well as feeding.

- Particularly at <32 weeks' gestation, spontaneous breathing will most likely be inadequate, as these babies have immature lungs which are deficient in surfactant.

- Pre-hospital clinicians should resuscitate/stabilise using the newborn life support algorithm and approach (refer to **Newborn Life Support**). Prioritise thermal care and airway breathing support. These babies require immediate transfer to the nearest emergency department (ED) with an obstetric unit.

- Premature babies can be born in good condition initially but may deteriorate quickly without support. Therefore, they require continuous monitoring, and clinicians need to be ready to intervene with airway/breathing support at any time.

Care of the Newborn

3.4.1 Extremely Preterm Birth: Survival-focused Care

- Ambulance clinicians may attend births at the extremes of prematurity and viability. These babies require intensive thermoregulation, ventilatory support and rapid transfer to hospital.

- **Newborn Life Support** outlines the survival-focused care that is justified in babies born above 22 weeks and those where the gestation is not known. Be aware that even an extremely premature neonate may initially have breathing efforts with a good heart rate but is at risk of rapid deterioration, so will require airway and breathing support with continuous monitoring until definitive care can be delivered in the hospital setting.

- Evident observed signs of life after birth include at least one of the following:
  - easily visible heartbeat seen through the chest wall,
  - visible pulsation of the cord,
  - breathing or sustained gasps and/or
  - definite movement of arms and legs.

- Short-lived fleeting reflex activity, including transient gasps, brief visible pulsation of the chest wall or brief twitches or involuntary muscle movement, can be observed in babies that have died shortly before birth, and so fleeting reflex activity observed only in the first minute after birth may not warrant classification as signs of life.[1]

- Where there are signs of life and the gestation is unknown, airway and breathing support with ventilation should be continued until a neonatal team can assess the gestation and weight of the baby. The team will then consider the ongoing management in the best interests of the baby and the family.

- Neither a midwife nor an ambulance clinician should discontinue resuscitative attempts; this decision should be made by the neonatal team.

3.4.2 Extremely Preterm Birth: Comfort Care

- Babies **known** to be born before 22 weeks are pre-viable and should receive comfort care. This includes:
  - Compassionately explaining to the parents that the baby has been born too early and will not be able to survive even with significant neonatal care. Express your condolences and sympathy. Give the parents time and be sensitive to the individualised needs of the parents.
  - Wrapping the baby sensitively and offering the baby to the parents to hold. Most parents will find this extremely challenging but very helpful within the grieving process.
  - Explaining to the parents that the baby may have the occasional movement or reflex but that the baby is not in pain or suffering and may continue to show signs of life for some time after birth.
  - The baby should be held firmly and can be cuddled but not receive too much stimulation.
  - Please see the following link for information for parents (SANDS Leaflet): https://www.sands.org.uk/sites/default/files/Sands_Bereavement_Book_June2021.pdf.

3.5 Congenital Abnormalities

- The outcome of babies born with congenital abnormalities varies but is improving with advancement in medical therapies and interventions. The abnormality may have been detected on antenatal scans or may have been undiagnosed until birth. All babies who are known to have a congenital abnormality should be transferred to hospital where the abnormality can be assessed and treated, even when the baby appears to be normal at birth.

- Where the abnormality involves a section of the internal organs being outside the body, use cling film to cover the defect to reduce fluid and heat losses and risk of infection. **Do not wrap the cling film circumferentially around the newborn's body as this may inhibit breathing**.

3.6 Early Onset Neonatal Sepsis

- Early onset neonatal sepsis can be life-threatening, and it is important that it is recognised and treated early.

- **If the mother has any of the following risk factors, the baby is more at risk of having early onset neonatal sepsis:**
  - Systemic antibiotic treatment given to the mother for confirmed or suspected invasive bacteria.
  - Group B Streptococcus (GBS) colonisation, bacteriuria or infection in CURRENT pregnancy.
  - A previous baby with invasive GBS infection.
  - Preterm, pre-labour rupture of membranes of any duration.
  - Suspected or confirmed intrapartum rupture of membranes >18 hours.

- If any of the following are recognised in the baby, early neonatal sepsis could be the cause:[13]
  - Hypoglycaemia.
  - Altered behaviour or responsiveness.
  - Altered muscle tone (e.g. floppiness).
  - Feeding difficulties (e.g. feed refusal).
  - Feed intolerance (including vomiting or abdominal distension).
  - Abnormal heart rate (bradycardia or tachycardia).
  - Signs of respiratory distress (including grunting, recession, tachypnoea).
  - Hypoxia (e.g. central cyanosis or reduced oxygen saturation level).

Care of the Newborn

- Jaundice within 24 hours of birth.
- Temperature abnormality (lower than 36°C or higher than 38°C) unexplained by environmental factors.

- Unexplained excessive bleeding.
- If risk factors, signs or symptoms are identified, the baby should be transferred to the nearest ED with an obstetric unit.

4. Assessment and Management

Normal observations in a newborn baby			
	Normal ranges	**How to measure**	**Further information**
Colour	Pink/centrally perfused mucous membranes	Observation: It is normal for a baby to be blue for the first couple of minutes after birth, but the baby should be centrally perfused at all times following this.	Babies may be blue at birth but should rapidly begin to go pink. Acrocyanosis (blue hands and feed) is normal in the first 48 hours of life.
Tone	Flexed	Observation: A baby born well-flexed and with good tone is normally well.	Babies who remain floppy require urgent medical attention.
Respiratory rate	40–60 breaths per minute	Observation: Count breaths over 1 minute. Irregular, abdominal breathing is normal in a neonate.	Observe for signs of increased work of breathing or inadequacy, such as grunting (noise on inspiration or expiration), intercostal recession, nasal flaring.
Heart rate	100–160 bpm	Auscultation: Listen to the heart rate for 1 minute with a stethoscope.	Palpating the cord is less accurate. Saturation and ECG monitoring (if suitable leads are available) can be effective but may not be available immediately after birth.
Temperature	36.5–37.5°C	Measure: Use an appropriately calibrated thermometer.	Maintain temperature throughout any assessment, resuscitation and transport.

TABLE 5.6 – ASSESSMENT and MANAGEMENT of: The Newborn
Place of Resuscitation
▪ Consider these factors in advance of birth if possible.
▪ Ensure room is warm and close doors and windows to minimise drafts.
Management of the Cord
▪ Unless there are concerns about mother or baby, the cord should remain intact until it has gone white (or for at least 60 seconds). It can then be clamped and cut approximately 5 cm from the umbilicus.
▪ If assessment indicates a need for immediate resuscitation of the newborn, clamp and cut the cord and move to the resuscitation area.
▪ If there is any evidence of a snapped cord, clamp the cord immediately and observe the baby for signs of hypovolaemia (for example, pale mucous membranes and respiratory issues).

Care of the Newborn

TABLE 5.6 – ASSESSMENT and MANAGEMENT of: The Newborn *(continued)*
Assess Need for Resuscitation at Birth (Refer to Newborn Life Support)
▪ Assess **colour**, **tone**, **breathing** and **heart rate** after birth and continue to observe until care is handed over to the maternity team.
▪ Undertake any necessary resuscitation/stabilisation according to **Newborn Life Support** guidance.

▪ Prioritise:
  – thermal care
  – airway and breathing
  – (circulation).

▪ Undertake a **TIME-CRITICAL** transfer to the nearest appropriate destination as agreed locally once available resources are secured. This may require transfer separately from the mother.
▪ Provide a pre-alert/information call detailing the neonatal emergency.
Thermoregulation
▪ Always optimise thermoregulation throughout.
▪ Ensure the newborn baby is dried thoroughly after birth, with particular attention to the head. Apply a hat, cover the baby with towels, foil wrap and increase the environmental temperature.
▪ Consider other adjuncts (plastic wrap/thermal mattress if required/available).
▪ If mother and baby are well, skin-to-skin contact can be used to optimise thermoregulation, but it is paramount to continuously monitor airway and breathing.
Preterm Babies
▪ Use **Newborn Life Support** guidelines to initiate resuscitation in babies ≥22 weeks or where the gestation is unknown and there are signs of life.
▪ Provide comfort care to babies known to be <22 weeks gestation.
▪ Be aware that preterm babies may often deteriorate quickly even if born in good condition, so be ready to ventilate at any point.
Meconium
▪ Babies born with thick meconium-stained amniotic fluid should receive the same care as all babies – stimulation, thermal care and resuscitation as required. If not responding to initial airway and breathing manoeuvres, inspection may be considered to exclude obstruction.
▪ It is important to inform hospital staff at handover so that accelerated monitoring of the baby can be initiated.
Suspected Hypoglycaemia
▪ Ensure early feeding and keep the baby warm to prevent hypoglycaemia.
▪ Transfer to hospital if the baby is at risk of hypoglycaemia or signs of hypoglycaemia are seen.
▪ IM glucagon will NOT work due to poor glycogen stores in the newborn. Buccal dextrose can be used.
Jaundice
▪ Jaundice babies require a timely assessment by an appropriate healthcare professional.
Safeguarding
▪ If there are safeguarding concerns on scene, these should instigate a referral as per local protocols. A woman who has had a BBA and declines transfer to hospital should not be left on scene with the baby without initiating discussions with safeguarding professionals (unless a midwife is present).

SECTION **5** Maternity Care

Care of the Newborn

4.1 APGAR score

- The APGAR score is used to retrospectively record the clinical condition of the baby at birth. The components of the APGAR score are important variables to help judge the health of the baby and it is typically recorded for the baby at 1, 5 and 10 minutes of age.

TABLE 5.7 – Apgar Score

Score	0	1	2
Appearance	Blue or pale all over	Blue at extremities, body pink	Body and extremities pink
Pulse rate	Absent	<100	≥100
Grimace or response to stimulation	No response to stimulation	Grimace/feeble cry when stimulated	Cry or pull away when stimulated
Activity or muscle tone	None	Some flexion	Flexed arms and legs that resist extension
Respiration	Absent	Weak, irregular, gasping	Strong, lusty cry

5. Interface with Maternity Care Providers

- History-taking and accessing maternity notes will support your on-scene decision making.
- Liaison with maternity services should occur within local recommended processes. If a mother and baby is well and there is a midwife en-route, it may be appropriate to wait for the midwife. Your clinical assessment on scene will help you decide whether you need to escalate the care.
- Any baby born with a midwife unavailable will require hospital admission with their mother to receive ongoing care from the maternity team. The mother and baby should be promptly transported to the nearest obstetric maternity unit. Apply a wristband label to the mother and baby if available.
- If the mother declines conveyance to hospital, the priority is to explain that pre-hospital clinicians cannot discharge a mother and newborn baby on scene without a midwife or doctor present. Follow local guidelines on assessing maternal capacity. Once born, the baby has rights of its own, so should receive medical care that is in its best interests.

KEY POINTS!

Care of the Newborn

- Ensure the environment is optimised; consider cord management and the need for additional resources.
- Dry baby thoroughly at birth and keep warm during assessment, resuscitation and transport using a hat, warm blankets and foil wrap/pod or other adjuncts (plastic wrap/thermal mattress) if available/necessary.
- The need for resuscitation can be determined from an assessment of the baby's condition at birth, including colour, tone, breathing and heart rate.
- Undertake any necessary resuscitation/stabilisation using the recommended Newborn Life Support approach.
- Preterm babies need extra vigilance, get cold quicker and even if demonstrating breathing efforts and adequate HR at birth may deteriorate, so be prepared to provide additional thermal, airway and ventilatory support. They will require further management in hospital.
- Consider and treat hypoglycaemia as soon as possible to prevent convulsions or long-term neurological damage.
- All babies with congenital abnormalities should be transferred to hospital for assessment.
- Identify jaundice and ensure that the neonate receives timely medical review.
- Be aware of risk factors in mother or baby, which might suggest a high risk of early onset neonatal sepsis.

Care of the Newborn

Bibliography

1. MBRRACE-UK. *Determination of Signs of Life Following Spontaneous Birth Before 24+0 Weeks of Gestation Where, Following Discussion with the Parents, Active Survival-focused Care Is Not Appropriate*. 2020. Available at: https://timms.le.ac.uk/signs-of-life/resources/signs-of-life-guidance-v1.2.pdf.

2. National Institute for Health and Care Excellence. *Neonatal Infection: Antibiotics for Prevention and Treatment* [NG195]. London: National Institute for Health and Clinical Excellence, 2021. Available from: https://www.nice.org.uk/guidance/ng195.

3. Beard L, Lax P, Tindall M. Physiological effects of transfer for critically ill patients. *Anaesthesia Tutorial of the Week* 2016, 330. Available from: http://anaesthesiology.gr/media/File/pdf/330-Physiological-effects-of-transfer-for-critically-ill-patients.pdf.

4. British Association of Perinatal Medicine. 2022. Available from: https://www.bapm.org/

5. Burakevych N, McKinlay CJD, Harris DL et al. Factors influencing glycaemic stability after neonatal hypoglycaemia and relationship to neurodevelopmental outcome. *Sci Rep* 2019, 9: 8132. Available from: https://doi.org/10.1038/s41598-019-44609-1.

6. Carter BS. Pediatric palliative care in infants and neonates. *Children (Basel, Switzerland)* 2018, 5(2): 21. Available from: doi:10.3390/children5020021.

7. Cornblath M, Hawdon JM, Williams AF, Aynsley-Green A, Ward-Platt MP, Schwartz R et al. Controversies regarding definition of neonatal hypoglycemia: suggested operational thresholds. *Pediatrics* 2000, 105(5): 1141–1145.

8. National Collaborating Centre for Women's and Children's Health. *Diabetes in Pregnancy* (CG63). London: National Institute for Health and Clinical Excellence, 2015.

9. Wyckoff MH, Wyllie J, Aziz K, de Almeida MF, Fabres J, Fawke J, Guinsburg R et al. and on behalf of the Neonatal Life Support Collaborators. *Neonatal Life Support: 2020 International Consensus on Cardiopulmonary Resuscitation and Emergency Cardiovascular Care Science with Treatment Recommendations* 2020, 142: S185–S221. Available from: https://doi.org/10.1161/CIR.0000000000000895Circulation.

10. National Institute for Health and Care Excellence. *Jaundice in Newborn Babies under 28 Days* [CG98]. London: National Institute for Health and Care Excellence, 2016. Available from: https://www.nice.org.uk/guidance/cg98

11. Polglase GR, Blank DA, Barton SK, Miller SL, Stojanovska V, Kluckow M, Gill AW, LaRosa D, Te Pas AB, Hooper SB. Physiologically based cord clamping stabilises cardiac output and reduces cerebrovascular injury in asphyxiated near-term lambs. *Arch Dis Child Fetal Neonatal Ed* 2018, 103: F530–F538. Available from: doi:10.1136/archdischild-2017-313657.

12. Madar J, Roehr CC, Ainsworth S, Ersdal H, Morley C et al. European Resuscitation Council Guidelines 2021: Newborn resuscitation and support of transition of infants at birth. *Resuscitation* 2021, 161: 291–326. Available from: doi:10.1016/j.resuscitation.2021.02.014.

13. Simonsen KA, Anderson-Berry AL, Delair SF, Davies HD. Early-onset neonatal sepsis. *Clin Microbiol Rev* 2014, 27(1): 21–47. Available from doi:10.1128/CMR.00031-13

14. Van de Voorde P, Turner NM, Djakow J et al. European Resuscitation Council Guidelines 2021: Paediatric Life Support. Available from: https://cprguidelines.eu/assets/guidelines/European-Resuscitation-Council-Guidelines-2021-Pa.pdf

SECTION **5** Maternity Care

Haemorrhage During Pregnancy (including Miscarriage and Ectopic Pregnancy)

1. Introduction

- This guidance is for the assessment and management of women with bleeding during early and late pregnancy (including miscarriage and ectopic pregnancy). For postpartum haemorrhage, refer to **Birth Imminent: Normal Birth and Birth Complications**. For complications associated with therapeutic termination ('abortion'), refer to **Vaginal Bleeding: Gynaecological Causes**.

- Any bleeding from the genital tract during pregnancy is of concern and in early pregnancy may indicate miscarriage or an ectopic pregnancy. This more commonly occurs in the first 3 months (weeks 1–12) but can also occur in the second trimester. Haemorrhage may:
  - present with evident vaginal loss of blood (e.g. miscarriage in early pregnancy and placenta praevia in late pregnancy)
  - occur mainly (or completely) within the abdomen (e.g. ruptured ectopic pregnancy) or uterus (e.g. concealed placental abruption). This presents with little or no external loss, but pain and signs of hypovolaemic shock. Pregnant women may appear well even with a large amount of concealed blood loss. Tachycardia may not appear until 30% or more of the circulating volume has been depleted.

- Bleeding in pregnancy is broadly divided into two timeframes: bleeding that occurs in the early part of pregnancy, such as miscarriage or ectopic pregnancy (less than 24 weeks), and that occurring in the late second and third trimesters of pregnancy, such as placenta praevia or placental abruption (i.e. after 24 weeks).

2. Haemorrhage in Early Pregnancy (≤24 weeks)

Haemorrhage in early pregnancy may indicate miscarriage or ectopic pregnancy

2.1 Incidence

Miscarriage is most common in the first 12 weeks of gestation. The mother will often be anxious as to what is happening and can be very concerned as to the health and well-being of her unborn baby.

2.2 Pathophysiology

- Miscarriage is the loss of pregnancy before 24 completed weeks. It is most commonly seen at 6–14 weeks of gestation but can occur after 14 weeks.

- Miscarriage occurs when some of the early fetal or placental tissue (known as 'products of conception') is partly passed through the cervix

and may become trapped, leading to continuing blood loss. If shock ensues, it may be out of proportion to the amount of blood loss (i.e. when there is an added vagal component due to tissues trapped in the cervix).

Risk factors – miscarriage
- Previous history of miscarriage.
- Previously identified potential miscarriage at scan.
- Smoker.
- Obesity.

Symptoms characteristic of miscarriage:

- Bleeding – light or heavy, often with clots and/or jelly-like tissue.
- Pain – central, crampy, suprapubic or backache.
- Signs of pregnancy may be subsiding, e.g. nausea or breast tenderness.
- Significant symptoms (including hypotension) without significant external blood loss may indicate 'cervical shock' due to retained miscarriage tissue stuck in the cervix. Symptomatic bradycardia may arise due to vagal stimulation.

Symptoms characteristic of a ruptured ectopic pregnancy:

- Usually presents at around 6–8 weeks gestation, so usually only one period has been missed.
- Acute lower abdominal pain.
- Slight bleeding or brownish vaginal discharge.
- Tachycardia and skin coolness can indicate significant hidden bleeding within the abdomen.

Other suspicious symptoms:

- Unexplained fainting.
- Shoulder-tip pain.
- Unusual bowel symptoms.
- Intra-uterine contraceptive device fitted.
- Previous ectopic pregnancy.
- Tubal surgery.
- Sterilisation or reversal of sterilisation.
- Endometriosis.
- Pelvic inflammatory disease.
- Subfertility (delay in conceiving).

2.3 Management of Pregnancy Loss and Fetal Tissue in Early Pregnancy (<22 weeks)

Ambulance clinicians are often called to attend women who may have miscarried before the clinicians' arrival, or during the episode of care. This

Haemorrhage During Pregnancy (including Miscarriage and Ectopic Pregnancy)

can be a very distressing time for the woman, her family and the ambulance clinicians involved.

Fetal tissue, including the baby, may be passed by the mother during the miscarriage. It may resemble blood-stained tissue, or demonstrate a discernible baby with placenta still attached. The management of fetal tissue must follow the principles below to ensure that all staff comply with the Human Tissue Act (March 2015).

- Where a woman has passed a pregnancy, whether miscarriage or following a medical induction, she may choose to handle the pregnancy remains herself; she should, however, have been given advice by the service provider (this is likely to be an early pregnancy unit or termination service). In **ALL** cases, offer the woman the opportunity to transfer the early pregnancy tissue/baby with her into the hospital.

Practical guidance:

- In **ALL** cases, inform the woman, and discuss her preferences about management of the fetal tissue or 'her baby'.

- Where it is difficult to identify fetal tissue, transport this tissue, using a soft item from the maternity pack.

- Where the baby is noticeably developed and small, the mother may wish to have the baby wrapped within a towel and placed with her during conveyance to hospital; this may be an important part of her grieving process.

- If the mother declines to see or hold the pregnancy tissue or baby, wrap it in a sensitive way using a towel or soft item from the maternity pack and convey to hospital.

- Where the pregnancy remains have been passed into a toilet and are no longer accessible, document the inspection undertaken.

- Where the mother is unable to make a decision, or is not able to articulate her wishes at that time, in order to act in the best interests of the mother, it is appropriate to remove the pregnancy remains from the toilet, wrapping them sensitively as detailed above.

- In **ALL** cases, document how the fetal tissue/baby was conveyed, and hand the fetal tissue/baby to the nurse or midwife at transfer of care.

3. Haemorrhage in Late Pregnancy

Antepartum or prepartum haemorrhage (>24 weeks) may indicate placenta praevia or placental abruption.

3.1 Incidence

Placenta praevia occurs in one in 200 pregnancies and usually presents at 24–32 weeks with small episodes of painless bleeding.

3.2 Pathophysiology

- **Placenta Praevia:** the placenta develops low down in the uterus and partially or completely covers the internal opening of the cervical canal, the internal cervical os. With the development and growth of the uterus, bleeding is inevitable. This can lead to severe haemorrhage during the pregnancy (i.e. painless bleeding) or when labour begins.

- **Placental Abruption:** Any vaginal bleeding in late pregnancy or during labour which is accompanied by severe/sudden continuous abdominal/back pain, or by signs of shock, may be due to placental abruption. Bleeding occurs between the placenta and the wall of the uterus, detaching an area of the placenta from the uterine wall. It can be associated with severe pregnancy-induced hypertension (PIH) and trauma. Placental abruption causes continuous severe/sudden abdominal/back pain, tightening of the uterus and/or signs of hypovolaemic shock, and puts the baby at immediate risk. There may be some external blood loss, but more commonly the haemorrhage is **concealed** behind the placenta. Where there is a combination of **revealed** (external) blood loss and concealed haemorrhage, this can be particularly dangerous, as it can lead to an underestimation of the amount of total blood lost. The woman's abdomen will be tender when felt and the uterus will feel rigid or 'woody' with no signs of relaxation.

NOTE:

Because the true amount of bleeding is concealed, placental abruption is also associated with disseminated intravascular coagulation (DIC), which can worsen the tendency to bleed.

TABLE 5.8 – ASSESSMENT and MANAGEMENT of: Haemorrhage During Pregnancy
Primary Survey
▪ If any **TIME-CRITICAL** features are present correct **<C>ABC** and transport to nearest suitable receiving hospital (refer to **Medical Emergencies in Adults – Overview** and **Medical Emergencies in Children – Overview**).
▪ Provide an alert/information call.
Monitor SpO$_2$
▪ If **oxygen** (O$_2$) <94% administer O$_2$ to aim for a target saturation within the range of 94–98%.

(continued)

Haemorrhage During Pregnancy (including Miscarriage and Ectopic Pregnancy)

TABLE 5.8 – ASSESSMENT and MANAGEMENT of: Haemorrhage During Pregnancy *(continued)*

Assess Volume of Blood Loss

- Obtain IV access – insert **LARGE BORE** (16G) cannula.
- Visually inspect sanitary towels if worn.
- A large sanitary towel can absorb 50 ml of blood. Blood loss will appear greater if mixed with amniotic fluid.

Four sanitary towels each soaked with 50 ml blood.

Life-threatening Haemorrhage and a Confirmed Diagnosis of Miscarriage

(e.g. where a patient has gone home with medical management and starts to bleed)

- Administer Syntometrine intramuscularly if available (refer to **Syntometrine**).
- If Syntometrine is **NOT** available or the woman is hypertensive (≥140/90), administer misoprostol 800 micrograms sublingually (four tablets) (refer to **Misoprostol**).

CAUTION: DO NOT administer Syntometrine or misoprostol with a fetus in situ.

Assess for Signs of Shock

(e.g. tachycardia >100 bpm, systolic <90 mmHg with cool sweaty skin)

- Undertake a capillary refill test.

NOTE: Hypovolaemia is manifested late in pregnant women; the woman may be very unwell and the fetus may be compromised; therefore **ADMINISTER** fluid replacement early (refer to **Intravascular Fluid Therapy in Adults** and **Intravascular Fluid Therapy in Children**).

- If >20 weeks, the gravid uterus may compress the inferior vena cava in a patient who is supine. Therefore, it is important to ensure adequate venous return before determining the need for fluid resuscitation; this can be achieved by using manual uterine displacement (see **Maternal Resuscitation**) or alternatively by placing the woman in a full lateral ('recovery') position or by lying her supine with lateral tilt (towards her left side where possible).
- Administer 250 ml of sodium chloride 0.9% IV to maintain SBP of 90 mmHg (refer to **Intravascular Fluid Therapy in Adults** and **Intravascular Fluid Therapy in Children**).
- Reassess vital signs prior to further fluid therapy.
- Take any blood-soaked pads to hospital.

NB: Symptoms of hypovolaemic shock occur very late in otherwise fit young women; tachycardia may not appear until 30% of circulating volume has been lost, by which stage the patient is very unwell.

Ask 'When Did You Last Feel the Baby Move?'

- Record when the mother last felt her baby move.

Haemorrhage During Pregnancy (including Miscarriage and Ectopic Pregnancy)

TABLE 5.8 – ASSESSMENT and MANAGEMENT of: Haemorrhage During Pregnancy *(continued)*

Secondary Survey

- If no **TIME-CRITICAL** features, perform a more thorough assessment with secondary survey including fetal assessment (refer to **Maternity Care (including Obstetric Emergencies Overview)**).

- Check the handheld maternity records for scan results confirming a 'low-lying' placenta.

Assess the Woman's Level of Pain

- Titrate pain relief against pain (refer to **Pain Management in Adults** and **Pain Management in Children**):
  - **Paracetamol**.
  - **Entonox**.
  - **Morphine**: **NOTE** administer cautiously if the woman is hypotensive.

- Nil by mouth.

- Symptomatic bradycardia due to vagal stimulation can be treated with atropine (refer to **Atropine Sulfate** and **Cardiac Rhythm Disturbance**).

- Adjust woman's position as required.

- If **TIME-CRITICAL** features are present, transfer to the nearest appropriate destination with a pre-alert stating the emergency.

- Dependent upon locally agreed pathways and the gestational age of the pregnancy, it may be necessary to take the woman directly to the nearest maternity unit.

KEY POINTS!

Haemorrhage During Pregnancy (including Miscarriage and Ectopic Pregnancy)

- **Haemorrhage during pregnancy is broadly divided into two categories, occurring in early and late pregnancy.**

- **Haemorrhage may be revealed (evident vaginal blood loss) or concealed (little or no obvious loss).**

- **Pregnant women may appear well even when a large amount of blood has been lost (tachycardia may not appear until 30% of circulating volume as symptoms of hypovolaemic shock occur very late, by which stage the woman is critically ill).**

- **Obtain venous access with large bore cannulae (16G).**

- **In the presence of a confirmed miscarriage, intramuscular Syntometrine administration should be considered.**

Bibliography

1. Soar J, Perkins GD, Abbas G, Alfonzo A, Barelli A, Bierens JJLM, et al. European Resuscitation Council Guidelines for Resuscitation 2010 Section 8: cardiac arrest in special circumstances: electrolyte abnormalities, poisoning, drowning, accidental hypothermia, hyperthermia, asthma, anaphylaxis, cardiac surgery, trauma, pregnancy, electrocution. *Resuscitation* 2010, 81(10): 1400–1433.

2. Woollard M, Simpson H, Hinshaw K, Wieteska S. Obstetric services. In *Pre-hospital Obstetric Emergency Training*. Oxford: Wiley-Blackwell, 2009: 1–6.

3. Woollard M, Hinshaw K, Simpson H, Wieteska S. Anatomical and physiological changes in pregnancy. In *Pre-hospital Obstetric Emergency Training*. Oxford: Wiley-Blackwell, 2009: 18–27.

4. Woollard M, Hinshaw K, Simpson H, Wieteska S. Structured approach to the obstetric patient. In *Pre-hospital Obstetric Emergency Training*. Oxford: Wiley-Blackwell, 2009: 38–52.

5. Woollard M, Hinshaw K, Simpson H, Wieteska S. Emergencies in early pregnancy and complications following gynaecological surgery. In *Pre-hospital Obstetric Emergency Training*. Oxford: Wiley-Blackwell, 2009: 53–61.

6. Woollard M, Hinshaw K, Simpson H, Wieteska S. Emergencies in late pregnancy. In *Pre-Hospital Obstetric Emergency Training*. Oxford: Wiley-Blackwell, 2009: 62–110.

7. Human Tissue Authority (2015) *Guidance on the Disposal of Pregnancy Remains Following Pregnancy Loss or Termination*. Available from: https://www.hta.gov.uk/sites/default/files/Guidance_on_the_disposal_of_pregnancy_remains.pdf, 2015.

8. Royal College of Nursing. *Managing the Disposal of Pregnancy Remains. RCN Guidance for Nursing and Midwifery Practice*. 2015. Available from: https://www2.rcn.org.uk/__data/assets/pdf_file/0008/645884/RCNguide_disposal_pregnancy_remains_WEB.pdf.

5 Maternity Care SECTION

Haemorrhage During Pregnancy (including Miscarriage and Ectopic Pregnancy)

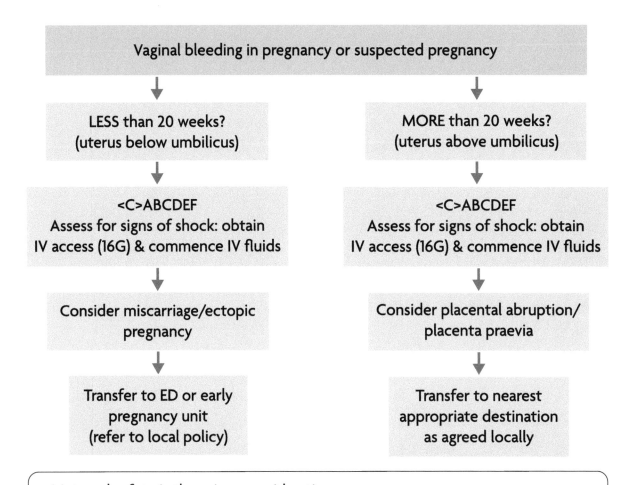

Figure 5.12 – Pre-hospital maternity emergency management – haemorrhage during pregnancy.

Maternal Resuscitation

1. Introduction

- As outlined by the Mother and Babies: Reducing Risk through Audits and Confidential Enquiries Across the UK (MBRRACE) report, 'for women in the United Kingdom, giving birth remains safer than ever – less than 9 in every 100,000 women die in pregnancy and around childbirth. Overall the maternal mortality rate in the UK continues to fall'.

- Between 2012 and 2014, deaths from 'indirect' causes were the largest group of deaths; these are deaths from conditions not directly due to pregnancy but due to existing conditions which are exacerbated by pregnancy, for example women with heart problems. Given the very gradual rate of decline and the complexity of medical conditions now experienced by women during pregnancy, achieving the Government's ambition to reduce maternal deaths by 20% by 2020 and 50% by 2030 presents a major challenge for the health service that will require co-ordination of care across multiple specialities.[1]

- A maternal death is defined internationally as the death of a woman during or up to 6 weeks (42 days) after the end of pregnancy (whether the pregnancy ended by termination, miscarriage or a birth, or was an ectopic pregnancy) through causes associated with, or exacerbated by, pregnancy.[2]

- A late maternal death is one that occurs between 6 weeks and 1 year after the end of pregnancy.

- Deaths are further subdivided on the basis of cause into:
  - direct deaths, from pregnancy-specific causes, such as pre-eclampsia
  - indirect deaths, from other medical conditions made worse by pregnancy, such as cardiac disease
  - coincidental deaths, where the cause is considered to be unrelated to pregnancy, such as road traffic accidents.

These definitions are summarised in Table 5.9.

TABLE 5.9 – Definitions of Maternal Deaths[2]

Maternal Death is the death of a woman while pregnant or within 42 days of the end of the pregnancy, including giving birth, ectopic pregnancy, miscarriage or termination of pregnancy, from any cause related to or aggravated by the pregnancy or its management, but not from accidental or incidental causes.

Direct Death	Resulting from obstetric complications of the pregnant state (pregnancy, labour and puerperium), from interventions, omissions, incorrect treatment or from a chain of events resulting from any of the above.
Indirect Death	Resulting from previous existing disease, or disease that developed during pregnancy and which was not the result of direct obstetric causes but which was aggravated by the physiological effects of pregnancy.
Late Death	Occurring between 42 days and 1 year after the end of pregnancy, including giving birth, ectopic pregnancy, miscarriage or termination of pregnancy, as the result of Direct or Indirect maternal causes.
Coincidental Death	From unrelated causes that happen to occur in pregnancy or the puerperium. Termed 'Fortuitous' in the International Classification of Diseases (ICD).

- It is important to recognise that there are two patients.

- Effective resuscitation of the mother may provide effective resuscitation of the fetus.

- Resuscitation of the mother is the primary concern.

- If there is no response to CPR after 5 minutes, undertake a **TIME-CRITICAL** transfer to the nearest emergency department (ED), ideally with an obstetric unit attached. Place a pre-alert as soon as possible to enable the ED team to organise a maternity team, as an immediate peri-mortem caesarean section (resuscitative hysterotomy) may be performed.

2. Cardiac Arrest

Undertake a TIME-CRITICAL transfer as soon as ventilation is achieved and CPR commenced.

2.1 Introduction

- The approach to resuscitating a pregnant woman is the same as that of any adult in cardiac arrest. However, from 20 weeks gestation onwards, the weight of the gravid uterus can cause 30% of cardiac output to be sequestered into the lower limbs with a woman lying supine.

- Immediately manually displace the uterus to the maternal left side (relieving pressure on the inferior vena cava (refer to Figure 5.13)).

Maternal Resuscitation

Figure 5.13 – Manual uterine displacement during resuscitation.

Maternal Resuscitation

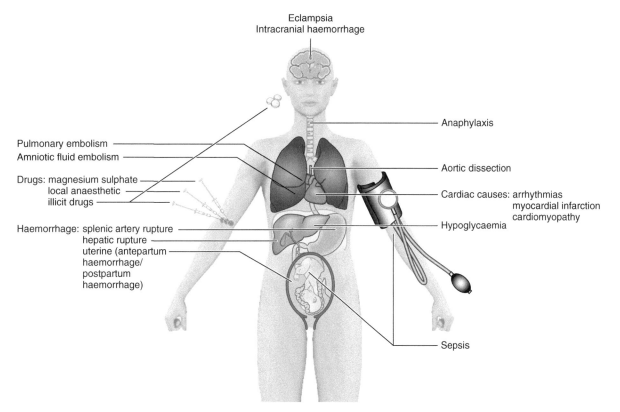

Eclampsia
Intracranial haemorrhage

Anaphylaxis

Pulmonary embolism
Amniotic fluid embolism

Aortic dissection

Drugs: magnesium sulphate
local anaesthetic
illicit drugs

Cardiac causes: arrhythmias
myocardial infarction
cardiomyopathy

Hypoglycaemia

Haemorrhage: splenic artery rupture
hepatic rupture
uterine (antepartum
haemorrhage/
postpartum
haemorrhage)

Sepsis

Figure 5.14 – Causes of maternal collapse.[3] Republished with kind permission of the Royal College of Obstetricians and Gynaecologists.

- CPR should not be terminated in the pre-hospital setting on a pregnant woman.

2.2 Pathophysiology

Cardiac arrest in pregnancy is very rare. Common causes of sudden maternal death include haemorrhage, embolism (thromboembolic and amniotic fluid) and hypertensive disorders. Figure 5.14 and Table 5.10 detail the common reversible causes of maternal collapse in the pregnant woman.

TABLE 5.10 – Reversible Causes of Maternal Collapse[3]

REVERSIBLE CAUSE		CAUSE IN PREGNANCY
4Hs	- Hypovolaemia	- Bleeding (may be concealed) (obstetric/other) or relative hypovolaemia of dense spinal block; septic or neurogenic shock.
	- Hypoxia	- Pregnant women become hypoxic rapidly.
	- Hypo/hyperkalaemia and other electrolyte disturbances	- Cardiac events: peripartum cardiomyopathy, myocardial infarction, aortic dissection, large-vessel aneurysms.
	- Hypothermia	- No more likely.
4Ts	- Thromboembolism	- Amniotic fluid embolus, pulmonary embolus, air embolus, myocardial infarction.
	- Toxicity	- Local anaesthetic, magnesium, other.
	- Tension pneumothorax	- Following trauma/suicide attempt
	- Tamponade (cardiac)	
	- Eclampsia and pre-eclampsia	- Includes intracranial haemorrhage.

Maternal Resuscitation

Figure 5.15 – Working as a team.

2.3 Modifications for Cardiac Arrest in Pregnancy

For the assessment and management of cardiac arrest during pregnancy, refer to Table 5.11.

Key points are listed below:

- Start resuscitation according to standard ALS guidelines, with manual displacement of the uterus to the maternal left to minimise inferior vena caval compression (spinal board will not achieve the required left lateral tilt).

- The hand position for chest compressions may need to be slightly higher (2–3 cm) on the sternum for patients with advanced pregnancy (e.g. >28 weeks).

- Consider using a tracheal tube 0.5–1.0 mm smaller than usual as the trachea can be narrowed by oedema and swelling. Supraglottic airway devices are a suitable alternative in the pre-hospital setting and may provide a more rapid means of oxygenation than potentially prolonged intubation attempts.[4]

- Defibrillation energy levels are as recommended for standard defibrillation. If large breasts make it difficult to place an apical defibrillator electrode, use an antero-posterior or bi-axillary electrode position.

- Establish IV or IO access as soon as possible, preferably at a level above the diaphragm.

- Identify and correct the cause of the arrest using 4Hs and 4Ts as appropriate.

- Administer 100% supplemental oxygen (refer to **Oxygen**).

- Undertake a **TIME-CRITICAL** transfer to the nearest ED, ideally with an obstetric unit attached. Place a pre-alert as soon as possible to enable the ED team to organise a maternity team, as an immediate peri-mortem caesarean section (resuscitative hysterotomy) may be performed.

Maternal Resuscitation

2.4 The Team Approach to Pre-hospital Resuscitation (Resuscitation Council 2015)

- Resuscitation requires a system to be in place to achieve the best possible chance of survival. The system requires technical and non-technical skills (teamwork, situational awareness, leadership, decision making) in the pregnant woman; this will also involve consideration for manual uterine displacement.

Allocation of Roles

- Appoint a team leader as early as possible; ideally they should be a paramedic or clinician experienced in pre-hospital resuscitation.

- The team leader should assign team members specific roles, which they clearly understand and are capable of undertaking. This will promote teamwork, reduce confusion and ensure organised and effective management of resuscitation.

- A minimum of four trained staff are required to deliver high-quality resuscitation. This will necessitate dispatch of more than one ambulance resource.

- Ensure there is 360° access to the patient ('Circle of Life'):
  - Position 1: Airway (at head of patient) – the person must be trained and equipped to provide the full range of airway skills.
  - Position 2: High-quality chest compressions and defibrillation if needed – at patient's left side. Be prepared to alternate with the operator at position 3 to avoid fatigue.
  - Position 3: High-quality chest compressions and access to the circulation (intravenous, intraosseous) – at patient's right side.
  - Position 4: Team leader – stand back and oversee the resuscitation attempt, only becoming involved if required. The team leader should have an awareness of the whole incident and ensure high-quality resuscitation is maintained and appropriate decisions made.

The team leader will need to allocate the role of manual uterine displacement and may need the involvement of additional resources where available.

TABLE 5.11 – ASSESSMENT and MANAGEMENT of: Cardiac Arrest During Pregnancy

Undertake a primary survey ABCDE

- At 20 weeks, the uterine fundus will be below the umbilicus.

- Manage as per standard advanced life support (refer to **Advanced Life Support**).

- Assess and exclude reversible causes (see Table 5.10).

- Caution – ventilation with a bag-valve-mask may lead to regurgitation and aspiration. A supraglottic airway device may reduce the risk of gastric aspiration and make ventilation of the lungs easier (refer to **Airway and Breathing Management**).

- If there is no response to CPR after 5 minutes, undertake a **TIME-CRITICAL** transfer to the nearest ED, ideally with an obstetric unit attached. Place a pre-alert as soon as possible to enable the ED team to organise a maternity team, as an immediate peri-mortem caesarean section (resuscitative hysterotomy) may be performed.

- For pregnant women at 20 weeks gestation or more, use manual uterine displacement (to the maternal left side) to avoid compression of the inferior vena cava.

- Manual displacement can be applied from either the maternal left or right side, with the assistant ensuring the uterus is displaced towards the maternal left (Resuscitation Council, 2015).

- Within the ambulance saloon, manual uterine displacement must be maintained.

- Establish IV or IO access as soon as possible, preferably at a level above the diaphragm.

> **KEY POINTS!**

Maternal Resuscitation

- **DO NOT withhold or terminate maternal resuscitation.**

- **ALWAYS manage pregnant women in cardiac arrest at greater than 20 weeks' gestation with manual displacement of the uterus to the maternal left.**

- **If resuscitation attempts fail to achieve ROSC within 5 minutes of the cardiac arrest, undertake a TIME-CRITICAL transfer to the nearest ED, ideally with an obstetric unit attached.**

- **Provide an early pre-alert to enable the ED team to summon the maternity team, as an immediate peri-mortem caesarean section (resuscitative hysterotomy) may be performed.**

5 Maternity Care

SECTION

Maternal Resuscitation

Further Reading

Further important information and evidence in support of this guideline can be found in the Bibliography.[5,6,7,8]

Bibliography

1. Knight M, Tuffnell D, Kenyon S, Shakespeare J, Gray R, Kurinczuk JJ (eds) on behalf of MBRRACE-UK. *Saving Lives, Improving Mothers' Care – Surveillance of maternal deaths in the UK 2011–13 and lessons learned to inform maternity care from the UK and Ireland Confidential Enquiries into Maternal Deaths and Morbidity 2009–13*. Oxford: National Perinatal Epidemiology Unit, University of Oxford, 2015.

2. World Health Organization. *International Classification of Diseases (ICD) 10.* Available from: http://apps.who.int/classifications/icd10/browse/2016/en#/XV, 2010.

3. Royal College of Obstetricians and Gynaecologists. *Maternal Collapse in Pregnancy and the Puerperium* (Green-top Guideline 56). London: RCOG, 2010, updated 2014. Available from: https://www.rcog.org.uk/globalassets/documents/guidelines/gtg_56.pdf.

4. Resuscitation Council. *Prehospital Resuscitation.* Available from: https://www.resus.org.uk/resuscitation-guidelines/prehospital-resuscitation, 2015.

5. Deakin CD, Nolan JP, Soar J, Sunde K, Koster RW, Smith GB, et al. European Resuscitation Council Guidelines for Resuscitation 2010 Section 4: adult advanced life support. *Resuscitation* 2010, 81(10): 1305–1352.

6. Koster RW, Baubin MA, Bossaert LL, Caballero A, Cassan P, Castren M, et al. European Resuscitation Council Guidelines for Resuscitation 2010 Section 2: adult basic life support and use of automated external defibrillators. *Resuscitation* 2010, 81(10): 1277–1292.

7. Soar J, Perkins GD, Abbas G, Alfonzo A, Barelli A, Bierens JJLM, et al. European Resuscitation Council Guidelines for Resuscitation 2010 Section 8: cardiac arrest in special circumstances: electrolyte abnormalities, poisoning, drowning, accidental hypothermia, hyperthermia, asthma, anaphylaxis, cardiac surgery, trauma, pregnancy, electrocution. *Resuscitation* 2010, 81(10): 1400–1433.

8. Deakin CD, Nolan JP, Sunde K, Koster RW. European Resuscitation Council Guidelines for Resuscitation 2010 Section 3: electrical therapies: automated external defibrillators, defibrillation, cardioversion and pacing. *Resuscitation* 2010, 81(10): 1293–1304.

Newborn Life Support

This section of the newborn guidance focuses on the resuscitation/stabilisation of a baby immediately after birth. The guideline will discuss recognition and management of a baby born in poor condition and the immediate actions that should be taken.

1. Introduction

- Passage through the birth canal is a hypoxic event for the fetus, since placental respiratory exchange is prevented for the 50–75 seconds' duration of the average contraction. Mature babies have energy stores to help cope with this.

- Most, but not all, infants adapt well to extra-uterine life, but some require help with stabilisation, and some require resuscitation. Up to 85% breathe spontaneously without intervention; a further 10% respond after drying, stimulation and airway opening manoeuvres; approximately 5% receive positive pressure ventilation. Intubation rates vary between 0.4% and 2%. Fewer than 0.3% of infants receive chest compressions and only 0.05% receive adrenaline.[1]

- The approach to Newborn Life Support comprises the following elements:
  - umbilical cord management
  - thermal care – drying and covering the baby to conserve heat
  - assessing the need for any intervention
  - opening the airway
  - lung aeration
  - ventilation breaths
  - chest compressions.

2. Assessment and Management

TABLE 5.12 – ASSESSMENT and MANAGEMENT of: Newborn Life Support

Environment

In all cases:

- Ensure the ambient temperature is as high as possible.
- Close windows and doors to reduce cold draughts.
- Prepare a firm, flat environment for potential resuscitation.
- Prepare equipment, including warm towels, and consider extra warming equipment if possible.
- Are additional resources required?

Cord Management

Delayed clamping of the cord improves haemodynamic stability and may have survival and longer-term benefits, especially in the preterm. Warm placental blood may improve thermal stability.

Planning is required:

- The cord can remain intact while the baby is assessed at birth. If the baby initiates breathing spontaneously and does not require immediate intervention, wait at least 60 seconds or ideally for the cord to become white as blood stops flowing from the placenta to the baby.
- If immediate resuscitation is required, then the cord should be clamped and cut, the baby moved to the resuscitation area and appropriate measures taken to stabilise the baby.
- Initial thermal measures and assessment can take place on the perineum with the cord intact. Do not leave the baby exposed in a cold environment.
- If there is any evidence of a snapped cord, clamp the cord immediately and observe the baby for signs of hypovolaemia (for example, pale mucous membranes and respiratory issues).

Thermal Care

Outcomes are poorer and mortality increased if babies get cold. Babies are born wet and can become cold very easily, particularly if they remain wet and exposed.

- Term and late preterm infants:
  - Dry the baby, ideally with pre-warmed towels, paying particular attention to the head; remove the wet towel, and cover with a dry towel.
  - Apply a hat – a lot of heat can be lost from the head.
  - A newborn that does not require resuscitation can be placed with the mother and skin-to-skin contact provided. Use a blanket covering the baby to protect from drafts.
- Preterm infants (<32 weeks):[2]
  - In the preterm infant, the same measures may be used. Where airway and breathing are stable, skin to skin can be an effective way of providing warmth.

(continued)

Newborn Life Support

TABLE 5.12 – ASSESSMENT and MANAGEMENT of: Newborn Life Support *(continued)*

With skin-to-skin care, continuous observations of the baby's airway position and breathing are needed, to ensure these are maintained. Where interventions are needed, this may not be practical.

Skin to skin affords the opportunity for early feeding to reduce the risk of hypoglycaemia. If available, other measures may be considered, such as:

- Plastic bag/[3,4] wrap:
  - There is evidence from hospital and low-resource settings that placing babies under 32 weeks' gestation undried into a plastic wrap or a bag with radiant heat can improve thermal stability.
  - A plastic wrap reduces evaporative heat loss and where a radiant heat source (exothermic mattress, skin to skin) is not available may still be used with conventional measures, such as wrapping in a towel. It is not necessary to dry the baby if a plastic wrap or bag is used in a timely manner.
  - **Babies must never be placed in plastic wrap and left exposed.**
- Thermal mattress:
  - Exothermic mattresses are an effective way of providing radiant heat to help keep babies warm and may be used in conjunction with plastic wrap and towels.
  - Activate in advance of the delivery according to manufacturer recommendations.
  - The heat is unregulated. Never place a baby directly onto a mattress, as this may cause burns; ensure the mattress and/or baby is wrapped with a towel.
- The use of such devices should be under specific agreed local guidance.
- Care needs to be taken in the unregulated environment of the pre-hospital setting and ambulance where monitoring of temperature may be more of a challenge.
- Record the temperature as soon as is practical. Check at regular intervals if able to do so without unwrapping the baby. Beware of overheating the baby.
- If in transit, ensure cabin temperature is high. (If uncomfortable for the attendants, then likely more appropriate for the baby.)

Assessment

The initial assessment should be carried out as soon as possible after the birth of the baby. It establishes whether interventions are required.

Assessment can be carried out with the cord intact and while measures are being undertaken to keep the baby warm.

- **Colour** – Babies are blue immediately after delivery but should then become pink. A baby that stays blue is of potential concern. A white baby is of immediate concern as this suggests significant stress.
- **Tone** – A flexed baby with muscle tone has a functioning nervous system. Of concern are floppy unconscious babies who need immediate help and who may not be able to maintain their airway.
- **Breathing** – If a baby is breathing with visible chest movement, this suggests the brain is working. Ensure the baby has an open airway – breathing efforts may be adequate or inadequate/absent, in which case support is required.
- **Heart rate** – Listen to the heart rate with a stethoscope – a fast heart rate (>100) suggests adequate oxygenation; a slower heart rate (60–100) suggests that there is a degree of hypoxia. A very slow HR (<60) indicates significant fetal hypoxic stress and a need to intervene.

Try not to expose the baby when checking the heart rate. A stethoscope is the best immediate tool.

Breathing and heart rate determine whether actions are required.

Pulse oximeter: If a suitable probe is available, then attaching to the right wrist using an infant probe can give an accurate heart rate and provides an indication of oxygenation. It does not provide immediate information at the time of birth but takes approximately 90 seconds to establish a satisfactory signal where the circulation is adequate. It can help guide subsequent interventions.

ECG leads can be used to monitor heart rate (see below).

Defibrillator pads are not required for newborn life support (NLS) and should not be used to monitor heart rate.

Airway

Having an open airway is critical. In the unconscious or floppy baby, the prominent occiput may lead to flexion and compromise of the airway of an infant on their back. Position rather than particulate matter is the commonest problem.

- Place the baby on their back with the head in a neutral position, neither flexed nor extended.

SECTION 5 Maternity Care

Newborn Life Support

TABLE 5.12 – ASSESSMENT and MANAGEMENT of: Newborn Life Support *(continued)*

- If the baby is very floppy, a chin support or jaw thrust may be required.
- A small pad (2 cm thick) can be placed under the shoulders to assist in maintaining the neutral position. Be careful not to over-extend.

Breathing

Inflation (aeration) of the lungs by delivery of air is essential to displace lung fluid in order to establish effective ventilation – longer breaths are delivered to achieve this.

If a baby is crying vigorously, this suggests an adequate airway and breathing effort. Feeble or intermittent cries or silence indicate that help may be required.

If the breathing is inadequate after initial assessment, it is necessary to support (use two people if resources permit).

- Select an appropriate (best-fit) mask and 500 ml paediatric bag-valve system.
- Start in air.
- Give five inflation breaths, sustaining the inflation pressure for 2–3 seconds with each breath.
- Be careful when squeezing the bag. Aim for consistent but not forceful delivery.
- Where it is possible to measure the inflation pressure, aim for 30 cm of water peak pressure for a term baby (25 cm initially for a preterm baby <32 weeks) – otherwise aim for enough pressure to see the chest rise gently.

Note – The first two or three breaths replace the fluid in the lungs with air without changing the volume in the chest. Therefore, you may not observe the chest wall rise until the fourth or fifth breath.

Reassess

- After any intervention, reassess.
- Check the **heart rate** and whether there is **chest movement**.

If the heart rate is fast (>100), assume lung aeration has been successful.

- If the baby does not breath spontaneously, then breathe for the baby.
- Deliver ventilation breaths – 30/minute.
- Reassess heart rate and chest movement every 30 seconds.
- Continue until the baby is breathing on their own.

If the heart is slow (60–100), very slow (<60) or absent, either lung aeration has not been adequate **or** the baby requires more than lung aeration alone.

- It is most likely that you have not aerated the lungs effectively.
- It is vital to achieve effective lung inflation and chest movement before moving on to chest compressions.

If the chest is **not** moving:

- Reposition
  - Is the head in the neutral position?
  - Do you need to do a jaw thrust?
- Repeat inflation breaths.
- Reassess **heart rate** and **chest movement**.

If there is no heart rate response and no visible chest movement:

- Consider:
  - Do you need help with the airway from a second person (if not used already)?
  - Is there obstruction in the oropharynx? (Where an appropriately sized laryngoscope is available with suction and where the clinician has the expertise, inspect the airway and remove any obvious obstruction under direct vision.)
  - An oropharyngeal airway can be used in babies >32 weeks' gestation but must be sized correctly.
  - Do you need to consider a supraglottic airway device? For babies of around 2 kg or more, an appropriate size laryngeal mask (e.g. size 1 i-gel) may be used.
  - Do you need a longer inflation time or higher pressure?
- Repeat five inflation breaths after each manoeuvre.

(continued)

TABLE 5.12 – ASSESSMENT and MANAGEMENT of: Newborn Life Support *(continued)*

- Reassess heart rate and chest movement.

If the chest is moving but the heart rate remains slow/very slow, ensure that the lungs have been successfully aerated:

- Ventilate for 30 seconds.
- Check the **heart rate** and confirm **chest movement**.

Cardiac Compressions

Should only be commenced after the lungs have been successfully inflated and the HR remains very slow or absent.

- **If the heart rate remains very slow or absent despite the chest moving and after 30 seconds of ventilation, commence cardiac compressions.**
- Ensure the baby is on a flat, hard surface (not a mattress or sofa).
- Encircle the lower chest with both hands in such a way that the two thumbs can compress the lower third of the sternum, at a point just below an imaginary line joining the nipples, with the fingers over the spine at the back.
- Compress the chest quickly and firmly in such a way as to reduce the antero–posterior diameter of the chest by a third.
- The ratio of compressions to inflations in newborn resuscitation is synchronised at 3:1 – 15 cycles in 30 seconds.
- If available, supplement oxygen 100% (flow approx. 6–8 l/min into reservoir bag).
- If baby is in a plastic bag, leave in the bag. Try and maintain the baby's temperature.

Reassess

Reassess every 30 seconds.

- If the heart rate increases and is greater than 60 bpm:
  - Stop cardiac compressions.
  - Continue ventilation unless the baby is breathing effectively.
  - Monitor the heart rate.
  - Wean oxygen if saturations are satisfactory (>95%).
- ECG complexes do not indicate the presence of a cardiac output and should not be the sole means of monitoring the infant. However, improving heart rate on ECG is likely to indicate successful ventilation and some cardiac output.
- If the heart rate continues to be very slow or absent:
  - Continue cardiac compressions and ventilation.
  - Consider next steps.

Next Steps

- Undertake a TIME-CRITICAL transfer.
- Provide a pre-alert and convey to the nearest appropriate destination, as agreed locally.
- Consider securing the airway if not done previously by placing a supraglottic airway device if the infant is of sufficient maturity/size and this will not significantly delay transport.

Venous Access and Drugs

- Attempting to gain IV/IO access must not distract from maintaining high-quality chest compressions and effective lung inflation, and it should only be undertaken when crew numbers and resources are sufficient.
- Early enhanced care support should be requested as per local procedures.
- Where fluid and drugs are required, they may be administered to the neonate as per **Page for Age.**
- Very rarely, the heart rate cannot increase because the infant has lost significant blood volume. If this is the case, there is often a history of blood loss from the infant, but not always. In the presence of hypovolaemia, a fluid bolus of 0.9% sodium chloride may be given over 10–20 seconds.[2] Refer to **Sodium Chloride.**

Newborn Life Support

TABLE 5.12 – ASSESSMENT and MANAGEMENT of: Newborn Life Support *(continued)*

Meconium

- Babies born with thick meconium-stained amniotic fluid should receive the same care as all babies – stimulation, thermal care and resuscitation as required. If not responding to initial airway and breathing manoeuvres, inspection may be considered to exclude obstruction.

Newborn life support

Team briefing and equipment check

APPROX 60 SECONDS

Preterm <32 weeks

Place undried newborn **in plastic wrap** and use heated mattress.

Use plastic wrap to reduce heat loss with towel and/or radiant heat (skin to skin/exothermic mattress).

NB Do **NOT** apply ECG electrodes (this is to prevent tissue damage).

Birth
Delay cord clamping if possible

Start clock/note time
Dry/wrap, stimulate, keep warm

Assess
Colour, tone, breathing, heart rate

Ensure an open airway and neutral head position

If gasping/not breathing
- **Give 5 inflations – start in air**
- Apply SpO$_2$ +/– ECG

Reassess
If no increase in heart rate, look for chest movement

If the chest is not moving
- Check mask, head and jaw position
- 2 person support
- Consider suction, laryngeal mask/iGel
- Repeat inflation breaths

Reassess
If no increase in heart rate, look for chest movement

Once chest is moving continue ventilation breaths for 30 seconds

If heart rate is not detectable or less than 60 beats per minute after 30 seconds of ventilation
- Synchronise 3 chest compressions to 1 ventilation
- Increase oxygen to 100%

Reassess heart rate and chest movement every 30 seconds

Transport to appropriate conveyance destination

Update parents and debrief team
Complete records

TITRATE OXYGEN TO ACHIEVE TARGET SATURATIONS

Figure 5.16 – Newborn life support algorithm – modified from the Resuscitation Council (UK) Guidelines 2021 algorithm (www.resus.org.uk).

Newborn Life Support

3. Resuscitation/Stabilisation of the Preterm Baby

This section of the newborn life support guidance focuses on the care of babies born at preterm and extreme preterm gestations. This includes the care of babies born at 22 weeks.

As stated within **Care of the Newborn**, a preterm infant is any baby born at <37 weeks' gestation. For the purpose of this guidance, an extreme preterm baby is any baby born at <32 weeks' gestation, in line with the UK Resuscitation Council guidelines. These babies are vulnerable and require an altered approach in resuscitation.

Why an altered approach?

- **Delayed cord clamping (DCC):** Many preterm babies do not need resuscitation but stabilisation to help them adapt to birth. DCC confers greater advantages in this vulnerable population and should be considered unless immediate intervention is required.

- **Size:** Babies born <32 weeks are smaller and can get cold very quickly. They also have fewer reserves and hypothermia will take effect sooner. It is vital that measures are taken to help them keep warm.

- **Fragile lungs:** Surfactant will not be present in the lungs and a preterm may not breathe effectively. Even if making breathing efforts or initially crying, preterm babies may still need help as the breathing efforts may be inadequate and they get tired. Care needs to be taken with smaller inflation volumes and gentle breaths.

- **Oxygen requirement:** These babies may require oxygen and ideally under pulse oximetry guidance. This can be difficult in the out-of-hospital setting without blenders.

- Clinicians should use the NLS algorithm (Figure 5.16) for resuscitation/stabilisation.

- It is not appropriate to resuscitate babies known to be at <22 weeks' gestation; however, in other situations the approach is towards 'survival-focused care' for the extreme preterm baby with measures as recommended above. Separate guidance exists for comfort care of the extreme preterm baby[2] (see Figure 5.17).

- Early communication with specialist teams is important to ensure destination and receiving teams are prepared for the arrival of the baby.

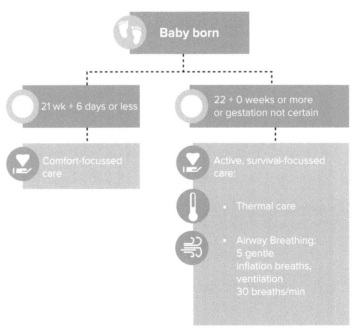

Figure 5.17 – Stabilisation versus non-intervention. Reproduced with permission from the British Association of Perinatal Medicine (BAPM) 2022 (www.bapm.org).

Newborn Life Support

Newborn Life Support

- Passage through the birth canal is a hypoxic event and some babies may require help to establish normal breathing after birth.

- Keep the environment as warm as possible, prepare an area for potential resuscitation/ stabilisation.

- Consider delayed cord clamping unless immediate resuscitation is required.

- Assess colour, tone, breathing and heart rate.

- Babies become cold very easily; dry the baby, remove any wet towels and wrap with dry ones. Use a hat and other thermal measures if required. Skin to skin for well babies. Preterm babies need extra help.

- If intervention is required, ensure the airway is open by placing the baby on their back with the head in a neutral position. If the baby is very floppy, apply jaw support/thrust.

- If the baby is not breathing adequately, give five 2–3-second inflation breaths.

- Check heart rate and chest movement.

- If the chest does not move and the heart rate is not fast/increasing, repeat airway manoeuvres and inflation breaths.

- Once lung aeration is achieved, if the baby is not spontaneously breathing, give 30 seconds of ventilation breaths – approx. 30 breaths/min – and confirm chest movement.

- Check heart rate and chest movement.

- If the chest is moving with ventilation breaths (no spontaneous breathing) and the heart rate is fast, continue ventilation.

- If the chest is moving but the heart rate remains very slow (< 60 breaths/min), chest compressions are necessary. Compress the chest quickly and firmly at a synchronised ratio of three compressions: one inflation ideally with two thumb encircling technique. Fifteen cycles per 30 seconds. 100% oxygen if available.

- On transfer, once in the ambulance keep the compartment as warm as possible.

- Liaise with the receiving unit to inform of situation of baby and mother.

Further Reading

Further important information and evidence in support of this guideline can be found in the Bibliography.[3,4]

Bibliography

1. Fawke J, Wyllie J, Madar J et al. *Newborn Resuscitation and Support of Transition of Infants at Birth*. London: Resuscitation Council UK, 2021. Available from: https://www.resus.org.uk/library/2021-resuscitation-guidelines/newborn-resuscitation-and-support-transition-infants-birth.

2. British Association of Perinatal Medicine. *Pre-hospital Management of the Baby Born at Extreme Preterm Gestation: A BAPM Framework for Practice.* 2022. Available from: https://www.bapm.org/.

3. Belsches TC, Tilly AE, Miller TR, Kambeyanda RH, Leadford A, Manasyan A, Chomba E et al. Randomised trial of plastic bags to prevent term neonatal hypothermia in a resource-poor setting. *Pediatrics* 2013, 132(3). Available from: http://pediatrics.aappublications.org/content/132/3/e656.

4. Leadford AE, Warren JB, Manasyan A, Chomba E, Salas AA, Schelonka R, Carlo WA. Plastic bags for prevention of hypothermia in preterm and low birth weight infants. *Pediatrics* 2013, 132(1). Available from: http://pediatrics.aappublications.org/content/132/1/e128.

5. Wyllie J, Bruinenberg J, Roehr CC, Rüdiger M, Trevisanuto D, Urlesberger B. European Resuscitation Council Guidelines for resuscitation 2015: Section 7. resuscitation and support of transition of babies at birth. *Resuscitation* 2015, 95: 249–263.

6. Wyllie J, Perlman JM, Kattwinkel J, et al. Part 7: neonatal resuscitation: 2015 International Consensus on Cardiopulmonary Resuscitation and Emergency Cardiovascular Care Science with Treatment Recommendations. *Resuscitation* 2015, 95: e169–201.

SECTION **5** Maternity Care

Pregnancy-induced Hypertension (including Eclampsia)

1. Introduction

- Pregnancy-induced hypertension (PIH) or gestational hypertension are generic terms used to define a significant rise in blood pressure after 20 weeks' gestation, in the absence of proteinuria or other features of pre-eclampsia.

- Collapse related to hypertension is rare and usually related to eclampsia. Treatment and resuscitation of the mother will also resuscitate the fetus.

2. Incidence

- Hypertension from all causes is a common medical problem affecting 10–15% of all pregnancies.

- Approximately 15% of women who present with pregnancy-induced hypertension will develop pre-eclampsia.

3. Severity and Outcome

- PIH is usually mild (i.e. blood pressure (BP) 140/90 mmHg) and there is only a 10% risk of developing pre-eclampsia with mild rises in BP beyond 37 weeks.

- Fetal outcomes are good; however, pre-eclampsia accounted for 13.6% of maternal deaths related to pregnancy causes.

4. Pathophysiology

4.1 Pre-eclampsia

- Pre-eclampsia is PIH associated with proteinuria. It commonly occurs beyond 24–28 weeks' gestation, but rarely can occur as early as 20 weeks.

- Although the underlying pathophysiology is not fully understood, pre-eclampsia is primarily a placental disorder associated with poor placental perfusion, which often results in a fetus that is growth-restricted (i.e. smaller than expected because of the poor placental blood flow).

- In the UK, the diagnosis of pre-eclampsia includes an increase in BP above 140/90 mmHg, oedema and detection of protein in the woman's urine.

- Pre-eclampsia is usually diagnosed at routine antenatal visits and may require admission to hospital and early delivery.

- The disease may be of mild, moderate or severe degree.

4.2 Severe Pre-eclampsia

- May present in a patient with known mild pre-eclampsia or may present with little or no prior warning.

4.3 Signs and Symptoms of Severe Pre-eclampsia

- Blood pressure is significantly raised and the diagnosis should be considered with a BP of 160/110 or more. There is proteinuria. Severe pre-eclampsia is usually associated with one or more of the following symptoms:
  - headache – severe and frontal
  - visual disturbances
  - epigastric pain – often mistaken for heartburn
  - right-sided upper abdominal pain – due to stretching of the liver capsule
  - muscle twitching or tremor
  - nausea
  - vomiting
  - confusion
  - rapidly progressive oedema.

- **Note** – the absence of these symptoms does not exclude severe pre-eclampsia and still requires critical assessment and management of the blood pressure alone.

- Agitation and restlessness may be signs of an underlying problem or impending deterioration in women with hypertension.

Pre-existing Risk Factors for Development of Pre-eclampsia

- Primiparity or first child with a new partner.
- Previous severe pre-eclampsia.
- Essential hypertension.
- Diabetes.
- Obesity.
- Twins or higher multiples.
- Renal disease.
- Advanced maternal age (over 35 years).
- Young maternal age (less than 16 years).
- Pre-existing cardiovascular disease.

Severe pre-eclampsia is:

- a 'multi-organ' disease; although hypertension is a cardinal feature, other complications include:
  - intracranial haemorrhage
  - stroke
  - renal failure
  - liver failure
  - abnormal blood clotting, e.g. disseminated intravascular coagulation (DIC).

Pregnancy-induced Hypertension (including Eclampsia)

5. Assessment and Management

- For the assessment and management of mild/moderate pre-eclampsia, refer to Table 5.13.
- For the assessment and management of severe pre-eclampsia, refer to Table 5.14.

TABLE 5.13 – ASSESSMENT and MANAGEMENT of: Mild/Moderate Pre-eclampsia

Definition – raised blood pressure >140/90 mmHg, detection of proteinuria and sometimes oedema.

- Any woman with a blood pressure >140 mmHg systolic or >90 mmHg diastolic on **TWO** occasions in labour or immediately after birth should be transferred to a consultant obstetric unit.
- Blood pressure of 150/100 in pregnancy, labour or immediately after birth **requires urgent treatment**, and therefore rapid transfer to a consultant-led obstetric unit should be arranged.

Undertake a Primary Survey ABCDE

- Assess for **TIME-CRITICAL** features (see definition and symptoms of severe pre-eclampsia below).
- If any time-critical features are present, correct **A** and **B** and transport to nearest suitable receiving hospital (refer to **Medical Emergencies in Adults – Overview** and **Medical Emergencies in Children – Overview**).
- Provide an alert/information call.

- If **NON-TIME-CRITICAL**, perform a more thorough assessment of the woman with secondary survey, including fetal assessment (refer to **Maternity Care (including Obstetric Emergencies Overview)** for guidance).

Measure Blood Pressure

Transfer to further care:

- If pregnant ≥20 weeks and systolic blood pressure is >140/90 mmHg, discuss management directly with the BOOKED OBSTETRIC UNIT or MIDWIFE.

TABLE 5.14 – ASSESSMENT and MANAGEMENT of: Severe Pre-eclampsia

Definition and symptoms – blood pressure of BP 160/110 or more, particularly with one or more of the following: headache (severe and frontal), visual disturbances, proteinuria, epigastric or RUQ pain twitching or tremor, nausea, vomiting, confusion, rapidly progressive oedema.

Undertake a Primary Survey ABCDEF

- Assess for signs of severe pre-eclampsia (see definition and symptoms above). Signs of severe pre-eclampsia are **TIME-CRITICAL FEATURES**.
- If any time-critical features are present, correct **A** and **B** problems (refer to **Medical Emergencies in Adults – Overview** and **Medical Emergencies in Children – Overview**) and transfer to a consultant-led obstetric unit. **NB** Caution with 'lights and sirens', as strobe lights and noise may precipitate convulsions.
- If the patient is convulsing, refer to Eclampsia, Table 5.15.
- TIME-CRITICAL transfer to nearest Obstetric unit.
- Administer **Magnesium Sulfate** if available.
- Provide an alert/information call.

Monitor SpO₂ (94–98%)

- Attach pulse oximeter; if SpO_2 <94%, administer O_2 to aim for a target saturation within the range of 94–98%.
- Obtain IV access – insert a LARGE BORE (16G) cannula en-route.
- **DO NOT** administer intravenous fluid boluses because of the risk of provoking pulmonary oedema.

Measure Blood Glucose Level

- Refer to **Glycaemic Emergencies in Adults and Children**.

Pregnancy-induced Hypertension (including Eclampsia)

SECTION 2 – Eclampsia

1. Introduction

- Eclampsia is generalised tonic/clonic convulsion and is identical to an epileptic convulsion.

- Many patients will have had pre-existing pre-eclampsia (of a mild, moderate or severe degree), but cases of eclampsia can present acutely with no prior warning – ONE THIRD of cases present for the FIRST TIME post-delivery (usually in the first 48 hours). **THE BP MAY ONLY BE MILDLY ELEVATED AT PRESENTATION** (i.e. 140/80–90 mmHg).

- Refer to **Convulsions in Adults** and **Convulsions in Children**.

2. Incidence

- Eclampsia occurs in approximately 2.7:10,000 deliveries, usually beyond 24 weeks.

3. Severity and Outcome

- Eclampsia is one of the most dangerous complications of pregnancy, and is a significant cause of maternal mortality, with a mortality rate of 2% in the UK.

- Convulsions are usually self-limiting, but may be severe and repeated.

- Other complications associated with eclampsia include renal failure, hepatic failure and DIC.

4. Pathophysiology

- The hypoxia caused during a tonic/clonic convulsion may lead to significant fetal compromise and death.

Risk Factors – Eclampsia
- Known pre-eclampsia.
- Primiparity or first child with a new partner.
- Previous severe pre-eclampsia.
- Essential hypertension.
- Diabetes.
- Obesity.
- Twins or higher multiples.
- Renal disease.
- Advanced maternal age (over 35 years).
- Young maternal age (less than 16 years).

5. Assessment and Management

- For the assessment and management of eclampsia and eclamptic convulsion, refer to Table 5.15.

TABLE 5.15 – ASSESSMENT and MANAGEMENT of: Eclampsia

Definition – generalised tonic/clonic convulsion and identical to an epileptic convulsion.

Undertake a Primary Survey ABCDEF

- Assess for **TIME-CRITICAL** features such as recurrent convulsions.

- Correct **A** and **B** and transport to a consultant-led obstetric unit (refer to **Medical Emergencies in Adults – Overview** and **Medical Emergencies in Children – Overview**).

- Obtain IV (LARGE BORE cannulae) or IO access. DO NOT administer fluid boluses because of the risk of provoking pulmonary oedema.

- Provide a pre-alert stating the obstetric emergency of eclampsia.

- If **NON-TIME-CRITICAL**, perform a more thorough assessment of the woman with secondary survey, including fetal assessment (refer to **Maternity Care (including Obstetric Emergencies Overview)** for guidance).

NOTE: Epileptic patients may suffer tonic/clonic convulsions.

- If ≥20 weeks gestation with a history of hypertension or pre-eclampsia, treat as for eclampsia – refer to Tables 5.13 and 5.14.

- If there is no history of hypertension or pre-eclampsia and blood pressure is normal, treat as for epilepsy (refer to **Convulsions in Adults** and **Convulsions in Children**).

- Protect the airway. Place the woman in a full lateral ('recovery') position – do not use the supine position with left lateral tilt. If formal resuscitation is required, use the supine position with manual uterine displacement (refer to **Maternal Resuscitation**).

Monitor SpO$_2$ (94–98%)

- Attach pulse oximeter; if SpO$_2$ <94%, administer O$_2$ to aim for a target saturation within the range of 94–98%.

Pregnancy-induced Hypertension (including Eclampsia)

TABLE 5.15 – ASSESSMENT and MANAGEMENT of: Eclampsia *(continued)*

Continuous or Recurrent Convulsion

- If the patient convulses for longer than 2–3 minutes or has a second or subsequent convulsion, administer diazepam IV/PR (refer to **Diazepam** for dosages and information).

NOTE: IV magnesium sulphate (4 g slow IV over 10 minutes) can be given if available and avoids the use of multiple drugs.

KEY POINTS!

Pregnancy-induced Hypertension (including Eclampsia)

- **Pregnancy-induced hypertension and pre-eclampsia commonly occur beyond 24–28 weeks' gestation but can occur as early as 20 weeks.**

- **Pre-eclampsia can present up to 6 weeks post-delivery.**

- **Diagnosis of pre-eclampsia includes an increase in blood pressure above 140/90 mmHg, oedema and detection of protein in the woman's urine.**

- **Eclampsia is one of the most dangerous complications of pregnancy.**

- **Only administer diazepam if the convulsions are prolonged or recurrent.**

- **Severe pre-eclampsia and eclampsia are TIME-CRITICAL EMERGENCIES for both mother and fetus.**

- **Administer Magnesium Sulfate en-route to hospital for eclampsia and severe pre-eclampsia.**

Bibliography

1. Soar J, Perkins GD, Abbas G, Alfonzo A, Barelli A, Bierens JJLM, et al. European Resuscitation Council Guidelines for Resuscitation 2010 Section 8: cardiac arrest in special circumstances: electrolyte abnormalities, poisoning, drowning, accidental hypothermia, hyperthermia, asthma, anaphylaxis, cardiac surgery, trauma, pregnancy, electrocution. *Resuscitation* 2010, 81(10): 1400–1433.

2. Centre for Maternal and Child Enquiries. Saving mothers' lives: reviewing maternal deaths to make motherhood safer: 2006–2008. *BJOG: An International Journal of Obstetrics & Gynaecology* 2011, 118 (suppl. 1).

3. Woollard M, Simpson H, Hinshaw K, Wieteska S. Obstetric services. In *Pre-hospital Obstetric Emergency Training.* Oxford: Wiley-Blackwell, 2009: 1–6.

4. Woollard M, Hinshaw K, Simpson H, Wieteska S. Anatomical and physiological changes in pregnancy. In *Pre-hospital Obstetric Emergency Training.* Oxford: Wiley-Blackwell, 2009: 18–27.

5. Woollard M, Hinshaw K, Simpson H, Wieteska S. Structured approach to the obstetric patient. In *Pre-hospital Obstetric Emergency Training.* Oxford: Wiley-Blackwell, 2009: 38–52.

6. Woollard M, Hinshaw K, Simpson H, Wieteska S. Emergencies in late pregnancy. In *Pre-Hospital Obstetric Emergency Training.* Oxford: Wiley-Blackwell, 2009: 62–110.

Trauma in Pregnancy

1. Introduction

- The management of pregnant women with traumatic injuries requires a special approach.

- Mechanism of injury may indicate possible trauma to enlarged internal organs and structures, especially trauma occurring in the third trimester. For example, trauma to the gravid uterus during domestic violence can be linked to placental abruption (refer to **Birth Imminent: Normal Birth and Birth Complications**).

- It is important to remember that resuscitation of the mother may facilitate resuscitation of the fetus.

2. Incidence

- In the UK, 5% of maternal deaths are as a result of trauma, with a high proportion related to domestic violence and road traffic collisions.

Mechanism of Injury

- Domestic violence.
- High-energy transfer (especially road traffic accidents).
- Fall from height.

3. Severity and Outcome

- Managing a pregnant woman with major trauma is rare; however, both blunt and penetrating trauma can cause catastrophic haemorrhage.

- Trauma can lead to major placental abruption (separation) with significant hidden blood loss within the uterus and no visible vaginal bleeding abruption (refer to **Birth Imminent: Normal Birth and Birth Complications**).

4. Pathophysiology

- There are a number of physiological and anatomical changes during pregnancy that may influence the management of the pregnant woman with trauma (refer to **Maternity Care (including Obstetric Emergencies Overview)**).

TABLE 5.16 – ASSESSMENT and MANAGEMENT of: Trauma in Pregnancy

Assess <C>ABCDEF

- Quickly assess the scene and the woman as you approach.

- Undertake a primary survey – specifically assess for:
  - abdominal pain – should be presumed to be significant and may be associated with internal concealed blood loss
  - vaginal blood loss
  - abruption may occur 3–4 days after the initial incident
  - stage of the pregnancy and impact on resuscitation if >20 weeks gestation
  - any medical problems with the pregnancy or relevant previous medical history
  - twins or multiple pregnancy
  - fetal movements (refer to **Maternity Care (including Obstetric Emergencies Overview)**).

- Review the maternity handheld record if available.

- If domestic violence is suspected, consider any other children/adults present who may be at risk (refer to **Safeguarding Adults at Risk** and **Safeguarding Children**).

- Control external catastrophic haemorrhage using direct and indirect pressure or tourniquets where indicated (refer to **Trauma Emergencies in Adults – Overview**).

- Refer to **Maternal Resuscitation** where cardiac/respiratory arrest is identified.

- Open, maintain and protect the airway in accordance with the woman's clinical need.

- Administer high levels of supplemental oxygen and aim for a target saturation within the range of 94–98% (refer to **Oxygen**). Provide assisted ventilation as indicated (refer to **Airway Management**).

- If the woman is unable to position herself (e.g. if she is unconscious), she should be positioned on the left (right side up) by using a spinal board and her airway should be monitored. Where resources allow, the uterus can be manually displaced to the maternal left side (and this must be recorded on the patient record form), as illustrated in Figure 5.1.

- Provide cervical spine protection as necessary (refer to **Spinal Injury and Spinal Cord Injury**).

Trauma in Pregnancy

TABLE 5.16 – ASSESSMENT and MANAGEMENT of: Trauma in Pregnancy *(continued)*
▪ Manage thoracic injuries (refer to **Thoracic Trauma**). **NB** The management of thoracic injuries is the same as for the non-pregnant woman.
▪ Insert a minimum of one large bore IV cannula (16G) – do not delay transfer.
▪ Administer intravascular fluids as indicated to maintain a systolic blood pressure above 90 mmHg (refer to **Intravascular Fluid Therapy in Adults**).
▪ Undertake a secondary survey **<C>ABCDEF.**
Assess the Woman's Level of Pain
▪ Pain management (refer to **Pain Management in Adults**). **NB** Administer morphine cautiously if the patient is hypotensive.
▪ Apply splints as appropriate, for example to pelvis (refer to **Major Pelvic Trauma**) or long bone fractures (refer to **Limb Trauma**).
Assess Blood Glucose
▪ Measure blood glucose en-route to the appropriate facility.
▪ Nil by mouth.
Assess for Burns and Scalds
▪ For the management of burns, treat as non-pregnant woman (refer to **Burns and Scalds** and **Intravascular Fluid Therapy in Adults**).

KEY POINTS!

Trauma in Pregnancy

▪ **All trauma is significant.**

▪ **If the pregnant woman is found in cardiac arrest or develops cardiac/respiratory arrest en-route, commence advanced life support and pre-alert the nearest ED with an obstetric unit.**

▪ **Resuscitation of the woman may facilitate resuscitation of the fetus.**

▪ **Compression of the inferior vena cava by the gravid uterus (>20 weeks) is a serious potential complication; manually displace the uterus to the maternal left. Maintain during transfer.**

▪ **Due to the physiological changes in pregnancy, signs of shock may be slow to appear following trauma, hypotension being an extremely late indication of volume loss. Signs of hypovolaemia during pregnancy are likely to indicate a 35% (class III) blood loss and must be treated aggressively.**

▪ **Abruption may occur 3–4 days after the initial incident.**

▪ **If sexual assault or domestic violence is suspected, consideration must be given to potential safeguarding issues and provision made to ensure safety is maintained (refer to Safeguarding Adults at Risk).**

Bibliography

1. Centre for Maternal and Child Enquiries. Saving mothers' lives: reviewing maternal deaths to make motherhood safer: 2006–2008. *BJOG: An International Journal of Obstetrics & Gynaecology* 2011, 118(suppl. 1).

2. Woollard M, Simpson H, Hinshaw K, Wieteska S. Obstetric services. In *Pre-hospital Obstetric Emergency Training.* Oxford: Wiley-Blackwell, 2009: 1–6.

3. Woollard M, Hinshaw K, Simpson H, Wieteska S. Anatomical and physiological changes in pregnancy. In *Pre-hospital Obstetric Emergency Training.* Oxford: Wiley-Blackwell, 2009: 18–27.

4. Woollard M, Hinshaw K, Simpson H, Wieteska S. Structured approach to the obstetric patient. In *Pre-hospital Obstetric Emergency Training.* Oxford: Wiley-Blackwell, 2009: 38–52.

5. Woollard M, Hinshaw K, Simpson H, Wieteska S. Emergencies in late pregnancy. In *Pre-Hospital Obstetric Emergency Training.* Oxford: Wiley-Blackwell, 2009: 62–110.

6. Woollard M, Hinshaw K, Simpson H, Wieteska S. Emergencies after delivery. In *Pre-hospital Obstetric Emergency Training.* Oxford: Wiley-Blackwell, 2009: 111–124.

7. Woollard M, Hinshaw K, Simpson H, Wieteska S. Management of non-obstetric emergencies. In *Pre-hospital Obstetric Emergency Training.* Oxford: Wiley-Blackwell, 2009: 136–165.

Vaginal Bleeding: Gynaecological Causes

1. Introduction

- A number of conditions can cause vaginal bleeding that is different from normal menstruation. Such conditions may result in a call to the ambulance service, including:
  - excessive menstrual period
  - normal or excessive menstrual period associated with severe abdominal pain
  - following surgical or medical therapeutic termination ('abortion') (**NB** bleeding often continues for up to 10 days after treatment)
  - following gynaecological surgery (e.g. hysterectomy) (**NB** heavy, ongoing bleeding commencing 7–14 days after surgery can indicate pelvic infection requiring antibiotics and may require hospital assessment)
  - colposcopy (**NB** slight bleeding may occur up to 10 days after a colposcopy). A colposcopy is an outpatient test where the cervix is inspected following an abnormal cervical smear. Treatment such as cone biopsy for the abnormal smear may have been undertaken. Heavy bleeding post-colposcopy affects very few women in this situation. Heavy, ongoing bleeding at 7–14 days post-procedure can indicate infection requiring antibiotics and may require hospital assessment
  - gynaecological cancers, either before diagnosis or after treatment (i.e. cervix, uterus or vagina), may present with heavy vaginal bleeding
  - trauma; this can include post-coital tears and may be caused by sexual assault/rape.
- This guideline provides guidance for the assessment and management of gynaecological vaginal bleeding. For causes of bleeding in early or late pregnancy, refer to **Haemorrhage During Pregnancy (including Miscarriage and Ectopic Pregnancy)**.

2. Incidence

- Women over 50 years old are more at risk of cancers of the uterus and cervix.

3. Severity and Outcome

- The majority of causes of vaginal bleeding do not compromise the circulation, but blood loss can be alarming.

Sexual Assault

- In sexual assault cases, there may be other injuries.
- When sexual assault is suspected (especially in a child or vulnerable adult), there are clear safeguarding issues (refer to **Safeguarding Children** and **Safeguarding Adults at Risk**).
- It is not the role of the ambulance service to investigate. This is a police matter.
- Remember that the victim of sexual assault has physical forensic evidence on their body and clothing, and represents a 'crime scene' (refer to **Sexual Assault**).

4. Assessment and Management

For the assessment and management of vaginal bleeding, refer to Table 5.17.

TABLE 5.17 – ASSESSMENT and MANAGEMENT of: Vaginal Bleeding
Assess \<C>ABCDEF
• Quickly assess the woman and scene as you approach.
• Undertake a primary survey.
• Evaluate whether the woman has any **TIME-CRITICAL** features or any signs of hypovolaemic shock.
• If any **TIME-CRITICAL** features are present, correct **A** and **B** and transport to nearest suitable receiving hospital (refer to **Medical Emergencies in Adults – Overview** and **Medical Emergencies in Children – Overview**).
• Provide an alert/information call.

Vaginal Bleeding: Gynaecological Causes

TABLE 5.17 – ASSESSMENT and MANAGEMENT of: Vaginal Bleeding *(continued)*

Assess Blood Loss

- Ask about clots, blood-soaked clothes, bed sheets and number of soaked tampons/towels/pads, and, where necessary, visibly inspect. **NB** Blood under the feet or between toes indicates significant bleeding.

- If **NON-TIME-CRITICAL**, perform a more thorough assessment of the woman with brief secondary survey for lower abdominal tenderness or guarding.

- Measure temperature and consider sepsis (refer to **Sepsis**).

- Check the woman's age:
  - \>50 years – more at risk of cancers of the uterus/cervix
  - <50 years – may be pregnant.

- Obtain IV access – insert a **LARGE BORE (16G)** cannula.

- If there is visible external blood loss >500 ml, refer to **Intravascular Fluid Therapy in Adults** and **Intravascular Fluid Therapy in Children**.

50 ml blood loss on various sanitary towels.

500 ml blood loss on maternity pad and 50 ml on maternity towel.

Monitor SpO$_2$ (94–98%)

- If oxygen (SpO$_2$) <94%, administer O$_2$ to aim for a target saturation within the range of 94–98%.

(continued)

Vaginal Bleeding: Gynaecological Causes

TABLE 5.17 – ASSESSMENT and MANAGEMENT of: Vaginal Bleeding *(continued)*
Assess the Woman's Level of Pain

▫ Titrate analgesia against pain (refer to **Pain Management in Adults** and **Pain Management in Children**):
   – Paracetamol
   – Entonox
   – Morphine – **NB** administer cautiously if the patient is hypotensive.

Assess the Woman's Comfort
▫ Nil by mouth.
▫ Adjust the woman's position as required.
▫ Transfer to further care.

KEY POINTS!

Vaginal Bleeding: Gynaecological Causes

- **The majority of vaginal bleeding episodes do not compromise circulation, but blood loss can be alarming.**

- **Following gynaecological surgical interventions, heavy, ongoing vaginal bleeding commencing 7–14 days post-procedure may indicate underlying infection.**

- **Assess blood loss; ask about number of soaked tampons/towels/pads and visually inspect.**

- **Provide analgesia where indicated.**

- **If you suspect a miscarriage or ectopic pregnancy, refer to Haemorrhage During Pregnancy (including Miscarriage and Ectopic Pregnancy).**

Bibliography

1. Centre for Maternal and Child Enquiries. Saving mothers' lives: reviewing maternal deaths to make motherhood safer: 2006–2008. *BJOG: An International Journal of Obstetrics & Gynaecology* 2011, 118(suppl. 1).

2. Woollard M, Hinshaw K, Simpson H, Wieteska S. Emergencies in early pregnancy and complications following gynaecological surgery. In *Pre-hospital Obstetric Emergency Training.* Oxford: Wiley-Blackwell, 2009: 53–61.

3. Woollard M, Hinshaw K, Simpson H, Wieteska S. Management of non-obstetric emergencies. In *Pre-hospital Obstetric Emergency Training.* Oxford: Wiley-Blackwell, 2009: 136–165.

6

Special Situations

Atropine for CBRNE

1. Presentation

- Pre-filled syringe containing 1 milligram atropine in 5 ml.
- Pre-filled syringe containing 1 milligram atropine in 10 ml.
- Pre-filled syringe containing 3 milligrams atropine in 10 ml.
- An ampoule containing 600 micrograms in 1 ml.
- Duodote® containing 2.1 milligrams of atropine sulphate.

2. Indications

Organophosphate (OP) poisoning.

Adults and children with a clinical diagnosis of poisoning by OP nerve agents, as an adjunct to maintenance of oxygenation.

Atropine should be administered for confirmed OP poisoning, or where features of OP poisoning develop. Clinical diagnosis of nerve agent poisoning (see below) is suggested by the characteristic features of nerve agent poisoning, associated with a history of possible exposure. Clinical features must include one or more of the following: bronchorrhoea, bronchospasm, severe bradycardia (<40 bpm).

3. Contra-Indications

Hypersensitivity to atropine sulphate or excipients in nerve agent poisoning.

4. Cautions

There are no other absolute criteria for the exclusion from administration of atropine in the treatment of OP poisoning, as the consequences of not instituting prompt treatment in poisoned patients will usually outweigh the risks associated with treatment. However, caution needs to be administered in the following:

- Patients with ulcerative colitis.
- Patients with risk of urinary retention.
- Patients with glaucoma.
- Patients with conditions characterised by tachycardia (e.g. thyrotoxicosis, heart failure).
- Patients with myasthenia gravis.

5. Side Effects

Reactions are mostly dose related and usually reversible, and include:

- Loss of visual accommodation.
- Photophobia.
- Arrhythmias, transient bradycardia followed by tachycardia.
- Palpitations.
- Difficulty in micturition.

6. Additional Information

Toxic doses may cause CNS stimulation manifesting as restlessness, confusion, ataxia, lack of coordination, hallucinations and delirium. In severe intoxication, CNS stimulation may give way to CNS depression, coma, circulatory and respiratory failure and death.

Characteristic Features of Nerve Agent Poisoning

- Miosis, excess secretions (e.g. lacrimation and bronchorrhoea).
- Respiratory difficulty (e.g. bronchospasm or respiratory depression).
- Altered consciousness, convulsions, together with a history of possible exposure.

6.1 Nerve Agent Poisoning

- Atropine must only be administered after the patient is adequately oxygenated.
- In OP poisoning there is no maximum dose and large doses (e.g. 20 milligrams) may be required to achieve atropinisation. Signs of atropinisation include dry skin and mouth and an absence of bradycardia (e.g. heart rate adult ≥80 bpm; heart rate child ≥100 bpm). **NB** DO NOT rely on reversal of pinpoint pupils as a guide to atropinisation.
- Administering large volumes intramuscularly could lead to poor absorption and/or tissue damage; therefore, administer the smallest volume possible and divide where necessary and practicable. Vary the site of injection for repeated doses; appropriate sites include buttock (gluteus maximus), thigh (vastus lateralis), lateral hip (gluteus medius) and upper arm (deltoid).

Atropine for CBRNE

Intravenous 1 milligram in 5 ml

Route: Intravenous/intraosseous/intramuscular (as appropriate).

NAME	AGE	ROUTE	INITIAL DOSE	REPEAT DOSE	DOSE INTERVAL	CONCENTRATION	VOLUME	MAX DOSE
Atropine for CBRNE	≥8 years	IV/IO/IM	2 milligrams	2 milligrams	5 minutes	1 milligram in 5 ml	10 ml	No limit
Atropine for CBRNE	12 months – 7 years	IV/IO/IM	600 micrograms	600 micrograms	5 minutes	1 milligram in 5 ml	3 ml	No limit
Atropine for CBRNE	Birth – <12 months	IV/IO/IM	200 micrograms	200 micrograms	5 minutes	1 milligram in 5 ml	1 ml	No limit

Intravenous 1 milligram in 10 ml

Route: Intravenous/intraosseous/intramuscular (administer the smallest volume possible and divide where necessary and practicable).

NAME	AGE	ROUTE	INITIAL DOSE	REPEAT DOSE	DOSE INTERVAL	CONCENTRATION	VOLUME	MAX DOSE
Atropine for CBRNE	≥8 years	IV/IO/IM	2 milligrams	2 milligrams	5 minutes	1 milligram in 10 ml	20 ml	No limit
Atropine for CBRNE	12 months – 7 years	IV/IO/IM	600 micrograms	600 micrograms	5 minutes	1 milligram in 10 ml	6 ml	No limit
Atropine for CBRNE	Birth – <12 months	IV/IO/IM	200 micrograms	200 micrograms	5 minutes	1 milligram in 10 ml	2 ml	No limit

SECTION **6** Special Situations

Atropine for CBRNE

Intravenous 3 milligrams in 10 ml

Route: Intravenous/intraosseous/intramuscular (as appropriate).

NAME	AGE	ROUTE	INITIAL DOSE	REPEAT DOSE	DOSE INTERVAL	CONCENTRATION	VOLUME	MAX DOSE
Atropine for CBRNE	≥8 years	IV/IO/IM	2 milligrams	2 milligrams	5 minutes	3 milligrams in 10 ml	6.7 ml	No limit
Atropine for CBRNE	12 months – 7 years	IV/IO/IM	600 micrograms	600 micrograms	5 minutes	3 milligrams in 10 ml	2 ml	No limit
Atropine for CBRNE	Birth – <12 months	IV/IO/IM	200 micrograms	200 micrograms	5 minutes	3 milligrams in 10 ml	0.6 ml	No limit

Intravenous 600 micrograms in 1 ml

Route: Intravenous/intraosseous/intramuscular.

NAME	AGE	ROUTE	INITIAL DOSE	REPEAT DOSE	DOSE INTERVAL	CONCENTRATION	VOLUME	MAX DOSE
Atropine for CBRNE	≥8 years	IV/IO/IM	2 milligrams	2 milligrams	5 minutes	600 micrograms in 1 ml	3.3 ml	No limit
Atropine for CBRNE	12 months – 7 years	IV/IO/IM	600 micrograms	600 micrograms	5 minutes	600 micrograms in 1 ml	1 ml	No limit
Atropine for CBRNE	Birth – <12 months	IV/IO/IM	200 micrograms	200 micrograms	5 minutes	600 micrograms in 1 ml	0.3 ml	No limit

Chemical Biological Radiological Nuclear (CBRN) Incidents Including Hazardous Materials

1. Introduction

- Chemical, biological, radiological and nuclear (CBRN) incidents require a different approach from other incidents. Priorities include ensuring that the duration of exposure to the hazardous environment or substance is kept to a minimum and that the responders do not themselves become casualties.

- Recognition that an incident may be CBRN involves the Safety Triggers for Emergency Personnel (STEP) 1-2-3 Plus approach. When it is safe to do so, the Initial Operational Response (IOR) aims to quickly reduce people's exposure to a hazardous agent.

- Once the responsible agent(s) have been identified, specific procedures and treatment plans can be instigated.

- Specialist teams such as the Hazardous Area Response Team (HART) and Specialist Operational Response Team (SORT) are trained to work in these environments.

2. Safety Triggers for Emergency Personnel (STEP) 1-2-3 Plus

To recognise that a situation requires IOR, follow the STEP 1-2-3 Plus flowchart (Figure 6.1).

- First responders presented with unexplained casualties should adhere to STEP 1-2-3 Plus as shown in Figures 6.1 and 6.2.

TABLE 6.1 – 1-2-3 STEP Plus for Non-specialists and Specialists

Non-specialists	Specialists (Hazardous Area Response Team (HART), Specialist Operational Response Team (SORT))
Do not approach a potentially contaminated casualty. Advise casualties using the Remove, Remove, Remove guidance (Figure 6.3).	Will deal with non-ambulant casualties within the hot/warm zones as part of the Specialist Operational Response (SOR), and will wear the appropriate personal protective equipment (PPE) to operate in a contaminated environment.
Apply STEP 1-2-3 Plus and seek expert advice early.	**HART** will provide casualty management in the hot zone and evacuate patients to decontamination.
Locate yourself upwind, ideally uphill, and maintain a safe distance from those contaminated.	**SORT** will provide clinical decontamination to those casualties affected.

STEP 1-2-3 PLUS

STEP 1	STEP 2	STEP 3
One person incapacitated with no obvious reason ● Approach using standard protocols	**Two people incapacitated with no obvious reason** ● Approach with caution using standard protocols	**Three or more people in close proximity, incapacitated with no obvious reason** ● Use caution and follow ➕ PLUS

➕ PLUS

PLUS means follow the CBRN First Responder Flow Chart to consider what actions can be undertaken to save life, using the following principles:

- **Evacuate** – Get people away from the scene of contamination.

- **Communicate and Advise** – Give immediate medical advice and reassurance that help is on its way.

- **Disrobe** – Remove clothing.

- **Decontamination** – Dry decontamination should be the default process.

Figure 6.1 – Step 1-2-3 Plus. Home Office: Initial Operational Response to a CBRN Incident (http://www.jesip.org.uk/uploads/media/pdf/CBRN%20JOPs/IOR_Guidance_V2_July_2015.pdf).

Chemical Biological Radiological Nuclear (CBRN) Incidents Including Hazardous Materials

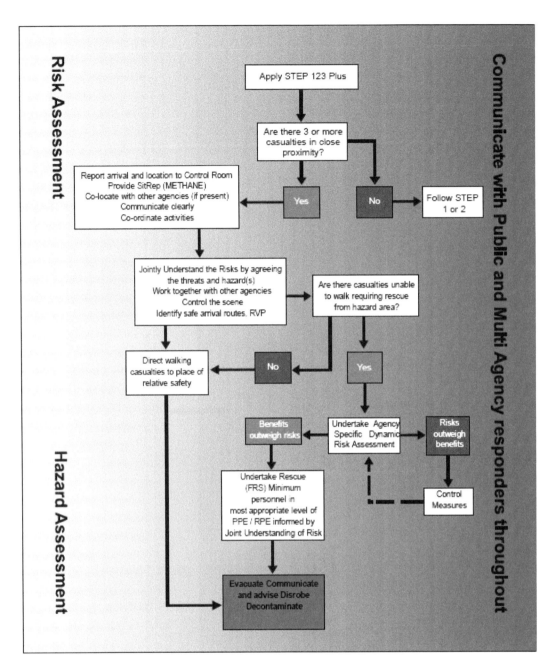

Figure 6.2 – IOR Guidance. NARU (https://naru.org.uk/videos/initial-operational-response-ior-for-nhs-ambulance-services/).

3. Initial Operational Response (IOR)

- IOR is a quick and effective way of helping people caught up in a CBRN incident.

- The people and area in the vicinity may have become contaminated. The longer the contaminant is in contact with a person (either in the air or on the person), the worse the effects will be. IOR looks to separate the person from the contaminant in the quickest possible time, to reduce the health effects on that person.

- Casualties should be advised to follow the instructions from first responders, who will direct their actions using the Remove, Remove, Remove guidance (see Figure 6.3).

- It also allows non-protected responders to safely help the public before the arrival of specialist CBRN personnel.

4. Recognition of Agent Involved

- In some cases, such as industrial incidents, the agent may already be known. In other cases, such as deliberate releases, the agent or agents may only be identified later using specialist equipment.

- Once casualties have been decontaminated, utilise the CBRN CRESS (consciousness, respiration, eyes, secretions, skin) tool (Figure 6.4) to identify what agent a casualty may have been exposed to, so the appropriate

Chemical Biological Radiological Nuclear (CBRN) Incidents Including Hazardous Materials

Figure 6.3 – Remove, Remove, Remove guidance.

initial clinical management can be provided. Ensure good communication so that once the agent(s) have been identified, any changes required to the treatment plan can be initiated, including for casualties who have already left the scene.

- If the agent has not been identified and the casualty presents with any of the above signs

and symptoms, seek specialist advice via internal process, such as NILO/Tac Ad. There are many drugs that can be used in the treatment of CBRN agent exposure, but it is imperative that the most appropriate drug is administered. This advice must be sought from specialists.

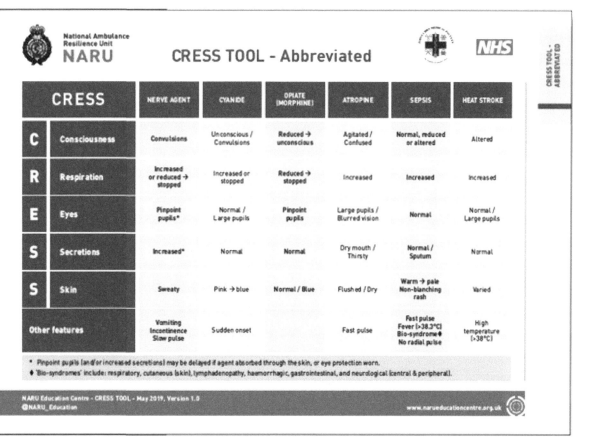

Figure 6.4 – CRESS Tool.

Chemical Biological Radiological Nuclear (CBRN) Incidents Including Hazardous Materials

5. Specific Agents

5.1 Nerve Agent

- The classic presenting features of nerve agent exposure are those for organophosphate poisoning. Organophosphates can be found in pesticides and some herbicides, and agricultural exposure or deliberate self-harm can result in toxicity.

- Where it is suspected or confirmed that a casualty has been poisoned with a nerve agent, the ambulance service's protocol is to administer a nerve agent countermeasure. The DuoDote® auto-injector is the countermeasure

of choice and should be administered as per local policy/training. This drug is under Schedule 19 Exemption of the Human Medicines Regulations (2012), and can be administered by any trained member of staff under a local medicines protocol.

- A number of DuoDote® doses are carried on every front-line ambulance vehicle, with additional supplies in mass casualty vehicles (MCVs) and HART supplies.

- Each DuoDote® auto-injector contains 2.1 mg atropine and 600 mg pralidoxime for intramuscular injection into a large muscle group. It is suitable for adults and children over 1 year old.

Figure 6.5 – CBRN Guideline: Nerve Agents. Courtesy of Surgeon Commander Steven Bland, Defence Specialist Advisor in CBRN Medicine.

Chemical Biological Radiological Nuclear (CBRN) Incidents Including Hazardous Materials

- Guidance on initial dose and any subsequent dosing can be taken from the NHSE CBRN Guidelines.

- Those patients with **severe** symptoms (unconsciousness, convulsions, respiratory arrest, severe respiratory distress, cyanosis or bradycardia <40 bpm) should have three doses of DuoDote® administered immediately, ideally into different large muscle groups to maximise absorption.

- Those patients with **moderate** symptoms (not walking, not obeying commands, confusion, excessive secretions, wheeze and incontinence) should have one dose of DuoDote® administered, with re-assessment every 15 minutes. If symptoms persist, a repeat dose should be given. If severe symptoms develop, administer an additional two doses to reach the total of three doses of DuoDote®.

- For **paediatric** patients, the dosing should be based on age. Those 12 years and over are managed as adults. DuoDote® is contraindicated in those under 1 year of age and atropine should be used instead.

TABLE 6.2 – Dosages of DuoDote®

Age	Initial Dose	Repeat Dose	Maximum Dose
12 years and over (Adult)	1–3 according to severity	1 every 15 minutes	3
8–11 years	1	1 after 15 minutes	2
1–7 years	1	N/A	1
Less than 1	Contraindicated. Use atropine (see below).	N/A	N/A

- Once DuoDote® has been administered, if able to do so, gain IV/IO access. Administer high-flow oxygen.

- If seizures are present, administer anticonvulsant diazepam (IV/IO) or midazolam (buccal) in accordance with local protocol.

- In those severely symptomatic patients in whom:
  - the maximum dose of DuoDote® has been reached and they remain severely symptomatic
  - there is no DuoDote® immediately available or
  - DuoDote® is contraindicated due to age

  Administer atropine via IV/IO route in accordance with guidance below. If IV/IO access cannot be achieved, IM is acceptable in extremis.

- In organophosphate and nerve agent poisoning, large doses of atropine may be required to adequately reverse the systemic effects (atropinisation), and the patient should be reassessed every 5 minutes with a view to repeat dose. Absence of bradycardia is the most reliable indicator of adequate effect, aiming for a heart rate over 80 bpm for adults and over 100 bpm for children under 12 years of age.

- Ensure the correct dose is administered, as presentations of atropine vary (3 mg in 10 ml, 1 mg in 10 ml, 1 mg in 10 ml and 600 mcg in 1 ml).

Refer to **Atropine for CBRNE**.

TABLE 6.3 – DuoDote® for Non-specialists and Specialists

Non-specialists	Specialists (Hazardous Area Response Team (HART))
Administer DuoDote® (as per instructions/training) to casualties who are showing signs and symptoms of nerve agent poisoning once they have been decontaminated.	Will administer DuoDote® to casualties in the hot/warm zone who have nerve agent poisoning.
Seek expert advice to identify countermeasures for biological agents and all other chemical agents.	Will seek specialist advice on appropriate countermeasures for casualties exposed to biological and all other chemical agents.
Use DuoDote® on themselves if they have signs and symptoms of nerve agent poisoning.	

Chemical Biological Radiological Nuclear (CBRN) Incidents Including Hazardous Materials

5.2 Cyanide

- Cyanide-containing substances are highly toxic and act at a cellular level by inhibiting the metabolism of oxygen to produce energy. So cellular hypoxia can result despite adequate inspired oxygen levels and SpO_2.

- Cyanide-containing substances can occur in solid (crystalline), liquid or gaseous forms and are used in several industrial processes. Cyanide-containing gases can be formed from burning plastics and are often present in house fires. Poisoning may be due to accidental or intentional exposure.

- Given the highly toxic nature, the onset of symptoms is often very rapid, within 20–30 seconds of exposure to toxic levels, and death can occur within 5–8 minutes. If a patient remains asymptomatic after 15 minutes, significant poisoning is unlikely unless there is ongoing exposure.

Treatment

- This should primarily focus on standard ABC approach, ensuring the safety of staff to prevent exposure. Specific antidotes for cyanide poisoning are available, though several of these are potentially toxic in their own right if administered when cyanide toxicity is not present.

- Hydroxycobalamin is emerging as the safest effective antidote, and is carried by some specialist pre-hospital care teams.

- If there is a suspicion of cyanide toxicity, ensure the safety of responders and seek expert advice urgently.

5.3 Opioids

- The classic features of opioid toxicity (respiratory depression, decreased level of consciousness and pin-point pupils) are well recognised from the administration of morphine as an analgesic and from patients with opiate addiction and a history of misuse.

- The management principles are fundamentally the same, with a focus on maintaining respiration and oxygenation. Synthetic opioids, such as fentanyl and carfentanil, are far more potent than morphine (80–1,000 times the potency of morphine). Therefore, toxic doses may be very small. Due to the potency, the period of respiratory depression may be prolonged, and cardiovascular collapse is more common. This potency often requires a higher dose and increased frequency of naloxone to achieve effective reversal of systemic effects.

- Synthetic opioids may be encountered in illicit drug laboratories (IDL), where those drugs are manufactured and are sometimes used for large

animal tranquilisation. They may be absorbed through skin exposure or inhalation of vapour.

- If you suspect significant toxicity from a high-potency synthetic opioid, ensure the safety of responders and seek expert advice on patient management.

5.4 Atropine

- The features of atropine toxicity are classic for anticholinergic toxidrome and are often seen in accidental and intentional medication overdoses, or exposure to some toxic plants. High temperature leading to hyperpyrexia can result in severe morbidity. The management is principally symptomatic, though specific antidotes are available in hospital. Severe anticholinergic toxicity can result in death. Seek expert advice and convey the patient to an appropriate receiving facility.

For more information regarding CBRN clinical management, visit:

https://narueducationcentre.org.uk/

https://www.gov.uk/government/publications/chemical-biological-radiological-and-nuclear-incidents-recognise-and-respond.

5.5 Corrosive Substances

- There has been a significant increase in both the profile and frequency of serious criminal assaults using acids and other corrosive materials across the UK.

- These cause significant harm to individuals. While the overall number of people impacted by this type of attack remains low, responders are advised to use the Remove, Remove, Remove guidance in the event they attend a victim of such an attack (see Figure 6.3).

- The key management principle for reducing harm from corrosive chemical exposure is irrigation with clean water. This is effective whether the corrosive chemical is strongly acidic or caustic alkali.

- When using high-volume irrigation on large areas of contamination, ensure measures to prevent the patient becoming hypothermic.

- There is emerging evidence of the benefits of amphoteric solutions, such as Diphoterine©. This is carried by some specialist services within police, fire and ambulance, and is kept in many emergency departments. However, if amphoteric solution is not immediately available, irrigation should NOT be delayed awaiting availability.

- Burns on large body-surface areas, chemical burns or those affecting special areas (eyes, face, hands and genitalia) should be transferred to an appropriate receiving facility in accordance with local guidelines.

Chemical Biological Radiological Nuclear (CBRN) Incidents Including Hazardous Materials

TABLE 6.4 – Dos and Don'ts for Corrosive Substances

Do	Don't
Exercise extreme caution if there appear to be multiple patients or an ongoing attack.	**Do not** approach containers or substance spillages.
Wear eye protection and gloves (double glove, nitrile gloves). Protect any exposed skin by wearing a jacket to provide a barrier.	**Do not** pull contaminated clothing over the head or remove clothing that is adhering to the skin.
Avoid becoming contaminated.	**Do not** delay on-scene time for patients with large burns or burns to the face, eyes or hands.
Advise HART if there are large numbers of patients or extensive contamination.	**Do not** apply any form of occlusive dressing (e.g. clingfilm).
Move to a ventilated area to minimise vapour hazards.	
Request fire and rescue service (FRS) assistance to provide copious amounts of water.	
Irrigate casualties freely with clean water for 20 minutes. Try to ensure any runoff does not come into contact with other uncontaminated parts of the body.	
Early and thorough irrigation of the face and eyes is particularly important to minimise the risk of long-term damage.	
Contaminated jewellery should be removed, rinsed and placed in bag/wrapped to avoid skin contact and given back to the patient.	
If possible, get the victim to do as much of the work themselves with direction – this may not always be practicable, but will greatly reduce exposure to first responders.	

5.6 Individual Chemical Exposure (ICE)

- Individual Chemical Exposure (ICE) events are frequently characterised by the use of a chemical, a mixture of chemicals or commercially available gases with the intent to self-harm predominantly via ingestion or inhalation.

- These events commonly occur in sealed or partially sealed environments, such as vehicles, residential bathrooms, hotel rooms, other enclosed areas or a bag over the casualty's head where a small amount of gas can quickly reach lethal concentrations. ICE events are usually single casualty or pairs rather than groups; for three or more casualties, follow STEPS 123 +.

- Any event involving exposure of an individual to chemicals or other hazardous substances may present a serious risk to the public, emergency services and to other health workers, such as hospital and mortuary staff, who may come into contact with the contaminated individual.

- ICE events are complex in nature and will require multi-agency response; specialist responders (HART) should be requested as a matter of urgency.

TABLE 6.5 – Individual Chemical Exposure for Non-specialists and Specialists

Non-specialists		Specialists
Do	**Don't**	**HART**
Be cautious if an ICE incident is suspected, and stay a safe distance from the scene.	**Do not** approach the scene if an ICE incident is suspected or confirmed.	Have appropriate PPE to enter the inner cordon to provide lifesaving interventions or to perform ROLE.
Call for HART immediately and provide a (M)ETHANE report to control.	**Do not** become exposed to any hazardous substances.	Will provide medical support to partner agencies who are committed to the inner cordon.

(continued)

TABLE 6.5 – Individual Chemical Exposure for Non-specialists and Specialists *(continued)*		
Seek specialist advice if required.	**Do not** attempt to perform resuscitation or medical treatment if there are clear signs of the casualties being contaminated. This should only take place if the responder is in appropriate PPE.	

For further information, visit: www.naru.org.uk.

5.7 Ionising radiation

There are four main types of ionising radiation:

- alpha
- beta
- gamma and X-rays
- neutrons.

There are two main types of hazards from radioactive material:

- **Radiation Hazard:** Where a solid or contained source is only emitting radiation, this is referred to as a 'radiation hazard'. The radiation travels from the fixed source, through the air, to the human body. The target absorbs the energy from the radiation but is not itself made 'radioactive'. An analogy to this may be the heat emitted by a lit open fireplace.

- **Contamination Hazard:** Contamination is a potential problem with any radioactive material, except electrically generated x-rays (which can be turned off). If a material that contains radioactive isotopes is in a form that is easily dispersed (i.e. dusts, powders, liquids, gases), the radioactive substance can become attached to the exterior of the body or other surfaces by direct contact or airborne dispersion (e.g. dust, spray, mist etc.). It may also enter the body through inhalation, ingestion or through an open cut or wound. In this sense, internal radioactive contamination poses much the same threat as any other chemical toxin or 'hazardous materials exposure'. Once inside the body, alpha-and beta-emitting materials, which are not considered high risk in terms of external radiation, may deliver damaging ionising radiation directly into tissue or travel around the body via normal biological mechanisms. An analogy to this may be the smoke and soot given off by a fire, travelling around the room. The patient will continue to receive a radiation exposure from any inhaled or ingested radioactive material until it is excreted or decays away.

Contamination cannot be destroyed or neutralised like a chemical or biological agent. It can, however, be removed. The aim of decontamination is to move radioactive contamination from the contaminated person or object onto something else, which can then be isolated and disposed of correctly.

It is important for emergency responders to make a distinction between sealed (closed) sources of radioactivity and unsealed (open) sources of radioactivity.

- **Sealed Sources** A sealed source is a radioactive source that is encapsulated into a solid material, usually metal. The encapsulation is intended to prevent the escape of the physical radioactive material, while allowing the radioactive energy to pass through. Because the radioactive source substance is encapsulated or plated onto a surface, sealed sources do not present a contamination hazard under normal conditions; however, they can still present a significant radiation hazard.

- **Unsealed Sources** Unsealed sources consist of powders, liquids or sometimes gases which contain radioactive elements and which could easily be released from their containers through leaks and spillages and dispersed into the environment. The main hazard with unsealed sources is contamination, although there may also be a significant irradiation hazard from the bulk material. Sealed sources may become unsealed in the event of explosion, intense fire or severe damage.

- **Special Form** Some sealed sources are designed to a standard known as 'special form', as defined by transport legislation. To meet it, the source capsule must remain intact after several rigorous tests, which include heating, bending and striking tests. The standard is intended to show that the radioactive material would not be released to form a contamination hazard, even in the event of major damage. It might still present a significant radiation hazard.

5.8 Decontamination

- Those that have been contaminated can be treated by non-specialist staff wearing clinical PPE using strict hygiene protocols. Contamination levels can easily be monitored with appropriate equipment.

Chemical Biological Radiological Nuclear (CBRN) Incidents Including Hazardous Materials

TABLE 6.6 – Treatment for Contaminated Patients	
P1	**P2 and P3**
Patients with life-threatening injuries should not have their treatment or transfer delayed for decontamination, other than the removal of clothing and personal belongings. (This should be undertaken during IOR.)	Patients should be decontaminated as far as reasonably practicable on scene, before approaching the ambulance for transport.
Any such clothing should be regarded as contaminated waste until proven otherwise, and so should be left in the scene where it can be appropriately removed.	If it is not practicable to decontaminate a patient before transfer to hospital, they may be wrapped in a sheet or blanket to prevent the spread of contamination.
Open wounds should be dressed, and the patient wrapped in sheets or blankets to stop the further spread of contaminant. The face and hands may be cleaned with wipes.	
Specialists (HART) will wear appropriate PPE to deal with non-ambulant patients in the inner cordon. Have detection, identification and monitoring (DIM) equipment to monitor radiation dose and amount of contamination on a casualty.	
SORT will provide clinical decontamination for mass casualties if required.	

5.9 Illicit Drugs Laboratories (IDLs)

- There is a risk in the UK from IDLs, which present many chemical hazards, explosive risk and fire hazards to the emergency services. They are places where illegal drugs have been or are being manufactured.

- Synthetic opioids (e.g. Fentanyl), methylamphetamines and their by-products are of concern. Fentanyl represents a significant health risk to responders when manufactured illicitly.

- If you come across or suspect a location to be an IDL, use Table 6.7.

TABLE 6.7 – IDL for Non-specialists and Specialists		
Non-specialists		**Specialists**
Do	**Don't**	**HART**
Evacuate immediately and stay a safe distance away.	**Do not** touch or otherwise disturb the substance.	Will wear appropriate PPE to enter the inner cordon to provide lifesaving interventions or to perform ROLE.
Provide control with a METHANE report.	**Do not** attempt to perform resuscitation or medical treatment if there are clear signs of the casualty(s) being contaminated. This should only take place if the responder is in appropriate PPE.	Will provide medical support to partner agencies who are committed to the inner cordon.
Seek expert advice.		

KEY POINTS!

CBRN incidents

- **Ensure Initial Operational Response (IOR) is followed.**
- **Follow Step 1-2-3 Plus guidance.**
- **Communicate METHANE.**
- **If unsure of agent involved, use the CRESS tool.**
- **Follow specific guidance for known agents.**

6 Special Situations

Major, Complex and High-Risk Incidents

1. Specialist Capabilities

- Ambulance services maintain a range of specialist capabilities to support the response to complex incidents. These capabilities are interoperable, which means they can be used locally or combined to provide a national response.

- When responding to a complex or high-risk incident, it is essential for ambulance staff to request these specialist services early. They can be easily stood down if not required.

- The specialist capabilities are summarised in Table 6.8.

TABLE 6.8 – Ambulance Service Specialist Capabilities

Core Capability	Tactical Options	
Hazardous Area Response Teams (HART)	Hazardous materials	▪ Working inside the inner cordon ▪ Industrial accidents ▪ High Consequence Infectious Disease (HCID) ▪ Complex transportation accidents
	Chemical, biological, radiological, nuclear (CBRN)	▪ Specialist operational response (SOR) ▪ Component part of wider CBRN capability
	Marauding terrorist attack (MTA)	▪ Specialist support to warm zone operations ▪ Component part of wider MTA capability
	Safe working at height (SWaH)	▪ Manmade structures ▪ Natural environments
	Confined space	▪ Substantially enclosed spaces ▪ Building collapse ▪ Compromised atmospheres ▪ Entrapments
	Unstable terrain	▪ Active rubble pile ▪ Rural access/difficult terrain
	Water operations	▪ Swift water rescue ▪ Urban and rural flooding ▪ Boat operations
	Support to security operations (SSO)	▪ Support to security operations ▪ Support to police operations ▪ Illicit drug laboratories ▪ VIP close protection support
Marauding terrorist attack (MTA)	▪ Working inside a ballistically unsafe area (warm zone) ▪ Siege/stronghold	
Chemical, biological, radiological, nuclear explosives (CBRN)	▪ Initial Operational Response (IOR) ▪ Specialist Operational Response Team (SORT) provided by HART & SORT ▪ Interim decontamination of casualties ▪ Full wet decontamination of casualties	

Major, Complex and High-Risk Incidents

Core Capability	Tactical Options
TABLE 6.8 – Ambulance Service Specialist Capabilities *(continued)*	
Command and control (C2)	▪ Strategic command of major and critical incidents ▪ Tactical command of major and critical incidents ▪ Operational command of major and critical incidents ▪ National Interagency Liaison Officers (NILOs) ▪ Strategic and tactical advisors ▪ Medical advisors
Mass casualties	▪ Capabilities to treat large numbers of casualties ▪ Casualty clearing stations (CCS) ▪ National coordination of patient transfers

2. Security

2.1 UK Threat Levels

▪ The UK threat level is set by the Joint Terrorism Analysis Centre (JTAC) and is advised by intelligence or probability relating to international or domestic terrorism activities.

▪ Threat levels are designed to give a broad indication of the likelihood of terrorist attack.
  - **LOW** means an attack is unlikely.
  - **MODERATE** means an attack is possible but not likely.
  - **SUBSTANTIAL** means an attack is a strong possibility.
  - **SEVERE** means an attack is highly likely.
  - **CRITICAL** means an attack is expected imminently.

▪ When the threat level is changed, particularly to **SEVERE** or **CRITICAL**, ambulance staff should seek specific advice from their own organisations. In general, staff should consider the following safety guidance:
  - For urgent information regarding suspicious activities, contact the police in the first instance.
  - For information regarding less imminent terrorist activities, contact the Anti-Terrorist Hotline: 0800 789 321.
  - For more information on UK threat levels, visit: https://www.mi5.gov.uk/threat-levels.

2.2 Personal Safety

If there is an increase in threat level or there is a heightened state of security, the following steps will help to ensure personal safety. However, these are also sensible precautions for clinicians to apply at all times:

▪ Challenge anyone on site who is not visibly displaying ID.

▪ Know the exits on all sites that are regularly visited or worked at.

▪ Consider means and routes for leaving the building or site.

▪ Beware of the surroundings. Look out for any suspicious or unusual behaviour, including unattended bags or packages.

▪ Vary routines, such as route to work or parking spot.

▪ Ensure your line manager knows where you are.

▪ Avoid travelling in uniform.

▪ Remove ID cards and vehicle car passes when leaving the workplace.

▪ Avoid drawing unnecessary attention to your occupation outside work.

▪ Update privacy settings on personal social media accounts so that information is only shared with known people. Never include operational or work information.

For more information regarding the Stay Safe campaign and other safety advice, visit:

▪ https://www.gov.uk/government/publications/stay-safe-film

▪ https://www.gov.uk/government/publications/recognising-the-terrorist-threat.

2.3 Protectively Marked Documents

▪ All information that the government needs to collect, store, process, generate or share to deliver services and conduct its business has intrinsic value and may require a degree of protection.

▪ Ambulance staff may come across protectively marked documents as part of routine work, especially work that may be associated with emergency preparedness. Failure to appropriately handle these documents (or associated materials) and the information contained within them can have serious consequences, including dismissal and potential criminal liability.

▪ Security classifications indicate the sensitivity of information and the need to protect it. There are three levels of classification:
  - **OFFICIAL:** The majority of information that is created or processed by the public sector.

SECTION **6** Special Situations

Major, Complex and High-Risk Incidents

This includes routine business operations and services, some of which could have damaging consequences if lost, stolen or published in the media, but are not subject to a heightened threat profile. Official classifications may be accompanied by a descriptor which will mandate special handling requirements. This includes 'Official – Sensitive'. If you receive material with an 'Official – Sensitive' descriptor, you must ensure you handle that material in accordance with the Government Protective Marking Scheme requirements.

- **SECRET:** Very sensitive information that justifies heightened protective measures to defend against determined and highly capable threat actors. For example, where compromise could seriously damage military capabilities, international relations or the investigation of serious organised crime.
- **TOP SECRET:** The government's most sensitive information requiring the highest levels of protection from the most serious threats. For example, where compromise could cause widespread loss of life or else threaten the security or economic wellbeing of the country or friendly nations.

2.4 Suspect Packages

- On discovery of a suspect package or if one is reported, follow these basic steps:

1. Report the matter to the police via the ambulance Emergency Operations Centre (EOC).

2. If possible, take a photograph of the package before withdrawing without touching or interfering with the package. If it is not possible to take a photograph, make a mental note of the size, location and any distinguishing features.

3. If the police or fire and rescue service (FRS) are not yet on scene, attempt to establish the following recommended minimum cordons:
   - small item (i.e. briefcase/rucksack) – 100 m
   - medium item (i.e. car) – 200 m
   - large item (i.e. van/lorry) – 400 m.

4. Be mindful of the risk of secondary devices or other devices.

- The police will be able to assess the device with known intelligence and risk factors to decide how best to manage the situation. If the device is deemed to be credible, it will require a specialist multi-agency response. From an ambulance service perspective, request HART support via the EOC.

2.5 Initial Actions for a Major Incident

- Each NHS ambulance trust has a major incident plan, which will define key actions that ambulance staff must take if they are faced with a major incident. First and foremost, follow the plan of your service.

- The *Civil Contingencies Act 2004* defines an emergency of this magnitude in the following terms:
   a. An event or situation which threatens serious damage to human welfare in a place in the United Kingdom.
   b. An event or situation which threatens serious damage to the environment in a place in the United Kingdom.
   c. War or terrorism which threatens serious damage to the security of the United Kingdom.

- An incident which requires a highly technical response or the utilisation of specialist capabilities could also be termed a **CRITICAL** incident.

- The first clinician on scene at incidents such as these should provide an initial report back to the EOC using the METHANE model, which has been approved for use by each of the emergency services under the Joint Emergency Services Interoperability Programme (JESIP).

- The major incident standard messages are:
   - **Major incident alert/standby** – The term used by any member of staff to prefix messages indicating that an incident with the potential to generate a large number of casualties has or may have occurred.
   - **Major incident confirmed/declared** – The term used by any member of staff to prefix a message to confirm that a major incident has occurred, indicating that the plan should be implemented and a full pre-determined attendance/response is required.
   - **Major incident cancel** – The term used by a commander to cancel a major incident alert.
   - **Ambulance major incident stop** – The term used by a commander to indicate that sufficient ambulance and/or medical resources are available at the scene and that no further assistance is required.
   - **Ambulance major incident scene evacuation complete** – The term used by a commander to indicate that the treatment and removal of casualties from the scene is complete.
   - **Ambulance major incident stand down** – The term used by a commander to indicate the conclusion of all ambulance service activity in connection with a declared major incident and a return to normal modes of operation.

- The early declaration of a major incident ensures that the appropriate resources are activated at the earliest opportunity. These messages should be part of a METHANE report, as outlined in Table 6.9.

Major, Complex and High-Risk Incidents

TABLE 6.9 – Methane Report Format	
M	Major incident standby or declared
E	Exact location of incident
T	Type of incident
H	Hazards (present and potential)
A	Access and egress routes
N	Number, severity and type of casualties
E	Emergency services present on scene and further resources required

- Now follow the Major Incident Action Cards of your ambulance trust.

2.6 Command and Control

- During a larger scale incident, a multi-agency command structure will form. The following information provides an overview of how the ambulance service will integrate in the wider command and control framework.

- There are NHS Standards for ambulance service command, to which local ambulance service plans are aligned. The ambulance service will work closely with other responding agencies using the joint working principles outlined in Figure 6.6.

- Important command decisions will be taken in the multi-agency setting using the joint decision model shown in Figure 6.7.

- Ambulance clinicians may be given a briefing by commanders. They may use the 'IIMARCH' model, outlined in Table 6.10.

CO-LOCATE

Co-locate with other responders as soon as practicably possible at a single, safe and easily identified location.

COMMUNICATE

Communicate using language which is clear, and free from technical jargon and abbreviations.

CO-ORDINATE

Co-ordinate by agreeing the lead organisation. Identify priorities, resources, capabilities and limitations for an effective response, including the timing of further meetings.

JOINTLY UNDERSTAND RISK

Jointly understand risk by sharing information about the likelihood and potential impact of threats and hazards, to agree appropriate control measures.

SHARED SITUATIONAL AWARENESS

Establish shared situational awareness by using M/ETHANE and the Joint Decision Model.

Figure 6.6 – Joint working principles for the emergency services.

SECTION **6** Special Situations

Major, Complex and High-Risk Incidents

Figure 6.7 – Joint decision model.

TABLE 6.10 – IIMARCH	
Initial	**Item**
I	Information: ▪ Where/what/how many? ▪ History (if applicable): use METHANE.
I	Intent: ▪ Why are we here? ▪ Strategy, tactical and operational plan.
M	Method: ▪ How are we going to do it? ▪ Tactical plan, policy, plans.
A	Administration: ▪ Command/media/dress code/ decision logs/welfare/food/ individual tasking/timing.
R	Risk assessment: ▪ Specific threat areas/PPE/filter changes.

TABLE 6.10 – IIMARCH *(continued)*	
Initial	**Item**
C	Communications: ▪ Confirm radio callsigns. ▪ Indicate other means of communication if required. ▪ Ensure staff understand inter-agency communications.
H	Human rights: ▪ Disclosure details.

▪ All ambulance clinicians attending a major or complex incident have a responsibility to support risk management at the scene. Clinicians must ensure that a dynamic risk assessment is undertaken. The situation must be regularly reviewed and any hazards that need to be considered by commanders should be reported, i.e. those hazards that present a risk to patients and responders.

▪ Figure 6.8 provides an overview of how commanders and responders will approach assessing and then controlling the hazards and risks present at the scene.

Major, Complex and High-Risk Incidents

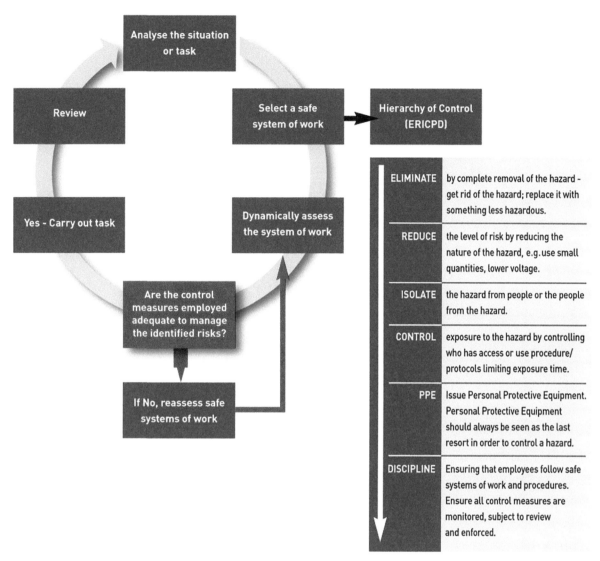

Figure 6.8 – Dynamic risk assessment/hierarchy of control.

- During a complex or major incident, ambulance responders may be assigned specific roles. This will include command roles and operational functions. Key roles are denoted by the nationally specified tabards shown in Figure 6.9.

- National guidance on command and control can be found on the NARU website: www.naru.org.uk.

- Refer to local trust plans and procedures.

2.7 Triage

- During the initial stages of an incident with large numbers of casualties, there are unlikely to be enough clinical responders to stay with each casualty and provide treatment. Therefore, the triage sieve tool shown in Figure 6.10 should be applied to ensure the best for everyone is achieved until such time that resources are sufficient to provide further care.

SECTION **6** Special Situations

Major, Complex and High-Risk Incidents

Tactical Commander (Ambulance Incident Commander)
White lower half with green & white checked shoulders.

Ambulance Operational Commander and any functional role not individually listed
Saturn yellow lower half and green & white checked shoulders. Insert as per role.

Airwave Tactical Advisor
Green & white check.

Ambulance Safety Officer (ASO)
Blue lower half with green & white checked shoulders.

Decontamination Officer
Purple lower half with green & white checked shoulders.

Doctor
Red lower half with green & white checked shoulders.

Strategic Advisor, Tactical Advisor or National Inter-Agency Liaison Officer (NILO)
Green lower half with green & white checked shoulders. Insert as per role.

Ambulance Entry Control Officer (ECO)
Green & yellow all over check.

Loggist
Orange lower half and green & white checked shoulders. All orange is any support function.

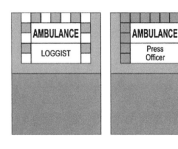

Figure 6.9 – National tabards for major incidents.

SECTION
6
Special Situations

Major, Complex and High-Risk Incidents

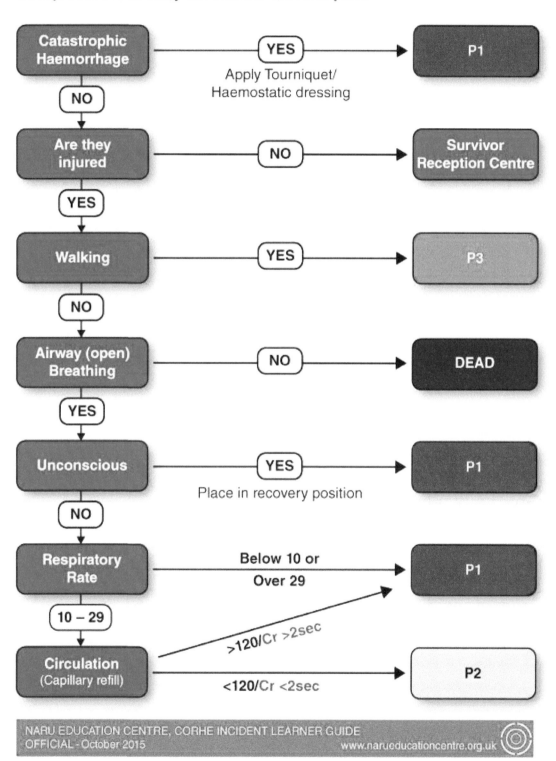

Triage Sieve

Best practice is to carry out TRIAGE SIEVE in pairs

Catastrophic Haemorrhage → YES → **Apply Tourniquet/ Haemostatic dressing** → P1

NO ↓

Are they injured → NO → Survivor Reception Centre

YES ↓

Walking → YES → P3

NO ↓

Airway (open) Breathing → NO → DEAD

YES ↓

Unconscious → YES → **Place in recovery position** → P1

NO ↓

Respiratory Rate → Below 10 or Over 29 → P1

10 – 29 ↓

Circulation (Capillary refill) → >120/Cr >2sec → P1

Circulation (Capillary refill) → <120/Cr <2sec → P2

NARU EDUCATION CENTRE, CORHE INCIDENT LEARNER GUIDE
OFFICIAL - October 2015   www.narueducationcentre.org.uk

Figure 6.10 – Triage sieve tool.

SECTION **6** Special Situations

Major, Complex and High-Risk Incidents

3. Incidents Involving Firearms and Weapons

- The prevalence of criminal or terrorism-related incidents is a significant risk to the public and emergency services personnel. In recent times, Europe, the UK and indeed many other countries have seen numerous actual or attempted attacks on their sovereign soil by non-State actors.

- In the UK, violent criminal attacks, using bladed and other types of weapons, are on the increase. Acts of terror have been conducted with varying degrees of sophistication, ranging from attacks using easily accessible items, such as knives and vehicles, to more complex incidents involving firearms, home-made explosives (HME) and improvised explosive devices (IEDs).

- It may not be obvious to responders (especially those first on scene) that an incident involving weapons has occurred and subsequently that there may still be a potential risk to the public and responders alike.

- Once on scene, incidents with mechanisms of injury (MOI) of penetrating and/or blast injury, particularly those with no apparent explanation, should be attended with caution. If either a criminal or terror-related act has occurred, then the safety of the responder(s) is paramount and unprotected responders should consider withdrawing from the area if they feel that their safety is compromised.

- The Home Office has issued specific advice to the public if they become caught up in an MTA or an active shooter event in the form of the Run, Hide, Tell campaign (Figure 6.11).

- While aspects of the Home Office campaign are applicable to the ambulance service, ambulance responders also owe a duty of care to reported casualties (refer to **Duty of Care**).

- The following guidance should be considered by ambulance personnel involved in an actual or suspected violent or terrorist attack:
  - Withdraw from the scene as quickly as possible. If possible, take casualties and mission-critical medical equipment.
  - Move in a direction away from the actual or perceived threat and avoid running in straight lines.
  - Move from point to point using hard cover as necessary and if available.
  - The distance to withdraw to is situationally dependent and individual judgement should be used.
  - If police and/or security services are present, they may give a specific distance to move to.
  - Safe distances in incidents involving firearms will depend on the type of weapon(s) being used. Some firearms have an effective range of as little as 50 m, while other types of weapon systems may have an effective range of up to 400 m.
  - When explosive devices are suspected to have been used or will be used, the minimum distance will again vary depending on the type and size of the device.
  - Once at a safe distance, responders should seek cover that gives physical protection and protection from view. Cover from ballistic or explosive threats could be a solid structure like a building, for example.
  - If physical cover is not achievable, then the responder should look for areas that will provide cover from view, for example a depression in the terrain.
  - Once in cover, plan an escape route.
  - Avoid isolated or obvious forms of cover, such as lone objects.

Figure 6.11 – Run, Hide, Tell. Source: Home Office, 2015.

Major, Complex and High-Risk Incidents

- Try to select cover that, while providing protection, also gives maximum fields of view.
- When in cover, scan the area for secondary threats and be prepared to move again if not satisfied with the area selected for cover.
- Stay calm and control breathing. Remain focused.
- Once it is safe to do so, it is imperative that the responders update the situation as soon as practicable using the METHANE reporting method.
- Ask for assistance from the police and the Hazardous Area Response Team (HART) if they are not already present or en-route.
- Continue to provide situational updates if practicable and safe to do so.
- Turn the volume down on the communication system and speak quietly. Where possible, use an earpiece.
- Turn other mobile devices to silent (turn OFF any vibrating alert) while still in danger.
- HART units and Specialist Operational Response Teams (SORTs) are specifically trained and equipped with ballistic personal protective equipment (PPE) to operate within a ballistic warm zone while responding to MTAs. HART also provide support to security operations (SSO). For any incidents of criminal attack involving weapons or terrorism, HART should be deployed as a matter of reflex. The deployment of SORT will normally be triggered by information received by the ambulance Emergency Operations Centre (EOC).
- Incidents involving different types of weapons result in different types and severities of injuries.

For specific guidance on treatment algorithms, refer to **Trauma Emergencies in Adults – Overview**, **Trauma Emergencies in Children – Overview**, **Head Injury** and **Thoracic Trauma**.

4. Water Rescue

- Ambulance responders are frequently called to incidents involving water. Non-specialists should not enter fast-moving water.
- Where patient(s) require lifesaving interventions, there are steps that can be taken by all ambulance staff prior to specialist teams arriving. Consider the following:
  - Carry out a dynamic risk assessment.
  - Inform the EOC of the situation.
  - Request specialist assistance, including HART assets, as soon as possible.
  - Wear a lifejacket if working within the warm zone (3 m from water's edge).
  - Shout at the patient to swim towards you.
  - If they are unable to do so, throw a safety buoy (or similar) for them to hold on to and pull them to safety.

- Do not carry out a task that is likely to cause you to enter the water unintentionally and become a casualty yourself.
- Only enter the water if it is shallow enough and, based on the risk assessment, you are competent to do so (i.e. a shallow pool in a recreational park as opposed to a canal, lake or fast-flowing river).
- Do not enter flood water without the support of specialist water responders.

- Ideally, non-specialists should not be working within the warm zone without appropriate training, equipment or PPE, but it is recognised that in some low-risk incidents it is unacceptable to delay life saving interventions awaiting specialist help. This must be managed appropriately within each trust.

5. High-consequence Infectious Disease

- Examples of high consequence infectious diseases are:
  - Ebola
  - Lassa fever
  - Marburg virus
  - pandemic influenza
  - other 'category 4' pathogens.

- It is crucial that the correct response to patient(s) with suspected/confirmed infectious disease is achieved to protect all those involved. The need for such a response will usually be pre-planned. Where this is not the case and an infectious disease is suspected, several precautions are needed.

- The patient should be isolated and further advice sought from a Tactical Advisor/NILO and trust protocols followed. Normally, universal precautions will be sufficient to protect ambulance responders. A more thorough history than normal will need to be obtained from the patient. Transfers of high-risk patients are usually completed by specialist HART staff who have access to additional protective equipment. If ambulance responders suspect they may have been exposed (i.e. needlestick injury), report and present for medical treatment immediately.

5.1 Pandemic Flu

- This is the highest-grade risk in the National Risk Register of Civil Emergencies. All ambulance responders should be familiar with their local trust's plans to respond to such patients. Universal precautions are normally appropriate. All ambulance responders should have access to FFP3 masks, or equivalent, and be appropriately fit tested. All ambulance responders are encouraged to receive an annual flu vaccination in order to protect themselves, their families and the public.

Major, Complex and High-Risk Incidents

6.1 Rail Incidents

Table 6.11 outlines how to manage rail incidents.

TABLE 6.11 – Management of Rail Incidents	
Non-specialists	**Specialists (HART)**
Do not approach the track without authorisation from the Ambulance Operational Commander (if on scene or via EOC if they are en-route) that the power is off and trains stopped as confirmed by Network Rail Route Control.	
Request HART support and provide a METHANE report to control.	Have appropriate PPE and specialist equipment to deal with such an incident.
	Will provide medical support to partner agencies responding to the incident.

Use the mnemonic POWER:

- **P**ower off and trains stopped confirmed by authorised person. When in doubt, contact EOC.
- **O**ff the tracks unless the patient appears viable.
- **W**ear PPE (minimum hi-vis jacket and helmet).
- **E**nsure EOC and ambulance commander knows clinicians are entering or leaving trackside.
- **R**apidly remove a viable patient and treat in the safest agreed area off the tracks.

Identify your location at track to Network Rail Control via Ambulance Control (EOC) (use signal; bridge or overhead line support number plates; quarter-mile posts at track side; station or level crossing nearby; electrical substation name plate).

6.2 Industrial Docks

- Report to the rendezvous point (RVP) to meet dock staff and be taken to the incident. If the activity is close to the water's edge, ensure HART attendance is requested early.

- Many docks contain structures that require staff to work at height or in confined spaces, i.e. ships, ISO containers and cranes. An early request for specialist resources who are equipped, trained and authorised to work in such environments is imperative. Request HART early.

- Local ambulance services may have site-specific plans and arrangements for large dockland areas. For further information, contact the EPRR Department.

6.3 Airports

- Each airport will have a site-specific plan for incidents and emergencies on their site. This will have been developed in conjunction with the emergency services, including ambulance services. When responding to an airport emergency, clinicians will usually be asked to report to a designed RVP, where they will be met and taken airside by airport staff. Identify relevant RVPs in advance. These will be contained in your local plans.

- Each ambulance service will also have a pre-determined attendance (PDA) for such incidents. For further information on airport incidents, contact the EPRR Department.

6.4 Carriageways and Motorways

General guidelines:

- Blue lights and hazard warning lights should be left ON, unless the scene has been secured and a major incident has been declared.

- Ensure hi-vis PPE is worn, and consider a helmet to provide protection from debris and during any extrication.

- Approach from the rear of the incident, if possible, at low speed.

- Identify hazards, consider parking position and identify a safe area of work.

- Request police/Highways England if not already present.

- Follow the flow of traffic unless directed otherwise by police or Highways England.

- Do not stop on the non-incident carriageway to gain access to an incident on the opposite side, irrespective of how urgent the situation appears on the affected carriageway or of the distance to the next junction or crossing point.

- In multiple vehicle collisions, it may be necessary to sectorise the scene to promote understanding and aid communication.

Actions on arrival:

- Ensure the road is closed or restricted.

- The first vehicle should park before the incident and additional vehicles should park beyond it, creating a boundary for a safe working area

Major, Complex and High-Risk Incidents

(except on motorways, where all vehicles should park beyond the incident in the obstructed lane).

- Exit the vehicle on the side away from moving traffic.
- Liaise with police, Highways England and the FRS.
- Ascertain the number and location of casualties trapped or injured and report to the control room.
- Ensure an operational commander is appointed to coordinate ambulance resources, and stand back to liaise with other agencies.
- Prioritise extrication and request further resources if required (i.e. HART for additional equipment and capabilities).
- Establish an inner and outer cordon around the scene of operations, if appropriate.
- Keep the working area clear by creating an equipment dump.
- Treat all non-activated SRS devices as live; high-voltage electrical systems should all be treated as live even when the engine is not running.
- Fires in an LPG-powered car will be treated by the FRS as a cylinder incident.

Agencies use Table 6.12 as a guide to help inform lane closures.

Leaving the incident:

- Do not move any vehicles, especially those providing the fend-off protection, before consulting with other emergency services.
- Maintain high visibility when moving away from the incident and re-joining traffic flows. Use warning lights until clear of the incident.

'All lane running':

- Some sections of the motorway may be utilised for 'all-lane running' (Figure 6.12). On these sections, the hard shoulder area may be used for live traffic at certain times. Lanes are then described as 1–4.

Incidents in tunnels:

- Attending resources should consider entering from both directions.
- Utilise both bores of the tunnel if possible and confirm that traffic has stopped.
- Utilise the non-incident bore for casualty treatment and loading if appropriate.
- Ensure that all responders are aware when operations are utilised in the non-incident bore.
- Consider toxic or hazardous fumes build-up in a protracted incident.

TABLE 6.12 – Lane Closures for Road Incidents

Incident location	Lane closures required
Two-way local roadway	Both lanes
Hard shoulder of the motorway or similar	Hard shoulder and lane 1
Lane 1 of a 3-lane roadway	Hard shoulder, lane 1 and lane 2
Lane 2 of a 3-lane roadway	Lanes 1, 2 and 3
Lane 3 of a 3-lane roadway	Lanes 2 and 3
Across the central reservation	Lanes 2 and 3 of both carriageways

Figure 6.12 – All-lane running.

Bibliography

1. Public Health England. *Chemical, Biological, Radiological and Nuclear Incidents: Recognise and respond.* 2018. Available from: https://www.gov.uk/government/publications/chemical-biological-radiological-and-nuclear-incidents-recognise-and-respond.

2. NHS England. *Clinical guidelines for major incidents and mass casualty events.* 2018. Available from: https://www.england.nhs.uk/publication/clinical-guidelines-for-major-incidents-and-mass-casualty-events/.

3. National Ambulance Resilience Unit. *Compliance & Quality Assurance: National Provisions for Interoperable Capabilities.* 2018. Available from: https://naru.org.uk.

SECTION **6** Special Situations

Police Incapacitants

- The deployment of police incapacitants (less lethal tactical options) on individuals and/or groups can lead to conditions requiring pre-hospital care.

- The aim of this guideline is to support clinical decision making for the management of patients following the deployment of:
  - Conducted Energy Devices (CED) previously termed Conducted Electrical Weapons (CEW). Predominantly in the UK, TASER™ products.
  - Irritant Sprays, previously termed incapacitant sprays, i.e. CS/PAVA.
  - Attenuating Energy Projectiles (AEP).
  - Batons.

- Not all patients exposed to police incapacitants will require hospital assessment; however, all patients should undergo a primary survey.

- Carry out a dynamic risk assessment; continually re-assess throughout the incident.

2. Conducted Energy Devices (CED)

CEDs are battery-operated hand-held devices which deliver up to 50,000 volts of electricity at low energy levels (0.1 J), in rapid pulses (~ 5 seconds), via two barbed electrodes. There are three variants of CED produced by TASER™ authorised for use by police forces within the UK. These are TASER™ X2, X26 and T7: the barb design varies according to type (refer to Figure 6.13).

- The barbs are designed to stick into skin or clothes and connect to the device by fine long copper wires, or via two probes directly applied to the skin or clothes.

- Firing the device results in pain and a transient loss of voluntary control of muscles, often causing the patient to fall. These devices are currently in use by all police forces in the United Kingdom.

- Before touching the patient, ensure the wires are disconnected from the device; the wires break easily by cutting with scissors.

There is an increased risk of combustion if a CED is deployed after the deployment of incapacitant sprays or following contact with flammable liquids such as petrol.

Assessment and management

- Most people incapacitated with a CED do not require hospital assessment; however, patients should undergo a primary survey especially assessing for the presence of:
  - Neck and back injuries. (Spinal fractures from muscle contraction have been described elsewhere.)
  - Secondary injuries as a result of the fall.
  - Cardiac symptoms.
  - Acute behavioural disturbance (ABD).
  - Attached electrodes.

- Death and severe injuries are rare, with most injuries associated with falling or probe penetration. Immediate cardiac dysrhythmia is very rare. Occasional cases of stroke, seizure and rhabdomyolysis have been reported.

- For the assessment and management of symptoms, conditions and injuries following deployment of CED, refer to Table 6.13.

Probe types:

X2	X26	T7

The actual barb length for the probes varies between 9.6 & 11.7mm depending on model

Figure 6.13 – CED (TASER™) barb types. Reproduced with permission from the Faculty of Forensic & Legal Medicines and the FFLM CED Hub https://fflm.ac.uk/cedhub

SECTION 6 Special Situations

Police Incapacitants

TABLE 6.13 – ASSESSMENT and MANAGEMENT: Following the Deployment of a CED
PRIMARY EFFECTS
Pain
Refer to **Pain Management in Adults** and **Pain Management in Children**.
Electrode Removal
The electrodes vary in length and have a 'fish hook'-type end which is designed to stick to clothes and into the skin. **NB** Although the lengths of the barbs may vary, the management principles remain the same. Probes very rarely penetrate beyond the dermis. Electrode removal for Taser™ X2 & X26: (For removal of the Taser™ T7, a cartridge safety clip is designed to aid removal. This is carried by police officers deploying the device along with instructions into use). ▪ Slightly stretch the skin around the electrode and pull sharply on the electrode. This usually only causes slight discomfort. ▪ The electrode is a biohazard and should be placed in a sealed container and may often be retained by the police for evidence. It can be disposed of as clinical waste if directed by the police. ▪ Clean the area. ▪ Cover the site with an adhesive dressing. ▪ Advise tetanus booster within 72 hours if not covered for tetanus. Antibiotics are not routinely required unless the patient is immunocompromised. **NB** If the electrode cannot be removed at the first attempt or breaks during attempted removal, leave in situ and transfer to definitive care. **DO NOT** attempt to remove the electrodes if they are: ▪ Attached to skin where blood vessels are close to the skin surface (e.g. neck and groin). ▪ Attached to one or both eye(s). ▪ Attached to the face. ▪ Attached to the genitalia. ▪ Attached to the mouth or throat or if the electrode has been swallowed. ▪ Firmly embedded in the scalp. ▪ Embedded in a joint (e.g. finger). ▪ Broken. In these circumstances, cut the wire close to the electrode, leaving approximately 4 cm attached to the electrode, and transfer to definitive care.
Burns
▪ Superficial burns are likely around the area where the electrode attached to the skin and electricity was delivered. ▪ Burns may also occur if a CED is deployed after the deployment of incapacitant sprays or following contact with flammable liquids such as petrol. ▪ Refer to **Pain Management in Adults**, **Pain Management in Children** and **Burns and Scalds**.
Cardiac Conditions/Symptoms

▪ Cardiac conditions have been reported following the deployment of a CED, including increases in heart rate, cardiac rhythm disturbance and cardiac arrest.
▪ ECGs are not needed for all patients. However, always undertake a 12-lead ECG and monitor blood pressure and oxygen saturation for patients:
  – Complaining of chest pain.
  – With cardiac symptoms (e.g. tachycardia, bradycardia).
  – With significant cardiac history (e.g. angina, arrhythmias or a myocardial infarction).
  – Fitted with pacemakers or cardioverter defibrillator. These patients should be transferred to definitive care for assessment.

SECTION **6** Special Situations

(continued)

Police Incapacitants

- Cardiac arrhythmia (refer to **Cardiac Rhythm Disturbance** for specific guidance).
- Cardiac arrest (refer to the appropriate **Resuscitation** guidelines).

Convulsions

- The deployment of a CED may elicit a convulsion or epileptic fit, though this is very rare.
- For specific guidance, refer to **Convulsions in Adults** and **Convulsions in Children**.

Obstetric and Gynaecological Conditions

- Spontaneous miscarriage has been reported following the deployment of CED.
- Refer to the appropriate **Maternity Care** guidelines.
- Any patient who is known to be pregnant and has been subject to CED discharge should be transferred to definitive care for assessment.

Soft Tissue Injury/Injuries

(Contusions, tendon damage, abrasions, dislocations, lacerations, puncture wounds)

- Abrasions, lacerations and puncture wounds:
  - Clean the area with an alcohol/antiseptic wipe.
  - Cover the site with an adhesive dressing.
  - Advise tetanus booster within 72 hours if not covered for tetanus.
- Contusions, damage to ligament and tendons: These injuries should be managed accordingly and transferred to definitive care.
- Puncture wounds around highly vascular areas should be assessed for significant pain, swelling or haematoma. If present, these patients should be transferred to definitive care for assessment.
- Puncture wounds around the neck and chest should be assessed for signs of subcutaneous emphysema. If present, these patients should be transferred to definitive care for assessment.

Head Injury

- Head injuries and loss of consciousness may also result from intracranial penetration of an electrode.
- For specific guidance, refer to **Head Injury** and **Altered Level of Consciousness**.

SECONDARY EFFECTS

Head, Neck and Back Injuries, Contusions, Abrasions and Lacerations

- The powerful muscular contractions caused by the deployment of a CED may result in vertebral fractures, usually thoracolumbar.
- The loss of voluntary control of the muscles caused by the deployment of a CED may result in falls, leading to injuries of the head, neck and back, contusions, abrasions, lacerations, ligament and tendon injury, etc.
- For specific guidance, refer to **Head Injury** and **Spinal Injury and Spinal Cord Injury**.

Contusions, abrasions, lacerations, ligament and tendon injury: Manage as per soft tissue injuries above.

COINCIDENTAL EFFECTS

Injuries and Conditions Unrelated to CED Deployment

- Injuries and/or conditions may be sustained or develop that are unrelated to the deployment of a CED, for example as the result of a physical struggle, the consumption of drugs or physical exhaustion.
- Assess and manage coincidental injuries as per condition, cognisant of the effects of drugs, dehydration or exhaustion.

Acute Behavioural Disturbance (ABD)

- A CED may be deployed on people in patients suffering from acute behavioural disturbance (ABD). People in this state may be at a greater risk of collapse, arrhythmias and sudden death. This may be unrelated to deployment of a CED – undertake a **TIME-CRITICAL** transfer and provide an alert/information call.
- For specific guidance, refer to **Acute Behavioural Disturbance**.

Police Incapacitants

3. Irritant Sprays

- Irritant sprays (Peripheral Chemosensory Irritants (PCSIs)) used within UK police forces include:
  - PAVA 'Pepper spray' (oleoresin, capsicum, pelargonic acid, vanillylamide). These are synthetic variants of capsicum products and dissolved in glycol, ethanol and water.
  - CS spray 2-chlorobenzalmalononitrile (O-chlorobenzylidene malononitrile). CS is solid at room temperature and dissolved in methyl isobutyl ketone (MIBK) as a solvent. When the solvent evaporates, the CS particles give their effect.

They have similar actions and the broad principles of management are the same. Severe injury, disability and death are very rare.

Actions

- The sprays cause irritation (burning sensation) when in contact with exposed skin and mucus membranes including eye, nose and mouth and respiratory tract, causing lacrimation (tearing), rhinorrhoea (runny nose), sialorrhoea (drooling), disorientation, dizziness, breathing difficulties, coughing and vomiting.
- The effects are usually short-lived (under 30 minutes), but some can persist for up to 2–6 hours.

Management

- Avoid entering a contaminated or closed environment.
- Avoid exposure to contaminated clothing.
- Wear gloves, apron and eye protection.
- Any irrigation may exacerbate symptoms transiently, and cool saline or water must be used to reduce risk of reactivating the irritant product.

Assessment and management

- Most people exposed to incapacitant sprays do not require hospital assessment.
- For the assessment and management of symptoms and conditions following deployment of incapacitant sprays, refer to Table 6.14.

4. Attenuating Energy Projectiles (AEP)

- Projectiles such as plastic bullets, rubber bullets or bean bags can cause sudden death (after strikes to the head, chest or abdomen), dislocations, fractures, joint damage, ligament and tendon damage, haemorrhage and haematoma, compartment syndrome, blunt intra-abdominal injury (splenic rupture, subcapsular liver/haematoma), blunt thoracic cavity injury (pneumothorax/haemothorax) and penetrating injuries to thorax, abdomen, eye, arm, leg and blood vessels.

TABLE 6.14 – ASSESSMENT and MANAGEMENT: Following the Deployment of Incapacitant Sprays

General Symptoms

Lacrimation, rhinorrhoea, sialorrhoea, dizziness, coughing and vomiting.

- Move the patient away from the source of the contamination.
- Expose to fresh air. This can be augmented by fanning.
- Remove contaminated clothing and place into sealed bags to prevent secondary exposure to patient or others.
- Reassure that effects will decrease rapidly after initial exposure.
- For patients with heavy contamination of the skin and eyes, irrigate with tap water.
- If skin symptoms persist for longer than 20 minutes, transfer to further care and consider irrigation with cool tap water.

Eye Symptoms

Lacrimation, blurred vision, stinging eyes, photophobia, blepharospasm, periorbital oedema, corneal injury.

Symptoms will usually resolve within 15–30 minutes.

- Move the patient away from the source of the contamination.
- Expose to fresh air. This can be augmented by fanning.
- Reassure that effects will decrease rapidly after initial exposure.
- Advise the patient not to rub their eyes for 2–3 hours.
- Encourage patient to remove any contact lenses.
- If the patient cannot open their eyes after 30 minutes, transfer to definitive care for assessment.
- If symptoms persist for longer than 60 minutes, consider irrigation with tepid sterile saline.

Breathing Difficulties

Shortness of breath and coughing are common and are usually self-limiting.

Bronchospasm and laryngospasm are rare.

- For specific guidance refer to **Dyspnoea**.
- The majority of symptoms should settle within 15–30 minutes.
- Those with pre-existing respiratory disease, such as asthma and COPD, are at increased risk of more severe effects.

SECTION **6** Special Situations

Police Incapacitants

- A sudden, single-blow blunt trauma to the front of the chest may on rare occasions lead to cardiac arrest due to the rhythm disturbance; this is the opposite of a pre-cordial thump for witnessed cardiac arrest. Refer to **Resuscitation** guidelines.

- Within police forces in the UK, the most common AEP is a soft-nosed 37 mm projectile. The nose cap has a hollow void to minimise the peak force, with the aim to deliver a high amount of kinetic energy while reducing the potential for life-threatening injury. The use is strictly regulated and restricted to accredited officers (Authorised Firearms Officers and Public Order Officers), and the training states the target area should be below the waist to minimise risk of injury to head, chest and abdomen.

5. Batons

- Baton strikes can cause:
  - dislocations
  - fractures
  - joint, ligament and tendon damage
  - haemorrhage and haematoma
  - compartment syndrome
  - death.

- Baton strikes to limbs will typically cause 'tramline bruising'; this is of no significant concern unless there is evidence of underlying fracture or neuromuscular condition.

- 'Police use of force' guidance within the UK advocates baton strikes avoiding head, neck, chest and groin to minimise the risk of serious and life-threatening injuries.

KEY POINTS!

Police Incapacitants

- **Ensure the wires are disconnected from the CED before touching the patient.**
- **DO NOT remove electrodes in any of the instances listed in Table 6.13.**
- **Patients may also sustain secondary injuries (e.g. head injuries and fractures following a fall).**
- **Transfer to definitive care any patient with one or more of the following: cardiac symptoms, neck and back injuries and ABD.**
- **The symptoms of patients exposed to irritant sprays should settle after exposure to air. If symptoms persist after 20–30 minutes, transfer to definitive care.**

SECTION

6 Special Situations

Index

Index

Index

pneumonia 252
primary survey 249
septic arthritis/osteomyelitis 252
source and severity 252
tachycardia 251
urinary tract infection 252
fire service, disclosure of information to 44
FLACC scale 36, 41
foreign body airway obstruction (FBAO) (child) 121
dyspnoea 242–243, 245
fractures
of femur 38
splintage as pain relief 37

gastritis 257
gastroenteritis (children)
dehydration 389–390
differential diagnosis 388
examination 389
key points 392
nutritional considerations 391
red flag symptoms 391
'safety netting' 391
gastrointestinal (GI) bleeding 257
assessment and management 258–259
differential diagnosis 258
diverticular disease 258
gastritis 257
haematemesis 257
haemorrhoids 258
inflammatory bowel disease 258
key points 260
lower gastrointestinal bleeding 258
Mallory-Weiss tears 257
melaena 257
mortality 257
oesophageal varices 257
oesophagitis 258
peptic ulcers 257
tumour 258
upper gastrointestinal bleeding 257
glycaemic emergencies in adults and children 261

haemorrhage
adult trauma 454
catastrophic 455
in pelvic trauma 511
haemorrhage during pregnancy (including miscarriage
and ectopic pregnancy) 572
haemorrhoids 258
headache 273
head injury 492
heart failure 278
heat related illness 286
assessment and management 287–288
factors 287
features 286
heat exhaustion 286

heat stress 286
heat stroke 286–287
key points 289
herpes simplex encephalitis 252
human factors 25
hypersalivation, and ketamine 38
hyperventilation syndrome (HVS) 292
assessment and management 294–296
key points 297
hypoglycaemia (adults)
and altered consciousness 463
hypoglycaemia (children)
convulsions 236
hypothermia 299
acute (immersion hypothermia) 299, 500
and large burns 37
assessment and management 300–301
chronic 299
clinical stages 300
definition of 299
diagnosis 299
key points 302
resuscitation 299
risk factors 299
subacute (exhaustion hypothermia) 299
hypoxia
immersion and drowning 499

immersion and drowning 499
airway and breathing 499
and trauma 499
aquatic rescue 499
assessment and management 500–501
bradycardia 500
chest compression 499
exacerbating factors 499
hypercapnia 499
hypothermia 500
hypoxia 499
intravascular fluid therapy 500
key points 502
laryngospasm 499
neck and back trauma 499
postural hypotension 499
risk assessment 499
survival and submersion 500
immersion, definition of 499
implantable cardioverter defibrillator (ICD) 304
assessment and management of patients fitted
with 306–308
ECG monitoring 305
key points 309
therapies 304
usual location 304
inflammatory bowel disease 258

Kawasaki's disease 252
ketamine 38

Index

Index

Index

2022